ADA Guide to

Dental Therapeutics

First Edition

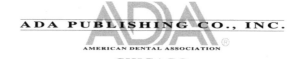

ADA PUBLISHING CO., INC.

AMERICAN DENTAL ASSOCIATION®

CHICAGO

ADA PUBLISHING CO., INC.
AMERICAN DENTAL ASSOCIATION

ADA Publishing Co., Inc.
211 East Chicago Avenue
Chicago, Illinois 60611-2678

E-Mail: adapco@ada.org
World Wide Web: http://www.ada.org/adapco/adapco/html

President and Publisher: Laura A. Kosden
Associate Publisher, Editorial: James H. Berry
Associate Publisher, Marketing and Operations: Gabriela Radulescu
Editorial Director: Lisbeth Maxwell
Director of Production: Beth Cox
Assistant Editor: Janyce Hamilton

The editor, authors, and publisher of the ADA Guide to Dental Therapeutics have used care to confirm that the drugs and treatment schedules set forth in this book are in accordance with current recommendations and practice at the time of publication. As the science of dental therapeutics evolves, changes in drug treatment and use become necessary. The reader is advised to consult the package insert for each drug to consider and adopt all safety precautions before use, particularly with new and infrequently used drugs. The reader is responsible for ascertaining the Food and Drug Administration clearance of each drug and device used in his or her practice.

The editor, authors, and publisher disclaim all responsibility for any liability, loss, injury or damage resulting directly or indirectly from the reader's use and application of the information in this book and make no representations or warranties with respect to such information, including the products described herein.

The editor, authors, and publisher have produced this book in their individual capacities and not on behalf or in the interest of any pharmaceutical companies or state or federal agencies.

Many of the proprietary names of the products listed in this book are trademarked and registered in the U.S. Patent Office.

Printed by R.R. Donnelley & Sons Company, Chicago, Illinois 60610

Design and composition by Perolio, Inc.

ISBN 1-891748-00-9

Introduction

Dentists are prescribing more medications today than ever before. Patients seeking dental care are using a wide range of medications for medical problems. And both dentists and patients have choices to make about the variety of nonprescription products available for treating various disorders of the mouth.

Dentists have been vocal about their need for a quick and accurate drug reference that is more than a dictionary and yet not a textbook of pharmacology. Encouragement to publish a new edition of the old Accepted Dental Therapeutics, which the ADA stopped publishing in 1984 with the 40th edition, has been widespread. The authors and I repeatedly heard from our lecture audiences across the country that they wanted a new version of ADT to carry them into the 21st century. The ADA has received a number of similar requests in the past few years and in 1992, its House of Delegates directed that a handbook on dental therapeutics be published.

Therefore, this new ADA Guide to Dental Therapeutics was not written as one person's view of what dentists need. Rather, it was prepared in response to what dentists themselves told all of us they wanted and needed to make their practices complete: concise and accurate information about the medications they use, information based on the science of pharmacology and provided in the form of a handbook rather than a treatise on individual drugs.

Pharmacology is the study of drugs—what they are, what effects they have, what happens to them in the body, how they are administered and how they work. This book provides all of this information, and it does so in a variety of innovative ways. It is not intended to replace textbooks of basic pharmacology. Instead, it is designed to build on the basic principles of pharmacology learned in dental school, and to apply these scientific principles in a practical way to the art of clinical practice. In that respect, the book can serve as a concise and reliable source of information essential to properly medicating patients. It also can serve as a useful resource for students and dentists in preparing for various board examinations.

Rational dental therapy requires the thorough understanding and careful selection of drugs used in dental practice. But we also must be aware that we and our patients are not islands unto ourselves. As dentists, we cannot limit our therapeutic knowledge only to the medications we prescribe; such action can compromise patient safety and the status of our profession. Because of our excellent recall programs, we tend to see patients on a more regular basis than physicians do—and, therefore, we need to be alert to the potential adverse effects of any medication our patients take, regardless of who prescribed it. This book has been developed to provide dentists with just such information.

A major strength of this book is that it was written by both academicians and clinicians in a team approach. As a result, the information is presented in a practical manner and is as valuable at chairside as are a mirror and explorer. The American Dental Association selected the writers based on their national and international reputations in dental therapeutics. The content is as up to the minute as is possible in publishing and, furthermore, is scheduled to be updated every two years. (An aside: We encourage readers to send us their suggestions for the second edition.)

The ADA Council on Scientific Affairs has reviewed all the material in this book, which is the only one of its kind that identifies medications—both prescription and nonprescription—that carry the ADA Seal of Acceptance. This Seal is designed to help the public and dental professionals make informed decisions about dental products. Backed by the knowledge of the Council—17 members, 20 staff members and more than 100 consultants—it provides an assurance of efficacy, safety and truth in advertising. Knowing which products carry the ADA Seal will enable all members of the dental team to select professional products knowledgeably and to discuss various toothpastes, mouthrinses and other nonprescription medications with their patients.

I wish to acknowledge the pioneering efforts of contributors to Accepted Dental Therapeutics, who laid the foundation for this book. I also wish to thank the authors, who applied their time and their broad talents generously to this task. I am grateful to my dean, Louis Goldberg, D.D.S., Ph.D., and to my wife, Marilyn, both of whom gave me the time and support needed to serve as editor. I would like to thank the following people for their editorial assistance: Arden Christen, D.D.S., M.S.D., M.A.; my son, Sebastian J. Ciancio, M.D.; Harold L. Crossley, D.D.S., Ph.D.; Michael Glick, D.M.D.; Jane Forsberg Jasek, R.D.H., M.P.A.; Michael Lynch, D.D.S.; S. William (Bill) Oberg; Mark Rubin, J.D.; Christine Ulrich, B.S. Finally, a special thanks is due to the staff of ADA Publishing Co., Inc.: to President and Publisher Laura Kosden for her visionary approach to this book; to the staff for helping me through the months of preparation; and especially to Editorial Director Lisbeth Maxwell and her assistant editor Janyce Hamilton, whose editing abilities and dedication helped make this a dental therapeutics book of excellence.

Sebastian G. Ciancio, D.D.S.
State University of New York at Buffalo
December 1997

Preface

The American Dental Association is proud to introduce the ADA Guide to Dental Therapeutics. Designed with the busy dental practitioner in mind, it aims to simplify one of the most important aspects of a dentist's practice—the appropriate and accurate use of therapeutic agents.

As a practical, easy-to-use chairside resource, the Guide offers quick access to crucial information about the drugs prescribed for and taken by dental patients—more than 800 generic drugs and 2,200 brand-name drugs in all. Every practicing dentist, dental educator, dental student and member of the dental team can profit from using this book.

Key Features of the Book

The Guide is unlike any other drug handbook available. It offers a host of benefits to the practicing dentist:

- clear, well-organized tables that offer rapid access to information on more than 900 drugs used in dentistry;
- crucial dosage, interaction and precaution data at the reader's fingertips;
- identification of adverse effects according to body system;
- brief but informative descriptions of drug categories that bridge the gap between drug handbooks and pharmacology texts;
- information on more than 1,100 drugs used in medicine, enabling dentists to knowledgeably communicate with other medical professionals about patients' medications and their dental side effects;
- identification of therapeutic products bearing the ADA Seal of Acceptance;
- a special section on drug-related issues that affect dental practice: substance abuse, smoking cessation, infection control.

Drugs Used in Dentistry

This book is arranged in three sections. The first focuses on drugs prescribed primarily by dentists, so that the practitioner can readily prescribe them with a full understanding of their actions, adverse effects and interactions. This section contains drug information essential to solving patients' dental problems. Throughout the Guide, dentists will be able to quickly locate dosages and, in italics, information of major clinical significance (interactions, adverse effects, precautions and contraindications). Drugs and products that have received the ADA Seal of Acceptance are identified with a blue star: ★. The names of drugs available in Canada are followed by [CAN].

In Section I, each chapter is organized by

- description of the general category of drugs and the accepted indications;
- listings of specific drugs by generic and trade name—including adult and child dosages, forms and strengths;

- special dental considerations—drug interactions, pertinent laboratory value alterations, drug cross-sensitivities and effects on pregnant and nursing women, children, elderly patients and other patients with special needs;
- adverse effects and precautions, arranged by body system;
- pharmacology;
- information for patient/family consultation.

If any of these categories or subcategories does not appear (for instance, laboratory value alterations), it is because it did not pertain to the particular type of drug or because there was no such information available.

In each chapter in Section I, the dosage information table (usually the first in the chapter) is based on the assumption that the dentist has determined—through taking a health history and interviewing the patient—that the patient is in general good health and is not taking any medications that may interact with the drug in question. Adverse effects and precautions/contraindications are arranged according to body systems, which are abbreviated as follows:

CV	cardiovascular
CNS	central nervous system
Endoc	endocrine
EENT	eye/ear/nose/throat
GI	gastrointestinal
GU	genitourinary
Hema	hematologic
HB	hepatobiliary
Integ	integumentary
Musc	musculoskeletal
Oral	oral
Resp	respiratory

Overall adverse effects and precautions/contraindications are listed under "General."

This book includes all ADA-accepted products in the various categories discussed. However, in some cases we have included only a representative sampling of products—ADA-accepted or not—in a category. Inclusion of a particular product in no way indicates that it is superior over others.

Drugs Used in Medicine

More and more dental patients are taking one or more prescription drugs. To assist the dentist, the second section of the book focuses on drugs prescribed primarily by physicians. This section presents drug information in a more abbreviated form, emphasizing each drug's effect on dental diagnosis and treatment planning. The information here will help the dentist interact intelligently with the patient's physician about the patient's medications, particularly when a modification of drug therapy is in question. Helpful dosage ranges enable dentists to anticipate potential side effects in patients at the upper end of the dosage range.

Drug Issues in Dental Practice

The book's third section focuses on issues related to dental pharmacology that affect the dentist's practice: cessation of tobacco use, patients with addictions, infection control, legal considerations in using drugs in dentistry. As part of the community of practitioners interested in patients as people and not just as "teeth and gums," dentists can use the information discussed here to build a successful and expanding practice. A highlight of this section is the chapter on oral manifestations of systemic medications. The topics presented in Section III are not addressed in most dental drug handbooks.

Appendixes and Indexes

The book also features several appendixes:
- FDA and Canadian schedules for controlled substances;
- pregnancy classifications;
- teratogens;
- the ADA's latest statements on medication-related issues such as prevention of bacterial endocarditis, the use of antibiotic

prophylaxis in patients with total joint replacements, the use of antibiotics in dentistry and the use of nitrous oxide in the dental office;
- normal laboratory values;
- weights and measures;
- a guide to calculating doses of local anesthetics and vasoconstrictors;
- a guide to antiretroviral medications used in treating patients with HIV;
- sample prescriptions and prescription abbreviations;
- a reporting form for adverse effects of medications.

Two indexes—a general index, which includes both generic and brand-name drugs, and an index of dental indications—make it even easier to find information quickly.

Editorial Board

Continued on next page

Authors (cont.)

Robert E. Mecklenburg, D.D.S., M.P.H.
Dental Coordinator
Smoking and Tobacco Control Program
National Cancer Institute (EPN 241)
Potomac, Maryland

Chris H. Miller, Ph.D.
Professor of Oral Microbiology
Director of Infection Control Research
 and Services
Associate Dean for Research and
 Graduate Education
School of Dentistry
Indiana University
Indianapolis, Indiana

Martha Somerman, D.D.S., Ph.D.
William K. and Mary Anne Najjar
 Endowed Professor
Professor and Chair
Department of
Periodontics/Prevention/Geriatrics
School of Dentistry
Professor of Pharmacology
School of Medicine
University of Michigan
Ann Arbor, Michigan

Kathleen M. Todd, J.D.
Associate General Counsel
Division of Legal Affairs
American Dental Association
Chicago, Illinois

Clay Walker, Ph.D.
Professor of Oral Biology
Periodontal Disease Research Center
Health Science Center
College of Dentistry
University of Florida
Gainesville, Florida

Jill Wolowitz, J.D.
Staff Attorney
Division of Legal Affairs
American Dental Association
Chicago, Illinois

John Yagiela, D.D.S., Ph.D.
Professor of Oral Biology
Coordinator of Anesthesia
 and Pain Control
University of California Los Angeles
School of Dentistry
Center for the Health Sciences
Los Angeles, California

Table of Contents

Section I. Drugs Used in Dentistry (cont.)

Section II. Drugs Used in Medicine: Treatment and Pharmacological Considerations for Dental Patients Receiving Medical Care

Section III. Drug Issues in Dental Practice

Appendixes

Indexes

Section I.

Drugs Used in Dentistry

Chapter 1.

Injectable and Topical Local Anesthetics

John Yagiela, D.D.S., Ph.D.; Stanley F. Malamed, D.D.S.

Injectable Local Anesthetics

Local anesthetics reversibly block neural transmission when applied to a circumscribed area of the body. Cocaine, the first local anesthetic (introduced in 1884), remains an effective topical agent, but it proved too toxic for parenteral use. Procaine, introduced in 1904, was the first practical local anesthetic for injection and contributed greatly to breaking the historic connection between dentistry and pain.

Vasoconstrictors are agents used in local anesthetic solutions to retard systemic absorption of the local anesthetic from the injection site. Although not active themselves in preventing neural transmission, vasoconstrictors such as epinephrine and related adrenergic amines can significantly increase the duration and even the depth of anesthesia. The vasoconstriction they produce also may be useful in reducing bleeding during intraoral procedures.

Chemistry and classification. Injectable local anesthetics consist of amphiphilic molecules; that is, they can dissolve in both aqueous and lipoid environments. A lipophilic ring structure on one end of the molecule confers fat solubility, and a secondary or tertiary amino group on the other permits water solubility. Local anesthetics intended for injection are prepared commercially as the hydrochloride salt.

Two major classes of injectable local anesthetics are recognized: esters and amides. They are distinguished by the type of chemical bond joining the two ends of the drug molecules.

Early local anesthetics, such as cocaine and procaine, were esters. Most local anesthetics introduced since 1940 have been amides.

The use of injectable local anesthetics in dentistry is almost exclusively limited to amide-type drugs. In fact, no ester agent is currently being marketed in dental cartridge form in the United States. Given the number of local anesthetic injections administered in dentistry (conservatively estimated at more than 300 million in the United States annually), a drug with a minimal risk of allergy is desirable. Amide anesthetics offer a significantly lower risk of allergy than ester anesthetics. Conversely, amides also have a somewhat greater risk of systemic toxicity than do esters. However, as toxic reactions usually are dose-related, adherence to proper injection techniques—including the use of minimal volumes of anesthetic—minimizes this risk. Amide formulations have also proved more effective than esters for achieving intraoral anesthesia. Thus, amide local anesthetics, as used in dentistry, offer the fewest overall risks and the greatest clinical benefits.

Selecting a local anesthetic. The selection of a local anesthetic for use in a dental procedure is based on four criteria:
- duration of the dental procedure;
- requirement for hemostasis;
- requirement for postsurgical pain control;
- contraindication(s) to specific anesthetic drugs or vasoconstrictors.

Duration. Local anesthetic formulations intended for use in dentistry are categorized by their expected duration of pulpal anesthesia as short-, intermediate- and long-acting drugs.

- Short-acting drugs, which typically provide pulpal and hard tissue anesthesia for up to 30 minutes after submucosal infiltration: 2% lidocaine, 3% mepivacaine and 4% prilocaine.
- Intermediate-acting agents, which provide up to 60 minutes of pulpal anesthesia: 4% articaine with 1:100,000 or 1:200,000 epinephrine, 2% lidocaine with 1:50,000 or 1:100,000 epinephrine, 2% mepivacaine with 1:20,000 levonordefrin and 4% prilocaine with 1:200,000 epinephrine.
- Long-acting drugs, which last up to 8 hours after nerve block anesthesia: 0.5% bupivacaine with 1:200,000 epinephrine and 1.5% etidocaine with 1:200,000 epinephrine.

Accepted Indications

Injectable local anesthetics are used to provide local or regional analgesia for surgical and other dental procedures.

They are also used for diagnostic or other therapeutic purposes via routes of administration specified in product labeling.

General Dosing Information

General dosing information is provided in Table 1.1. In addition, standard textbooks provide information on the appropriate dosage (both concentration and injection volume) of local anesthetic to be used for specific injection techniques and dental procedures.

The dosage depends on
- the specific anesthetic technique and operative procedure;
- tissue vascularity in the area of injection;
- individual patient response.

In general, the dentist should administer the lowest concentration and volume of anesthetic solution that provide adequate anesthesia.

Maximum Recommended Doses

Table 1.1 lists the maximum recommended doses for local anesthetic formulations per procedure or appointment, as approved by

the U.S. Food and Drug Administration (FDA). Additional anesthetic may be administered only after sufficient time is allowed for elimination of the initial dose.

Dosage Adjustments

The actual maximum dose for each patient must be individualized depending on his or her size, age and physical status; other drugs he or she may be taking; and the anticipated rate of absorption of the local anesthetic from the injected tissues. Reduced maximum doses are often indicated for pediatric and geriatric patients, patients who have serious illness or disability and patients who have medical conditions or are taking drugs that alter responses to local anesthetics or vasoconstrictors.

Table 1.1 presents specific limits for local anesthetic doses in pediatric patients.

Vasoconstrictors

A vasoconstrictor added to a local anesthetic may significantly prolong the anesthetic's duration of action by reducing blood flow around the injection site. This, in turn, may reduce the local anesthetic's peak plasma concentration and the risk of adverse systemic reactions.

Repeated injection of vasoconstrictors in local anesthetics also may decrease blood flow sufficiently to cause anoxic injury in the local tissue, leading to delayed wound healing, edema or necrosis. The use of local anesthetic solutions containing vasoconstrictors may be restricted or contraindicated in patients who have advanced cardiovascular disease or who are taking medications that increase the activity of the vasoconstrictor.

Special Dental Considerations

Drug Interactions of Dental Interest

Drug interactions and related problems involving local anesthetics (Table 1.2) and vasoconstrictors (Table 1.3) are potentially of clinical significance in dentistry. Table 1.4 itemizes potential cross-sensitivity considerations.

Table 1.1

Injectable Local Anesthetics: Dosage Information*

Generic name	Brand name(s)	Maximum adult dosage (lower maximum doses for extra margin of safety)	Maximum child dosage	Pregnancy risk category	Content/form
Articaine hydrochloride with epinephrine [CAN]	Septanest N, Septanest SP, Ultracaine, Ultracaine Forte	7 mg/kg	5 mg/kg	B (estimated)	Articaine HCl, 40 mg/mL; epinephrine, 5, 10 µg/mL
Bupivacaine hydrochloride with epinephrine	Marcaine with Epinephrine ★	90 mg	**Age < 12 y:** Not established	C	Bupivacaine HCl, 5 mg/mL; epinephrine, 5 µg/mL
Etidocaine hydrochloride with epinephrine	Duranest with Epinephrine ★	8 (5.5) mg/kg up to 400 mg	Not established	B	Etidocaine HCl, 15 mg/mL; epinephrine, 5 µg/mL
Lidocaine hydrochloride	Alphacaine, Lignospan, Octocaine, Xylocaine ★	4.5 mg/kg up to 300 mg	Same as adult	B	20 mg/mL
Lidocaine hydrochloride with epinephrine	Alphacaine with Epinephrine, Lignospan Standard ★, Lignospan Forte ★, Octocaine with Epinephrine ★, Xylocaine with Epinephrine ★; Octocaine-100 [CAN], Octocaine-50 [CAN]	7 (6.6) mg/kg up to 500 (300) mg	Same as adult (4-5 mg/kg up to a maximum of 100-150 mg)	B	Lidocaine HCl, 20 mg/mL; epinephrine, 10, 20 µg/mL
Mepivacaine hydrochloride	Arestocaine, Carbocaine ★, Isocaine ★, Polocaine ★, Scandonest ★	6.6 mg/kg up to 400 (300) mg	Same as adult (6.6 mg/kg up to a maximum of 270 mg)	C	30 mg/mL
Mepivacaine hydrochloride with levonordefrin	Arestocaine with Levonordefrin, Carbocaine with Neo-Cobefrin ★, Isocaine with Levonordefrin ★, Polocaine with Levonordefrin ★	6.6 mg/kg up to 400 mg	Same as adult (6.6 mg/kg up to a maximum of 180 mg)	C	Mepivacaine HCl, 20 mg/mL; levonordefrin, 50 µg/mL
Prilocaine hydrochloride	Citanest ★	8 mg/kg up to 600 (400) mg	Same as adult	B	40 mg/mL
Prilocaine hydrochloride with epinephrine	Citanest Forte ★	8 mg/kg up to 600 (400) mg	Same as adult	B	Prilocaine HCl, 40 mg/mL; epinephrine, 5 µg/mL

★ indicates a drug bearing the ADA Seal of Acceptance.
[CAN] indicates a drug available only in Canada.
*Dosages are the maximum recommended doses approved by the U.S. Food and Drug Administration. Dosages in parentheses are the more restrictive usual prescribing limits listed in the U.S. Pharmacopeia Dispensing Information. For conversion purposes, one cartridge delivers 1.8 mL of anesthetic solution (1.7 mL for articaine).

Table 1.2

Local Anesthetics: Possible Interactions with Other Drugs*

Drug taken by patient	Interaction with local anesthetics	Dentist's action
Amiodarone, cimetidine, β-adrenergic blocking agents (propranolol, metoprolol)	Hepatic metabolism of lidocaine and probably other amide local anesthetics may be depressed by competition for hepatic enzymes and possibly by decreased liver blood flow	Use local anesthetics cautiously, especially with regard to repeated dosing
Antiarrhythmic drugs, Class I (mexiletine, tocainide)	Additive CNS and cardiovascular depression	Use local anesthetics cautiously— as low a dose as possible to achieve anesthesia
CNS depressants: alcohols, antidepressants, antihistamines, antipsychotics, barbiturates, benzodiazepines, centrally acting antihypertensives and muscle relaxants, general anesthetics, opioids, parenteral magnesium sulfate	*Possible additive or supraadditive CNS and respiratory depression*	Consider limiting the maximum dose of local anesthetics, especially with opioids
Cholinesterase inhibitors: antimyasthenics, muscle paralysis reversal drugs, antiglaucoma agents, organophosphate insecticides	Antimyasthenic dosage may require adjustment because local anesthetic inhibits neuromuscular transmission May inhibit metabolism of ester local anesthetics	Consult with physician (dose reduction may be necessary) Use ester agents cautiously
Sulfonamides	Therapeutic effect may be blocked by ester local anesthetics that release para-aminobenzoic acid on hydrolysis	Avoid concurrent use of sulfonamides and ester local anesthetics

Italics indicate information of major clinical significance.
Avoid storing anesthetic cartridges in disinfectant solutions because leakage into anesthetic cartridge and injection into tissue may cause severe local tissue damage.

Table 1.3

Vasoconstrictors: Possible Interactions With Other Drugs

Drug taken by patient	Interaction with vasoconstrictors	Dentist's action
α-adrenergic blockers (phenoxyben-zamine, prazosin), antipsychotic drugs (haloperidol, thioridazine)	Blockade of α-adrenergic receptors may lead to hypotensive responses to large doses of epinephrine	Use vasoconstrictors cautiously—as low a dose as feasible for the procedure
Cocaine	*Increases effects of vasoconstrictor* *Can result in cardiac arrest*	Avoid using vasoconstrictors in patient under the influence of cocaine
Digitalis glycosides (digoxin, digitoxin)	*Increase risk of cardiac arrhythmias*	Use vasoconstrictors cautiously—as low a dose as feasible for the procedure—in consultation with physician
Hydrocarbon inhalation anesthetics (halothane, enflurane)	*Sensitization of the heart may lead to cardiac arrhythmias*	Inform anesthesiologist of intended use of vasoconstrictors
Levodopa, thyroid hormones (levothyroxine, liothyronine)	Large doses of levodopa or thyroid hormone (beyond replacement amounts) may increase risk of cardiac toxicity	Use vasoconstrictors cautiously—as low a dose as feasible for the procedure
Maprotiline, tricyclic antidepressants (amitriptyline, doxepin, imipramine)	*May enhance the systemic effects of vasoconstrictor*	Avoid the use of levonordefrin or norepinephrine; use epinephrine cautiously—as low a dose as feasible for the procedure
Methyldopa, adrenergic neuronal blocking drugs (guanadrel, guanethi-dine, reserpine)	May enhance systemic responses to the vasoconstrictor	Use vasoconstrictors cautiously—as low a dose as feasible for the procedure
Nonselective β-adrenergic blockers (propranolol, nadolol)	*Blockade of β-adrenergic receptors in skeletal muscle may lead to hypertensive responses to the vasoconstrictor, especially epinephrine*	Use vasoconstrictors cautiously and monitor blood pressure after initial local anesthetic injection

Italics indicate information of major clinical significance.

Table 1.4

Local Anesthetics: Potential Cross-Sensitivity with Other Drugs

A person with a sensitivity to	May also have a sensitivity to
Para-aminobenzoic acid (PABA) or paraben preservative	Procaine, chloroprocaine, benzocaine, butamben, tetracaine, other local anesthetic solutions containing paraben preservatives (as in multidose vials)
Any ester local anesthetic	Other ester local anesthetics
Any amide local anesthetic	Other amide local anesthetics (rarely)
Sulfites	Any local anesthetic with an adrenergic vasoconstrictor (sulfites are included with vasoconstrictors as antioxidants)

Cross-Sensitivity

Table 1.4 describes potential cross-sensitivity considerations.

Special Patients

Pregnant and nursing women

Local anesthetics readily cross the placenta and enter the fetal circulation. Although retrospective investigations of pregnant women receiving local anesthesia during the first trimester of pregnancy have found no evidence of fetal toxicity, animal investigations indicate a potential for birth defects—albeit at enormous doses—with some local anesthetics.

Considerations of risk/benefit suggest that purely elective treatment be delayed until after delivery and that other dental care be performed, if possible, during the second trimester. Lidocaine and, probably, other local anesthetics are distributed into breast milk; again, however, no problems with injected local anesthetics have been documented in humans.

Table 1.1 lists the FDA pregnancy category classifications for injectable local anesthetics used in dentistry.

Pediatric, geriatric and other special patients

Although there are some data to suggest that adverse reactions to local anesthetics may be more prevalent in pediatric and geriatric populations, studies involving mepivacaine and other local anesthetics have found no age-specific problem that would limit use. However, overdosage is more likely to occur in young children because of their small size and the commensurately low margin for error. Increased variability of response to the local anesthetic or vasoconstrictor is likely to be encountered in elderly patients and in those with significant medical problems. Lower maximum doses (as shown in parentheses in Table 1.1) in these patients provides an extra margin of safety.

Patient Monitoring: Aspects to Watch

- State of consciousness
- Respiratory status
- Cardiovascular status

Adverse Effects and Precautions

The incidence of adverse reactions to local anesthetic agents is low. Many reactions (headache, palpitation, tremor, nausea, dyspnea, hyperventilation syndrome, syncope) result from the perceived stress of injection and are not caused by the agents themselves. Toxic systemic reactions generally are associated with high plasma concentrations of the local anesthetic or vasoconstrictor, or both, after an accidental intravascular injection, administration of drug in a manner that causes rapid absorption, administration of a true overdosage or selection of a drug formulation inappropriate for the specific patient.

Idiosyncratic and allergic reactions account for a small minority of adverse responses. In addition, a small subset of asthmatic patients intolerant of inhaled or dietary sulfites may develop bronchospasm after injection of local anesthetic solutions containing sulfite antioxidants.

Systemic reactions to local anesthetics may occur immediately on administration or may be delayed for up to 30 min or more. Oxygen, resuscitative equipment and drugs necessary to treat systemic emergencies must be immediately available whenever a local anesthetic is administered. The adverse effects listed in Tables 1.5 and 1.6 apply to all routes of administration.

Table 1.5
Local Anesthetics: Adverse Effects, Precautions and Contraindications

Body system	Adverse effects	Precautions/contraindications
General	Allergic reactions, including contact dermatitis, skin rash, urticaria, erythema, itching, swelling of injection site, lips, tongue, eyelids and throat; may be accompanied by nausea with or without vomiting; much more likely to occur with esters than with amides Serious anaphylactoid reactions, including shock (rare) Numbness and tingling possible in area affected by injection; long-lasting or permanent paresthesia (rare) Trismus after nerve block injection (inferior alveolar, posterior superior alveolar nerves) Methemoglobinemia, *common with prilocaine overdose,* but rarely observed with other local anesthetics; cyanosis, symptomless with mild reactions, possibly accompanied by respiratory distress, tachycardia, headache, fatigue, dizziness and cardiopulmonary collapse	*Inflammation or infection in the region of injection or in the area to be anesthetized may decrease or eliminate anesthetic effect* *Contraindicated in patients who have history of drug sensitivity to the anesthetic being considered for use, to any preservative or other component of the anesthetic solution and to chemically related agents; it is not known whether a small test dose can predict the risk of allergic reaction* *Methemoglobinemia, congenital or acquired, contraindicates the use of prilocaine*
CV	Cardiovascular depression may be caused by excessive doses of local anesthetics, especially bupivacaine and etidocaine, but is usually secondary to respiratory depression; if not treated promptly, may cause or worsen hypoxia and acidosis and may lead to heart block and cardiac arrest	*Cardiovascular disease or impairment, especially serious forms of heart block and hypotension, may increase responsiveness to the cardiovascular depressant effects of local anesthetics*
CNS	Stimulation, including anxiety, minor twitching and tonic-clonic convulsions *(especially in children);* may be transient after intravascular injection or administration of large toxic doses Depression, including drowsiness, unconsciousness and respiratory depression; may follow initial stimulant phase or occur by itself (*especially in children* and with lidocaine)	None of significance to dentistry
GI	Nausea, vomiting	None of significance to dentistry

Italics indicate information of major clinical significance.

Continued on next page

Table 1.5 (cont.)
Local Anesthetics: Adverse Effects, Precautions and Contraindications

Body system	Adverse effects	Precautions/contraindications
GU	None of significance to dentistry	Local anesthetic metabolites may accumulate in patients with renal disease
HB	None of significance to dentistry	Any condition that involves decreased hepatic blood flow or function (congestive heart failure, cirrhosis, other hepatic disorders) may impair amide metabolism in the liver Decreased synthesis of plasma cholinesterase may reduce ester metabolism

Table 1.6
Vasoconstrictors: Adverse Effects, Precautions and Contraindications

Body system	Adverse effects	Precautions/contraindications
General	Asthma and other allergiclike reactions may be caused by the sulfite antioxidant used to prevent oxidation of the vasoconstrictor Local tissue damage; ischemia from decreased blood flow and increased oxygen demand may lead to delayed healing, edema or necrosis of injected tissue	History of nonallergic sulfite sensitivity, especially in systemic corticosteroid-dependent patient, may increase risk of asthmatic reaction Multiple injections at the same tissue site increase likelihood of local tissue damage *Contraindicated in patients with history of true allergic reaction to sulfites*
CV	Cardiac stimulation; may result in increased blood pressure, headache, palpitation, tachycardia, arrhythmias, angina pectoris and heart attack Peripheral vasoconstriction; may result in acute hypertension and reflex bradycardia, arrhythmias, angina pectoris, heart attack and stroke	Vasoconstrictor may acutely lower plasma potassium concentration in hypokalemic patient, increasing potential for arrhythmias *Cardiac defects (aortic stenosis, septal hypertrophy), disease (coronary atherosclerosis) or arrhythmias (atrial fibrillation, ventricular arrhythmias) increase potential for cardiac toxicity* *Cardiovascular toxicity is more likely in patients with poorly controlled hypertensive disease, pheochromocytoma or uncontrolled hyperthyroidism, or from interaction with antihypertensive medications* Exaggerated vascular responsiveness in patients with peripheral vascular disease may lead to hypertension or hypoxic injury to local tissues
CNS	CNS stimulation, including anxiety, nervousness, restlessness, tremor	None of significance to dentistry
GI	Nausea, vomiting	None of significance to dentistry
Resp	Dyspnea, pulmonary edema	None of significance to dentistry

Italics indicate information of major clinical significance.

Pharmacology

Local Anesthetics

Local anesthetics bind to sodium channels in the nerve membrane and prevent the entry of sodium ions in response to the membrane's depolarization. Propagation of the action potential is inhibited in the area of injection, and nerve conduction fails when an adequate length of nerve is exposed to a sufficient concentration of local anesthetic. Nerve conduction is restored as the anesthetic diffuses away from the injection site and is absorbed into the systemic circulation. Systemic effects, should they occur, are largely the result of the local anesthetic's inhibiting other excitable tissues. Systemic reactions are minimized when metabolism of the local anesthetic is able to inactivate the drug as it is absorbed into the bloodstream.

The rate of absorption of a local anesthetic is governed by several factors, including the drug, its concentration and dose, the vascularity of the injection site and the presence of a vasoconstrictor. Generally, peak concentrations are achieved in 10 to 30 min.

Most amide anesthetics are metabolized in the liver. Prilocaine is unusual in that it is metabolized in the kidneys to some extent.

Most esters are hydrolyzed by plasma esterase to inactive products; some metabolism also occurs in the liver. Although classified as an amide local anesthetic, articaine is inactivated by plasma esterase, which cleaves a vital side chain from the drug.

Small amounts of local anesthetics (2%-20%) and the various metabolites are eventually excreted into the urine.

Vasoconstrictors

Epinephrine, levonordefrin and other adrenergic amine vasoconstrictors help retard absorption of the local anesthetic by stimulating α-adrenergic receptors in the local vasculature. The resultant reduction in tissue blood flow gives the local anesthetic more time to reach its site of action in the nerve membrane.

Systemic effects of vasoconstrictors are associated with stimulation of both α- and β-adrenergic receptors. The intensity and duration of these effects parallel the rate of absorption of the vasoconstrictor from the injection site. Stimulation of β receptors results in cardiac stimulation and vasodilation in skeletal muscle (β_2 receptors only). Stimulation of α receptors causes constriction of resistance arterioles throughout the body as well as capacitance veins in the legs and abdomen, which increases peripheral vascular resistance and venous return to the heart. Both α- and β-receptor effects contribute to the potential for cardiac arrhythmias.

The adrenergic vasoconstrictors used in dentistry are quickly inactivated (plasma half-life of 1-2 min) by the enzyme catechol-O-methyltransferase. Additional metabolism of epinephrine by monoamine oxidase may occur, and the products are then excreted in the urine.

Patient Advice

- Injury to the anesthetized tissues may occur without any resulting sensation.
- To prevent injury, patients should not test for anesthesia by biting the lip or tongue, nor should they eat or chew anything until the anesthetic effect has dissipated.
- Children should be warned not to bite their lip or tongue and be monitored by their parents to prevent injury.

Suggested Readings

Butterworth JF IV, Strichartz GR. Molecular mechanisms of local anesthesia: a review. Anesthesiology 1990;72(4):711-34.

Jastak JT, Yagiela JA, Donaldson D. Local anesthesia of the oral cavity. Philadelphia: Saunders; 1995.

Malamed SF. Handbook of local anesthesia. 4th ed. St. Louis: Mosby–Year Book; 1996.

Persson G. General side-effects of local dental anaesthesia. Acta Odontol Scand 1969;27(Supplement 53):1-141.

Topical Local Anesthetics

Topical local anesthetic preparations used on oral mucosa differ in several respects from injectable preparations. Topical agents are selected for their ability to penetrate the oral mucosa and depend on diffusion to reach their site of action. Many of the anesthetics effective for nerve block or infiltration do not adequately cross the mucosa and, therefore, are not used for topical anesthesia.

In contrast to their injectable counterparts, topical ester-type agents are important for producing anesthesia, and some drugs used for mucosal anesthesia are neither esters nor amides. Life-threatening allergic reactions are extremely unlikely with topical anesthetics, regardless of type, and the inclusion of paraben preservatives in some topical amide formulations reduces the disparity in risk of allergy among these preparations.

Topical anesthetics are manufactured in a variety of forms. Gels, viscous gels and ointments are best used to limit the area of coverage of the topical anesthetic; aerosol sprays and solution rinses are best used for widespread application; lozenges, pastes and film-forming gels are specifically formulated to provide prolonged pain relief.

Table 1.7

Topical Anesthetics: Duration of Action

Drug	Duration of anesthetic action
Benzocaine	10-20 min
Cocaine	20-40 min
Dyclonine	20-40 min
Lidocaine	10-20 min*
Tetracaine	20-60 min

Duration can be extended up to 45 min if lidocaine transoral delivery patch is applied for 15 min.

Several drugs used as topical anesthetics are so insoluble in water that they cannot be prepared in aqueous solutions. They are soluble in alcohol, propylene glycol, polyethylene glycol, volatile oils and other vehicles suitable for surface application. Included in this group of anesthetics are benzocaine and lidocaine base. The poor water solubility of benzocaine in particular makes it safe for topical use on abraded or lacerated tissue.

To facilitate diffusion, the concentration of anesthetic used for surface application is usually much higher than that of injectable preparations. As a consequence, the potential toxicity of these preparations can be significant if large quantities are absorbed or even ingested. Systemic absorption of some topical anesthetics applied to the mucosa can be rapid, and blood concentrations approaching those with intravenous infusion may be achieved with tetracaine, depending on the area of coverage and method of application.

The rate of onset for topical anesthesia varies from 30 s to 5 min, depending on the anesthetic agent. Optimum effectiveness may be delayed for as much as 10 min (as in the case of dyclonine). The mucosa should be dried before application to improve local uptake. The duration of topical anesthesia is generally shorter than with injected anesthesia. Table 1.7 indicates the approximate durations of action of the various topical anesthetics for mucosal anesthesia.

An occlusive dressing preventing the loss of agent can extend the duration; removing the residual agent and rinsing the mouth can shorten it. Topical preparations do not contain adrenergic vasoconstrictors.

Generally, mucosal anesthesia is only about 2 mm deep and is poor or nonexistent in the hard palate. Lidocaine and prilocaine prepared in a eutectic mixture have been shown to improve anesthetic depth; however, no preparation for intraoral use has been marketed at this time.

The FDA recently approved a mucoadhesive patch containing lidocaine—DentiPatch

Lidocaine Transoral Delivery System—for use in the mouth. It is applied directly to the mucosa in the area where anesthesia is desired so that the lidocaine's effect is maximized and the flow and dilution of the medication is limited. Anesthetic effect begins in 2.5 min and the patch can be left in place for up to 15 min.

Accepted Indications

Topical local anesthetics are used to provide mucosal analgesia before local anesthetic injection; to facilitate dental examination, the taking of radiographs and other relatively noninvasive dental procedures by minimizing pain and the gag reflex; and to provide temporary symptomatic relief of toothache, oral lesions and wounds, as well as irritation caused by dentures and other appliances.

Additional uses for diagnostic and therapeutic purposes are described in product labeling.

General Dosing Information

The dosage of topical anesthetics depends on the anesthetic preparation selected, the area to be anesthetized, the ability to maintain the anesthetic agent on the area of application, the vascularity of the administration site and the patient's age, size and health status. Physical removal of the anesthetic and rinsing of the mouth once the need for topical anesthesia has passed preclude further absorption of the drug.

Maximum Recommended Doses

Table 1.8 lists the usual dose and the maximum recommended dose for topical anesthetic formulations per application and, where appropriate or available, the application interval.

Dosage Adjustments

The actual maximum dose for each patient must be individualized depending on his or her size, age and physical status; other drugs he or she may be taking; and the anticipated rate of absorption of the topical anesthetic from the application site. Reduced maximum doses are often indicated for pediatric and geriatric patients, people who have serious illness or disability and patients who have medical conditions or are taking drugs that alter responses to topical anesthetics.

Specific limits for topical anesthetic use in pediatric patients appear in Table 1.8.

Special Dental Considerations

Drug Interactions of Dental Interest

Drug interactions and related problems involving topical anesthetics are in general the same as those listed in Table 1.2. Interactions specific to cocaine (rarely used in dentistry) are listed in Table 1.9.

Cross-Sensitivity

The potential for cross-sensitivity of topical local anesthetics is addressed in Table 1.4.

Special Patients

Pregnant and nursing women

Once absorbed into the systemic circulation, topical anesthetics can cross the placenta to enter the fetal circulation. Table 1.8 includes the FDA pregnancy category classifications for topical anesthetics used in dentistry. Considerations of risk/benefit suggest that purely elective treatment should be delayed until after delivery and that other dental care should be performed, if possible, during the second trimester. Lidocaine and probably other topical anesthetics are distributed into breast milk, but no problems have been documented in humans, except with cocaine. Cocaine intake by infants during nursing has led to overt toxicity, including convulsions and cardiovascular derangements.

Pediatric, geriatric and other special patients

Adverse reactions to topical anesthetics are rare in dentistry but may be more prevalent in pediatric and geriatric populations. Overdosage is more likely to occur in young children because of their small size and the commensurately low margin of error. Methemoglobinemia with use of benzocaine is largely limited to young children. Increased

Table 1.8
Topical Anesthetics: Dosage Information*

Generic name	Brand name(s)	Usual adult dosage	Maximum adult dosage	Usual child dosage	Pregnancy risk category	Content/form
Benzocaine	**Aerosol:** Hurricaine ★, Super-Dent ★, Topex ★ **Film-forming gel:** Oratect, Zilactin-B **Gel:** Anbesol (several forms), Anbocaine, Baby Orabase ★, Gingicaine ★, Hurricaine ★, Numzident, Num-Zit, Orabase, Orajel (several forms), Rid-A-Pain Dental, SensoGARD, Super-Dent ★, Topex ★, Topicale ★; Xylonor; Topicaine [CAN] **Lozenges:** Chloraseptic Pediatric, Spec-T Sore Throat Anesthetic **Ointment:** Benzodent ★, CoraCaine ★, Kank-a ★, Dentapaine, Topicale ★ **Paste:** Orabase-B with Benzocaine ★ **Solution:** Anbesol Maximum Strength, Dent-Zel-Ite, Gingicaine ★, Hurricaine ★, Kank-a, Num-Zit Lotion, Topex ★, Topicale ★; Baby Orajel [CAN], Dentocaine [CAN], Oragel [CAN]	**Aerosol:** 1-s spray tid-qid **Lozenges:** 10-mg lozenge q 2 h or 5-mg lozenge q h **Other forms:** Amount needed to cover area to be anesthetized; in home use, tid-qid for no more than 2 days	Not established	**Most forms:** Dosage must be individualized up to 2 y of age (6 y for paste) **Ointment:** Dosage not established	C	**Aerosol:** 200 mg/mL **Film-forming gel:** 100, 150 mg/mL **Gel:** 63, 75, 100, 150, 180, 200 mg/mL **Lozenges:** 5, 10 mg **Ointment:** 161, 200 mg/mL **Paste:** 200 mg/mL **Solution:** 2, 50, 200 mg/mL; 65 [CAN], 75 [CAN] mg/mL
Benzocaine and menthol	**Lozenges:** Chloraseptic	1 lozenge q 2 h	No information available	**Age ≤ 2 y:** Dosage must be individualized	C	Benzocaine, 6 mg; menthol, 10 mg
Benzocaine and phenol	**Gel:** Anbesol Regular Strength, Anbesol Gel [CAN] **Solution:** Anbesol Regular Strength, Anbesol Maximum Strength; Anbesol [CAN]	Amount needed to cover area to be anesthetized; in home use, should not be used more than 2 days	No information available	**Age ≤ 2 y:** Dosage must be individualized	C	**Gel:** benzocaine, 63 mg/mL, 64 [CAN] mg/mL; phenol, 0.5% **Solution:** benzocaine, 63 mg/kg, 65 [CAN], 200 [CAN] mg/kg; phenol, 0.5%, 0.45 % [CAN]

Drug	Brand/Forms	Usual adult dosage	Maximum adult dose*	Pediatric dosage	Pregnancy category	Available forms
Benzocaine, butamben and tetracaine hydrochloride	**Aerosol, gel and ointment: Cetacaine ★**	**Aerosol:** 1-s spray	**Aerosol:** 2-s spray **Other forms:** 1 mL (20 mg tetracaine)	Dosage not established	C	Benzocaine, 140 mg/mL; butamben, 20 mg/mL; tetracaine HCl, 20 mg/mL
Cocaine hydrochloride†	**Powder, solution and tablets:** (generic)	**Solution:** 1% to 4% given by spray, instillation or topical application; 1-2 applications	400 mg	**Age < 12 y:** Dosage not established	C	**Powder:** 5, 25 g **Solution:** 40, 100 mg/mL **Tablets:** 135 mg
Dyclonine hydrochloride	**Lozenges:** Sucrets **Solution:** Dyclone ★	**Lozenges:** 1 lozenge q 2 h **Solution:** 0.5%; 1 application	**Solution:** 300 mg	Dosage not established (exception: 1.2-mg lozenge for ages ≥ 2 y)	C	**Lozenges:** 1.2, 2, 3 mg **Solution:** 5, 10 mg/mL
Lidocaine	**Aerosol:** Xylocaine **Ointment:** Xylocaine ★ **Patch:** DentiPatch **Solution:** Xylocaine ★	**Aerosol:** 2 sprays (20 mg) per quadrant **Ointment:** 1-2 applications, 50-200 mg **Patch:** 1 application **Solution:** 1-2 applications, 50-200 mg	**Aerosol:** 3 sprays (30 mg) per quadrant q 30 min **Ointment:** 5 g (250 mg lidocaine base)/dose or 20 g/day **Solution:** Up to 250 mg/day	**Aerosol:** 3 mg/kg **Patch:** Safety and effectiveness not established for ages < 12 y **Other forms:** 4.5 mg/kg	B	**Aerosol:** 10 mg/metered spray **Ointment:** 50 mg/mL **Patch (2 cm long/1 cm wide/2 mm thick):** 23, 46.1 mg/patch **Solution:** 25, 50 mg/mL
Lidocaine HCl	**Oral topical solution: Xylocaine Viscous ★** **Solution:** Xylocaine ★	**Oral topical solution:** q 3 h **Solution:** 4%	4.5 mg/kg up to 300 mg; not to exceed 8 doses/day	**Oral topical solution:** 25 mg up to age 3 y; 4.5 mg/kg for ages ≥ 3 y **Solution:** Dosage must be individualized	B	**Oral topical solution:** 20 mg/mL **Solution:** 40 mg/mL
Tetracaine [CAN]	**Aerosol:** Supracaine	2 sprays (1.4 mg) per site	20 mg (~28 sprays)	Dosage not established	C	**Aerosol:** 0.7 mg/metered spray

★ indicates a drug bearing the ADA Seal of Acceptance
[CAN] indicates a drug available only in Canada.
*Dosages are the maximum recommended doses approved by the U.S. Food and Drug Administration or listed in the USPDI.
†Cocaine is a Schedule II drug and rarely used in dentistry because there are safer alternatives.

Table 1.9

Cocaine: Possible Interactions With Other Drugs

Drug taken by patient	Interaction with cocaine	Dentist's action
Monoamine oxidase inhibitors (furazolidone, phenelzine)	*May increase stimulant effects of cocaine*	Avoid use of cocaine within 2 w of last use of monoamine oxidase inhibitor
Sympathomimetic drugs (epinephrine, levonordefrin, dopamine)	*Effects of the sympathomimetic drug are increased*	Avoid concurrent use of cocaine and sympathomimetic drugs
Digitalis glycosides (digoxin, digitoxin), tricyclic antidepressants (amitriptyline, doxepin, imipramine), nitrates (nitroglycerin, isosorbide dinitrate)	Risk of cardiac toxicity is increased	Use cautiously and in restricted doses
Hydrocarbon inhalation anesthetics (halothane, enflurane)	*Sensitization of the heart by anesthetic may lead to cardiac arrhythmias*	Inform anesthesiologist of intended use
Levodopa, methyldopa, thyroid hormones (levothyroxine, liothyronine)	Risk of cardiac toxicity may be increased in patients taking large doses of these agents	Use cautiously and in restricted doses
CNS stimulants (amphetamine, methylphenidate)	*Additive CNS stimulation possible*	Avoid concurrent use of cocaine and CNS stimulants
Adrenergic neuronal blocking drugs (guanadrel, guanethidine, reserpine)	May enhance systemic responses to cocaine; therapeutic effects of the blocking drugs may be reduced	Use cautiously
β-adrenergic blockers (propranolol, nadolol)	β-blocking effects on the heart may be attenuated by cocaine; blockade of β-adrenergic receptors in skeletal muscle by nonspecific β-adrenergic blockers may lead to hypertensive responses	Use cautiously and in restricted doses

Italics indicate information of major clinical significance.

variability of response to local anesthetics is likely to be encountered in elderly patients and in those with significant medical problems. Lower maximum doses in these patients provides an extra margin of safety.

Patient Monitoring: Aspects to Watch

- State of consciousness
- Respiratory status
- Cardiovascular status

Adverse Effects and Precautions

Systemic reactions may occur when local anesthetics are applied topically. Systemic absorption of these agents should be minimized by limiting the concentration of the drug, the area of application, the total amount of agent applied and the time of exposure for drugs that can be removed once the effect has been achieved. To minimize absorption, special caution is needed when applying topical agents to severely traumatized mucosa or to areas of sepsis.

Several topical anesthetic preparations are marketed in pressurized spray containers. It is difficult to control the amount of drug expelled with unmetered spray devices and to confine the agent to the desired site. Thus, a patient may inadvertently inhale sufficient quantities of the aerosol spray to provoke an adverse reaction. Therefore, caution is advised when using any spray device, and metered spray devices are preferred because they dispense a set amount of drug.

Adverse effects and precautions in addition to those included in Table 1.5 are listed in Table 1.10.

Pharmacology

Topical local anesthetics provide anesthesia by anesthetizing the free nerve endings in the mucosa. The mechanism of action is identical to that described in the previous section for injectable local anesthetics. Cocaine, however, has a distinct pharmacology. In addition to its local anesthetic action, cocaine blocks the reuptake of released adrenergic neurotransmitters (norepinephrine, dopamine) back into the nerve terminal. This action gives cocaine its vasoconstrictor and CNS stimulant properties, as well as its addictive potential and increased risk of cardiovascular toxicity.

The rate of absorption of a topical anesthetic depends on the dose administered, the duration of exposure, the area of coverage, the mucosa's permeability, the mucosa's intactness and the vascularity of the tissue. Benzocaine is unique in its poor solubility in water and is the least absorbed into the bloodstream.

A considerable portion of topical anesthetics administered intraorally is swallowed. Although absorption from the gastrointestinal tract occurs, extensive metabolism of the drug in the hepatic-portal system prevents toxic blood concentrations except with excessive doses. The metabolic fate and excretion of these drugs is covered in the first part of this chapter, in the section on injectable local anesthetics.

Patient Advice

- Injury to the anesthetized tissues may occur without any resulting sensation.
- To prevent pulmonary aspiration, patients who have undergone topical anesthesia of the pharynx should use caution when

Table 1.10

Topical Anesthetics: Adverse Effects, Precautions and Contraindications

Body system	Adverse effects	Precautions/contraindications
General	Methemoglobinemia, rare but occasionally observed with benzocaine in small children	Benzocaine should be used cautiously in patients with congenital or acquired methemoglobinemia
CV	Stimulation with cocaine	Cocaine should be used cautiously in patients with cardiovascular disease, hyperthyroidism, cerebrovascular disease
CNS	Stimulation with cocaine	Cocaine should be used cautiously in patients with Tourette's syndrome or seizure history Cocaine use contraindicated in patients with history of cocaine abuse
Oral	Numbness of throat; may impair swallowing and increase risk of aspiration; slight irritation at application site (rarely)	None pertinent to dentistry

Italics indicate information of major clinical significance.

eating or drinking until normal sensation has returned.

- To prevent injury, patients should not test for anesthesia by biting the lip or tongue, nor should they eat or chew anything until the anesthetic effect has dissipated.
- Children should be warned not to bite their lips or tongue and be monitored by their parents to prevent injury.
- Patients using topical anesthetics to manage toothache, intraoral conditions or ill-fitting dental appliances should seek professional dental care for definitive treatment.

Suggested Readings

Jastak JT, Yagiela JA, Donaldson D. Local anesthesia of the oral cavity. Philadelphia: Saunders; 1995.

Malamed SF. Handbook of local anesthesia. 4th ed. St. Louis: Mosby–Year Book; 1996.

Middleton RM, Kirkpatrick MB. Clinical use of cocaine. A review of the risks and benefits. Drug Safety 1993;9(3):212-7.

Vickers ER, Punnia-Moorthy A. Pulpal anesthesia from an application of a eutectic topical anesthetic. Quintessence Int 1993;24(8):547-51.

Chapter 2.

Conscious Sedation and Agents for the Control of Anxiety

B. Ellen Byrne, R.Ph., D.D.S., Ph.D.

Outpatient anesthesia for relatively short surgical procedures must achieve a difficult balance between adequate relief of patient pain and quick, uncomplicated recovery from the anesthetic. Regional and local anesthetic techniques offer only a partial solution to this problem, providing analgesia but no amelioration of anxiety, no amnesia and no blunting of stress responses. Conscious sedation appears to offer the remainder of the solution for many patients and procedures.

Conscious sedation is a minimally depressed level of consciousness that retains the patient's ability to independently and continuously maintain an airway and respond appropriately to physical stimulation and verbal command that is produced by a pharmacological or nonpharmacological method or a combination thereof.

The most common pharmacological methods for sedation and control of anxiety involve the use of the benzodiazepines, barbiturates, opioid analgesics and opioid agonists/antagonists. The level of sedation may vary from lighter sedation (conscious sedation) to levels approaching unconsciousness (deep sedation). Although certain drugs are more apt to produce profound sedation than others, any of these drugs can produce overly deep sedation. The nonpharmacological methods used for the management of pain and anxiety include hypnosis, acupuncture, acupressure, audioanalgesia, biofeedback, electroanesthesia (TENS) and electrosedation.

Conscious sedation lies on a dose-dependent continuum leading from no anesthesia to deep general anesthesia (Figure 2.1). The definition emphasizes the patient's ability to respond rationally to commands and the ability to maintain airway patency. (For further information, consult the American Dental Association's Guidelines for the Use of Conscious Sedation, Deep Sedation and General Anesthesia in Dentistry, adopted by the ADA House of Delegates in 1996.)

Complications are relatively minor and of low incidence compared to those associated with general anesthesia. Extensive use of conscious sedation in dental outpatient clinics over the past 20 years has shown this to be a safe, effective technique in the hands of experienced practitioners. Proper monitoring is essential. It is important for the clinician to establish vocal rapport with the patient before beginning the surgical procedure. Routine monitoring, required for parenteral sedation, includes checking the heart rate, blood pressure and respiration using a precordial stethoscope. The use of a digital pulse oximeter is standard practice to monitor both pulse rate and the level of oxygen in the blood.

Figure 2.1

The Spectrum of Pain and Anxiety Control

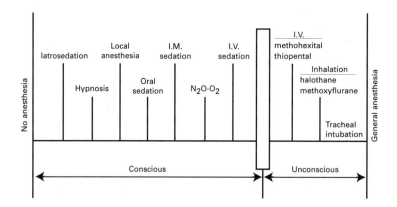

Figure 2.1. The continuum of techniques for the management of patients' pain and anxiety, ranging from no anesthesia to general anesthesia. The vertical bar represents the loss of consciousness.

Benzodiazepines

The benzodiazepines are among the most popular classes of drugs available today. They have been used since the late 1950s for effective and safe treatment of a variety of anxiety states as well as for epilepsy (diazepam, clonazepam) and sleep disorders (flurazepam, temazepam, triazolam). In addition to their use in anxiety, the benzodiazepines have extensive clinical applications in anesthesia procedures (diazepam, midazolam) and as muscle relaxants (diazepam).

Although the benzodiazepines have a wide margin of safety, they are not without adverse effects. Their time course of action is variable among patients as well as among various agents. Although all benzodiazepines are effective, there are significant differences among them. Diazepam and flurazepam are among the most rapidly absorbed, whereas oxazepam is one of the most slowly absorbed. Intramuscular, or IM, routes of administration for benzodiazepines often produce erratic and poor absorption. Most of the benzodiazepines are poorly soluble in water and are not available for intravenous, or IV, use. However, diazepam and midazolam, the two agents most commonly used for conscious sedation, can be administered intravenously. Anterograde amnesia is strongly associated with this class of drugs. The level of amnesia varies with agent and route of administration.

All benzodiazepines in use are bound 50% or more to plasma proteins. Their distribution to tissue depends on their lipid solubility.

The metabolism and excretion of the benzodiazepines are complex. Clorazepate is a prodrug converted by metabolism to the active form; others are inactivated by metabolism; still others are biotransferred to metabolites that retain activity. Many of the metabolites of benzodiazepines have longer half-lives than the parent compound and so accumulate to a greater extent. It is important to recognize that some of these compounds have the potential for extremely long durations of action. Thus, benzodiazepine half-lives vary from a few hours to as long as a week.

The imidazopyridine sedative hypnotic zolpidem is included in this section of the chapter because while it is structurally dissimilar to the benzodiazepines, many of its actions are explained by its action on the benzodiazepine receptor.

Antagonist. The benzodiazepines have a specific antagonist that reverses the CNS effects of benzodiazepines, including respiratory depression. Flumazenil is administered intravenously. Its duration of action may be as brief as 30 minutes, so treatment with it requires continuous monitoring of the patient and possibly repeated administration.

Accepted Indications

Benzodiazepines are used for the treatment of anxiety, insomnia and epilepsy. They are also used in the treatment of panic disorders and alcohol withdrawal. As adjuncts in anesthesia they are used as a preanesthetic medication to produce sedation, relieve anxiety and produce anterograde amnesia.

General Dosing Information

All benzodiazepines have similar pharmacologic actions. Their different clinical uses are often based on pharmacokinetic differences and availability of clinical use data. Optimal dosage of benzodiazepines varies with diagnosis and patient response. The minimum effective dose should be used for the shortest period of time. Prolonged use (for weeks or months) may result in psychological or physical dependence. Following prolonged administration, benzodiazepines should be withdrawn gradually to prevent withdrawal symptoms.

For parenteral dosing, after administration of the drug, patients should be kept under observation until they have recovered sufficiently to return home. Too-rapid intravenous administration may result in respiratory depression, apnea, hypotension, bradycardia and cardiac arrest. When parenteral benzodiazepines are administered intravenously, equipment necessary to secure and maintain an airway should be immediately available.

Table 2.1 provides benzodiazepine dosing information.

Dosage Adjustments

Geriatric or debilitated patients, children and patients with hepatic or renal function impairment should receive a lower initial dosage, as elimination of benzodiazepines may be slower in these patients, resulting in impaired coordination, dizziness and excessive sedation.

Special Dental Considerations

Drug Interactions of Dental Interest

Table 2.2 lists possible interactions of the benzodiazepines and zolpidem with other drugs.

Cross–Sensitivity

There may be cross-sensitivity between benzodiazepines.

Special Patients

Pregnant and nursing women

See Table 2.1 for pregnancy risk categories.

Benzodiazepines are reported to increase the risk of congenital malformations when used during the first trimester; chronic use may cause physical dependence in the neonate, resulting in withdrawal symptoms and CNS depression.

Benzodiazepines and their metabolites may distribute into breast milk, thus creating feeding difficulties and weight loss in the infant.

Pediatric, geriatric and other special patients

Children (especially the very young) and geriatric patients are usually more sensitive to the CNS effects of benzodiazepines. In the neonate, prolonged CNS depression may be produced because of the newborn's inability to metabolize the benzodiazepine into inactive products. In the geriatric patient, the dosage should be limited to the smallest effective dose and increased gradually to minimize ataxia, dizziness and oversedation.

Table 2.1

Benzodiazepines: Dosage Information

Generic name	Brand name(s)	Usual adult dosage	Maximum adult dosage	Usual child dosage	Maximum child dosage	Pregnancy risk category	Content/form
Alprazolam	**Solution:** Alprazolam Intensol **Tablets:** Xanax; Apo-Alpraz [CAN]; Novo-Alprazol [CAN]; Nu-Alpraz [CAN] ; Xanax [CAN]	**Antianxiety:** 0.25-0.5 mg tid	4 mg/day	Not established	Not established	D	**Tablets:** 0.25, 0.5, 1, 2 mg **Oral solution:** 1 mg/ 1 mL; 0.1 mg/1 mL
Bromazepam	Lectopam [CAN]	6-30 mg q day in divided doses	Up to 60 mg/day	Not established	Not established	Not established	**Tablets:** 1.5, 3 mg; 6 mg [CAN]
Chlordiazepoxide	Libritabs, Librium; Apo-Chlordiazepoxide [CAN], Novopoxide [CAN], Solium [CAN]	**Antianxiety—oral:** 5-25 mg tid or qid **Sedative-hypnotic:** 50-100 mg **Elderly patients:** 5 mg bid-qid **Antianxiety—IM or IV:** 50-100 mg initially, then 25-50 mg tid-qid **Preoperative—IM:** 50-100 mg 1 h before surgery	Up to 300 mg/ day **In alcohol withdrawal:** Up to 400 mg/day, then reduce to maintenance level	**Ages < 6 y:** Safety and efficacy not established **Ages ≥ 6 y:** 5 mg bid or qid	Not established	D	**Tablets:** 5, 10, 25 mg **Capsules:** 5, 10, 25 mg; 10, 25 mg [CAN] **Solution:** Sterile chlordiazepoxide HCl, 100 mg with 2 mL special IM diluent

Drug	Brand names	Adult dose		Pediatric dose		Pregnancy category	Dosage forms
Clonazepam	Klonopin; Rivotril [CAN], Syn-Clonazepam [CAN]	**Antianxiety:** 0.5 mg tid **Anticonvulsant:** 0.5 mg tid	Up to 20 mg q day	**Antianxiety:** 0.01-0.03 mg/kg in 2-3 divided doses **Anticonvulsant:** 0.01-0.03 mg/kg in 2-3 divided doses	0.05 mg/kg in 2-3 divided doses	C	**Tablets:** 0.5, 1, 2 mg; 0.5, 2 mg [CAN]
Clorazepate	Gen-XENE, Tranxene-T-Tabs, Tranxene-SD, generic; Apo-Clorazepate [CAN], Novo-Clopate [CAN], Tranxene [CAN]	**Antianxiety:** 7.5-15 mg bid-qid **Sedative-hypnotic:** 30 mg initially, then 15 mg bid-qid, then tapering off **Anticonvulsant:** 7.5 mg tid	90 mg q day	Not established	Not established	Not established	**Capsules:** 3.75, 7.5, 15 mg **Tablets:** 3.75, 7.5, 11.25, 15, 22.5 mg
Diazepam	Valium, generic; Apo-Diazepam [CAN], Novodipam [CAN], Valium [CAN], Vivol [CAN]	**Anxiety/sedation/skeletal muscle relaxation—oral:** 2-10 mg bid-qid **IM, IV:** 2-10 mg; may repeat in 3-4 h if needed **Status epilepticus—IV:** 5-10 mg every 10-20 min, up to 30 mg in an 8-h period; may repeat in 2-4 h if necessary *Continued on next page*	Not established	**Conscious sedation for procedures—oral:** 0.2-0.3 mg/kg (maximum: 10 mg) 45-60 min before procedure **Sedation, muscle relaxation or anxiety—oral:** 0.12-0.8 mg/kg/day in divided doses q 6-8 h *Continued on next page*	Not established	D	**Tablets:** 2, 5, 10 mg

[CAN] indicates a drug available only in Canada.

Continued on next page

Chapter 2. Conscious Sedation and Agents for the Control of Anxiety

Table 2.1 (cont.)

Benzodiazepines: Dosage Information

Generic name	Brand name(s)	Usual adult dosage	Maximum adult dosage	Usual child dosage	Maximum child dosage	Pregnancy risk category	Content/form
Diazepam (cont.)		**Elderly, for anxiety— oral:** 1-2 mg 1-2 times/day, initially; increase gradually as needed (rarely need to use > 10 mg/day) **Skeletal muscle relaxant:** 2-5 mg bid-qid		**IM, IV:** 0.04-0.3 mg/kg/dose every 2-4 h to a maximum of 0.6 mg/kg within an 8-h period **Adolescents: Conscious sedation for procedures —oral:** 10 mg **IV:** 5 mg, may repeat with 1/2 dose if needed			
Diazepam, extended release capsule	Valrelease	**Oral:** 15 or 30 mg once a day	Not established	Not established	Not established	Not established	**Extended-release capsules:** 15 mg **Tablets:** 2, 5, 10 mg
Diazepam, oral solution	Diazepam Intensol, generic; PMS-Diazepam [CAN]	2-10 mg bid-qid	Not established	**Age ≤ 6 mo:** Not recommended **Age > 6 mo:** 1-2.5 mg, 0.04-0.2 mg/kg tid-qid	**Age ≤ 6 mo:** Not recommended **Age > 6 mo:** 1-2.5 mg, 0.04-0.2 mg/kg tid-qid	D	**Intensol oral solution:** 5 mg/mL **Generic oral solution:** 5 mg/5 mL **PMS-Diazepam oral solution:** 1 mg/mL
Diazepam, injection	D-Val, Valium, Zetran, generic; Valium [CAN]	**Antianxiety:** 5-10 mg	Not established	Not established	Not established	D	5 mg/mL
Diazepam, sterile emulsion	Diazemuls [CAN]	**Antianxiety:** 10 mg 1-2 h before surgery	Not established	Not established	Not established	D	5 mg/mL

Estazolam	ProSom	Sedative-hypnotic—oral: 1 mg (2 mg may be necessary in some patients)	Not established	Not established	Not established	Not established	X	Tablets: 1, 2 mg
Flurazepam	Dalmane, generic; Apo-Flurazepam [CAN], Novoflupam [CAN]	Sedative-hypnotic—oral: 15-30 mg	Not established	Not established	Not established	Not established	X	Capsules: 15, 30 mg
Halazepam	Paxipam	Antianxiety—oral: 20-40 mg tid or qid	Not established	Not established	Not established	Not established	Not established	Tablets: 20, 40 mg
Ketazolam	Loftran [CAN]	Antianxiety—oral: 15 mg 1-2 times a day	Not established	Not established	Not established	Not established	Not established	Capsules: 15, 30 mg
Lorazepam	Ativan, Lorazepam Intensol Concentrated Solution, generic; Apo-Lorazepam [CAN], Ativan [CAN], Novo-Lorazem [CAN], Nu-Loraz [CAN]	**Antianxiety—oral:** 1 to 3 mg bid-tid **Sedation, hypnotic—oral:** 2-4 mg at bedtime **Antianxiety—IM:** 50 µg per kg, maximum 4 mg **Antianxiety—IV:** 44 µg per kg, maximum 2 mg **Antianxiety—sublingual:** 2-3 mg/day in divided doses **Sedative-hypnotic—oral:** 5-10 mg at bedtime	Not established	**Age > 18 y—injection:** Safety and efficacy not established for patients under age 18 y **Age < 12 y—oral, solution:** Not established for patients under age 12 y **Age < 6 y—oral, sublingual tablets:** Not recommended **Age 6-18 y—oral, sublingual tablets:** Not established	**Age < 12 y:** Not established	D	**Injection:** 2 mg/mL, 4 mg/mL; 4 mg/mL [CAN] **Oral solution:** 2 mg/mL [CAN] **Sublingual tablets:** 0.5, 1, 2 mg **Tablets:** 0.5, 1, 2 mg

[CAN] indicates a drug available only in Canada.

Continued on next page

Table 2.1 (cont.)

Benzodiazepines: Dosage Information

Generic name	Brand name(s)	Usual adult dosage	Maximum adult dosage	Usual child dosage	Maximum child dosage	Pregnancy risk category	Content/form
Midazolam	Versed	**Preoperative sedation—IM:** 0.07-0.08 mg/kg 30-60 min presurgery; usual dose 5 mg **Conscious sedation—IV:** Initially, 0.5-2 mg slow IV over at least 2 min; slowly titrate to effect by repeating doses every 2-3 min if needed; usual total dose 2.5-5 mg **Unpremedicated patient aged <55 y, anesthesia:** 0.2-0.35 mg/kg over 20-30 s, allowing 2 min for effect; if need to complete induction, increments of approximately 25% of patient's initial dose may be used; in resistant case, up to 0.6 mg/kg total dose may be used for induction, but with such large doses, recovery may be prolonged	Not established	**Preoperative sedation—IM:** 0.07-0.08 mg/kg 30-60 min presurgery **Preoperative sedation—IV:** 0.035 mg/kg/dose; repeat over several minutes as required up to a total dose of 0.1-0.2 mg/kg **Adjunct to general anesthesia:** must be individualized, but 0.05-0.2 mg/kg **Conscious sedation during mechanical ventilation—IV:** Loading dose 0.05-0.2 mg/kg, followed by initial continuous infusion of 1-2 µg/kg/min; titrate to desired effect; usual range 0.4-6 µg/kg/min	Not established	D	**Injection:** 1 mg/mL, 5 mg/mL; 5 mg/mL [CAN]

Midazolam (cont.)	**Unpremedicated patient aged > 55 y, for anesthesia:** Usually require less of the drug; 0.15-0.3 mg/kg is recommended	**Conscious sedation for procedures—oral, intranasal:** 0.2-0.4 mg/kg (maximum: 15 mg) 30-45 min before procedure
	Unpremedicated patient with systemic disease, for anesthesia: 0.2-0.25 mg/kg; in some cases, 0.15 mg/kg may suffice	**Conscious sedation for procedures—IV:** 0.05 mg/kg 3 min before procedure
	Premedicated patients, for anesthesia: 0.15-0.35 mg/kg; in average adult aged <55 y, give 0.25 mg/kg over 20-30 s and allow 2 min for effect	**Adolescents > 12 years—IV:** 0.5 mg q 3-4 min until effect achieved
	Surgical patients aged > 55 y, for anesthesia: Use 0.2 mg/kg for good-risk (ASA 1 and II) surgical patients; in patients with severe systemic disease or debilitation, 0.15 mg/kg may suffice	

Continued on next page

Table 2.1 (cont.)

Benzodiazepines: Dosage Information

Generic name	Brand name(s)	Usual adult dosage	Maximum adult dosage	Usual child dosage	Maximum child dosage	Pregnancy risk category	Content/form
Midazolam (cont.)		**Healthy adults < 60 years:** May respond to doses as low as 1 mg; administer no more than 2.5 mg within 2 min; dentist may administer additional doses after waiting 2 min and evaluating sedation after each dose; total dose > 5 mg generally not needed; reduce dose by 30% if narcotics or other CNS depressants administered concomitantly					
Nitrazepam	Mogadon [CAN]	**Sedative-hypnotic—oral:** 5-10 mg at bedtime	Not established	Not established	Not established	Not established	**Tablets:** 5 mg, 10 mg
Oxazepam	Serax, generic; Apo-Oxazepam [CAN], Novoxapam [CAN]	**Antianxiety—oral:** 10-30 mg tid or qid / **Sedative-hypnotic—oral:** 15-30 mg tid or qid	Not established	Not established	Not established	C	**Tablets and capsules:** 10, 15, 30 mg
Prazepam	Centrax, generic	**Antianxiety—oral:** 10 mg tid	Not established	Not established	Not established	C	**Capsules:** 5, 10, 20 mg / **Tablets:** 5, 10 mg

Quazepam	Doral	**Sedative-hypnotic—oral:** 15 mg initially, then reduce to 7.5 if needed	Not established	Not established	Not established	X	**Tablets:** 7.5, 15 mg
Temazepam	Restoril, generic	**Sedative-hypnotic—oral:** 15 mg	Not established	Not established	Not established	X	**Capsules:** 7.5, 15, 30 mg **Tablets:** 15, 30 mg
Triazolam	Halcion; Apo-Triazo [CAN], Gen-Triazolam [CAN], NovoTriolam [CAN], Nu-Triazo [CAN], generic [CAN]	**Sedative-hypnotic—oral:** 125–250 µg	Not established	Not established	Not established	X	**Tablets:** 125, 250 µg (0.125, 0.250 mg)
Zolpidem (IV)	Ambien	10 mg at bedtime; limit use to 7-10 days	20 mg/day	Not established	Not established	B	**Tablets:** 5, 10 mg

[CAN] indicates a drug available only in Canada.

Table 2.2

Benzodiazepines and Zolpidem: Possible Interactions With Other Drugs

Drug taken by patient	Interaction with benzodiazepines	Dentist's action
Alcohol or CNS depressants	*Concurrent use may increase CNS depressant effects of either medication*	Watch for increased response to CNS depression; decrease dose of benzodiazepine if necessary
Chlorpromazine	**With zolpidem:** Concurrent use may prolong elimination half-life of chlorpromazine	None significant to dentistry
Cimetidine	Inhibition of hepatic metabolism may increase serum levels of some benzodiazepines; may enhance certain actions, especially sedation	Monitor for enhanced response to benzodiazepine
Disulfiram	May inhibit hepatic metabolism of benzodiazepines that undergo oxidation, increasing the benzodiazepine's CNS depressant effect	Monitor for enhanced benzodiazepine response
Erythromycin, troleandomycin, clarithromycin	May decrease the metabolism of certain benzodiazepines, increasing the benzodiazepines' CNS depressant effect	Watch for increased response to benzodiazepines
Imipramine	**With zolpidem:** concurrent use may increase drowsiness and risk of anterograde amnesia; may also decrease peak concentrations of imipramine	None significant to dentistry
Omeprazole	Inhibits the oxidative metabolism of benzodiazepines, thus increasing or prolonging the benzodiazepines' CNS depressant effects	Monitor for enhanced benzodiazepine response
Oral contraceptives	May inhibit metabolism of benzodiazepines that undergo oxidation	Watch for evidence of increased response to benzodiazepines that undergo oxidative metabolism
Theophyllines	May antagonize sedative effects of benzodiazepines	Monitor for decreased benzodiazepine response

Italics indicate information of major clinical significance.

Patient Monitoring: Aspects to Watch

- Respiratory status
- Patient requests for benzodiazepines (all of which are Schedule IV controlled substances in United States)
- Possible abuse and dependence

Adverse Effects and Precautions

Table 2.3 lists adverse effects, precautions and contraindications related to benzodiazepines.

Pharmacology

Benzodiazepines depress all levels of the CNS, resulting in mild sedation, hypnosis or coma, depending on the dose. It is believed that benzodiazepines enhance or facilitate the inhibitory neurotransmitter action of γ-aminobutyric acid (GABA). After oral administration, benzodiazepines are absorbed well from the gastrointestinal tract. After intramuscular injection, absorption of lorazepam and midazolam is rapid and complete, whereas that of chlordiazepoxide and diazepam may be slow and erratic. Rectal absorption of diazepam is rapid. The benzodiazepines are metabolized by the liver to inactive or other active metabolites. During repeated dosing with long–half-life benzodiazepines, there is accumulation of the parent compound and/or active metabolites. During repeated dosing with short– to intermediate–half-life benzodiazepines, accumulation is minimal.

Patient Advice

- Avoid concurrent use of alcohol and other CNS depressants.
- Until CNS effects are known, avoid activities needing good psychomotor skills. Someone should drive the patient to and from dental appointments.
- These drugs may cause physical or psychological dependence.
- These drugs may cause dry mouth. Patients may be advised to suck on sugarless candy, chew sugarless gum or use a commercially available saliva substitute.

Table 2.3

Benzodiazepines: Adverse Effects, Precautions and Contraindications

Body system	Adverse effects	Precautions/contraindications
General	Variable per patient medication	Low serum albumin predisposes patients to a higher incidence of side effects
CV	Cardiac arrest, hypotension, tachycardia, local phlebitis, pain with injection, venous thrombosis	None of significance to dentistry
CNS	*Drowsiness, ataxia, amnesia, confusion, slurred speech, paradoxical excitement, fatigue, lightheadedness, insomnia, headache, anxiety, depression, hallucinations*	*Should be used with caution in patients using other CNS depressants or who have a history of drug abuse or dependence* *Pre-existing mental depression: suicidal tendencies may be present* *May exacerbate sleep apnea*
Endoc	Decreased libido, menstrual irregularities	None of significance to dentistry
EENT	*Blurred vision, diplopia*	*Narrow-angle glaucoma (benzodiazepines have an anticholinergic effect)*
GI	Constipation, nausea, vomiting, diarrhea, abdominal or stomach cramps	None of significance to dentistry
HB	Hepatic dysfunction	None of significance to dentistry
Integ	Allergic reaction or rash	None of significance to dentistry

Italics indicate information of major clinical significance.

Continued on next page

Table 2.3 (cont.)

Benzodiazepines: Adverse Effects, Precautions and Contraindications

Body system	Adverse effects	Precautions/contraindications
Musc	Impaired coordination, rigidity, tremor, muscle cramps	*May exacerbate myasthenia gravis* Long-acting benzodiazepines have been associated with falls in elderly patients
Oral	Dry mouth, increased thirst	None of significance to dentistry
Resp	*Decrease in respiratory rate, apnea, laryngospasm, nasal congestion, hyperventilation*	*Severe chronic obstructive pulmonary disease*

Italics indicate information of major clinical significance.

Benzodiazepine Antagonist: Flumazenil

Accepted Indications

Flumazenil is used to reverse the pharmacological effects of benzodiazepines used in anesthesia and to manage benzodiazepine overdose.

General Dosing Information

Flumazenil selectively reverses the pharmacologic effects of benzodiazepines used in anesthesia and for the management of benzodiazepine overdose. Flumazenil does not antagonize CNS depressants except for zolpidem. See Table 2.4.

Special Dental Considerations

Drug Interactions of Dental Interest

Table 2.5 lists the possible interactions of flumazenil with other drugs.

Cross-Sensitivity

There may be cross-sensitivity to benzodiazepines.

Special Patients

Pregnant and nursing women

Caution should be used in administering flumazenil to a nursing woman because it is not known whether flumazenil is excreted in human milk.

Pediatric, geriatric and other special patients

Flumazenil is not recommended for use in children, either for the reversal of sedation, the management of overdose or resuscitation of newborns.

The pharmacokinectics of flumazenil have been studied in elderly people and are not significantly different from those in younger patients.

Patient Monitoring: Aspects to Watch

- Respiratory status
- Patient alertness
- Possible resedation
- Possible seizure activity

Adverse Effects and Precautions

Table 2.6 lists adverse effects, precautions and contraindications related to flumazenil.

Pharmacology

Flumazenil, an imidazobenzodiazepine derivative, antagonizes the actions of benzodiazepines on the CNS. Flumazenil competitively inhibits the activity at the benzodiazepine recognition site on the benzodiazepine-GABA receptor-chloride ionophore complex. Flumazenil is a weak partial agonist in some animal models of activity, but has little or no agonist activity in humans.

The onset of reversal is usually evident 1 to 2 min after the injection is completed.

Table 2.4

Flumazenil: Dosage Information

Generic name	Brand name(s)	Usual adult dosage	Maximum adult dosage	Child dosage	Pregnancy risk category	Content/ form
Flumazenil	Romazicon	**For reversal of conscious sedation, initial dose—IV:** 0.2 mg over 15 s; if desired level of consciousness is not obtained, 0.2-mg dose may be repeated at 1-min intervals; most patients respond to dose of 0.6-1 mg **For suspected benzodiazepine overdose—IV:** 0.2 mg over 30 s initially, then 0.5 mg over 30 s, repeated at 1-min intervals	**For reversal of conscious sedation:** Up to 1 mg at any one time or 3 mg/h **For suspected benzodiazepine overdose:** Maximum total cumulative dose 5 mg	Not established, but may be used in ranges from 0.01 mg/kg for reversing sedation to 0.1 mg/kg for life-threatening overdose up to maximum cumulative dose of 1 mg	C	**Injection:** 0.1 mg/mL

Table 2.5

Flumazenil: Possible Interactions With Other Drugs

Drug taken by patient	Interaction with flumazenil	Dentist's action
Benzodiazepines taken chronically, especially with tricyclic or tetracyclic antidepressants	Effect is reversed by flumazenil; this may cause excitatory effects such as convulsions	Monitor patient for seizure activity

Eighty percent response will be reached within 3 min, with peak effect occurring at 6 to 10 min. The duration and degree of reversal are related to the plasma concentration of the sedating benzodiazepine as well as the dose of flumazenil given. Resedation is possible if a large single or cumulative dose of benzodiazepine has been given in the course of a long procedure and is least likely in cases where flumazenil is administered to reverse a low dose of a short-acting benzodiazepine.

Suggested Readings

American Dental Association. The use of conscious sedation, deep sedation and general anesthesia in dentistry. Adopted by the ADA House of Delegates, October 1996.

American Dental Association. Guidelines for the use of conscious sedation, deep sedation and general anesthesia for dentists. Adopted by the ADA House of Delegates, October 1996.

American Dental Association Council on Dental Education. Guidelines for teaching the comprehensive control of pain and anxiety in dentistry. Chicago: ADA; 1992.

Giangrego E. Conscious sedation: benefits and risks. JADA 1984;109:546-57.

Kallar SK, Dunwiddie WC. In: Wetchler BV, ed.

Table 2.6

Flumazenil: Adverse Effects, Precautions and Contraindications

Body system	Adverse effects	Precautions/contraindications
CV	Cutaneous vasodilation (sweating, flushing, hot flashes) Arrhythmias (atrial, nodal, ventricular extrasystoles), bradycardia, tachycardia, hypertension, chest pain	Should be used cautiously with patients who have increased left ventricular end-diastolic pressure
CNS	Confusion (difficulty in concentrating) delirium, convulsions, somnolence (stupor), agitation, anxiety, dizziness, emotional lability (crying, euphoria, depression, paranoia)	Should not be used in cases of suspected heterocyclic antidepressant overdose, with patients physically dependent on benzodiazepines or with patients maintained on benzodiazepines for control of potentially life-threatening situations (for example, seizure disorder) Whether for reversal or conscious sedation or for suspected benzodiazepine overdose, administer through a freely running IV infusion into a large vein to minimize pain at the injection site
EENT	Abnormal vision, diplopia	None significant to dentistry
GI	Nausea, vomiting, hiccups	None significant to dentistry
Oral	Dry mouth	None significant to dentistry
Resp	Dyspnea, hyperventilation	None significant to dentistry

Italics indicate information of major clinical significance.

Problems in anesthesia. Philadelphia: JB Lippincott Co; 1988:93–100.

Malamed SF. Sedation: A guide to patient management. 3rd ed., St. Louis: Mosby; 1995.

Miller RD. Clinical Therapeutics 1992; 14(Special Supplemental Section): 861–995.

Barbiturates

The barbiturates were the first drugs truly effective for the management of anxiety. The barbiturates are generalized CNS depressants, depressing the cerebral cortex, the limbic system, and the reticular activating system. These actions produce a reduction in the anxiety level, decreased mental acuity and a state of drowsiness. Barbiturates are capable of producing any level of CNS depression ranging from light sedation through hypnosis, general anesthesia, coma and death. Intravenous barbiturate compounds can be infused in subhypnotic doses to produce sedation.

The barbiturates used for conscious sedation are classified as sedative hypnotics and are categorized by their duration of clinical action following an average oral dose.

Short-acting barbiturates (with 3 to 4 h duration of action), most notably pentobarbital and secobarbital, are better suited for dental situations. The ultra–short-acting barbiturates are classified as general anesthetics and are described in Chapter 3. The long-acting (for 16 to 24 h) and the intermediate-acting (for 6 to 8 h) barbiturates produce clinical levels of sedation for too long a period of time for the usual dental or surgical appointment. The long-acting barbiturates, such as phenobarbital, are commonly used as anticonvulsants or when long-term sedation is necessary. The intermediate-acting barbiturates occasionally are used as "sleeping pills" for some types of insomnia.

Accepted Indications

Barbiturates have been used in the short-term treatment of insomnia, routine sedation to relieve anxiety, tension and apprehension; however, these agents have generally been replaced with the benzodiazepines for these treatments. Barbiturates are used as adjuncts in anesthesia to reduce anxiety and facilitate induction of anesthesia. They are also used in the treatment of epilepsy.

General Dosing Information

Dosage of the barbiturates must be individualized in patients with impaired hepatic function; lower dose should be used initially. Tolerance and physical dependence occurs with repeated administration. These agents are controlled substances in the United States and Canada. See Table 2.7.

Special Dental Considerations

Drug Interactions of Dental Interest

Possible drug interactions and/or related problems of clinical significance in dentistry are shown in Table 2.8.

Special Patients

Pregnant and nursing women
Barbiturates readily cross the placenta and increase the risk of fetal abnormalities. Use during the third trimester may result in physical dependence and respiratory depression in newborns.

Barbiturates distribute into the breast milk and may cause CNS depression in the infant.

Patient Monitoring: Aspects to Watch

• Respiratory status

Adverse Effects and Precautions

Adverse effects and precautions related to barbiturates are listed in Table 2.9.

Pharmacology

Barbiturates can produce all levels of CNS mood alteration, from excitation to sedation, hypnosis and coma. In sufficient therapeutic doses, barbiturates induce anesthesia and overdose can produce death. These agents depress the sensory cortex, decrease motor activity, alter cerebellar function and produce drowsiness, sedation and hypnosis. Barbiturates are respiratory depressants and the degree of respiratory depression is dose-dependent. All barbiturates exhibit anticonvulsant activity.

Barbiturates are enzyme-inducing drugs. This class of drugs can enhance the metabolism of other agents. The onset of this enzyme induction is gradual and depends on the accumulation of the barbiturate and the synthesis of the new enzyme, while offset depends on elimination of the barbiturate and decay of the increased enzyme stores.

Absorption varies depending on the route of administration: oral or rectal, 20 to 60 min; IM, slightly faster than oral or rectal; IV, immediate to 5 min. The sodium salts of the barbiturates are more rapidly absorbed than the free acids because they dissolve rapidly. The rate of absorption is increased if the agents are taken on an empty stomach. The barbiturates are weak acids and distribute rapidly to all tissues, with high concentrations initially in the brain, liver, lungs, heart and kidneys. The more lipid-soluble the drug, the more rapidly it penetrates all tissues of the body. The barbiturates are metabolized by the liver; phenobarbital is partially excreted unchanged in the urine.

Table 2.7

Barbiturates: Dosing Information

Generic name	Brand name(s)	Usual adult dosage	Maximum adult dosage	Usual child dosage	Maximum child dosage	Pregnancy risk category	Content/form
Amobarbital (II*,C†)	Amytal sterile solution	**Sedative—IV/IM:** 30-50 mg bid-tid **Hypnotic—IV/IM:** 65-200 mg	**Oral:** Not available **IM:** 500 mg/dose **IV:** 1 g/dose	**Age < 6 y, hypnotic—IM:** 2-3 mg/kg **Age ≥ 6 y, hypnotic—IM:** 2-3 mg/kg **Age ≥ 6 y, hypnotic—IV:** 65-500 mg/dose **Age ≥ 6 y, sedative, preoperative—IV:** 65-500 mg or 3-5 mg/kg/dose	Not established	D	**Sterile solution:** 500 mg
	Amytal, generic	**Hypnotic—oral:** 65-200 mg **Sedative, daytime—oral:** 50-300 mg/day divided doses **Preoperative:** 200 mg 1-2 h before therapy	Not established	Not established	Not established	Not established	**Capsules:** 200 mg
	Amytal [CAN]	**Hypnotic:** 65-200 mg at bedtime **Preoperative:** 2-6 mg/kg 1-2 h before therapy **Sedative:** 50-300 mg a day in divided doses	Not established	**Hypnotic:** dosage not established **Sedative:** 2 mg/kg **Preoperative—oral:** 100 mg/dose	Not established	Not established	**Tablets:** 100 mg [CAN]

Generic (Controlled Substance)	Brand/Forms						Available Forms
Aprobarbital (III*)	Alurate	Hypnotic—oral: 40-160 mg at bedtime / Sedative—oral: 40 mg tid	Not established	Not established	Not established	D	Elixir: 40 mg/5 mL
Butabarbital (III*; C†)	Elixir: Busodium, Butalan, Butisol, generic / Tablets: Busodium, Butisol, generic	Hypnotic: 50-100 mg at bedtime / Sedative—oral: 15-30 mg tid-qid / Preoperative—oral: 50-100 mg 60-90 min before surgery	Not established	Sedative—oral: 2-6 mg per kg of body weight per day / Preoperative—oral: 2-6 mg/kg, 100 mg/dose	Not established	D	Elixir: 30 mg/5 mL / Tablets: 15, 30, 50, 100 mg; 15, 30, 100 mg [CAN]
Mephobarbital (IV*; C†)	Mebaral	Anticonvulsant—oral: 200 mg at bedtime to 600 mg/day in divided doses / Sedative-hypnotic, daytime—oral: 32-100 mg tid-qid	Not established	Anticonvulsant: up to age 5 y, 16-32 mg tid-qid / Sedative-hypnotic—daytime: 16-32 mg tid-qid	Not established	D	Tablets: 30, 100 mg; 32, 50, 100 [CAN]
Pentobarbital (II*; C†)	Capsules: Nembutal, generic; Novopentobarb [CAN] / Elixir: Nembutal / Parenteral: Nembutal	Hypnotic: 100 mg at bedtime / Sedative, oral elixir: 20 mg tid-qid / Sedative, preoperative, capsules: 100 mg / Hypnotic—IM: 150-200 mg / Continued on next page	Hypnotic—IV: 50 mg total	Sedative—oral: 2-6 mg/kg / Preoperative—oral: 2-6 mg/kg, up to maximum of 100 mg/dose / Hypnotic—IM: 2-6 mg per kg up to 100 mg maximum / Hypnotic—IV: 50 mg initially, then small doses after 1 min	Sedative—oral: 2-6 mg/kg / Preoperative—oral: 2-6 mg/kg, up to maximum of 100 mg/dose / Hypnotic—IM: 2-6 mg/kg up to 100 mg maximum / Continued on next page	D	Capsules: 50, 100 mg; 100 mg [CAN] / Elixir: 20 mg/5 mL pentobarbital sodium (18.2 mg pentobarbital) / Injection: 50 mg/mL / Suppositories: 30, 60, 120, 200 mg; 25, 50 mg [CAN]

Continued on next page

[CAN] indicates a drug available only in Canada.
*Controlled substance in the United States; see Appendix A for complete description of schedule.
†Controlled substance in Canada; see Appendix A for complete description of schedule.

Table 2.7 (cont.)
Barbiturates: Dosing Information

Generic name	Brand name(s)	Usual adult dosage	Maximum adult dosage	Usual child dosage	Maximum child dosage	Pregnancy risk category	Content/form
Pentobarbital (II*, C†) *(cont.)*		**Hypnotic—IV:** 100 mg initially, then after 1 min small doses at 1-min intervals			**Hypnotic—IV:** 50 mg initially, then small doses after 1 min **Age 1-4 y, preopera-tive—rectal:** 30 or 60 mg **Age 5-12 y, preopera-tive—rectal:** 60 mg **Age 12-14 y, preopera-tive—rectal:** 60 or 120 mg	Not established	**Sterile solution:** 500 mg **Suppositories:** 25, 50 mg
	NovaRectal [CAN]	**Preoperative—IM:** 150-200 mg **Hypnotic—rectal:** 120-200 mg at bedtime **Sedative—rectal:** 30 mg bid-qid	**Age 1-4 y, preop-erative—rectal:** 30 or 60 mg **Age 5-12 y, preoperative—rectal:** 60 mg **Age 12-14 y, preoperative—rectal:** 60 or 120 mg	Not established	Not established		
Phenobarbital (IV*, C†)	**Capsules:** Solfoton, Barbita **Tablets:** Barbita, Solfoton, generic **Injection:** Luminal, generic **Sterile solution:** generic	**Hypnotic—oral:** 100-320 mg at bedtime **Sedative—oral:** 30-120 mg in 2 or 3 divided doses/day	Not available	**Preoperative—oral:** 1-3 mg/kg **Preoperative—IM or IV:** 1-3 mg/kg 60-90 min before surgery	Not established	D	**Tablets:** 8, 15, 30, 60, 100 mg; 15, 30, 60, 100 mg [CAN] **Capsules:** 15 mg **Elixir:** 20 mg/5 mL

Generic name (schedule)	Brand names		Adult dosage		Child dosage		Availability
			Preoperative—IM: 120-200 mg 60-90 min before surgery				**Phenobarbital sodium injection USP:** 30, 60, 65, 130 mg/mL; 30, 120 mg/mL [CAN] **Sterile phenobarbital sodium USP:** 120 mg
Secobarbital (II*; oral, C†)	Seconal; Novosecobarb [CAN]	Not available	**Preoperative—oral:** 200-300 mg 1-2 h before surgery **Hypnotic—oral:** 100 mg at bedtime **Sedative—oral:** 30-50 mg tid-qid	Not available	**Preoperative—oral:** 2-6 mg/kg, up to maximum of 100 mg/dose 1-2 h before surgery **Sedative—oral:** 2 mg/kg tid **Preoperative—IM:** 4-5 mg/kg	D	**Capsules:** 100 mg; 50, 100 mg [CAN] **Injection:** 50 mg/mL
Secobarbital and amobarbital (II*; C†)	Tuinal	Not available	1 capsule at bedtime or preoperatively	Not established	Not established	D	**Capsules:** 50 mg secobarbital and 50 mg amobarbital; 100 mg secobarbital and 100 mg amobarbital

[CAN] indicates a drug available only in Canada.
*Controlled substance in the United States; see Appendix A for complete description of schedule.
†Controlled substance in Canada; see Appendix A for complete description of schedule.

Table 2.8
Barbiturates: Possible Interactions With Other Drugs

Drug taken by patient	Interaction with barbiturates	Dentist's action
Acetaminophen	Risk of increased hepatotoxicity may exist with large or chronic barbiturate doses	Monitor liver enzymes Avoid prolonged high dosage use
Alcohol	*Concurrent use may increase the CNS depressant effects of either agent*	Patients receiving a barbiturate and another CNS depressant should be monitored for additive effects
Anticoagulants: coumarin oral anticoagulants	*Barbiturates can increase metabolism of anticoagulants, resulting in a decreased response*	No barbiturate therapy should be started or stopped without considering the possibility of readjustment to the anticoagulant dose
Carbamazepine	*Plasma concentrations may decrease owing to increased metabolism that results from induction of hepatic enzymes*	No special precautions appear necessary, but be aware that carbamazepine plasma concentrations may be lower
Charcoal	Charcoal reduces the absorption of barbiturates	Advise patient to avoid large amounts of food cooked over charcoal
Chloramphenicol	Chloramphenicol may inhibit phenobarbital metabolism; barbiturates may enhance chloramphenicol metabolism	Advise patient that sedative effect of phenobarbital may be prolonged Limit use of barbiturates and be aware that anticonvulsant effect of clonazepam may be reduced
Clonazepam	Increased clonazepam clearance may occur, which can lead to lower steady-state levels and less efficacy	
Contraceptives, oral	*Reliability may be reduced because of accelerated estrogen metabolism caused by barbiturates' induction of hepatic enzymes*	Suggest alternate form of birth control
Corticosteroids	Barbiturates may enhance corticosteroid metabolism through induction of hepatic microsomal enzymes	
Doxycycline	Phenobarbital decreases doxycycline's half-life and serum levels	Dose of doxycycline may have to be increased
Griseofulvin	Phenobarbital appears to interfere with the absorption of oral griseofulvin	Dose of griseofulvin may have to be increased
Hydantoins	Effect of barbiturates on metabolism of hydantoins is unpredictable	Advise patient that anticonvulsant effect may be reduced

Italics indicate information of major clinical significance.

Continued on next page

Table 2.8 (cont.)
Barbiturates: Possible Interactions With Other Drugs

Drug taken by patient	Interaction with barbiturates	Dentist's action
MAO-I	MAO-I may enhance the sedative effects of barbiturates	Reduced dosage of barbiturate should be considered
Methoxyflurane	Enhanced renal toxicity may occur	
Metronidazole	Antimicrobial effectiveness of metronidazole may be decreased	Dose of metronidazole may have to be increased
Narcotics	May increase the toxicity of meperidine and reduce the effect of methadone	Monitor for excessive meperidine effect; dose of methadone may have to be increased
Phenylbutazone	Elimination half-life of phenylbutazone may be reduced	Consultation with patient's physician may be needed
Quinidine	Phenobarbital may significantly reduce serum levels and half-life of quinidine	Dose of phenobarbital may have to be reduced
Rifampin	Rifampin induces hepatic microsomal enzymes and may decrease the effectiveness of barbiturates	Increased dose of barbiturates may be necessary
Theophylline	Barbiturates decrease theophylline levels, possibly resulting in decreased effects	Consultation with patient's physician may be needed
Valproic acid	*Concurrent use may decrease the metabolism of barbiturates, resulting in increased plasma concentrations*	Monitor for excessive phenobarbital effect
Verapamil	Clearance of verapamil may be increased and its bioavailability decreased	

Italics indicate information of major clinical significance.

Table 2.9

Barbiturates: Adverse Effects, Precautions and Contraindications

Body system	Adverse effects	Precautions/contraindications
General	Local pain on IM injection	None significant to dentistry
CV	Hypotension, cardiac arrhythmias, bradycardia, gangrene with inadvertent intra-arterial injection, thrombophlebitis with IV use	Should be used cautiously in patients with congestive heart failure
CNS	Dizziness, lightheadedness, "hangover" effect, drowsiness, lethargy, CNS excitation or depression, impaired judgment, confusion, depression, insomnia, nightmares	Should be used cautiously with patients who have history of drug abuse, suicidal tendencies Use caution when administering to patients with acute or chronic pain, because of paradoxical excitement Contraindicated in patients with preexisting CNS depression
GI	Nausea, vomiting, constipation	None significant to dentistry
Hema	Agranulocytosis, megaloblastic anemia, thrombocytopenia, porphyria	Should be used cautiously in patients with anemia
Integ	Exfoliative dermatitis, Stevens-Johnson syndrome, rash	None significant to dentistry
Resp	Apnea (especially with rapid IV use), respiratory depression, laryngospasm	Should be used cautiously in patients with asthma Contraindicated in patients with severe respiratory disease involving dyspnea or obstruction

Opioids

The term "opioid" is used in a broad sense to include both opioid agonists and opioid agonists/antagonists. The opioids are administered from their analgesic properties and are considered excellent drugs for the relief of moderate to severe pain. The parenteral dosage forms of this class of drugs are also used as general anesthesia adjuncts in conjunction with other drugs, such as the benzodiazepines, neuromuscular blocking agents and nitrous oxide for the maintenance of "balanced" anesthesia. All opioid narcotic agents are classified as controlled substances in the U.S. and Canada.

General Dosing Information

Narcotic drugs are used to produce mood changes, provide analgesia and elevate the pain threshold. Opioid analgesics may not provide sufficient analgesia when used with nitrous oxide for the maintenance of balance anesthesia. Narcotic agents can be used in combination with other agents such as benzodiazepines, antihistamines, ultrashort-acting barbiturates and a potent hydrocarbon inhalation anesthetic. Dosage and dosing intervals should be individualized for the patient based on duration of action of the specific drug, other medications the patient is currently taking, the patient's condition and the patient's response. See Tables 2.10 and 2.11.

Table 2.10
Opioids: Types

Agonists	Antagonists	Mixed agents
Alfentanil	Naloxone	Buprenorphine
Codeine	Naltrexone	Butorphanol
Fentanyl		Nalbuphine
Hydrocodone		Pentazocine
Hydromorphone		
Levorphanol		
Meperidine		
Methadone		
Morphine		
Oxycodone		
Oxymorphone		
Sufentanil		

Special Dental Considerations

Drug Interactions of Dental Interest
Possible drug interactions of clinical significance in dentistry are shown in Table 2.12.

Laboratory Value Alterations
- Opioids delay gastric emptying, thereby invalidating gastric emptying studies.
- In hepatobiliary imaging, delivery of technectium Tc99m disofenin to small bowel may be prevented because opioids may constrict sphincter of Oddi; this results in delayed visualization and resembles an obstruction in the common bile duct.
- Cerebrospinal fluid may be increased secondary to respiratory depression–induced carbon dioxide retention.
- Plasma amylase activity may be increased.
- Plasma lipase activity may be increased.
- Serum alanine aminotransferase may be increased.
- Serum alkaline phosphatase may be increased.
- Serum aspartate aminotransferase may be increased.
- Serum bilirubin may be increased.
- Serum lactate dehydrogenase may be increased.

Cross-Sensitivity
Patients hypersensitive to fentanyl may be hypersensitive to the chemically related alfentanil or sufentanil.

Special Patients
Pregnant and nursing women
Risk-benefit must be considered because opioid analgesics cross the placenta.

Pediatric, geriatric and other special patients
Geriatric patients are more susceptible to the effects of opioids, especially respiratory depression. Clearance of opioid analgesics can be reduced in the geriatric patient, which leads to a delayed postoperative recovery. Children aged up to 2 y may be more susceptible to opioids' effects, especially respiratory depression. Paradoxical excitation is especially likely to occur in the pediatric population.

Patient Monitoring: Aspects to Watch
- Respiratory status
- State of consciousness
- Heart rate
- Blood pressure

Table 2.11
Opioids: Dosage Information

Generic name	Brand name(s)	Usual adult dosage	Maximum adult dosage	Usual child dosage	Maximum child dosage	Pregnancy risk category	Content/form
Alfentanil	Alfenta	**Incremental injection:** 3-5 µg/kg for procedures < 30 min; 5-15 µg/kg for procedures 30-60 min **Continuous infusion:** 0.5-1.5 µg/kg/min **Anesthetic induction for procedures ≥ 45 min:** 0.13–0.245 mg/kg total **Maintenance of anesthesia for procedures < 30 min:** loading dose, 8-20 µg/kg; then either 3-5 µg/kg doses as required or continuous infusion of 0.5-1 µg/kg/min **Maintenance of anesthesia for procedures > 30 min:** loading dose, 20-75 µg/kg; then 5-15 µg/kg doses as required or 0.5-4 µg/kg/min	Not established	**Incremental injection:** 10-15 µg/kg **Continuous infusion:** 0.5-1.5 µg/kg/min **Anesthetic induction:** 0.03-0.05 µg/kg/min	Not established	C	500 mg (0.5 mg/mL)
Butorphanol	Stadol	**Preoperative—IV:** usually 2 mg 60-90 min before surgery	Not established	Not established	Not established	C	**With preservative:** 2 mg/mL **Without preservative:** 1 mg/mL, 2 mg/mL

Generic name	Trade names	Adult dose		Pediatric dose	Maximum dose	Pregnancy category	Preparations
Fentanyl	Sublimaze, generic	**Sedation for local anesthesia adjunct:** 0.07-1.14 µg/kg **Sedation for minor procedures:** 2 µg/kg	Not established	**Ages 2 to 12 y—IV:** 2-3 µg/kg	Not established	C	**Without preservative:** 50 µg/mL
Meperidine	Demerol, generic	**Preoperative—IM or SC:** 50-100 mg 30-90 min before anesthesia **IV:** repeated slow injection of fractional doses of a solution diluted to 10 mg/mL **IV:** infusion, as a solution diluted to 1 mg/mL	Not established	**Preoperative—IM or SC:** 1-2.2 mg/kg q 3-4 h	Not to exceed 100 mg	Not classified	**Solution with preservative:** 25, 50, 75, 100-mg/mL solution; 50, 100 mg/mL [CAN] **Solution without preservative:** 10, 25, 50, 75, 100 mg/mL; 10, 25, 50, 75, 100 mg/mL [CAN]
Morphine	Astramorph PF, Duramorph, generic; Epimorph [CAN], Morphine Forte [CAN], Morphine Extra Forte [CAN], Morphine HP [CAN]	**Analgesic—IM or SC:** 5-20 mg q 4 h **Analgesic—IV:** 4-10 mg in 4-5 mL water, administered slowly	Not established	**Preoperative—IM:** 0.05-1 mg/kg	Not to exceed 10 mg/dose	C	**Injection with preservative:** 1, 2, 4, 5, 8, 10, 15 mg/mL; 1, 2, 5, 10, 15 mg/mL [CAN] **Injection without preservative:** 0.5, 1, 25 50 mg/mL; 0.5, 1, 25, 50 mg/mL [CAN]
Nalbuphine	Nubain	**Balanced anesthesia—IV:** 300 µg-3 mg/kg administered over 10-15 min period **Supplemental—IV:** 250-500 µg/kg as required	20-mg single dose; 160 mg/day	Not established	Not established	C	**Solution with preservative:** 10, 20 mg/mL; 10, 20 mg/mL [CAN]

[CAN] indicates a drug available only in Canada.

Continued on next page

Table 2.11 (cont.)
Opioids: Dosage Information

Generic name	Brand name(s)	Usual adult dosage	Maximum adult dosage	Usual child dosage	Maximum child dosage	Pregnancy risk category	Content/form
Pentazocine lactate	Talwin	**Analgesic—IM, IV, SC:** 30 mg q 3-4 h	Up to 360 mg/days	Not established	Not established	C	**Injection:** 30 mg/mL
Sufentanil citrate	Sufenta	**General anesthesia adjunct, low dose—IV:** 0.0005-0.001 mg/kg initially, then doses of 0.01-0.025 mg as needed **General anesthesia adjunct, moderate dose (for major surgical procedures)—IV:** 0.002-0.008 mg/kg initially, then doses of 0.01-0.05 mg as needed	Not available	Not available	Not available	C	**Injection:** 0.05 mg/mL

Table 2.12

Opioids: Possible Interactions With Other Drugs

Drug taken by patient	Interaction with opioids	Dentist's action
Barbiturate anesthetics (methohexital, thiamylal, thiopental)	Dose of thiopental required to induce anesthesia may be reduced in presence of narcotic analgesics Apnea may occur	No additional precautions other than those routinely used in anesthesia appear necessary
Benzodiazepines	*Increased respiratory depression* *Increased recovery time* *Increased risk of hypotension*	Monitor for excess sedation
Cimetidine	Actions of narcotic analgesics may be enhanced, resulting in toxicity	If significant CNS depression occurs, withdraw the drugs; if warranted, administer a narcotic antagonist such as naloxone
CNS depressants	*Increased CNS depression*	Monitor for excess sedation
Diuretics/antihypertensives	Hypotensive effects increased by opioids	Monitor blood pressure
MAO-inhibitors	*With meperidine: agitation, seizures, fever, coma, apnea, death*	Avoid this combination
Phenothiazines	Increased or decreased effects of opioid analgesic supplements Hypotension may occur when phenothiazine is administered with meperidine	Avoid concurrent use of meperidine and phenothiazines

Italics indicate information of major clinical significance.

Table 2.13

Opioids: Adverse Effects, Precautions and Contraindications

Body system	Adverse effects	Precautions/contraindications
General	Bradycardia; physical dependence, with or without psychological dependence, may occur with chronic administration	Emotional instability, suicide attempts
CV	Hypotension, peripheral circulatory collapse, cardiac arrest	Cardiac arrythmias
CNS	Weakness, tiredness, drowsiness, dizziness, confusion, nervousness, headache, restlessness, malaise, increased intracranial pressure, paradoxical CNS stimulation	History of convulsions, head injury, increased intracranial pressure, intracranial lesions

Continued on next page

Table 2.13 (cont.)

Opioids: Adverse Effects, Precautions and Contraindications

Body system	Adverse effects	Precautions/contraindications
EENT	Miosis	None of significance to dentistry
GI	*Nausea, vomiting, constipation, dry mouth, biliary spasm, paralytic ileus*	*Diarrhea associated with pseudomembranous colitis, poisoning* *In inflammatory bowel disease: risk of toxic megacolon may be increased*
GU	Ureteral spasms, decreased urination	Renal function impairment—risk of convulsions because opioids and/or their metabolites are excreted via the kidney Prostatic hypertrophy
HB	None of significance to dentistry	Hepatic function impairment (opioids metabolized by the liver)
Oral	All opioids may cause oral dryness, which can lead to caries, periodontal disease, oral candidiasis and discomfort with prolonged use	None of significance to dentistry
Resp	*Shortness of breath, troubled breathing, rigid chest syndrome*	*Respiratory depression, chronic respiratory disease, Asthma, acute attack*

Italics indicate information of major clinical significance.

Adverse Effects and Precautions

Table 2.13 lists adverse effects, precautions and contraindications related to opioids.

Pharmacology

Opioid analgesics bind to receptors within the central nervous system and peripheral nervous system. This interaction affects both the perception of pain and the emotional response to pain. There are at least five types of opioid receptors—mu (μ), kappa (K), sigma (σ), delta (Δ) and epsilon (ε)—located throughout the body that may be activated by exogenous or endogenous opioid-like substances (endorphins). The action of various opioids at the various receptors determine the agents' specific actions and side effects (Table 2.14). Based on their actions at these receptors, the commercially available opioids may be divided into three groups: pure agonists, pure antagonists and mixed agents (agonists/antagonists or partial agonists) (Table 2.10).

All opioids are respiratory depressants. By exerting a depressant action on respiratory center neurons in the medulla, they decrease respiratory rate, tidal volume and minute ventilation. They may increase arterial CO_2 tensions. All opioids affect the cardiovascular system by their actions on the autonomic nervous system. Hypotension may result from arteriolar and venous dilation as a result of either histamine release or decreased sympathetic nervous system tone. Bradycardia results from vagal stimulation. Finally, all opioids disorganize GI function, causing increased tone and muscle spasm but delayed emptying and decreased motility and secretions.

Table 2.14

Opioids: Effect on Types of Nerve Receptors

Receptor	Effect
mu$_1$(μ_1)	Supraspinal analgesia
mu$_2$(μ_2)	Respiratory depression
	Bradycardia
	Hypothermia
	Euphoria
	Moderate sedation
	Physical dependence
	Miosis
kappa (K)	Spinal analgesia
	Heavy sedation
	Miosis
sigma (σ)	Dysphoria
	Tachycardia
	Tachypnea
	Mydriasis
delta (Δ)	Modulation of μ receptor
epsilon (ε)	Altered neurohumoral functions

Opioid (Narcotic) Antagonist: Naloxone

Like the benzodiazepines, the opioids have a specific antagonist that reverses the pharmacologic effects caused by the opioid drugs.

Accepted Indications

Naloxone is used for the complete or partial reversal of narcotic depression, such as respiratory depression induced by opioids including natural and synthetic narcotics. Naloxone is also used for the diagnosis of suspected acute opioid overdose.

General Dosing Information

Varying amounts of naloxone may be needed to antagonize the effects of different agents. Lack of significant improvement of CNS depression and/or respiration after administration of an adequate dose (10 mg) of naloxone may indicate that the condition is due to a nonopioid CNS depressant. Naloxone reverses the analgesic effects of the opioid and may precipitate withdrawal symptoms in physically dependent patients. See Table 2.15.

Dosage Adjustments

Repeat dosing may be required within 1- or 2-h intervals depending on the amount and type (that is, short- or long-acting) of narcotic and the interval since the last administration of the narcotic. Supplemental IM doses can produce a long-lasting effect.

Special Dental Considerations

Drug Interactions of Dental Interest

A possible drug interaction of clinical significance in dentistry is shown in Table 2.16.

Special Patients

Pregnant and nursing women

Naloxone crosses the placenta and may precipitate withdrawal in the fetus as well as the mother. Breast-feeding problems in humans have not been documented.

Pediatric, geriatric and other special patients

Studies performed in pediatrics have not shown problems that would limit the usefulness of naloxone in children. Geriatric-specific problems do not seem to limit the usefulness of this medication in elderly patients.

Patient Monitoring: Aspects to Watch

- Cardiac status
- State of consciousness
- Respiratory status

Adverse Effects and Precautions

Adverse effects, precautions and contraindications related to naloxone are listed in Table 2.17.

Pharmacology

Naloxone reverses the CNS and respiratory depression associated with narcotic overdose. It also reverses postoperative opioid

---

Table 2.15

Naloxone: Dosage Information

Generic name	Brand name(s)	Adult dosage	Child dosage	Pregnancy risk category	Content/form
Naloxone	Narcan ★	Dose must be individualized **Opioid toxicity—IV, IM or SC:** 0.4-2 mg in a single dose; repeat at 2- to 3-min intervals **Postoperative opioid depression—IV:** 0.1-0.2 mg q 2-3 min until adequate ventilation and alertness without pain are obtained	**Opioid toxicity —IV, IM or SC:** 0.01 mg/kg, repeated every 2-3 min for 1 or 2 additional doses **Postoperative opioid depression—IV:** 0.005 to 0.01 mg q 2-3 min until adequate ventilation and alertness without pain are obtained	B	**Solution with preservative:** 20 µg/mL, 400 µg/mL, 1 mg/mL **Solution without preservative:** 20 µg/mL, 400 µg/mL, 1 mg/mL; 20 µg/mL, 400 µg/mL [CAN]

★ indicates a drug bearing the ADA Seal of Acceptance.
[CAN] indicates a drug available only in Canada.

Table 2.16

Naloxone: Possible Interactions With Other Drugs

Drug taken by patient	Interaction with naloxone	Dentist's action
Narcotic analgesics	*Effect decreased by naloxone*	Monitor patient for withdrawal

Italics indicate information of major clinical significance.

Table 2.17

Naloxone: Adverse Effects, Precautions and Contraindications

Body system	Adverse effects	Precautions/contraindications
CV	Sweating, hypertension, hypotension, tachycardia, ventricular arrhythmias	Contraindicated in patients with hypersensitivity to naloxone
CNS	Insomnia, irritability, anxiety, convulsions	None significant to dentistry
EENT	Blurred vision	None significant to dentistry
GI	Nausea and vomiting	None significant to dentistry

depression. Naloxone competes with and displaces narcotics at narcotic receptor sites.

Because of naloxone's short half-life, a continuous infusion may be required to maintain alertness. A patient should never be released soon after receiving naloxone because the ingested narcotic may have a longer half-life than naloxone, and its toxic effects—such as respiratory depression—may break through.

Chloral Hydrate

Choral hydrate is an oral sedative-hypnotic that is used when providing dental treatment to the uncooperative preschool child.

Accepted Indications

Accepted indications for chloral hydrate are nocturnal sedation; preoperative sedation to lessen anxiety; in postoperative care and control of pain as an adjunct to opiates and analgesics.

General Dosing Information

Deaths have been associated with the use of chloral hydrate, especially in children. Repetitive dosing of chloral hydrate is not recommended owing to the accumulation of the active metabolite trichloroethylene. As with any sedation procedure, this sedative should be administered where there can be

proper monitoring. Practitioners must know how to properly calculate and administer the appropriate dose. See Table 2.18.

Special Dental Considerations

Drug Interactions of Dental Interest

Drug interactions between chloral hydrate and other drugs are listed in Table 2.19.

Laboratory Value Alterations

- Chloral hydrate may interfere with the copper sulfate test for glucosuria (confirm suspected glucosuria by glucose oxidase test) and with fluorometric tests for urine catecholamines (do not administer medication for 48 h preceding the test).

Special Patients

Pregnant and nursing women
Chloral hydrate crosses the placenta. Chronic use of chloral hydrate during pregnancy may cause withdrawal symptoms in the neonate; chloral hydrate is distributed into breast milk; use by nursing mothers may cause sedation in the infant.

Pediatric, geriatric and other special patients
Chloral hydrate is not recommended for use in infants and children in cases in which repeated dosing would be necessary. With repeated dosing, accumulation of trichloroethanol and trichloroacetic acid metabolites may increase the potential for excessive CNS depression.

No information is available on the rela-

Table 2.18

Chloral Hydrate: Dosage Information

Generic name	Brand name(s)	Usual adult dosage	Maximum adult dosage	Usual child dosage	Maximum child dosage	Pregnancy risk category	Content/form
Chloral hydrate	**Capsules:** generic; Novo-Chlorhydrate [CAN] **Syrup:** generic; PMS–Chloral Hydrate [CAN], generic [CAN] **Suppositories:** Aquachloral Supprettes, generic	**Sedative hypnotic—oral:** 500 mg–1 g 15–30 min before bedtime **Sedative, daytime—oral:** 250 mg tid after meals **Preoperative—oral:** 500 mg–1 g 30 min before surgery	2 g/day	**Sedative-hypnotic premedication before procedure:** 50 mg/kg, up to maximum of 1 g per single dose; doses of 25–100 mg/kg may be used in individual patients; total dose should not exceed 100 mg/kg or 2 g	100 mg/kg or 2 g	C	**Capsules:** 250, 500 mg; 500 mg [CAN] **Oral solution:** 250, 500 mg/5 mL; 500 mg/5 mL [CAN] **Suppositories:** 325, 500, 650 mg

[CAN] indicates a drug available only in Canada

Table 2.19

Chloral Hydrate: Possible Interactions With Other Drugs

Drug taken by patient	Interaction with chloral hydrate	Dentist's action
Alcohol or other CNS depressants	*Concurrent use may increase CNS depressant effects of either medication*	Monitor for excessive CNS depression
Anticoagulants, coumarin or indandione-derivative	*Displacement of the anticoagulant from its plasma protein increases the anticoagulant effect*	Avoid use
Catecholamine	Large doses of chloral hydrate may sensitize cardiac tissues to catecholamine	Avoid treating chloral hydrate overdose with adrenergic vasoconstrictor
Furosemide (IV)	Flushing, diaphoresis and blood pressure changes	Avoid use

Italics indicate information of major clinical significance.

Table 2.20

Chloral Hydrate: Adverse Effects, Precautions and Contraindications

Body system	Adverse effects	Precautions/contraindications
General	None of significance to dentistry	Should be used with caution in patients with history of drug or alcohol abuse Contraindicated for patients with hypersensitivity to chloral hydrate or any component
CV	None of significance to dentistry	Contraindicated for patients with severe cardiac disease
CNS	Clumsiness, hallucinations, drowsiness, "hangover" effect, disorientation, sedation ataxia, paradoxical excitement, dizziness, fever, confusion	None of significance to dentistry
GI	Gastric irritation, flatulence, nausea and vomiting, diarrhea	Contraindicated for patients with gastritis or ulcers
Hema	Leukopenia, eosinophilia	None of significance to dentistry
HB	None of significance to dentistry	Contraindicated for patients with hepatic or renal impairment Should be used with caution in patients who have porphyria

tionship of age to the effects of chloral hydrate in geriatric patients. Elderly patients are more likely to have age-related hepatic function impairment and renal function impairment. Dose reduction may be required.

Patient Monitoring: Aspects to Watch
- Respiratory status
- Possible abuse and dependence
- Blood pressure

Adverse Effects and Precautions
Table 2.20 lists adverse effects, precautions and contraindications related to chloral hydrate.

Pharmacology
The mechanism of action of chloral hydrate is unknown; however, it is believed that the CNS depressant effects are due to its active metabolite, trichloroethanol. It is rapidly absorbed from the gastrointestinal tract following oral administration and is metabolized in red blood cells in the liver to the active metabolite. Its onset of action is usually within 30 min and its duration of action is 4-8 h.

Patient Advice
- Swallow the capsule whole; do not chew because of unpleasant taste.
- Take with a full glass of water or juice to reduce gastric irritation.
- For syrup dose: Mix with glassful of juice or water to improve flavor and reduce gastric irritation.
- For suppository form: If too soft for insertion, chill suppository in refrigerator for 30 min before removing foil wrapper.

Other Sedative-Hypnotics: Ethchlorvynol

Ethchlorvynol is a sedative hypnotic used for the short-term management of insomnia. This medication has been replaced with other safer sedative-hypnotic agents. Remember the following principles when using sedative-hypnotics like ethchlorvynol:
- never sedate any patient with any technique of sedation without an assistant present in the room;
- provide assistance when escorting patient due to possibility of dizziness;
- reposition supine patient slowly to avoid orthostatic hypotension.

Accepted Indications
Ethchlorvynol is used as a sedative and a hypnotic.

General Dosing Information
Give the smallest effective dose to elderly and debilitated patients. Do not prescribe for longer than 1 w. See Table 2.21.

Special Dental Considerations

Drug Interactions of Dental Interest
Possible drug interactions with ethchlorvynol are listed in Table 2.22.

Special Patients
Pregnant and nursing women
Ethchlorvynol crosses the placenta and produces CNS depression in the neonate. It is not known if ethchlorvynol is excreted in breast milk.

Table 2.21
Ethchlorvynol: Dosage Information

Generic name	Brand name(s)	Usual adult dosage	Maximum adult dosage	Child dosage	Pregnancy risk category	Content/ form
Ethchlorvynol	Placidyl, generic	500 mg-1 g at bedtime	1 g	Not established	C	**Capsules:** 200, 500, 750 mg

Table 2.22

Ethchlorvynol: Possible Interactions With Other Drugs

Drug taken by patient	Interaction with ethchlorvynol	Dentist's action
Alcohol or CNS depressant medications	Increased CNS depressant effects	Dosage of one or both medications should be reduced
Antidepressants	Transient delirium	
Anticoagulants	Decreased effect due to ethchlorvynol's increased metabolism of anticoagulant (through enzyme induction in the liver)	Anticoagulant dosage adjustments may be necessary

Table 2.23

Ethchlorvynol: Adverse Effects

Body system	Adverse effects
CV	Bradycardia
CNS	Dizziness, weakness, clumsiness, confusion, daytime drowsiness, excitement
GI	Indigestion, nausea, stomach pain, unpleasant aftertaste
HB	Cholestatic jaundice
Musc	Trembling

Pediatric, geriatric and other special patients
Safety and efficacy have not been established in the pediatric population. Elderly patients are more sensitive to the effects of ethchlorvynol.

Adverse Effects

Adverse effects related to ethchlorvynol are listed in Table 2.23.

Pharmacology

The mechanism of action of ethchlorvynol is unknown. Absorption is rapid from the gastrointestinal tract, with onset of action in 15-60 min and a duration of action of 5 h.

Meprobamate

Meprobamate is an antianxiety agent used for the management of anxiety disorders. It is not indicated for the treatment of anxiety or tension associated with everyday life. Prolonged use of meprobamate may decrease or inhibit salivary flow, thus contributing to the development of caries, periodontal disease, oral candidiasis and discomfort.

Accepted Indications

Meprobamate is used for management of anxiety disorders.

Table 2.24

Meprobamate: Dosage Information

Generic name	Brand name(s)	Usual adult dosage	Maximum adult dosage	Child dosage	Pregnancy risk category	Content/ form
Meprobamate	**Tablets:** Equanil, Miltown, Trancot; Apo-Meprobamate [CAN], Equanil [CAN], Miltown [CAN] **Extended-release capsules:** Meprospan 200, Meprospan 400; Meprospan 400 [CAN]	**Tablets:** 400 mg tid-qid or 600 mg bid **Capsules:** 400-800 mg tid	2.4 g/day	**Age < 6 y:** Dosage not established **Age 6-12 y—oral:** 100-200 mg bid-tid	D	**Tablets:** 200, 400, 600 mg; 400 mg [CAN] **Extended-release capsules:** 200, 400 mg; 400 mg [CAN]

[CAN] indicates a drug available only in Canada.

Table 2.25

Meprobamate: Possible Interactions With Other Drugs

Drug taken by patient	Interaction with meprobamate
Alcohol or CNS-depression–producing medication	Increased CNS depressant effects

General Dosing Information

Dosing information for meprobamate is listed in Table 2.24.

Special Dental Considerations

Drug Interactions of Dental Interest

Drug interactions with meprobamate are listed in Table 2.25.

Cross-Sensitivity

Patients sensitive to other carbamate derivatives (carbromal, carisoprodol, mebutamate or tybamate) may be sensitive to this medication.

Special Patients

Pregnant and nursing women

Meprobamate crosses the placenta and has been associated with congenital malformations. It is excreted in the breast milk in a con-centration of 2 to 4 times maternal plasma concentration and may cause sedation in the infant.

Pediatric, geriatric and other special patients

No pediatric-specific problems have been documented. Elderly patients are more sensitive to the effects of meprobamate.

Adverse Effects and Precautions

Adverse effects and precautions related to meprobamate are listed in Table 2.26.

Pharmacology

Mechanism of action of meprobamate is unknown. It is well absorbed from the gastrointestinal tract, with an onset of action within 1 h.

Table 2.26

Meprobamate: Adverse Effects, Precautions and Contraindications

Body system	Adverse effects	Precautions/contraindications
General	None of significance to dentistry	Physical and psychological dependence may occur
CNS	Drowsiness, ataxia, clumsiness, dizziness, paradoxical excitement, confusion, slurred speech, headache, chills	None of significance to dentistry
EENT	Blurred vision	None of significance to dentistry
GI	Nausea and vomiting, stomatitis	None of significance to dentistry
HB	None of significance to dentistry	Should be used cautiously for patients with hepatic impairment
Renal	None of significance to dentistry	Should be used cautiously for patients with renal impairment
Resp	Wheezing	None of significance to dentistry

Suggested Readings

Briggs GG, Freeman RK, Vaffe SJ. Drugs in pregnancy and lactation. 4th ed. Baltimore: Williams & Wilkins; 1994.

Jastak JT, Donaldson D. Nitrous oxide. Anesth Prog 1991; 38:142-53.

Kallar SK, Dunwiddie WC. Problems in anesthesia: outpatient anesthesia. In: Wetchler BV, ed. Conscious sedation. Philadelphia: JB Lippincott Co.; 1988: 93-100.

Malamed SF. Sedation: A guide to patient management. 3rd ed. St. Louis: Mosby; 1994.

Chapter 3

General Anesthetics

John Yagiela, D.D.S., Ph.D.; Stanley F. Malamed, D.D.S.

General Anesthetics

General anesthesia can be defined as an induced state of unconsciousness accompanied by loss, partial or complete, of protective reflexes—among them the ability to independently maintain an airway and respond purposefully to physical stimulation or verbal command. General anesthesia has been an integral part of dental practice since 1844, when Dr. Horace Wells first used nitrous oxide to induce the loss of consciousness in patients. General anesthesia was for many years a major part of the pain control armamentarium of dentists, primarily because other pain control techniques were less well developed. The introduction of local anesthetics in the clinical setting in 1884 and their steady improvement throughout this century, however, has decreased the need for general anesthesia as a primary means of achieving pain control in dentistry. Furthermore, the introduction of sedation techniques has lessened the need for general anesthesia in managing patients' fear and apprehension. Despite dentists' decreasing need to rely on general anesthesia, its use may be indicated for patients who

- are extremely anxious and fearful;
- are mentally or physically challenged, or both;
- are too young to cooperate with the dentist;
- fail to respond to local anesthesia; or
- are undergoing stressful, traumatic procedures.

Inhalation anesthetics provided the first reliable means of producing controlled unconsciousness. Originally including only nitrous oxide and ether, inhalation anesthetics now comprise a number of easily volatilized halogenated hydrocarbons.

Various injectable agents, including the ultrashort-acting barbiturates, several opioid and benzodiazepine anesthetics and miscellaneous drugs, are also available. Injectable anesthetics have been used alone, in combination with each other and in conjunction with inhalation anesthetics for inducing and maintaining general anesthesia. In lower doses, dentists administer them to produce deep sedation, an induced state of depressed consciousness accompanied by a partial loss of protective reflexes such as those mentioned earlier.

The techniques of general anesthesia and deep sedation cannot be taught in a short course. Dentists who are contemplating using any anesthetic technique in which the patient's airway or protective reflexes could be impaired should have extensive training; this training is outlined in Part 2 of the *Guidelines for Teaching the Comprehensive Control of Pain and Anxiety in Dentistry*, published by the ADA Council on Dental Education. All states and Canada now regulate dentists' use of general anesthesia and deep sedation.

This section includes a discussion of the following drugs: the inhalation anesthetics, ultrashort-acting barbiturates, etomidate, propofol, ketamine and droperidol/fentanyl.

The benzodiazepines and opioids, which are used for general anesthesia and deep sedation, can also be used to produce conscious sedation. These drugs are discussed in Chapter 2, and opioids are discussed further in Chapter 4.

Accepted Indications

Inhalation and injectable anesthetics are used to induce and maintain general anesthesia. Selected agents such as nitrous oxide, methoxyflurane, enflurane, droperidol/fentanyl, thiopental and propofol have also been approved for use in providing sedation and analgesia for specific procedures that do not require general anesthesia. The product literature describes additional indications for specific agents.

General Dosing Information

General anesthetics have a narrow margin of safety, and their administration must be individualized (titrated) according to the desired depth of anesthesia, the concomitant use of other medications and the patient's physical condition, age, size and body temperature. Table 3.1 provides general dosing guidelines for inducing and maintaining anesthesia.

Maximum Recommended Doses

Because of the inherent danger of general anesthetics and significant variations in patients' responsiveness, maximum recommended doses do not guarantee a safe upper limit and have not been identified for most drugs. The risk of hypoxia limits the maximum concentration of nitrous oxide to 70%. Excitation of the CNS restricts the amount of enflurane that can be used to a maximum final induction dose of 4.5% and a maintenance dose of 3%. The following usual maximum doses apply to injectable anesthetics: 4 g of thiopental (rectal), 4.5 mg/kg IV and 13 mg/kg IM of ketamine and 0.05 (children) and 0.1 mL/kg (adults) IV of droperidol/fentanyl.

Dosage Adjustments

The patient's size and physical status and the procedure being performed determine the actual dose. Infants, geriatric patients and people with medical conditions or who are on drug therapy that can alter responses to general anesthetics often require reduced doses, even after correcting for the usual variables of size and physical status. Conversely, children and adolescents are resistant to CNS depressants and require increased doses of inhalation anesthetics and propofol.

Special Dental Considerations

Drug Interactions of Dental Interest

Table 3.2 lists the drug interactions and related problems involving general anesthetics that are potentially of clinical significance in dentistry.

See Chapter 2 (Table 2.12) for drug interactions specific to the fentanyl component of droperidol/fentanyl. Table 3.3 itemizes potential cross-sensitivity considerations.

Laboratory Value Alterations

- Liver function tests (aminotransferases, lactate dehydrogenase) are abnormal with volatile anesthetics.
- Blood glucose is increased with desflurane and sevoflurane.
- Blood urea nitrogen and serum creatinine are increased with sevoflurane.
- Leukocyte count is increased with desflurane and sevoflurane.
- Serum fluoride is increased with methoxyflurane, enflurane and sevoflurane.

Cross-Sensitivity

Table 3.3 lists the potential cross-sensitivities between general anesthetics and other substances.

Special Patients

Pregnant and nursing women

General anesthetics cross the placenta and enter the fetal circulation. Although retrospective investigations of pregnant women receiving general anesthetics during pregnancy have found no evidence of fetal toxicity, investigations using animals indicate that with some agents—namely, nitrous oxide,

Table 3.1

General Anesthetics: Dosage Information

Generic name	Brand name(s)	Usual adult dosage	Usual child dosage	Pregnancy risk category	Content/form
		Inhalation			
Desflurane	Suprane	**Inhalation:** Must be individualized—0.5%-3% initially, to be increased by 0.5%-1% every 2-3 breaths or as tolerated until onset of anesthesia **Maintenance:** 2.5-8.5%	**Induction:** Use not recommended **Maintenance:** Individualized, usually 5.2-10%	B	**Liquid:** 240-mL bottles
Enflurane	Ethrane	**Inhalation:** Must be individualized **Maintenance:** 0.5-3%	Must be individualized	B	**Liquid:** 125-, 250-mL bottles
Halothane	Fluothane, Somnothane [CAN]	**Induction:** Must be individualized (usually 0.5-3%) **Maintenance:** 0.5-1.5%	Must be individualized	C	**Liquid:** 125-, 250-mL bottles
Isoflurane	Forane	**Inhalation:** 1.5-3% **Maintenance:** 1-3.5%	Must be individualized	B	**Liquid:** 100-mL bottles
Methoxyflurane	Penthrane	**Induction:** Up to 2% with ≥ 50% nitrous oxide and oxygen **Maintenance:** Not to exceed 4 h of 0.25% or 2 h of 0.5% **Analgesia:** Intermittent inhalation of 0.3-0.8%	Must be individualized	C	**Liquid:** 15-, 125-mL bottles

	(generic)				
Nitrous oxide	(generic)	**Induction:** 70% with 30% oxygen **Maintenance:** 30-70% with oxygen **Sedation/analgesia:** 25-50% with oxygen	Must be individualized	Not classified	**Pressurized liquid:** Steel cylinders
Sevoflurane	Ultane, Sevorane [CAN]	**Inhalation:** Must be individualized **Maintenance:** 0.5-3%	Same as adult	B	**Liquid:** 250-mL bottles

IM/IV

Droperidol/fentanyl citrate (II, N)*	Innovar	**Induction:** 0.1 mL/kg slowly or rapid drip of 10 mL in 250 mL 5% dextrose solution until somnolence **Premedication—IM:** 0.5-2 mL 45-60 min before procedure	**Induction and maintenance:** Up to 0.05 mL/kg (not established for children aged < 2 y) **Premedication—IM:** 0.025 mL/kg 45-60 min before procedure	C	**Injection (2.5 mg/mL droperidol and 0.05 mg/mL fentanyl citrate):** 2-, 5-mL ampules
Etomidate	Amidate	**Induction—IV:** 0.2-0.6 mg/kg **Maintenance—IV:** Smaller increments with doses individualized	Same as adult (not established for children aged < 10 y)	C	**Injection (2 mg/mL):** 10-, 20-mL ampules and 20-mL syringes
Ketamine HCl	Ketalar	**Induction—IV:** 1-4.5 mg/kg **Induction—IM:** 6.5-13 mg/kg **Maintenance:** Increments are one-half to full dose	Same as adult	Not classified	**Injection (10 mg/mL):** 20-, 25-, 50-mL vials **Injection (50 mg/mL):** 10-mL vials **Injection (100 mg/mL):** 5-mL vials

Continued on next page

[CAN] indicates a drug available only in Canada.
*Controlled substances (United States, Canadian classifications).

Table 3.1 (cont.)

General Anesthetics: Dosage Information

Generic name	Brand name(s)	Usual adult dosage	Usual child dosage	Pregnancy risk category	Content/form
		IM/IV (cont.)			
Methohexital Na (IV, F)*	Brevital, Brietal [CAN]	**Induction—IV:** 1-2.0 mg/kg **Induction—IM:** 5-10 mg/kg **Maintenance—IV:** 0.25-1 mg/kg increments or continuous drip of 0.2% solution with flow rate individualized	**Induction:** Not established **Maintenance:** Not established **Rectal basal anesthesia:** 15-30 mg/kg as a 5-10% solution	B	**Powder:** 500-mg, 2.5-, 5-g vials
Propofol	Diprivan	**Adults ≤ age 55 y, induction—IV:** 2-2.5 mg/kg **Adults > age 55 y, induction—IV:** 1-1.5 mg/kg **Adults ≤ age 55 y, maintenance—IV:** Increments of 25-50 mg or continuous infusion of 100-200 μg/kg/min, beginning in upper range and decreasing to lower range during next 30 min **Adults > age 55 y, maintenance—IV:** Increments of 25-50 mg or continuous infusion of 50-100 μg/kg/min, beginning in upper range and decreasing to lower range during next 30 min	**Induction:** 2.5-3.5 mg/kg (not established for children under age 3 y) **Maintenance—IV:** Continuous infusion of 125-300 μg/kg/min, beginning in upper range and decreasing to lower range during next 30 min	B	**Injection (10 mg/mL):** 50-, 100-mL vials and 20-mL ampules

Thiopental Na (III, F*)	Pentothal	**Induction—IV:** 3-5 mg/kg **Maintenance —IV:** 25-100 mg increments or continuous drip of 0.2-0.4% solution **Rectal sedation:** 30 mg/kg **Rectal narcosis:** 9 mg/kg	**Induction—IV:** Same as adult **Maintenance—IV:** 1 mg/kg increments **Rectal sedation/narcosis:** Same as adult	C	**Powder:** 250-, 400-, 500-mg vials and syringes; 0.5-, 1-, 2.5-, 5-, 10-g kits **Suspension (400 mg/g):** 2-g rectal syringes

Adults ≤ age 55 y, conscious sedation—IV: 0.5 mg/kg over 3-5 min followed by continuous infusion of 25-75 µg/kg/min

Adults > age 55 y, conscious sedation—IV: Same as for adults ≤ age 55 y, with 20% lower infusion rates

[CAN] *indicates a drug available only in Canada.*
Controlled substances (United States, Canadian classifications).

Table 3.2

General Anesthetics: Possible Interactions With Other Drugs

Drug taken by patient	Interaction with general anesthetics	Dentist's action
Adrenergic amines, cocaine, doxapram, *levodopa,* methylxanthines	Coadministration of volatile anesthetics, especially *halothane,* potentiates arrhythmogenic action of these drugs	Limit concurrent use, especially with halothane anesthesia
Aminoglycosides, capreomycin, clindamycin, neuromuscular blockers, polymyxins, tetracyclines	Increased skeletal muscle weakness with volatile anesthetics	Monitor neuromuscular function and respiratory status
Antimyasthenic cholinesterase inhibitors: ambenonium, neostigmine, pyridostigmine	Volatile anesthetics may antagonize antimyasthenic effects postoperatively	Monitor neuromuscular function and respiratory status
CNS depressants: *alcohols, antidepressants, antihistamines, antipsychotics, barbiturates, benzodiazepines, centrally acting antihypertensives and muscle relaxants, local anesthetics, opioids, parenteral magnesium sulfate*	*Summation of drug effects may lead to increased CNS depression, respiratory depression or cardiovascular depression. Anesthetic dosage requirements may be decreased significantly and recovery times prolonged*	Avoid overmedicating patient by carefully titrating inhalation and IV agents to the desired effect and by reducing dosages of drugs administered IM or rectally
Hepatic enzyme inducers: alcohol, barbiturates, carbamazepine, glutethimide, griseofulvin, isoniazid, phenytoin, rifampin	Increased metabolism of volatile anesthetics may increase the risk of hepatitis (halothane, enflurane, methoxyflurane) or renal toxicity (methoxyflurane, enflurane, sevoflurane)	Use cautiously
Hypotension-producing drugs: adrenergic neuron blockers, α- and β-adrenergic blockers, amiodarone, angiotensin-converting enzyme inhibitors, centrally acting antihypertensives, calcium channel blockers, diuretics, ganglionic blockers, levodopa, vasodilators	Summation of drug effects may lead to significant hypotension	Monitor patient's blood pressure at regular intervals; ensure proper hydration and adjust anesthetic dosage as necessary
Hypothermia-producing drugs: CNS depressants, α- and β-adrenergic blockers, insulin, vasodilators	Increased tendency toward hypothermia	Monitor core temperature during general anesthesia for other than brief cases
Nephrotoxic drugs: aminoglycosides, nonsteroidal anti-inflammatory drugs, cyclosporine	*With methoxyflurane, increased risk of renal toxicity*	Avoid concurrent or sequential use
Thyroid hormones	Increased cardiovascular stimulation with ketamine	Recognize minimal risk with replacement therapy only; otherwise avoid concurrent use
Volatile anesthetics	Decreased elimination of ketamine	Use cautiously

Italics indicate information of major clinical significance.

Table 3.3
General Anesthetics: Potential Cross-Sensitivity With Other Substances

A person with a sensitivity to	May also have a sensitivity to
Barbiturates	Thiopental or methohexital
Droperidol or fentanyl-type opioids	Droperidol/fentanyl
Egg phosphatide (lecithin), soybean oil	Propofol (its emulsion vehicle)
Volatile anesthetics or other halogenated hydrocarbons	Other volatile anesthetics

halothane, etomidate, ketamine and propofol (although at greater than usual doses or exposure times or both)—can pose the risk of birth defects. Table 3.1 lists the U.S. Food and Drug Administration pregnancy category classifications for general anesthetics. Considerations of the risks versus the benefits suggest that purely elective treatment be delayed until after delivery and that other dental care be delayed, if possible, until the second trimester. Halothane, thiopental, methohexital, propofol and, it is presumed, other general anesthetics are distributed into breast milk, although no problems associated with general anesthetics have been documented in humans.

Of special concern to the dental profession is the link between occupational exposure to nitrous oxide and reproductive toxicity in exposed females and spontaneous abortion in the spouses of exposed males. Because no health risks were observed when scavenging inhalation circuits were used to minimize nitrous oxide pollution, it is believed that existing technologies, when used appropriately, permit nitrous oxide to be administered with minimal risk to both the patient and the dental team.

Pediatric, geriatric and other special patients
Pediatric patients. Specific approved dosage recommendations for pediatric patients are not available either for inhalation anesthetics or for the following injectable drugs: etomidate (in children aged < 10 y), propofol (in children aged < 3 y) and droperidol/fentanyl (in children aged < 2 y). Although children aged > 1 y tend to be relatively resistant to drugs administered on the basis of weight—because of higher clearance rates, more active homeostatic mechanisms and other variables—differences in metabolic rates, oxygen consumption and cardiovascular responses can complicate the treatment of reactions to an overdose. Qualitative differences in responses to general anesthetics can also occur. Excitement is more likely to occur in response to subanesthetic doses of these agents; however, disturbing hallucinations with ketamine are less problematic. Because of their behavior, young children and mentally challenged patients may cause difficulties when the dentist is trying to induce anesthesia with inhalation or an IV injection. In these cases, alternative methods of drug delivery, such as IM injection or rectal suppositories, should be considered.

Geriatric patients. Separate geriatric dosage guidelines for most general anesthetics have not been published. Age-related limitations of respiratory function may slow the onset of and recovery from inhalation anesthesia. Recovery from IV anesthesia is also commonly delayed due to a decreased total body clearance and altered volume of distribution in these patients. Lower induction doses and a reduced maintenance schedule for many injectable agents should be used with geriatric patients. Elderly patients are more susceptible to cardiovascular instability, such as orthostatic hypotension, during and after general anesthesia.

Other special patients. IV drugs that pose the potential for abuse may be inappropriate for certain patients, such as those who have a history of drug abuse. Mentally challenged patients are more likely than other patients to exhibit excitement reactions.

Patient Monitoring: Aspects to Watch

- Cardiovascular status: arterial blood pressure, heart rate, electrocardiogram
- Respiratory status: oxygenation and ventilation
- Core body temperature

Adverse Effects and Precautions

General anesthetics differ from each other in the incidence and severity of their adverse effects. Most adverse effects are dose-related and are extensions of the normal pharmacology of the drug—for example, exaggerated CNS responses or cardiovascular depression. Idiosyncratic and allergic reactions account for a small minority of adverse responses to general anesthetics. Appropriate resuscitative and endotracheal intubation equipment, oxygen and medications for preventing and treating anesthetic emergencies must be immediately available.

The adverse effects and precautions/contraindications listed in Tables 3.4 and 3.5 apply to all routes of administration.

Table 3.4

Inhalation General Anesthetics: Adverse Effects, Precautions and Contraindications

Body system	Adverse effects	Precautions/contraindications
General	*Malignant hyperthermia*	*Muscular dystrophy is associated with increased risk of malignant hyperthermia*
		Nitrous oxide increases pressures of enclosed air spaces, as with pneumothorax, acute intestinal obstruction, middle ear infections, air-containing cysts, air emboli and pneumoencephalography
		Personal or family history of malignant hyperthermia contraindicates use of inhalation agents other than nitrous oxide
		History of drug sensitivity to the volatile anesthetic considered for use
CV	Cardiac arrhythmias (fast, slow or irregular heartbeat)	Preexisting cardiovascular disease or pheochromocytoma predisposes patient to cardiovascular effects, *especially with halothane and desflurane*
	Hypotension from myocardial depression and/or peripheral vasodilatation (minimal with nitrous oxide)	Ensure proper fluid replacement before anesthesia in patients who are dehydrated or have had a blood loss
CNS	Increased intracranial pressure	*Patients with head injuries, increased intracranial pressure or intracranial tumors are at increased risk of intracranial hypertension; barbiturates help reduce intracranial pressure*
	Excitatory effects during induction; electrical convulsive activity with enflurane	
		Hyperventilation

Italics indicate information of major clinical significance.

Continued on next page

Table 3.4 (cont.)

Inhalation General Anesthetics: Adverse Effects, Precautions and Contraindications

Body system	Adverse effects	Precautions/contraindications
GI	Nausea and vomiting	Employ dietary restrictions and consider use of antiemetic agents to minimize risk of nausea and vomiting
GU	Decreased renal blood flow, glomerular filtration and urine production	Risk of renal toxicity is increased in patients with preexisting renal disease or impairment Ensure proper hydration before anesthesia *Methoxyflurane is contraindicated in patients with renal disease*
HB	Hepatitis, both reversible and fulminant (most common with halothane)	Preexisting hepatic disease increases risk of hepatotoxicity *Repeated use of halothane in adults is contraindicated*
Musc	None of significance to dentistry	Postoperative weakness is possible with volatile anesthetics in patients with myasthenia gravis, muscular dystrophy or related disorders
Resp	*Respiratory depression, hypoxemia and hypercarbia* Increased secretions, coughing, breath-holding, laryngospasm Pulmonary aspiration Loss of airway patency	*Maintain inspired oxygen tension $\geq 30\%$ and use nitrous oxide or inhalation anesthesia delivery systems equipped with fail-safe and minimum oxygen flow devices* *Avoid use of desflurane for mask induction* *Use dietary restrictions to minimize risk of aspiration, which increases with a full stomach, obesity, alcohol intake and gastric reflux disorders*

Italics indicate information of major clinical significance.

Pharmacology

General anesthetics produce their effects through a variety of actions, some of which may be unique to individual drugs. Because of their respective routes of administration, inhalation and injectable anesthetics should be considered separately. Within each group there are also some important similarities, as well as differences, with respect to the mechanism of action and pharmacologic profile.

Inhalation anesthetics. Inhalation anesthetics are believed to produce general anesthesia by interacting with the nerve cell membrane. The anesthetic potency of these agents increases in direct correlation with the oil:gas partition coefficient, a measure of hydrophobicity. Recent findings suggest that inhalation agents interact directly with membrane proteins to cause general anesthesia. Postsynaptic inhibition of the brain stem and midbrain is believed to account for most anesthetic actions. With drugs such as nitrous oxide and enflurane, certain areas of the brain may become disinhibited and demonstrate increased electrical activity.

Some inhalation anesthetics have specific analgesic actions; in the case of nitrous oxide, an interaction with the endogenous opioid system has been proposed. Respiratory depression is a common feature of all inhalation anesthetics; it is often moderated when a

Table 3.5

Injectable General Anesthetics: Adverse Effects, Precautions and Contraindications

Body system	Adverse effects	Precautions/contraindications
General	Allergic reactions, including anaphylaxis *Infection, sometimes fatal, after injection of contaminated propofol solution* Vascular irritation, including pain on injection, phlebitis and thrombophlebitis; pain most likely with etomidate, propofol and methohexital	*Use proper aseptic technique in the handling and administration of propofol, including individual patient use of unit doses and discarding unused drug after 6 h* *Contraindicated in patients with history of drug sensitivity to the injectable anesthetic being considered for use or to any component of the selected preparation*
CV	Cardiac arrhythmias (fast, slow, or irregular heartbeat); tachycardia more likely to occur with barbiturates and ketamine; bradycardia with propofol and droperidol/fentanyl Hypotension from myocardial depression and/or peripheral vasodilatation; more likely to occur with barbiturates and propofol Hypertension from ketamine Transient venous pain at injection site	Hypotension and arrhythmias are more likely to occur in patients with preexisting cardiovascular disease Ensure proper fluid replacement before anesthesia in patients with dehydration or blood loss *Avoid intra-arterial injection;* venous sequelae less likely when drugs are infused slowly into large vein with rapid IV drip *Ketamine is contraindicated in patients with severe hypertension or cardiovascular disease, or a recent (within last 6 mo) stroke or heart attack*
CNS	Excessive CNS depression Postoperative drowsiness, confusion, depression CNS excitation, hyperactivity, anxiety, hallucinations, dysphoria Extrapyramidal signs and symptoms (dystonia, akathisia) with droperidol/fentanyl Increased intracranial pressure with ketamine	Avoid too-rapid IV injection Avoid multiple repeated injections or prolonged infusion leading to drug accumulation (exception: propofol) Excitatory reactions are more likely with ketamine and in patients with psychiatric disorders Ensure adequate anesthesia intraoperatively; minimize aversive, intensive stimuli in the recovery period *Ketamine is contraindicated in patients with head injuries, increased intracranial pressure, intracranial tumors or history of stroke or intracranial hemorrhage*
EENT	Elevation of intraocular pressure, diplopia and nystagmus with ketamine	Ketamine increases risk of eye injury in patients with open eye wound, increased intraocular pressure
GI	Nausea and vomiting	*Employ dietary restrictions* and consider the use of antiemetic agents with ketamine or etomidate to minimize risk of nausea and vomiting
GU	None of significance to dentistry	CNS depressant effects may be prolonged in patients with renal function impairment

Italics indicate information of major clinical significance.

Continued on next page

Body system	Adverse effects	Precautions/contraindications
HB	Porphyria after repeated doses of barbiturates	Prolonged CNS depressant effects of barbiturates and fentanyl/droperidol may occur in patients with impaired hepatic function Barbiturates are contraindicated with history of acute intermittent porphyria or porphyria variegata
Musc	Skeletal muscle movements; unilateral movements may occur in response to noxious stimuli; bilateral movements, possibly a manifestation of disinhibition of cortical activity, may include tonic and clonic movements resembling seizure activity Muscle rigidity with ketamine	None of significance to dentistry
Resp	*Respiratory depression, hypoxemia and hypercarbia* Increased secretions, coughing, breath-holding and laryngospasm, especially with ketamine Pulmonary aspiration Loss of airway patency	*Avoid manipulation of the airway in the lightly anesthetized patient* Consider administering an antisialogogue when using ketamine *Use dietary restrictions to minimize risk of aspiration, which increases with a full stomach, obesity, alcohol intake and gastric reflux disorders*

Italics indicate information of major clinical significance.

reduced dose of volatile anesthetic is administered with nitrous oxide. Cardiovascular depression is an effect shared by all volatile inhalation agents in common use but not by nitrous oxide. Some drugs, most notably halothane, reduce blood pressure by direct myocardial depression, whereas some (such as isoflurane) induce peripheral vascular relaxation and still others (such as enflurane) produce both effects. Volatile agents produce varying degrees of muscle relaxation; nitrous oxide tends to increase muscle tone in anesthetic concentrations.

The pharmacokinetics of inhalation anesthetics are strongly governed by the blood:gas partition coefficient. As indicated in Table 3.6, drugs with a low partition coefficient equilibrate very quickly between the inspired tension and the brain concentration. The irritating odor of desflurane, the least soluble inhalation anesthetic, negates much of the drug's potential benefit, especially in children, because of breathing disturbances (such as breath-holding, coughing and laryngospasm) that limit ventilation. Metabolism plays a minor role in the pharmacokinetics of all the inhalation agents except methoxyflurane. However, the metabolism of halothane helps speed recovery, as does (in short cases) the redistribution of volatile agents from the brain to other tissues. The metabolic release of fluoride and other potentially toxic metabolites has severely limited the use of methoxyflurane and is of potential concern for the use of sevoflurane and enflurane.

Injectable anesthetics. Injectable anesthetics also depress CNS function by binding to specific membrane receptors. Ultrashort-acting barbiturates bind to receptor sites on the γ-aminobutyric acid (GABA)–activated

Table 3.6

Inhalation General Anesthetics: Pharmacokinetic Parameters

Drug	Blood: gas partition coefficient	Onset of action	Recovery time	Metabolism (%)
Desflurane	0.42	Very rapid*	Very rapid	0.02
Enflurane	1.91	Rapid*	Rapid	2.4
Halothane	2.3	Rapid	Rapid	up to 20
Isoflurane	1.43	Rapid*	Rapid	0.17
Methoxyflurane	13	Slow	Slow	65
Nitrous oxide	0.47	Very rapid	Very rapid	0
Sevoflurane	0.69	Rapid	Rapid	5

*The pungent odor of these drugs, especially desflurane, may cause breath-holding and laryngospasm and limit the onset of anesthesia.

chloride channel to enhance responsiveness to GABA, increase membrane conductance of chloride and hyperpolarize the cell. Inhibition of certain glutamate receptor responses may be a secondary mechanism. The ultrashort-acting agents etomidate and propofol appear to exert similar effects. Other receptors are involved in the actions of ketamine and droperidol-fentanyl.

The pharmacology of the ultrashort-acting barbiturates, etomidate and propofol share important similarities. They produce unconsciousness and decrease cerebral blood flow but cause no specific analgesia or muscle relaxation. They are rapidly redistributed from the brain and other highly perfused organs (liver, kidneys, heart) to muscle and later to fatty tissues. Induction doses depress laryngeal reflexes and often cause brief periods of apnea (shortest with etomidate, longest with propofol). Etomidate also produces minimal changes in cardiovascular status, whereas propofol generally depresses myocardial contractility and arterial blood pressure. Thiopental and methohexital each reduce myocardial contractility, but arterial pressures are usually well maintained unless the patient

is hypovolemic or the drug is used in combination with opioids. Decreases in renal and cerebral blood flow commonly occur with all four induction anesthetics. Pain on injection is common with etomidate and propofol, less so with methohexital and infrequent with thiopental. Involuntary movements follow a similar pattern of incidence.

Ketamine and droperidol/fentanyl are not simple CNS depressants. The "dissociative" anesthetic state produced by ketamine is notable for its profound analgesia, nystagmus, increased muscle tone, relative lack of respiratory depression, maintenance of laryngeal reflexes and cardiovascular stimulation. Excitatory reactions are made manifest by involuntary motor movements, vivid dreams or frank hallucinations and emergence delirium. The adverse excitatory effects of ketamine can be minimized by coadministration of diazepam or midazolam; glycopyrrolate is useful in blunting the secretory stimulation caused by ketamine. Ketamine acts rapidly after IV injection and is one of the fastest agents for inducing anesthesia after IM injection. Droperidol/fen-

Table 3.7

Injectable General Anesthetics: Pharmacokinetic Parameters

Drug	Elimination half-life (h)	Onset of action	Duration of action (min)	Plasma protein binding (%)
Droperidol	1.7 to 2.2	3 to 10 min	120 to 240	Not available
Etomidate	1.25	< 60 s	3 to 5	76
Ketamine	2 to 3	30 s	5 to 10	12
Methohexital	1.5 to 5	< 60 s	5 to 7	73
Propofol	24 to 72	< 40 s	3 to 5	95-99
Thiopental	10 to 12	30 to 60 s	10 to 30	72-86

tanyl produces a quiescent state known as "neuroleptanalgesia." As with ketamine, there is indifference to the environment and analgesia. Droperidol reduces peripheral vascular tone by blocking α-adrenergic receptors; fentanyl tends to lower the heart rate. In contrast to ketamine, droperidol produces an antiemetic effect and reduces motor activity.

All of the injectable anesthetics are metabolized to inactive products, and the liver plays the predominant role. However, Table 3.7 illustrates the independence between the elimination half-life and the duration of action of these drugs. After multiple injections or continuous infusion, the redistribution sites become saturated with the drug, and the duration of action becomes progressively longer. Propofol, which has an enormous capacity for redistribution, is an important exception. Because of the extended duration of droperidol, attributed to that drug's tight binding to its receptor, repeated injections are rarely administered. Pharmacokinetic aspects of fentanyl are discussed in the opioid section of Chapter 2.

Patient Advice

- Because of the possibility of psychomotor impairment following the use of anesthetics, driving or other tasks requiring alertness and coordination should be avoided or performed with added caution, as appropriate, for the first 24 h after anesthesia.
- Use of alcohol or other CNS depressants should be avoided during the first 24 h after anesthesia except as directed by the dentist or physician.
- Patients should be aware of the potential for delayed side effects, especially mood or mental changes, nightmares or unusual dreams and blurred vision.

Suggested Readings

American Dental Association. Guidelines for the use of conscious sedation, deep sedation and general anesthesia for dentists. Chicago: American Dental Association; 1996.

American Dental Association Council on Dental Education. Guidelines for teaching the comprehensive control of pain and anxiety in dentistry. Chicago: American Dental Association; 1992.

Franks NP, Lieb WR. Molecular and cellular mechanisms of general anaesthesia. Nature 1994;367:607-14.

McGlothlin JD, Crouch KG, Mickelsen RL. Control of nitrous oxide in dental operatories. Cincinnati: U.S. Department of Health and Human Services, Public Health Service, Centers for Disease Control and Prevention, National Institute for Occupational Safety and Health, 1994; DHEW publication no. 94-129.

Stoelting RK. Pharmacology and physiology in anesthetic practice. 3rd ed. Philadelphia: Lippincott; 1995.

Neuromuscular Blocking Drugs

Muscle relaxation during general anesthesia is often desirable and sometimes required for surgical procedures. Endotracheal intubation is also greatly facilitated by paralysis of the vocal cords. Although varying degrees of muscle relaxation can be produced by the volatile general anesthetics, the dosages required are generally excessive compared to those needed to produce unconsciousness and unresponsiveness to noxious stimuli. Neuromuscular blocking drugs, beginning with the clinical introduction of tubocurarine in 1942, are commonly used whenever flaccidity of skeletal muscle is sought, and are among the most important adjuncts in general anesthesia.

With the exception of succinylcholine, which is a classified as a "depolarizing" blocker because it acts like acetylcholine in stimulating muscle nicotinic receptors, the neuromuscular blocking drugs competitively inhibit the binding of acetylcholine to its receptor on the motor endplate and are thus characterized as "competitive" or "nondepolarizing" blockers.

Accepted Indications

Neuromuscular blocking drugs are used for the induction and maintenance of skeletal muscle relaxation during general anesthesia and to facilitate the management of patients receiving mechanical ventilation.

General Dosing Information

Table 3.8 lists the usual IV doses for induction of paralysis (intubation) and for maintenance of neuromuscular blockade. The clinician should individualize the actual maintenance dosage, using a peripheral nerve stimulator to monitor motor responsiveness.

Dosage Adjustments

When nondepolarizing neuromuscular blocking agents are administered concurrently with inhalation general anesthetics other than nitrous oxide, the dosage of the neuromuscular blocker should be reduced by up to 50%, as determined with a peripheral nerve stimulator. A reduced dosage may also be indicated for patients with neuromuscular disorders and severe electrolyte disturbances.

Special Dental Considerations

Drug Interactions of Dental Interest

The following drug interactions and related problems involving neuromuscular blocking agents (Table 3.9) are potentially of clinical significance in dentistry (interactions of major importance are italicized).

Table 3.10 itemizes potential cross-sensitivity considerations.

Laboratory Value Alterations

- Serum potassium concentrations: succinylcholine may temporarily increase these

Cross-Sensitivity

Table 3.10 lists potential cross-sensitivities between neuromuscular blocking drugs and other substances.

Special Patients

Pregnant and nursing women

Neuromuscular blocking agents cross the placenta in small amounts to enter the fetal circulation. Table 3.8 lists the FDA pregnancy risk category classifications for neuromuscular blocking agents. Considerations of risk/benefit suggest that purely elective treatment should be delayed until after delivery and that other dental care be performed, if possible, during the second trimester. Problems related to breast-feeding have not been reported in humans.

Pediatric, geriatric and other special patients
Pediatric patients. Many side effects of succinylcholine are noted in children. Of major concern is an increased sensitivity to the vagal effects of succinylcholine, with profound bradycardia and asystole, which occasionally occurs after a standard dose. Administration of atropine is often

Table 3.8

Neuromuscular Blocking Drugs: Dosage Information*

Generic name	Brand name(s)	Usual adult dosage	Usual child dosage	Pregnancy risk category	Content/form
Atracurium besylate	Tracrium	0.4–0.5 mg/kg initially and 0.08-0.1 mg/kg as needed	**Age > 2 y:** Same as adult dose	C	**Injection, 10 mg/mL:** in 5-mL ampules and 10-mL vials
Cisatracurium besylate	Nimbex	0.15-0.20 mg/kg initially and 0.03 mg/kg as needed or infusion of 1-3 μg/kg/min as needed	**Age 2-12 y:** 0.1 mg/kg initially and then same as adult dose	B	**Injection, 2 mg/mL:** in 5-, 10-mL vials **Injection, 10 mg/mL:** in 20-mL vials
Doxacurium chloride	Nuromax	50 μg/kg initially and 5-10 μg/kg as needed	Same as adult dose	C	**Injection, 1 mg/mL:** in 5-mL vials
Gallamine triethiodide	Flaxedil	1 mg/kg initially and 0.5-1 mg/kg as needed, not to exceed 100 mg per dose†	Same as adult dose	Not classified	**Injection, 20 mg/mL:** in 10-mL vials
Metocurine iodide	Metubine Iodide	0.2-0.4 mg/kg initially and 0.5-1 mg as needed	Not established	C	**Injection, 2 mg/mL:** in 20-mL vials
Mivacurium chloride	Mivacron	0.15 mg/kg initially and 0.10 mg/kg as needed	**Age 2-12 y:** 0.2 mg/kg initially and 0.1 mg/kg as needed	C	**Infusion, 0.5 mg/mL:** in 50-mL containers **Injection, 2 mg/mL:** in 5-, 10-mL vials

Continued on next page

*All medications are given IV.
†Intubation doses (4-6 mg/kg) for gallamine are generally not used. Strong vagolytic activity of gallamine restricts normal initial dose to 1 mg/kg; with tubocurarine, histamine release is prominent, and doses such as 0.16mg/kg are generally recommended.

Table 3.8 (cont.)

Neuromuscular Blocking Drugs: Dosage Information*

Generic name	Brand name(s)	Usual adult dosage	Usual child dosage	Pregnancy risk category	Content/form
Pancuronium bromide	Pavulon	60-100 µg/kg initially and 10 µg/kg as needed	**Age > 1 mo:** Same as adult dose	C	**Injection, 1 mg/mL:** in 10-mL vials **Injection, 2 mg/mL:** in 2-, 5-mL ampules
Pipecuronium bromide	Arduan	70-85 µg/kg initially and 10-15 µg/kg as needed	**Age > 1 mo:** Same as adult dose †	C	**Powder, 10 mg:** in 10-mL vials
Rocuronium bromide	Zemuron	0.6 mg/kg initially and 0.1-0.2 mg/kg as needed	Same as adult dose †	B	**Injection, 10 mg/mL:** in 5-, 10-mL vials
Succinylcholine chloride	Anectine, Quelicin, Sucostrin, Sux-Cert	0.3-1.1 mg/kg initially and 0.04-0.07 mg/kg as needed or infusion of 0.5-1.0 mg/min as needed ‡	**Infants and small children:** 2 mg/kg **Older children and adolescents:** 1 mg/kg‡	C	**Injection, 20 mg/mL:** in 10-mL vials **Injection, 50 mg/mL:** in 10-mL ampules **Injection, 100 mg/mL:** in 10-mL vials **Powder, 100 mg:** in 5-mL vials **Powder:** in 500-mg, 1-g vials

Tubocurarine chloride	(generic); Tubarine [CAN]	0.5-0.6 mg/kg initially and 3 mg as needed §	Age > 1 mo: 0.5-0.6 mg/kg initially and 0.1 mg/kg as needed	C	Injection, 3 mg/mL: in 5-mL syringes and 10-, 20-mL vials
Vecuronium bromide	Norcuron	80-100 µg/kg initially and 10-15 µg/kg as needed	Age > 1 y: Same as adult dose†	C	Powder, 10 mg: in 5-, 10-mL vials

[CAN] indicates a drug available only in Canada.

* All medications are given IV.

† Children aged 1 y to puberty may be less sensitive to neuromuscular blockade and need increased dosage and/or more frequent administration.

‡ May also be given IM (adults, 2.5 mg/kg; children, 2.5-4 mg/kg; not to exceed 150 mg). The routine use of succinylcholine in children, particularly by continuous infusion, is considered unsafe because of sudden death linked to ventricular dysrhythmia and malignant hyperthermia.

§ Intubation doses (4-6 mg/kg) for gallamine are generally not used. Strong vagolytic activity of gallamine restricts normal initial dose to 1 mg/kg; with tubocurarine, histamine release is prominent, and doses such as 0.16mg/kg are generally recommended.

recommended before administration of succinylcholine to prevent vagally induced arrhythmias. Cardiac arrest associated with acute muscle destruction (rhabdomyolysis) and hyperkalemia has occurred in children with undiagnosed skeletal muscle disorders. Malignant hyperthermia may be a related condition. For these reasons, succinylcholine is no longer recommended for routine use in children.

Geriatric patients. Neuromuscular blocking agents, except for doxacurium, have shown no significant differences in effectiveness, safety or dosage requirements when given to healthy elderly and younger patients. With doxacurium, the neuromuscular blockade has a slower onset, is more variable and has a longer duration in older patients. Elderly patients are more likely to have impaired renal function, however, which may decrease the clearance of doxacurium, gallamine, metocurine, mivacurium, pancuronium, pipecuronium or tubocurarine from the body and prolong their effects.

Patient Monitoring: Aspects to Watch
- Cardiovascular status (arterial blood pressure, heart rate, electrocardiogram)

Table 3.9

Neuromuscular Blocking Drugs: Possible Interactions With Other Drugs

Drug taken by patient	Interaction with neuromuscular blocking drugs	Dentist's action
Anticholinesterases, including antimyasthenics, organophosphate insecticides, nerve gases and eye drops and hexafluorenium, thiotepa, cyclophosphamide	*Antimyasthenic agents and edrophonium antagonize effect of competitive blockers and vice versa; duration of action of succinylcholine and mivacurium may be prolonged by anticholinesterases* and anticancer drugs *that reduce cholinesterase activity*	Avoid concurrent use in myasthenic patients if possible; otherwise, use a short-acting agent such as cisatracurium or rocuronium that is not metabolized by esterases and monitor patient carefully Anticholinesterases such as edrophonium and neostigmine are used to reverse the action of competitive blockers Hexaflurenium has been used to prolong the action of succinylcholine Avoid concurrent use of other agents with succinylcholine and mivacurium
Digitalis glycosides	*May increase cardiac effects when used concurrently with succinylcholine and, to a lesser extent, with pancuronium, possibly resulting in cardiac arrhythmias*	Avoid concurrent use
Local anesthetics (large doses), aminoglycosides, clindamycin, lincomycin, capreomycin, polymyxins, procainamide, quinidine, lithium, β-adrenergic blockers, magnesium salts (parenteral), calcium channel blockers	*May increase respiratory depression or paralysis (apnea); incomplete reversal of neuromuscular blockade at the end of surgery may significantly increase possibility of inadequate ventilation*	Carefully monitor patient and reduce dosage of neuromuscular blocker in accordance with clinical response
Methotrimeprazine	May stimulate CNS, evoke extrapyramidal reactions and cause hypotension with tachycardia when used with succinylcholine	Avoid concurrent use

Italics indicate information of major clinical significance.

Continued on next page

Table 3.9 (cont.)

Neuromuscular Blocking Drugs: Possible Interactions With Other Drugs

Drug taken by patient	Interaction with neuromuscular blocking drugs	Dentist's action
Neuromuscular blockers	Competitive blockers produce additive effects when used with each other; prior administration of a competitive blocker reduces activity of succinylcholine initially but may prolong effect of repeated administrations; prior administration of succinylcholine may increase duration of competitive blocker	Adjust dosage in accordance with actual or predicted clinical response
Opioid analgesics	CNS depressant effects may increase respiratory depressant effects of neuromuscular blockers; hypotension also more likely, except with vagolytic drugs such as gallamine and pancuronium, which may cause tachycardia and hypertension Histamine release by meperidine or morphine-like opioids may add to effects of histamine-releasing neuromuscular blockers (tubocurarine, atracurium, metocurine, succinylcholine)	Carefully monitor patient; consider use of antihistamines to prevent or treat histamine responses
Potassium-depleting drugs such as thiazide and high-efficacy diuretics, corticosteroids, carbonic anhydrase inhibitors, amphotericin B	Enhances blockade produced by nondepolarizing neuromuscular blocking agents	Reduce dosage of neuromuscular blocker in accordance with clinical response
Volatile inhalation anesthetics	Enhances neuromuscular blockade, especially with nondepolarizing neuromuscular blocking agents	Reduce dosage of neuromuscular blocker in accordance with clinical response

Table 3.10

Neuromuscular Blocking Drugs: Potential Cross-Sensitivity With Other Substances

A person with a sensitivity to	May also have a sensitivity to
Bromides	Bromide salts of pancuronium, pipecuronium, rocuronium or vecuronium
Iodine or iodides	Iodide salts of gallamine or metocurine
Para-aminobenzoic acid (PABA) or paraben preservative	Neuromuscular blocker preparations containing paraben preservatives
Sulfites	Neuromuscular blocker preparations containing sulfite antioxidants

- Core body temperature
- Neuromuscular responsiveness (peripheral nerve stimulator)
- Respiratory status (oxygenation and ventilation)

Adverse Effects and Precautions

Adverse effects, precautions and contraindications related to the use of neuromuscular blocking agents are presented in Table 3.11.

Neuromuscular blocking agents do not alter consciousness or the perception of pain; therefore, adequate general anesthesia must be ensured when these drugs are used during surgery. Since neuromuscular blocking agents commonly induce respiratory depression or respiratory arrest, they should be used only by dentists experienced in the techniques of tracheal intubation, artificial respiration and the administration of oxygen under positive pressure; in addition, facilities for these procedures should be immediately available.

Succinylcholine, the only depolarizing neuromuscular blocker in clinical use, is associated with a unique set of side effects. Myalgia, malignant hyperthermia, hyperkalemia and profound bradycardia are related to succinylcholine's ability to excite acetylcholine receptors in skeletal muscle and the heart. The likelihood of each of these effects is increased in special groups of patients with the following disorders:

- myalgia in ambulatory patients;
- malignant hyperthermia in patients with a family history of malignant hyperthermia or young males with dystrophic muscle disorders;
- hyperkalemia in patients with neurologic disorders or recent history of severe trauma or burns;
- bradycardia in patients with increased vagal sensitivity, including young children and patients receiving a second dose of succinylcholine.

Pharmacology

Nondepolarizing neuromuscular blocking drugs cause muscle relaxation by blocking the ability of acetylcholine to activate its receptors at the motor endplate. In order of increasing resistance to blockade are the levator muscles of the eyelids, muscles of mastication, limb muscles, trunk muscles, muscles of the glottis, intercostal muscles and the diaphragm. Doses that cause paralysis of the respiratory muscles are commonly used, and mechanical ventilation of the patient is necessary. Reversal of paralysis can be achieved by administration of a suitable anticholinesterase, such as edrophonium or neostigmine, which increases the amount of acetylcholine at the neuromuscular junction. Atropine or glycopyrrolate is also administered to block the unwanted muscarinic side effects of the acetylcholine.

Succinylcholine, the only depolarizing neuromuscular blocking drug used in clinical practice, produces a prolonged activation of acetylcholine receptors. A short period of uncoordinated muscle contraction, evident by the fasciculation of surface muscles of the neck and shoulders, is followed by muscle relaxation, in which the cell membrane becomes refractory to the continued depolarization of the motor endplate. Administration of anticholinesterase potentiates the depolarizing block. With repeated administration or continuous infusion of succinylcholine, the motor endplate repolarizes gradually, probably as a result of receptor inactivation, and the blockade takes on some characteristics of a competitive block.

Cardiovascular responses to neuromuscular blocking drugs are common but are usually of minor consequence. Mild hypotension may follow muscle flaccidity and mechanical ventilation. Contributing to the pharmacology of some neuromuscular blockers is their propensity to release histamine from storage cells.

Table 3.11

Neuromuscular Blocking Drugs: Adverse Effects, Precautions and Contraindications

Body system	Adverse effects	Precautions/contraindications
General	*Malignant hyperthermia after succinylcholine* Allergy-induced hypotension, bronchospasm, edema, erythema, skin rash and hives—all are rarely noted; similar reactions are more common with drugs (tubocurarine, metocurine, mivacurium, succinylcholine and atracurium) that cause histamine release	*Muscular dystrophy is associated with increased risk of malignant hyperthermia* Premedication with antihistamine may blunt or eliminate allergiclike responses in patients with increased sensitivity to histamine *Personal or family history of malignant hyperthermia contraindicates use of succinylcholine* *Contraindicated in patients with history of drug sensitivity to the neuromuscular blocker considered for use*
CV	Hypotension, especially after large doses of tubocurarine, metocurine or atracurium; hypertension with gallamine Tachycardia with gallamine, pancuronium or rocuronium Bradycardia, arrhythmias, cardiac arrest with succinylcholine, *especially in children and after second dose*	Cardiovascular reactions are more likely in patients with preexisting cardiovascular disease *Hyperkalemia, severe trauma or burns, spinal cord injury or neuromuscular disease increases the risk of cardiac reaction to succinylcholine* *Atropine should be administered before second dose of succinylcholine*
EENT	Increased intraocular pressure immediately after injection of succinylcholine	*Succinylcholine contraindicated in patients with open eye injury*
GU	Myoglobinuria after succinylcholine, especially in children	Renal function impairment may lead to prolonged neuromuscular blockade; *absolute contraindication for gallamine* and relative contraindication for other competitive blockers excreted renally
HB	None of significance to dentistry	Effect of vecuronium and rocuronium may be increased in patients with decreased hepatic function Decreased cholinesterase synthesis may prolong action of succinylcholine and mivacurium
Musc	Persisting muscle weakness Fasciculation and postoperative myalgia with succinylcholine	Prolonged muscle weakness may follow administration of succinylcholine or mivacurium in patients with acquired pseudocholinesterase deficiency (as from severe hepatic disease, anemia, dehydration or malnutrition) *Myasthenia gravis*, electrolyte disturbances, hypotension and hyperthermia increase risk of postoperative weakness Muscle fasciculation may worsen tissue damage associated with fractures *Continued on next page*

Italics indicate information of major clinical significance.

Continued on next page

Table 3.11 (cont.)

Neuromuscular Blocking Drugs: Adverse Effects, Precautions and Contraindications

Body system	Adverse effects	Precautions/contraindications
Musc (cont.)		Myalgia, likely in ambulatory patients, may be prevented by a defasciculating dose of nondepolarizing blocker *Succinylcholine and mivacurium are contraindicated in patients with congenital pseudocholinesterase deficiency*
Resp	*Respiratory depression and arrest* Excessive salivation with succinylcholine or pancuronium	Decreased pulmonary function, bronchogenic carcinoma or *myasthenia gravis* increases risk of postoperative respiratory complications

Italics indicate information of major clinical significance.

Table 3.12

Neuromuscular Blocking Drugs: Pharmacokinetic Properties

Drug	Onset time (min)*	Time to peak effect (min)	Duration of peak effect (min)	Time to recovery (min)	Primary route of elimination
Atracurium	2-2.5	3-5	35-45	60-70	Plasma†
Cisatracurium	1.5-2	4-6	55-60	75-100	†
Doxacurium	4-5	2.5-13	40-230	90-280	Kidneys
Gallamine ‡	1-2	3-5	90-120	Not available	Kidneys
Metocurine	1-4	3-5	60-120	> 360	Kidneys
Mivacurium	2-2.5	2.5-3.5	15-20	25-30	Plasma
Pancuronium	2-3	3-5	60-120	100-160	Kidneys/liver
Pipecuronium	2.5-3	3-5	60-120	90-150	Kidneys
Rocuronium	1-1.5	2-3	20-30	60	Kidneys/liver
Succinylcholine	0.5-1	1-2	4-10	12-15	Plasma
Tubocurarine ‡	1-2	2-5	60-100	Not available	Kidneys/liver
Vecuronium	2.5-3	3-5	25-40	45-65	Kidneys/liver

Time required for muscle relaxation to become sufficient to permit endotracheal intubation.
†*Cisatracurium, one of the isomers in atracurium, undergoes spontaneous inactivation (Hofmann elimination).*
‡ *Intubation doses generally are not used.*

The release of histamine is most prominent with tubocurarine but also occurs clinically with succinylcholine, metocurine, atracurium and mivacurium. Hypotension and skin erythema are the most common responses. Large doses of tubocurarine may also reduce blood pressure by blocking autonomic ganglia. Conversely, the vagolytic effects of rocuronium, pancuronium and, especially, gallamine may increase the heart rate.

The muscle depolarization caused by succinylcholine results in significant potassium efflux and even hyperkalemia in burn patients and patients with recent traumatic injuries, especially those involving the spinal cord.

Neuromuscular blocking drugs are selected according to their freedom from side effects, their route of elimination and their pharmacokinetic properties. Table 3.12 reviews some of the salient pharmacokinetic characteristics of these drugs. The duration of effect and the recovery time after a single administration strongly depend on the dose. Recovery after repeated doses with some agents, such as tubocurarine, metocurine, gallamine, rocuronium and succinylcholine, may be prolonged.

Suggested Readings

Savarese JJ, Miller RD, Lien CA, Caldwell JE. Pharmacology of muscle relaxants and their antagonists. In: Miller RD, ed. Anesthesia. 4th ed. New York: Churchill Livingstone; 1994: 417-88.

Stoelting RK. Pharmacology and physiology in anesthetic practice. 3rd ed. Philadelphia: Lippincott; 1995.

Chapter 4

Analgesics: Opioids and Nonopioids

Steven Ganzberg, D.M.D., M.S.

The use of systemically acting medications to reduce pain perception is an integral part of dental practice. Analgesic medications in dentistry are indicated for the relief of acute pain, postoperative pain and chronic pain, as well as for adjunctive intraoperative pain control. In addition, these medications can be given preoperatively to decrease expected postoperative pain. There are two general categories of analgesic medications: opioid and nonopioid.

Opioid Analgesics

Accepted Indications

Moderate to Moderately Severe Pain

Opioid medications are generally reserved for moderate to moderately severe pain. Codeine, hydrocodone, dihydrocodeine and oxycodone, in combination preparations that contain aspirin, acetaminophen or ibuprofen, are commonly prescribed to manage acute orodental and postoperative pain in dental practice. This type of pain is generally considered to be moderate to moderately severe in intensity. Based on the amount of drug needed to produce a specific analgesic effect, oxycodone is a more potent analgesic than these other medications, but an equianalgesic dose can be found with any of the other agents. At an equianalgesic dose, opioid side effects of sedation, nausea, vomiting, constipation, respiratory depression and pupillary constriction are relatively similar. Table 4.1 lists the commonly prescribed combination

opioids, along with oral dosages and schedule of dosing. For severe pain, opioids such as morphine and methadone are available without a nonsteroidal anti-inflammatory drug (NSAID) or acetaminophen.

Table 4.2 lists commonly prescribed opioids not in combination with other analgesics, along with oral dosages and schedule of dosing.

Cancer and Chronic Nonmalignant Pain

Long-acting opioid analgesics, such as MS Contin, Oramorph, Oxycontin, methadone, levorphanol and fentanyl patches, are available for treating cancer pain and selected cases of chronic nonmalignant pain. These agents are not indicated for acute pain relief and should be prescribed only for people who can tolerate short-acting opioids. Only practitioners who are skilled in the management of chronic pain should prescribe these agents. Tramadol (Ultram), which acts as a mu (μ) agonist and a serotonin reuptake blocker, has recently been introduced. The latter effect, which would be expected to be helpful for chronic pain conditions, may also produce analgesia. The intravenous use of opioid medications for intraoperative sedation is discussed in Chapters 2 and 3.

General Dosing Information

Analgesic medications should be prescribed in a manner that affords the patient the greatest degree of comfort within a high margin of safety. If the dentist suspects that a patient will have pain for 24-48 h after a

Table 4.1

Opioid Combination Analgesics for Moderate or Moderate-to-Severe Pain: Dosage Information

Generic name	Brand name(s)	Narcotic component	Non-narcotic component	Usual adult dosage	Child dosage	Pregnancy risk category
			Codeine combinations			
Codeine with aceta-minophen (II*;N†)	Tylenol #1	Codeine 7.5 mg	Acetaminophen 300 mg	1-2 tablet(s) q 4 h	Must adjust according to codeine content **Age 2-6 y:** 2.5-5 mg q 4-6 h, maximum 60 mg/24 h **Age 6-12 y:** 5-10 mg q 4-6 h, maximum 60 mg/24 h	C
	Tylenol #2	Codeine 15 mg	Acetaminophen 300 mg	1-2 tablet(s) q 4 h	Must adjust according to codeine content **Age 2-6 y:** 2.5-5 mg q 4-6 h, maximum 60 mg/24 h **Age 6-12 y:** 5-10 mg q 4-6 h, maximum 60 mg/24 h	C
	Tylenol #3	Codeine 30 mg	Acetaminophen 300 mg	1-2 tablet(s) q 4 h	Must adjust according to codeine content **Age 2-6 y:** 2.5-5 mg q 4-6 h, maximum 60 mg/24 h **Age 6-12 y:** 5-10 mg q 4-6 h, maximum 60 mg/24 h	C

Continued on next page

*Controlled substance in the United States; see Appendix A for complete description of schedule.
†Controlled substance in Canada; see Appendix A for complete description of schedule.

Table 4.1 (cont.)

Opioid Combination Analgesics for Moderate or Moderate-to-Severe Pain: Dosage Information

Generic name	Brand name(s)	Narcotic component	Non-narcotic component	Usual adult dosage	Child dosage	Pregnancy risk category
		Codeine combinations (cont.)				
Codeine with aceta-minophen (II*;N†) *(cont.)*	Tylenol #4	Codeine 60 mg (MDD‡ 360 mg)	Acetaminophen 300 mg (MDD‡ 4,000 mg)	1 tablet q 4 h	Must adjust according to codeine content **Age 2-6 y:** 2.5-5 mg q 4-6 h, maximum 60 mg/24 h **Age 6-12 y:** 5-10 mg q 4-6 h, maximum 60 mg/24 h	C
	Capital with Codeine, Tylenol with Codeine Elixir; PMS-Acetaminophen with Codeine [CAN]	Codeine 12 mg	Acetaminophen 5 mL	**Elixir/solution:** 15 mL q 4 h	Must adjust according to codeine content **Age 2-6 y:** 2.5-5 mg q 4-6 h, maximum 60 mg/24 h **Age 6-12 y:** 5-10 mg q 4-6 h, maximum 60 mg/24 h	C
Codeine with aceta-minophen, caffeine and butalbitol § (II*;N†)	Fioricet #3	Codeine 30 mg	Acetaminophen 325 mg, butalbitol† 50 mg, caffeine 40 mg	1-2 tablet(s) q 4 h, maximum 6/day	Not established	C
Codeine with aspirin (II*;N†)	Empirin #2	Codeine 15 mg	Aspirin 325 mg	1-2 tablet(s) q 4 h	Not established	C
	Empirin #3	Codeine 30 mg	Aspirin 325 mg	1-2 tablet(s) q 4 h	Not established	C

Codeine with aspirin, caffeine and butalbitol§ (II*;N†)	Empirin #4	Codeine 60 mg (MDD‡ 360 mg)	Aspirin 325 mg (MDD‡ 4,000 mg)	1 tablet q 4 h	Not established	C
	Ascomp with codeine, butalbitol compound with codeine, Butinal with codeine, Fiorinol #3, Idenal with codeine, Isollyl with codeine; Fiorinal-C1/2 or C1/4 [CAN], Tecnal-C1/2 or C1/4 [CAN]	Codeine 30 mg	Aspirin 325 mg, butalbitol§ 50 mg, caffeine 40 mg	1-2 tablet(s) q 4 h, maximum 6/day	Not established	C
Dihydrocodeine combinations						
Dihydrocodeine bitartrate with acetaminophen and caffeine (III*)	DHC Plus	Dihydrocodeine 16 mg	Acetaminophen 356.4 mg, caffeine 30 mg (MDD‡ 4,000 mg acetaminophen)	2 capsules q 4 h, maximum 6/day	Not recommended	Not classified
Dihydrocodeine bitartrate with aspirin and caffeine (III*)	Synalgos DC	Dihydrocodeine 16 mg	Aspirin 356.4 mg Caffeine 30 mg (MDD‡ 4,000 mg aspirin)	2 capsules q 4 h, maximum 6 capsules/day	Not recommended	Not classified
Hydrocodone combinations						
Hydrocodone bitartrate with acetaminophen (III*; N†)	Lortab 2.5/500	Hydrocodone 2.5 mg	Acetaminophen 500 mg	1-2 tablet(s) q 4-6 h	Not recommended	C

[CAN] indicates a drug available only in Canada.
*Controlled substance in the United States; see Appendix A for complete description of schedule.
†Controlled substance in Canada; see Appendix A for complete description of schedule.
‡ Maximum daily dose.
§Butalbitol is a barbiturate. This medication may be more sedating than other combination products.
Barbiturate drug interactions and contraindications should be observed.

Continued on next page

Table 4.1 (cont.)

Opioid Combination Analgesics for Moderate or Moderate-to-Severe Pain: Dosage Information

Generic name	Brand name(s)	Narcotic component	Non-narcotic component	Usual adult dosage	Child dosage	Pregnancy risk category
			Hydrocodone combinations (cont.)			
Hydrocodone bitartrate with acetaminophen (III*; N†) (cont.)	**Capsules:** Allay, Anolar DH5, Bancap-HC, Dolacet, Dolagesic, Hycomed, Hyco-pap, Hydroset, Hydrogesic, Loret-HD, Margesic-H, Panlor, Polygesic, Stagesic, T-Gesic, Ugesic, Vendone, Zydone, generic **Tablets:** Anexsia 5/500, Co-gesic, Duocet, Hy-phen, Lortab 5/500, Oncet, Panacet 5/500, Vanacet, Vicodin ★, generic	Hydrocodone 5 mg	Acetaminophen 500 mg	1-2 tablets or capsules q 4-6 h, 2 q 6 h	Not recommended	C
	Lortab 7.5/500, generic	Hydrocodone 7.5 mg	Acetaminophen 500 mg	1 tablet q 4-6 h, 2 q 6 h	Not established	C
	Anexsia 7.5/650, Lorcet Plus	Hydrocodone 7.5 mg	Acetaminophen 650 mg	1 tablet q 4-6 h, 2 q 6 h	Not established	C
	Vicodin ES	Hydrocodone 7.5 mg	Acetaminophen 750 mg	1 tablet q 4-6 h	Not established	C
	Lortab 10/500, Lorcet 10/650	Hydrocodone 10 mg	Acetaminophen 500/650 mg (MDD‡ 4,000 mg)	1 tablet q 4-6 h, maximum 6/day	Not established	C
	Lortab	Hydrocodone 2.5 mg/5 mL	Acetaminophen 167 mg/5 mL	**Elixir/solution:** 5-15 mL q 4-6 h	Not established	C

Oxycodone combinations						
Oxycodone with acetaminophen (II*; N†)	**Tablets:** Endocet, Percocet ★, Roxicet, generic **Oral solution:** Roxicet	**Tablets:** Oxycodone 5 mg **Oral solution:** Oxycodone 5 mg/mL	**Tablets:** Acetaminophen 325 mg **Oral solution:** Acetaminophen 325 mg/5 mL	**Tablets:** 1 q 4-6 h **Oral solution:** 5-10 mL q 4-6 h	Not recommended	C
	Capsules: Roxilox, Tylox **Tablets:** Roxicet 5/500, generic	**Capsules:** Oxycodone 5 mg **Tablets:** Oxycodone 5 mg	**Capsules:** Acetaminophen 500 mg (MDD‡ 4,000 mg) **Tablets:** Acetaminophen 500 mg (MDD‡ 4,000 mg)	**Capsules:** 1 capsule q 4-6 h **Tablets:** 1 tablet q 4-6 h	Not established	C
	Percocet-Demi [CAN]	2.5 mg oxycodone	325 mg acetaminophen	Not established; do not use in children	Not established	C
Oxycodone with aspirin (II*; N†)	Percodan-Demi ★	Oxycodone 2.5 mg	Aspirin 325 mg	1-2 tablet(s) q 4-6 h	Not established	Not classified
	Percodan ★, Roxiprin	Oxycodone 5 mg	Aspirin 325 mg (MDD‡ 4,000 mg)	1 tablet q 4-6 h	Not established	Not classified

Continued on next page

★ indicates a drug bearing the ADA Seal of Acceptance.
[CAN] indicates a drug available only in Canada.
*Controlled substance in the United States; see Appendix A for complete description of schedule.
†Controlled substance in Canada; see Appendix A for complete description of schedule.
‡ Maximum daily dose.

Table 4.1 (cont.)

Opioid Combination Analgesics for Moderate or Moderate-to-Severe Pain: Dosage Information

Generic name	Brand name(s)	Narcotic component	Non-narcotic component	Usual adult dosage	Child dosage	Pregnancy risk category
Pentazocine combinations						
Pentazocine with aceta-minophen (IV*; N†)	Talacen	Pentazocine 25 mg	Acetaminophen 650 mg (MDD‡ 4,000 mg)	1 tablet q 4 h, maximum 6/day	Not established	C
Pentazocine with aspirin (IV*; N†)	Talwin Compound	Pentazocine 12.5 mg	Aspirin 325 mg (MDD‡ 4,000 mg)	2 tablets tid/qid	Not established	Not classified
Propoxyphene combinations						
Propoxyphene HCl or napsylate with acetaminophen (IV*; N†)	E-Lor, Wygesic	Propoxyphene HCl 65 mg	Acetaminophen 650 mg	1 tablet q 4 h	Not established	Not classified
	Darvocet N-50 ★	Propoxyphene napsylate 50 mg	Acetaminophen 325 mg	1-2 tablet(s) q 4 h	Not established	Not classified

	Darvocet N-100 ★	Propoxyphene napsylate 100 mg	Acetaminophen 650 mg (MDD‡ 4,000 mg)	1 tablet q 4 h	Not established	Not classified
Propoxyphene HCl with aspirin and caffeine (IV*; N†)	Darvon Compound-65, PC-Cap, Propoxyphene Compound-65, generic; 692 [CAN]	Propoxyphene 65 mg (MDD‡ 390 mg)	Aspirin 389 mg Caffeine 32.4 mg (MDD‡ 4,000 mg aspirin)	Capsules: 1 q 4 h Tablets [CAN]: 1 q 4 h	Not established	Not classified

★ indicates a drug bearing the ADA Seal of Acceptance.

[CAN] indicates a drug available only in Canada.

*Controlled substance in the United States; see Appendix A for complete description of schedule.

†Controlled substance in Canada; see Appendix A for complete description of schedule.

‡ Maximum daily dose.

Table 4.2

Opioid Noncombination Analgesics: Dosage Information

Generic name	Brand name(s)	Narcotic component	Adult dosage	Maximum child dosage	Pregnancy risk category
Butorphanol (agonist-antagonist)	Stadol	Butorphanol 1, 2 mg/mL; 1 mg/dose	**IM:** 1-4 mg q 3-4 h **IV:** 0.5-2 mg q 3-4 h **Nasal spray:** 1-2 doses q 4-6 h	Not established	C
Codeine phosphate (II*; C†)	generic	30, 60 mg; 15, 30 mg [CAN]	**Tablets:** 15-60 mg (usually 30 mg) q 3-6 h up to 120 mg/day maximum	**Premature infants:** Not recommended **Newborn infants and children:** Not established	C
	generic	30, 60 mg; 30, 60 [CAN]	**Injection:** 15-60 mg (usually 30 mg) q 4-6 h	**Premature infants:** Not recommended **Newborn infants and children:** Not established	C
	generic	30, 60 mg	**Soluble tablets:** 15-60 mg (usually 30) q 4-6 h	**Premature infants:** Not recommended **Newborn infants and children:** Not established	C
Codeine sulfate (II*; C†)	generic	15, 30, 60 mg	**Tablets:** 15-60 mg (usually 30 mg) q 3-6 h up to 120 mg/day	**Premature infants:** Not recommended **Newborn infants and children:** Not established	C

Continued on next page

Drug	Brand/generic	Strengths	Dosage	Pediatric	Schedule
Hydromorphone HCl (II*; C†)	generic	30, 60 mg	**Soluble tablets:** 15-60 mg (usually 30 mg) q 4-6 h	**Premature infants:** Not recommended **Newborn infants and children:** Not established	C
	Dilaudid, Hydrostat IR; PMS Hydromorphone [CAN], generic	**Dilaudid:** 2, 4, 8 mg; 1, 2, 4, 8 mg [CAN] **Hydrostat IR:** 1, 2, 3, 4 mg **PMS Hydromorphone:** 1, 2, 4, 8 mg **Generic:** 2, 4 mg; 2, 4 mg [CAN]	**Tablets:** 2 mg q 3-6 h	Not available	C
	Dilaudid-5, Dilaudid; PMS-Hydromorphone Syrup [CAN]	5 mg/mL	**Oral solution:** 2.5-10 mg q 3-6 h	Not available	C
	Dilaudid, generic	**Dilaudid with preservatives:** 2 mg/mL; 2 mg/mL [CAN] **generic with preservatives:** 1, 2, 3, 4 mg/mL **Dilaudid without preservatives:** 1, 2, 4 mg/mL; 2 mg/mL [CAN] **Dilaudid-HP without preservatives:** 10 mg/mL; 10 mg/mL [CAN]	**Injection:** 1-2 mg q 3-6 h; if severe, 3-4 mg q 4-6 h	Not available	C

[CAN] indicates a drug available only in Canada.
*Controlled substance in the United States; see Appendix A for complete description of schedule.
†Controlled substance in Canada; see Appendix A for complete description of schedule.

Table 4.2 (cont.)
Opioid Noncombination Analgesics: Dosage Information

Generic name	Brand name(s)	Narcotic component	Adult dosage	Maximum child dosage	Pregnancy risk category
Meperidine (II*; C†)	Demerol, generic	**Tablets:** 50, 100 mg **Syrup:** 50 mg/mL **Solution for injection:** 25, 50, 75, 100 mg/mL; 100 mg/mL [CAN]	**Tablets, syrup:** 50-150 mg q 3-4 h **Analgesic, solution—IM or SC:** 50-150 mg q 3-4 h **Analgesic, solution—IV infusion:** 15-35 mg/h as required **Anesthesia adjunct, preoperative, solution—IM or SC:** 50-100 mg 30-90 min prn to anesthesia **Anesthesia adjunct, preoperative, solution—IV:** By repeated slow injection of fractional doses of a solution diluted to 10/mg/mL **Anesthesia adjunct, preoperative, solution—IV infusion:** As a solution diluted to 1 mg/mL	**Tablets, syrup:** 1.1-1.76 mg/kg, not to exceed 100 mg q 3-4 h as needed **Analgesic, solution—IM or SC:** 1.1-1.76 mg/kg, not to exceed 100 mg q 3-4 h **Analgesic, solution, preoperative—IM or SC:** 1-2.2 mg/kg, not to exceed 100 mg, 30-90 min prior to anesthesia	Not classified
Morphine HCl (II*; C†)	**Syrup:** Morphitec; M.O.S. [CAN] **Tablets:** M.O.S. [CAN] **Extended-release tablets:** M.O.S.-S.R. [CAN] **Suppositories:** M.O.S. [CAN]	**Syrup:** 1, 5, 10, 20, 50 mg/mL **Tablets:** 10, 20, 40, 60 mg **Extended-release tablets:** 30, 60 mg **Suppositories:** 10, 20, 30 mg	**Syrup:** 10-30 mg q 4 h **Tablets:** 10-30 mg q 4 h **Extended-release tablets:** Established by physician **Suppositories:** 20-30 mg q 4-6 h	**Syrup:** Not available **Tablets:** Not available **Extended-release tablets:** Not available **Suppositories:** Not available	

Morphine sulfate (II*, C†)	Capsules: MSIR	Capsules: 15, 30 mg	Capsules: 10-30 mg q 4 h	Not established	C
	Extended-release capsules: M-Eslon [CAN]	Extended-release capsules: 10, 30, 60, 100 mg	Extended-release capsules: Initially, 30 mg q 12 h		
	Oral solution: Rescudose, Roxanol UD, MSIR, MS/L, MS/L Concentrate, OMS Concentrate, Roxanol, Roxanol 100, generic; Statex drops [CAN]	Oral solution: 10 mg/2.5 mL, 10 mg/5mL, 20 mg/5 mL, 20 mg/mL, 30 mg/1.5 mL, 100 mg/5 mL; 2, 4, 50 mg/mL [CAN]	Oral solution: Initially, 30 mg q 12 h		
	Syrup: Statex [CAN]	Syrup: 1, 5, 10 mg/mL	Syrup: Initially, 30 mg q 12 h		
	Tablets: MSIR, MSIR [CAN], Statex [CAN], generic	Tablets: 15, 30 mg; 5, 10, 20, 25, 50 mg [CAN]	Tablets: Initially, 30 mg q 12 h		
	Injection: Astramorph PF, Duramorph, generic; Epimorph [CAN], Morphine Extra-Forte [CAN], Morphine Forte [CAN], Morphine H.P. [CAN]	Injection: 0.5, 1, 2, 4, 5, 8, 10, 15, 25, 50 mg/mL	Injection, IM or SC: 5-20 initially, then q 4 h		
	Soluble tablets: generic	Soluble tablets: 10, 15, 30 mg	Soluble tablets: 5-20 mg initially, then q 4 h		
	Suppositories: MS/S, RMS Inserts, Roxanol, generic; MSIR [CAN], Statex [CAN]	Suppositories: 5, 10, 20, 30 mg	Suppositories: 10-30 mg q 4 h		
Oxycodone HCl (II*, C†)	Oral solution: Roxicodone, Roxicodone Intensol	Oral solution: 5 mg/5 mL, 20 mg/mL	Oral solution: 5 mg q 3-6 h; may be increased if severe pain is present	Not available	Not classified
	Tablets: Roxicodone; Supeudol [CAN]	Tablets: 5 mg; 10 mg [CAN]	Tablets: 5 mg q 3-6 h or 10 mg q 6-8 h; may be increased if severe pain is present		
	Suppositories: Supeudol [CAN]	Suppositories: 10; 20 mg [CAN]	Suppositories: 10-40 mg tid-qid		

[CAN] indicates a drug available only in Canada.
*Controlled substance in the United States; see Appendix A for complete description of schedule.
†Controlled substance in Canada; see Appendix A for complete description of schedule.

surgical procedure, it is prudent to prescribe either opioid or NSAID analgesics on a regularly scheduled basis for at least 24-36 h rather than on an as-needed or prn basis. The rationale for this approach is to provide as continuous a plasma level of medication as possible. If a patient waits until an analgesic medication loses effect and then takes another dose, he or she will be in pain for an additional 30-60 min. Further, it requires more analgesic medication to overcome pain than to maintain pain relief once it has been established. Therefore, the clinician needs knowledge of a specific analgesic's duration of action to prescribe appropriately.

Likewise, it is well-established that if an NSAID or an opioid is given preoperatively, pain relief can be more easily achieved with postoperative analgesics. Similarly, analgesic medication should be started before cessation of local anesthetic activity to achieve a sufficient plasma level of medication before the onset of pain perception.

All opioid medications can cause tolerance, a reduced drug effect that results from continued use and the need for higher doses to produce the same effect. These medications can also cause physical dependence, the physiological state associated with discontinuation of the drug after prolonged use (withdrawal), and psychological dependence, which is an intense craving for the drug and compulsive drug-seeking behavior. Because the pain commonly encountered in dental practice is of the acute type, tolerance of, and physical and psychological dependence on, opioids are so rare as to be of little concern, because such drugs are used only over the short term. The dentist should use opioid medications in sufficiently large doses for high-quality management of acute pain without fear that patients will develop dependence. The one exception may be patients with a history of drug abuse. For these patients, nonopioid analgesics or perhaps an agonist-antagonist opioid should be

prescribed initially. The majority of important drug interactions involve the possibility of sedative and gastrointestinal side effects, among others. A complete listing of these is provided in Table 4.3.

Maximum Recommended Doses
Adult
Recommended doses for the combination products are listed in Table 4.1. The combination opioid products are generally limited by the dosage of the nonopioid product (for example, 4,000 mg per day for acetaminophen or aspirin). In general, there is no maximum dose of an opioid alone if proper titration has occurred other than the dose at which side effects are not tolerated. The use of noncombination opioids in this way is generally reserved for the management of severe acute pain and selected chronic pains.

Pediatric
Generally, in pediatric patients, codeine and acetaminophen would be used for pain not responsive to acetaminophen alone. The maximum dosages for codeine with acetaminophen are shown in Table 4.1.

Geriatric
Geriatric patients may develop exaggerated sedative effects with opioid medications. Consider starting at lower dose ranges.

Dosage Adjustments
Adjust dosage based on patient response. If duration of analgesia is insufficient, a shorter period between doses (for example, q 3 h vs. q 4 h) or a higher dosage (for example, 7.5 mg vs. 5 mg of hydrocodone) is appropriate. If analgesia itself is insufficient, a higher dosage of pain medication is appropriate. For short-term acute pain conditions, dependence on opioids is generally not of concern and efforts should be made to provide adequate postoperative analgesia.

Dosage Forms
Opioid medications are available for oral,

intravenous, intramuscular, transnasal or transdermal use. The dentist will likely use oral forms (capsule, tablet or elixir—see Tables 4.1 and 4.2) or perhaps butorphanol, which is available in a nasal spray form.

Available Strengths
Table 4.1 lists the available strengths of oral medications that dentists would be most likely to prescribe.

Special Dental Considerations
Opioids may decrease salivary flow. Consider opioid use in the differential diagnosis of caries, periodontal disease or oral candidiasis.

Drug Interactions of Dental Interest
The most common drug interactions of concern for dentistry involve the potential sedative side effects, which are exaggerated in patients taking other CNS depressants (see Table 4.3).

Table 4.3
Standard Opioids: Possible Drug Interactions With Other Drugs

Drug taken by patient	Interaction with standard opioids	Dentist's action
Agonist-antagonist drugs (nalbuphine, butorphanol, pentazocine)	Can lead to withdrawal syndrome or loss of analgesia with hypertension, tachycardia	Never prescribe agonist-antagonist opioids with conventional agonist opioids
Alcohol	Sedative side effects	Advise patients to never drink alcohol when taking opioids
Amphetamines	With meperidine: hypotension, respiratory collapse	Dentist should not prescribe meperidine to a patient taking amphetamines
Anticholinergics	Constipation	Prescribe opioids only for short periods of time; consider physician consultation
Antidiarrheals	Constipation	Prescribe opioids only for short periods of time; consider physician consultation
Antihypertensives and vasodilators	Potentiation of hypotensive effects	Advise patients to notify dentist if postural hypotension or dizziness occurs
Barbiturates	Sedative side effects	Alert patient to possible additive side effects and to notify dentist if not tolerated
Carbamazepine	With propoxyphene: Increased carbamazepine levels	Dentists should not prescribe propoxyphene to patients taking carbamazepine
CNS depressants	Sedative side effects	Alert patient to possible additive side effects and to notify dentist if not tolerated

Continued on next page

Table 4.3 (cont.)

Standard Opioids: Possible Drug Interactions With Other Drugs

Drug taken by patient	Interaction with standard opioids	Dentist's action
Coumarin anticoagulants	With propoxyphene: Increased anticoagulant effects	Dentists should not prescribe propoxyphene to patients taking coumarin anticoagulants
Hydroxyzine	Sedative side effects	Alert patient to possible additive side effects and to notify dentist if not tolerated
Hypnotics (sedative)	Sedative side effects	Alert patient to possible additive side effects and to notify dentist if not tolerated
MAO inhibitors	With meperidine: severe hypertension	Dentist should not prescribe meperidine to a patient taking MAO inhibitors
Metoclopramide	Can antagonize metoclopramide	Prescribe opioids only for short periods of time; consider physician consultation
Other opioids	Sedative side effects	Dentist should avoid prescribing two opioids at one time unless for chronic pain
Tobacco	With propoxyphene: May decrease the effect of propoxyphene	Advise patient to stop smoking; dentist should not prescribe propoxyphene to tobacco users

Cross-Sensitivity

Possible cross-sensitivity is possible with opioids. It is important for the dentist to distinguish whether a true allergic reaction occurred, as most opioids can produce nausea and/or vomiting and release histamine. These reactions are typically referred to as "allergic" by patients. Consider using a nonopioid analgesic in these patients. Switching to a different opioid may produce fewer side effects.

Special Patients

Opioids should be used with extreme caution in patients with chronic obstructive pulmonary disease, such as emphysema or chronic bronchitis, due to possible respiratory compromise.

Likewise, patients with severe cardiac disease, such as advanced congestive heart failure, may not tolerate hypotensive side effects. Due to constipating effects, opioids should be used with caution in patients with severe inflammatory bowel disease. If mentally challenged patients are prescribed opioids, they should be closely monitored by an appropriate caregiver. Opioids should be prescribed cautiously for a patient with emotional instability, suicidal ideation or attempts, or a previous history of substance abuse.

Pregnant and nursing women

Opioids should not be prescribed for a pregnant or nursing patient without consultation with the patient's physician.

Patient Monitoring: Aspects to Watch

- Respiratory depression and sedation: the patient should contact the dentist if these side effects are observed.

Adverse Effects and Precautions

The majority of important drug interactions involve the possibility of sedative and gastrointestinal side effects; a more complete listing is provided in Tables 4.3 and 4.4.

Table 4.4
Opioids: Adverse Effects, Precautions and Contraindications

Body system	Adverse effects	Precautions/contraindications
General	None of significance to dentistry	Contraindicated in those with a history of allergy to agent
CV	Hypotension	None of significance to dentistry
CNS	Cough suppression, pupillary constriction, sedation, mental clouding, hallucinations, dependence with chronic use	History of or current drug abuse or dependence, intracranial conditions Emotional instability, suicidal ideation
GI	Constipation, increased biliary duct pressure, hepatic toxicity, xerostomia	Chronic GI disease in which constipation would not be desirable Gallbladder disease Contraindicated in patients with diarrhea secondary to colitis Contraindicated in patients using antibiotics, such as penicillins, cephalosporins, lincomycin Contraindicated with use of toxic materials Contraindicated in some acute GI conditions
GU	Urine retention	Prostatic hypertrophy Renal function impairment
Hema	Histamine release or itching, or both; true allergic reaction	None of significance to dentistry
Oral	Xerostomia	None of significance to dentistry
Resp	Respiratory depression, asthma attack	Asthma, especially when opioids are given through the IV route with histamine-releasing opioids Contraindicated in patients with chronic respiratory impairment, such as chronic obstructive pulmonary disease and acute respiratory depression

Pharmacology

Opioid medications produce analgesia by interaction at specific receptors in the central nervous system, mimicking the effect of endogenous pain-relieving neurochemicals (for example, dynorphin, enkephalin and β-endorphin). These receptors are present in higher brain centers such as the hypothalamus and periaqueductal gray regions, as well as in the spinal cord and trigeminal nucleus. The result of this interaction is a decrease in pain transmission to higher thalamocortical centers and a corresponding decrease in pain perception. Recent evidence suggests a possible peripheral effect of opioid analgesics.

Opioids undergo hepatic transformation generally to inactive metabolites, which are excreted in the urine and/or bile. These drugs are subdivided into agonist, agonist-antagonist or antagonist compounds based on their receptor effects.

Agonists

The opioid medications typified by morphine act primarily in the CNS through varied activity on specific opioid receptor subgroups. Although there is activity at all opioid receptors, morphine and related agents—such as codeine, hydrocodone, dihydrocodeine and oxycodone, as well as meperidine and the fentanyl derivatives—provide analgesia chiefly through agonist activity at the μ receptor.

Agonist-antagonists

Another group of opioid analgesics, the agonist-antagonists—including pentazocine, nalbuphine and butorphanol—are agonists at the kappa (κ) receptor, and antagonists at the μ receptor.

Antagonists

Specific competitive opioid antagonist medications—namely, naloxone and naltrexone—have also been developed. Naloxone's main use in dentistry is reversal of excessive opioid IV sedation. Naltrexone is used to treat former opioid abusers and recently has been used for individuals with certain CNS disorders.

Patient Advice

- Avoid use of alcohol or other CNS depressant medications unless physician or dentist gives approval.
- Inform dentist if nausea, vomiting, excessive dry mouth, dizziness or lightheadedness occurs.
- Exercise caution when getting up suddenly from a lying or sitting position.
- Avoid driving a motor vehicle or operating heavy machinery, especially if sedative side effects are present.

Suggested Readings

Dionne RA, Snyder J, Hargreaves KM. Analgesic efficacy of flurbiprofen in comparison with acetaminophen, acetaminophen plus codeine, and placebo after impacted third molar removal. J Oral Maxillofac Surg 1994;52(9):919-24.

Forbes JA, Bates JA, Edquist IA, et al. Evaluation of two opioid-acetaminophen combinations and placebo in post-operative oral surgery pain. Pharmacotherapy 1994;14(2):139-46.

Hargreaves KM, Troullos ES, Dionne RA. Pharmacologic rationale for the treatment of acute pain. Dent Clin North Am 1987;31(4):675-94.

Neidle EA, Yagiela JA, eds. Pharmacology and therapeutics for dentistry. St. Louis: Mosby; 1989.

The United States Pharmacopeial Convention, Inc. USP Dispensing Information. Drug information for the health care professional. Vol. I. 17th ed. Rockville, Md.: The United States Pharmacopeial Convention, Inc.; 1997.

Nonopioid Analgesics

This group of analgesics includes the nonsteroidal anti-inflammatory drugs and acetaminophen. The site of action of these drugs is primarily peripheral (that is, outside the CNS).

Nonsteroidal Anti-inflammatory Drugs

Although NSAIDs influence a number of systems, a primary effect is the inhibition of the synthesis of prostaglandins, which are potent vasodilators and mediators of the inflammatory response. Prostaglandins also decrease the threshold needed for nerves conducting pain information to signal the CNS. By decreasing the production of prostaglandins, NSAIDs depress the inflammatory response. This decrease in prostaglandin concentration also raises the threshold for pain-conducting nerves to discharge, thus providing an analgesic effect. NSAIDs also reduce fever by decreasing the concentration of prostaglandins in the hypothalamus, a brain center regulating body temperature.

The NSAIDs consist of several basic groups of drugs with different structures but similar actions. They are primarily indicated for the relief of mild to moderate pain. Although no individual NSAID has been found to be significantly superior for pain relief in all patients, NSAIDs do differ in duration of action and side-effect profile. If one NSAID is ineffective for pain control, the dentist should keep in mind that another from a different structural group may be effective. Many NSAIDs have a ceiling dose for analgesia and require a higher dose for the anti-inflammatory effect. For instance, ibuprofen, at 200 mg taken qid, provides close to a maximum analgesic effect, but a dose of 2,400-3,200 mg per day may be required for the anti-inflammatory effect. NSAIDs with an easier dosing schedule, such as bid or tid, may provide better patient compliance and result in a more pain-free patient. Some NSAIDs may be better analgesics while others are better anti-inflammatories. Table 4.5 presents a list of acetaminophen and NSAIDs by structural group, indicating dosing schedule, maximum daily dose and drugs that may be more analgesic than others.

Acetaminophen

Acetaminophen's mechanism of action is poorly understood. Its analgesic and antipyretic properties are similar to those of aspirin, but acetaminophen has poor anti-inflammatory action.

Accepted Indications

NSAIDs are indicated for use as analgesics for mild to moderate pain, including pain of acute dental origin or for postoperative dental pain. These drugs are also indicated for pain of inflammatory origin, especially for rheumatic conditions and primary nonrheumatic inflammatory conditions. These drugs may also be used as antipyretics (ibuprofen and naproxen) and for treatment of primary dysmenorrhea. Although most NSAIDs possess all these properties, FDA-approved indications vary from drug to drug.

NSAIDs may be indicated for longer-term use in patients with chronic orofacial pain, especially pain with an inflammatory component such as temporomandibular joint synovitis. If these medications are prescribed for an extended time, appropriate laboratory studies—including CBC, renal function tests and liver function tests—are appropriate. Recent indentification of specific subtypes of the cyclooxygenase enzyme may lead to the development of NSAIDs with considerably less prominent side effects. Regardless, the long-term use of these agents should be undertaken only by those skilled in chronic pain management.

General Dosing Information

It appears that many NSAIDs have a ceiling effect for analgesia. For instance, 200 mg of ibuprofen may provide maximum analgesic efficacy, while higher doses are required for an anti-inflammatory effect. Depending on the condition treated, the dentist may consider higher or lower dosages. For chronic conditions, one NSAID may be ineffective while another provides excellent pain relief. The dentist may consider switching NSAIDs, perhaps to one from a different structural category, to obtain desired results.

As a general rule, analgesic medications should be prescribed in a manner that affords the patient the greatest degree of comfort

Table 4.5

NSAIDs and Acetaminophen: Dosage Information

Generic name	Brand name(s)	Adult dosage	Maximum adult dosage	Maximum child dosage	Pregnancy risk category	Content/form
Aminophenol						
Acetaminophen	Tylenol (various brand names)	325-500 mg q 4-6 h	4,000 mg q day short-term; 2,600 mg q day long-term unless monitored	**Age < 6 mo/1 y:** 15-60 mg/dose q 4-6 h; do not exceed 65 mg/kg/day **Age 1-2 y:** 120 mg/dose q 4 h **Age 2-3 y:** 160 mg/dose q 4 h **Age 3-4 y:** 180 mg/dose q 4 h **Age 4-5 y:** 240 mg/dose q 4 h **Age 5-10 y:** 325 mg/dose q 4 h **Age 6-11 y:** Not to exceed 1,625 mg in 24 h **Age > 12 y:** Not to exceed 4,000 mg per 24 h	B	**Capsules:** 325, 500 mg **Elixir:** 120, 160, 325 mg/5mL **Granules:** 80, 120, 160 mg **Solution:** 100 mg/mL, 80 mg/5 mL, 120 mg/5 mL, 130 mg/5 mL **Suspension:** 48 mg/mL, 160 mg/5 mL, 100 mg/mL; 80 mg/mL [CAN], 80 mg/5 mL [CAN] **SOC (infant drops):** 100 mg/1 mL, 120 mg/2.5 mL **Suppositories:** 120, 125, 325, 650 mg **Tablets, chewable:** 80, 160 mg
Fenamates						
Meclofenamate sodium †	Meclomen	50-100 mg tid-qid	400 mg	Not established	Not established	**Capsules:** 10, 20 mg
Mefenamic acid	Ponstan, Ponstel	500 mg initially then 250 mg qid	1,500 mg (maximum 7 days)	Not established	C	**Capsules:** 250 mg

Generic Name	Brand Name(s)	Usual Dosage	Maximum Dose	Pediatric Dosage	Pregnancy Category	Availability
Etodolac †	Lodine ★	200-400 mg tid	1,200 mg	Not established	C	Capsules: 200, 300 mg Tablets: 400 mg
Indomethacin	Indocid, Indocin, Apo-Indomethacin, Novo-Methacin, Nu-Indo	25-50 mg tid	200 mg	1.5-2.5 mg/kg/day in 3-4 doses, up to maximum of 4 mg/kg/day or 150-200 mg/day, whichever is less	Not established	Capsules: 25, 50 mg Oral suspension: 25 mg/5 mL Suppositories: 50 mg
Indomethacin, sustained release	Indocin SR	75 mg q day or bid	150 mg	Not established	Not established	Capsules: 75 mg
Ketorolac tromethamine †	Toradol	Oral: 20 mg initially, then 10 mg qid IM: 30 mg q 6 h IV: 30 mg q 6 h OR loading dose 15-30 mg IV/IM, then 10 mg qid oral	Oral: Not to exceed 40 mg/day, maximum use 5 days IM: 20 doses over 5 days (120 mg/day) IV: 20 doses over 5 days (120 mg)	Not established	C	Tablets: 10 mg Parenteral: 15 mg/mL, 30 mg/mL
Sulindac	ApO-Sulin, Clinoril, Novo-Sundac	150-200 mg bid	400 mg	Not established	Not established	Tablets: 150, 200 mg
Tolmetin sodium	Tolectin	200-600 mg tid	2,000 mg	15-30 mg/kg/day in divided doses	C	Capsules: 400 mg Tablets: 200, 600 mg

Continued on next page

★ indicates a product bearing the ADA Seal of Acceptance.
* Drugs with the prefixes Apo-, Novo- and Nu- are available only in Canada.
† indicates a medication possessing good analgesic properties.

Table 4.5 (cont.)
NSAIDs and Acetaminophen: Dosage Information

Generic name	Brand name(s)*	Adult dosage	Maximum adult dosage	Maximum child dosage	Pregnancy risk category	Content/form
Oxicams						
Piroxicam	Apo-Piroxicam, Feldene, Novo-Pirocam, Nu-Pirox, PMS-Piroxicam	20 mg q day or 10 mg bid	20 mg	Not established	C	**Capsules:** 10, 20 mg
Phenylacetic acids						
Diclofenac + potassium	Cataflam; Voltaren Rapide [CAN]	50 mg tid	150 mg	Not established	B	**Tablets:** 25, 50 mg
Diclofenac sodium†	Voltaren (delayed release); Apo-Diclo, Novo-Difenac, Novo-Difenac SR, Nu-Diclo, Voltaren (delayed release), Voltaren SR	50 mg tid-qid; 75 mg bid; 100 mg q day	150 mg	Not established	B	**Tablets:** 25, 50, 75 mg
Propionic acids						
Fenoprofen	Nalfon, Nalfon 200	200-300 mg 300-600 mg tid-qid	3,200 mg	Not established	Not established	**Capsules:** 200, 300 mg **Tablets:** 600 mg
Flurbiprofen †	Ansaid, Apo-Flurbiprofen, Froben, Novo-Flurprofen, Nu-Flurbiprofen	50-100 mg bid-tid	300 mg	Not established	B	**Tablets:** 50, 100 mg

Drug	Brand names	Adult dose	Maximum dose	Pediatric dose	Pregnancy category	Available forms
Ibuprofen †	Apo-Ibuprofen, Dolgesic, Ibu, Ibu-4, Ibuprohm, Ibu-Tab, Motrin, Novo-Profen, Nu-Ibuprofen, Rufen OTC 200 mg: Advil★, Bayer Select Ibuprofen, Cramp End, Excedrin IB, Genpril, Haltran, Ibu-200, Ibuprin, Ibuprohm, Ibu-Tab, Medipren, Midol, Motrin, Nuprin, Pamprin, Q-profen, Trendar	200, 400, 600, 800 mg tid-qid	3,600 mg	**Age 6 mo-12 y, usual dose:** 5-10 mg/kg q 4-6 h **Maximum pediatric dose:** 40-50 mg/kg/day	Not established	**Oral suspension:** 40 mg/mL, 100 mg/5 mL **Tablets:** 100, 200, 300, 400, 600, 800 mg **Tablets, chewable:** 50 mg, 100 mg
Ketoprofen †	Apo-Keto, Orudis, Rhodis OTC 12.5 mg: Actron, Orudis KT	25, 50, 75 mg tid/qid	300 mg	Not established	B	**Capsules:** 25, 50, 75 mg **Tablets:** 12.5 mg
Ketoprofen, sustained relief	Apo-Keto-E, Novo-Keto-EC, Orudis-E, Oruvail, Rhodis-EC	100, 150, 200 mg q day	200 mg	Not established	B	**Capsules:** 100, 150, 200 mg
Naproxen †	Naprosyn, Apo-Naproxen, Naxen, Novo-Naprox Sodium, Nu-Naprox	**Tablets:** 250, 375 q 6-8 h; 500 mg bid **Elixir:** 125 mg/5 mL	1,250 mg	10 mg/kg/day in 2 doses	B	**Tablets:** 250, 375, 500 mg **Oral suspension:** 125 mg/5 mL
Naproxen sodium †	Anaprox, Anaprox DS, Apo-Napro-Na, Novo-Naprox Sodium, Synflex OTC 220 mg: Aleve	275 q 8 h, 550 mg q 12 h	1,375 mg	Not recommended	B	**Tablets:** 220, 275, 550 mg
Oxaprozin	Daypro	600 mg bid or 1,200 mg q day	1,800 mg or 26 mg/kg, whichever is lower	Not established	C	**Tablets:** 600 mg

Continued on next page

★ indicates a drug bearing the ADA Seal of Acceptance.
* Drugs beginning with the prefixes Apo-, Novo-, Nu- and PMS- are available only in Canada.
† indicates a medication possessing good analgesic properties.

Table 4.5 (cont.)

NSAIDs and Acetaminophen: Dosage Information

Generic name	Brand name(s)	Adult dosage	Maximum adult dosage	Maximum child dosage	Pregnancy risk category	Content/form
			Naphtylalkanone			
Nabumetone	Relafen	1,000 mg q day-bid	2,000 mg	Not established	C	**Tablets:** 500, 750 mg
			Salicylates			
Aspirin	(generic)	325-500 mg q 4-6 h	4,000 mg	40-100 mg/kg/day in divided doses q 4-6 h prm	D	**Capsules:** 325, 500 mg **Cream; gum:** 227.5 mg **Suppositories:** 60, 120, 125, 130, 195, 200, 300, 325, 600, 650 mg, 1.2 g **Tablets:** 65, 81, 325, 500, 690, 975 mg **Tablets, chewable:** 81 mg **Tablets, time-release:** 650 mg
Choline and magnesium trisalicylate	Trilisate	500, 750, 1,000 mg tid	4,000 mg	**Weight ≤ 37 kg:** 50 mg/kg/day in 2 doses **Weight > 37 kg:** 2,250 mg/day in 2 doses	C	**Liquid:** 500 mg/5 mL **Tablets:** 500, 750, 1,000 mg
Diflunisal*	Dolobid	1g initially, then 250, 500 mg q 8-12 h	1,500 mg	Not established	C	**Tablets:** 250, 500 mg
Salsalate	Disalcid	500, 750 tid	3,000 mg	Not established	C	**Capsules/tablets:** 500, 750 mg

indicates a medication possessing good analgesic properties.

within a high margin of safety. If the dentist suspects that a patient will have pain for 24-48 h after a surgical procedure, it is prudent to prescribe either opioid or NSAID analgesics on a regularly scheduled basis for at least 24-36 h rather than on an as-needed basis. The rationale for this approach is to provide as continuous a plasma level of medication as possible. If a patient waits until an analgesic medication loses effect and then takes another dose, the patient will be in pain for an additional 30-60 min. Further, it requires more analgesic medication to overcome pain than to maintain pain relief once it has been established. Therefore, the clinician needs knowledge of a specific analgesic's duration of action to prescribe appropriately.

Likewise, it is well-established that if an NSAID is given preoperatively, pain relief can be more easily achieved with postoperative analgesics. Similarly, analgesic medication should be started before cessation of local anesthetic activity to allow a sufficient plasma level of medication to be achieved before the onset of pain perception.

Owing to the possible gastrointestinal side effects, NSAIDs should be prescribed with meals.

Maximum Recommended Doses

Adults
See Table 4.5.

Pregnant women
NSAIDs are generally contraindicated during pregnancy. Some Pregnancy Category B NSAIDs may be used during the first trimester of pregnancy with somewhat less risk. Regardless, the use of NSAIDs should be considered contraindicated in dental practice for all pregnant patients, unless prescribed in consultation with the patient's obstetrician. Acetaminophen, although generally acceptable, should be prescribed in consultation with the patient's obstetrician if there are any questions about the appropriateness of its use in an individual case.

Pediatric and geriatric patients
As with most medications, dosages should be reduced for children and the elderly. Owing to their possible gastrointestinal side effects, NSAIDs should be prescribed with meals.

Dosage Forms
NSAIDs and acetaminophen are available for oral use except for ketorolac tromethamine, which is also available in an intravenous/intramuscular preparation. Elixir, liquid and rectal preparations are available for aspirin and acetaminophen. Liquid forms of ibuprofen are also available.

Special Dental Considerations
In the differential diagnosis of appropriate conditions, dentists should take into consideration that NSAIDs may cause soreness or irritation of the oral mucosa. Although rare, some NSAIDs may cause leukopenia and/or thrombocyopenia.

Drug Interactions of Dental Interest
Major drug interactions with NSAIDs stem from the effect of these drugs on platelet, gastrointestinal and renal function.

Laboratory Value Alterations
- There are no laboratory tests whose results are specifically altered by NSAIDs and acetaminophen.
- The effect of these drugs on platelet function will likely increase bleeding times.
- There may also be changes in renal and hepatic function, especially with long-term NSAID use.

Cross-Sensitivity
All NSAIDs and aspirin may exhibit cross-sensitivity. Any of these drugs should be used with extreme caution, if at all, in patients who have developed signs and symptoms of allergic reaction to any NSAID, including aspirin. It should also be noted that patients with a history of nasal polyps and asthma have an increased risk of sensitivity, including allergic reactions, to aspirin, particularly, but also to other NSAIDs.

Table 4.6

NSAIDs: Possible Interactions With Other Drugs

Drug taken by patient	Interaction with NSAIDs	Dentist's action
Alcohol	Increased risk of ulceration	Avoid if possible
Anticoagulants (oral)	Increased risk of bleeding	Contraindicated with concurrent use
Antihypertensives	Effect decreased by NSAIDs	Avoid if possible or monitor blood pressure
Aspirin	Increased risk of ulceration Increased risk of bleeding	Contraindicated with concurrent use
NSAIDs other than aspirin	Increased risk of ulceration Increased risk of bleeding	Avoid this combination
Colchicine	Increased risk of bleeding	Contraindicated with concurrent use
Corticosteroids	Increased risk of ulceration	Avoid if possible
Cyclosporine	Can cause nephrotoxicity	Avoid if possible
Digitalis	Increased digitalis levels	Avoid if possible
Diuretics (especially triamterene)	Effect decreased by NSAIDs	Avoid if possible or monitor blood pressure/excessive fluid retention
Heparin	Increased risk of bleeding	Contraindicated with concurrent use
Hypoglycemics (oral)	Effect increased by NSAIDs	Patient should monitor blood glucose carefully
Lithium	Concentration increased by NSAIDs	Contraindicated unless approved by physician
Methotrexate (when plasma level is increased)	Increased risk of bleeding	Contraindicated with concurrent use
Potassium supplements	Increased risk of ulceration	Avoid if possible
Valproic acid	Increased risk of ulceration Increased risk of bleeding	Avoid if possible

Special Patients

Pregnant and nursing women

NSAIDs should not be prescribed by dentists for pregnant or nursing women. Acetaminophen may be prescribed in consultation with the patient's physician.

Pediatric, geriatric and other special patients

Only acetaminophen, aspirin and ibuprofen are approved for pediatric use. Aspirin may cause Reye's syndrome in children infected with influenza virus. Reye's syndrome is a serious medical condition that can lead to severe hepatic and CNS disease, as well as death. Because other drugs are available that do not manifest this concern, the dentist should consider avoiding use of aspirin in all children with fever.

Geriatric patients may be more susceptible to the gastrointestinal and renal side effects of NSAIDs. Start at lower dosages and avoid longer-acting agents that may accumulate.

Patient Monitoring: Aspects to Watch

- Short-term NSAID therapy: no laboratory monitoring generally necessary, but patient should notify dentist of symptoms of dyspepsia or fluid retention
- Long-term NSAID therapy: hematologic parameters, renal and hepatic function require periodic evaluation

Adverse Effects and Precautions

These drugs have numerous drug interactions (Table 4.6) and side effects (Table 4.7). For short-term use, gastrointestinal side effects such as dyspepsia, diarrhea and abdominal pain are the most common. Longer-term use can lead to gastrointestinal ulceration, bleeding or perforation. As a precaution, NSAIDs should be taken with meals. Various drugs have been developed to counteract some of the gastrointestinal side effects of NSAIDs, and NSAIDs that have fewer gastrointestinal side effects are listed later in this section. NSAIDs are contraindicated in patients who have active peptic ulcer disease and should be prescribed with extreme caution to patients who have a history of peptic ulcer disease.

Renal complications can also occur as idiosyncratic reactions with short-term use or as renal failure with long-term use. These medications are metabolized by the liver and should be prescribed cautiously to people who have liver disease.

It is important to note that NSAIDs can increase bleeding through their reversible inhibition of platelet aggregation by their effect on a platelet aggregating agent, thromboxane A_2. This is the case with all NSAIDs except aspirin, which irreversibly inhibits platelet aggregation for the entire life of the platelet (11 days). If major oral surgery is planned,

- discontinue aspirin for 4-5 days before surgery;
- for NSAIDs that require dosing of 4-6 times per day, stop NSAID use 1-2 days before surgery;
- for NSAIDs that require bid-tid dosing, stop NSAID use 2-3 days before surgery;
- for q day NSAIDs, stop NSAID use 3-4 days before surgery to avoid excessive bleeding.

Drug interactions are presented in Table 4.6. An important contraindication involves the use of aspirin in children, which can lead to Reye's syndrome. Hypersensitivity reactions, such as anaphylactoid reactions, also have occurred with NSAIDs, especially aspirin. Patients with a history of bronchospastic disease and/or nasal polyps have an increased risk of having hypersensitivity reactions. If a patient's medical history indicates that this type of reaction could be encountered, it is prudent not to prescribe NSAIDs unless the patient has taken one of these drugs without complication after a prior hypersensitivity reaction.

Some NSAIDs have potentially fewer gastrointestinal complications. The following drugs may cause less gastrointestinal irritation in a patient who, for instance, has a previous history of peptic ulcer disease and no longer requires ulcer medication but for whom an NSAID is indicated:

- choline magnesium trisalicylate;
- diflunisal;
- lodine;
- nabumetone;
- salsalate;
- sulindac.

Pharmacology

Although NSAIDs influence a number of systems, a primary effect is the inhibition of the breakdown of arachidonic acid by the enzyme cyclo-oxygenase. One of the by-products of this breakdown is prostaglandins, which are potent vasodilators and mediators of the inflammatory response. Prostaglandins also decrease the threshold needed for nerves conducting pain information to signal the CNS. By decreasing the production of prostaglandins, NSAIDs depress the inflammatory response. This decrease in prostaglandin concentration also raises the threshold for pain-conducting nerves to discharge, thus providing an analgesic effect. NSAIDs also reduce fever, in part by decreasing the concentration of prostaglandins in the hypothalamus, a brain center regulating body temperature.

Table 4.7

NSAIDs: Adverse Effects, Precautions and Contraindications

Body system	Adverse effects	Precautions/contraindications
General	Drowsiness, angioedema, weight loss	None of significance to dentistry
CV	May cause fluid retention, tachycardia	Severe cardiac disease Patients taking diuretics Phenylbutazone is contraindicated in patients with severe cardiac disease
CNS	Dizziness, headache, sedation, tinnitus, photophobia, decreased hearing	May have additive effects with other CNS depressants
GI	Abdominal pain, diarrhea, dyspepsia, peptic ulcer, ulcerated bowel, diarrhea, nausea, vomiting	History of GI disease History of chronic alcohol abuse History of tobacco use Patients with diabetes Contraindicated in patients with active peptic ulcer disease Contraindicated in patients with diverticulitis Contraindicated in patients with ulcerative colitis
GU	Impaired renal function, renal disease, dysuria, polyuria, cystitis	Patient taking diuretics Contraindicated in severe renal disease
Hema	Increased bleeding time Rare blood dyscrasia Petechia	*Stop NSAID use for 3-4 half-lives and aspirin for 4-5 days before procedures that may involve significant bleeding* Contraindicated in patients receiving anticoagulation therapy

Italics indicate information of major clinical significance.

Continued on next page

Table 4.7 (cont.)

NSAIDs: Adverse Effects, Precautions and Contraindications

Body system	Adverse effects	Precautions/contraindications
HB	Elevated enzyme activity	Severe hepatic disease Phenylbutazone is contraindicated in patients with severe hepatic disease
Integ	Dermatitis, Stevens-Johnson syndrome, stomatitis, petechia	*Unusual hypersensitivity reactions*
Musc	*Muscle weakness*	None of significance to dentistry
Oral	Stomatitis, glossitis, gingival ulceration	None of significance to dentistry
Resp	Anaphylaxis, angioedema, bronchospasm	Children may develop Reye's syndrome precipitated by use of aspirin Relatively contraindicated in patients with history of bronchospasm, nasal polyps and asthma Contraindicated in patients with allergic reaction to aspirin or other NSAIDs

Italics indicate information of major clinical significance.

Cyclo-oxygenase metabolism of arachidonic acid also produces thromboxane A_2, which increases platelet aggregability. NSAIDs decrease the production of thromboxane A_2; this decreases platelet aggregation and causes an increased tendency toward bleeding. NSAID inactivation of cyclo-oxygenase, and thus increased bleeding tendency, is reversible for all drugs except aspirin, which binds cyclo-oxygenase irreversibly for the life of the platelet (11 days).

Patient Advice

- Patients should be cautioned regarding the gastrointestinal side effects of these medications.
- These medications preferably should be taken with or after meals with a full glass of water to prevent lodging of the capsule or tablet in the esophagus.
- The patient should notify the dentist of any side effects that occur after starting use of the medication.

Suggested Readings

Brandt KD. The mechanism of action of non-steroidal antiinflammatory drugs. J Rheumatol 1991;27(Supplement):120-1.

Dionne RA, Gordon SM. Nonsteroidal anti-inflammatory drugs for acute pain control. Dent Clin North Am 1994;38(4):645-67.

Joris J. Efficacy of nonsteroidal antiinflammatory drugs in post-operative pain. Acta Anaesthesiol Belg 1996;47(3):115-23.

Lawton GM, Chapman PJ. Diflunisal—a long acting non-steroidal anti-inflammatory drug. A review of its pharmacology and effectiveness in management of dental pain. Aust Dent J 1993;38(4):265-71.

Neidle EA, Yagiela JA, eds. Pharmacology and therapeutics for dentistry. St. Louis: Mosby; 1989.

The United States Pharmacopeial Convention Inc. USP Dispensing Information. Drug information for the health care professional. Vol. I. 17th ed. Rockville, Md.: The United States Pharmacopeial Convention Inc.; 1997.

Woolf CJ, Chong MS. Preemptive analgesia—treating postoperative pain by preventing the establishment of central sensitization. Anesth Analg 1993;77(2)362-79.

Chapter 5

Hemostatics, Astringents and Gingival Retraction Cords

Kenneth H. Burrell, D.D.S., S.M.

Hemostatics

Sometimes normal blood clotting mechanisms are insufficient to stop blood flow during or after surgery. This is when a hemostatic must be used. Mechanical devices, cold applications, substances that cause the aggregation of platelets, agents that can counter systemic fibrinolysis and vitamin K to treat or prevent prothrombin deficiency all are examples of hemostatics. This chapter discusses selected agents useful in arresting small vessel blood flow and modifying blood coagulation.

The most common cause of abnormal surgical and postsurgical bleeding is local factors such as a severed, unligated or cauterized blood vessel. In some cases, it is the result of a hemostatic defect. The medical history usually will reveal a congenital bleeding disorder and, in most cases, the presence of or the cause for suspecting an acquired bleeding disorder. The preoperative examination can also offer evidence of the potential for abnormal bleeding. The presence of petechiae, ecchymoses and hematomas may suggest that such a condition exists.

Accepted Indications

If blood flow is profuse, mechanical aids such as a compress, hemostatic forceps, a modeling compound splint or ligatures should be used. For slow blood flow and oozing, a combination of hemostatics can be used. The three kinds of hemostatics to be noted here are absorbable hemostatic agents, agents that modify blood coagulation and vasoconstrictors. Vasoconstrictors act by constricting or closing blood vessels. They are used to a limited extent to control capillary bleeding. Vasoconstrictors are described in detail in Chapter 1 (Tables 1.3, 1.6). See Table 5.1 for a comparison of various hemostatics useful in dentistry.

Absorbable Gelatin Sponge

The absorbable gelatin sponge consists of a tough, porous matrix prepared from purified pork skin gelatin, granules and water for injection that is indicated as a hemostatic device for control of capillary, venous or arteriolar bleeding when pressure, ligature or other conventional procedures are either ineffective or impractical. It can be used in extraction sites and is resorbed in 4-6 w.

Oxidized Cellulose

Oxidized cellulose is a chemically modified form of surgical gauze or cotton that is used to control moderate bleeding by forming an artificial clot when suturing or ligation is impractical and ineffective. Because it is friable, oxidized cellulose is difficult to place and retain in extraction sockets, but can be used as a sutured implant or temporary packing. The cotton or gauze can be removed before dissolution is complete by irrigation with saline or a mildly alkaline solution.

Absorption of oxidized cellulose ordinarily

occurs between the second and seventh day after implantation of material, but complete absorption of large amounts of blood-soaked material may take six weeks or longer.

Oxidized Regenerated Cellulose

Oxidized regenerated cellulose is prepared from alpha-cellulose by reaction with alkali to form viscose, which is then spun into filaments and oxidized. This process results in greater chemical purity and uniformity of physical structure than oxidized cellulose. It is a sterile, absorbable, knitted fabric that is strong enough to be sutured or cut. It has less tendency to stick to instruments and gloves and is less friable than oxidized cellulose.

Oxidized regenerated cellulose is used to control capillary, venous and small arterial hemorrhage when ligature, pressure, or other conventional methods of control are impractical or ineffective. The product can be used as a surface dressing because it does not retard epithelialization. It is bactericidal against numerous gram-negative and gram-positive microorganisms, both aerobic and anaerobic.

It can be placed over extraction sites.

Microfibrillar Collagen Hemostat

Microfibrillar collagen hemostat is a hemostatically active agent prepared from bovine deep flexor tendon (Achilles tendon) as a water-soluble, partial-acid salt of natural collagen. It reduces bleeding from cancellous bone, gingival graft donor sites and other surgical procedures. It should not be left in infected or contaminated spaces because it may prolong or promote infection and delay healing.

Collagen Absorbable Hemostat

Collagen absorbable hemostat is composed of purified and lyophilized bovine dermal collagen. Used as an adjunct to hemostasis, collagen absorbable hemostat can be sutured into place. It reduces bleeding when ligation and other conventional methods are ineffective or impractical. Excess material should be removed before the wound is closed.

Vitamin K

Vitamin K therapy is required when hypoprothrombinemia results from inadequately available vitamins K_1 and K_2. This occurs when there is decreased synthesis by intestinal bacteria, inadequate absorption from the intestinal tract or increased requirement by the liver for normal synthesis of prothrombin.

Vitamin K, in its various forms, is an essential component of blood coagulation. Vitamins K_1, K_2 or menadione (Vitamin K_3) are required for the production of the functional forms of six coagulation proteins: prothrombin, factors VII, IX and X and proteins C and S. Vitamin K_4 is converted to Vitamin K_3 in the liver.

Phytonadione (vitamin K_1)

Phytonadione—known as vitamin K_1—is used for

- anticoagulant–induced prothrombin deficiency;
- prophylaxis and therapy of hemorrhagic disease of the newborn;
- hypoprothrombinemia resulting from oral antibacterial therapy;
- hypoprothrombinemia secondary to factors limiting absorption or synthesis of vitamin K such as obstructive jaundice, biliary fistula, sprue, ulcerative colitis, celiac disease, intestinal resection, cystic fibrosis of the pancreas and regional enteritis;
- other drug-induced hypoprothrombinemia such as that which results from salicylate use.

Menadiol sodium diphosphate (vitamin K_4)

Menadiol sodium diphosphate is effective as a hemostatic agent only when bleeding results from prothrombin deficiency.

Menadione (vitamin K_3)

This requires normal flow of bile into the intestine; otherwise, the administration of bile salts is needed, as menadione (vitamin K_3) must be converted to vitamin K_2 by the liver.

Thrombin

Thrombin is useful as a topical local hemo-

Table 5.1

Hemostatics: Dosage Information

Generic name	Brand name(s)	Usual adult dosage	Pregnancy risk category	Form
		Absorbable hemostatic agents		
Absorbable gelatin sponge	Gelfoam ✶	Absorbable gelatin sponge may be cut into various sizes; may be applied to bleeding surfaces in amounts sufficient to cover area	Not available	**Dental packing blocks:** 20X20X7mm **Powder:** 1 g
Oxidized cellulose	Oxycel	Hemostatic effect is greater when material is applied dry as opposed to moistened with water or saline	Not available	**Pad:** 3X3 in **Pledget:** 2X1X1 in **Strip:** 18X2, 5X½, 36X½ in
Oxidized regenerated cellulose	Surgicel Absorbable Hemostat ✶, Surgicel Nu-Knit Absorbable Hemostat	Can be laid over socket for control of bleeding from extraction sites; minimal amounts of the material should be placed on bleeding site; otherwise, it may be held firmly against tissue	Not available	**Surgicel sheets:** 2X14 in, 4X8 in, 2X3 in, ½X2 in **Surgicel Nu-Knit sheets:** 1X1 in, 3X4 in, 6X9 in
Microfibrillar collagen hemostat	Collacote ✶, Collaplug, Collatape ✶, Instat MCH	Is applied topically and adheres firmly to bleeding surfaces	Not available	**Instat MCH:** Coherent fibers packaged in 0.5- and 1.0-g containers **Collacote, Collaplug, Collatape:** 1X3, ¾X1½, ⅜X¾ in
Collagen absorbable hemostat	Instat	Should be applied directly to the bleeding surface with pressure; is more effective when applied dry, or may be moistened with sterile saline or thrombin solution, and may be left in place as necessary; is absorbed 8-10 w after placement	Not available	**Pads:** 1X2, 3X4 in

Systemic agents that modify blood coagulation

Vitamin K_1 or phytonadione	AquaMephyton, Konakion, Mephyton	Not available	**Anticoagulant-induced prothrombin deficiency (except heparin)—oral:** 2.5-10 mg or up to 25 mg (rarely 50 mg) **Anticoagulant-induced prothrombin deficiency (except heparin)—IM, aqueous dispersion:** 5-10 mg initially, up to 20 mg **Anticoagulant-induced prothrombin deficiency (except heparin)—SC or IM, aqueous colloidal solution:** 2.5-10 mg or up to 25 mg (rarely 50 mg) **Hypoprothrombinemia owing to other causes and factors limiting absorption or synthesis—SC or IM, aqueous colloidal solution:** 2.5-25 mg or more (rarely up to 50 mg) **Hypoprothrombinemia owing to other causes and factors limiting absorption or synthesis—IM, aqueous dispersion:** 2-20 mg **Hypoprothrombinemia owing to other causes and factors limiting absorption or synthesis—oral:** 0.5-25 mg or more (rarely up to 50 mg)	**Aqueous colloidal solution (AquaMephyton):** 2, 10 mg/mL **Aqueous dispersion (Konakion):** 2, 10 mg/mL **Tablets (Mephyton):** 5 mg
Vitamin K_4 or menadiol sodium diphosphate	Synkayvite	Not available	**Oral:** 5 mg q day, 4-7 days **Injection:** 5-10 mg q day, 4-7 days	**Tablets:** 5 mg **Injection:** 5, 10, 37.5 mg/mL

Continued on next page

★ indicates a product bearing the ADA Seal of Acceptance.

Table 5.1 (cont.)

Hemostatics: Dosage Information

Generic name	Brand name(s)	Usual adult dosage	Pregnancy risk category	Form
Systemic agents that modify blood coagulation (cont.)				
Vitamin K₃ or menadione	generic	2-10 mg/day, 4-7 days before surgery	Not available	**Powder**
Thrombin (topical agent)				
Thrombin	Thrombinar, Thrombogen, Thrombostat	**For profuse bleeding—solution:** 1,000-2,000 units/mL **For bleeding from skin or mucosa—solution:** 100 units/mL	C	**Powder:** 1,000, 5,000, 10,000, 20,000 units; 50,000 units (Thrombinar only) **Powder with isotonic saline diluent:** 5,000-, 10,000- and 20,000-unit containers with 5-, 10-, and 20-mL of isotonic saline **Thrombostat:** Also contains 0.02 mg/mL phemerol as a preservative

static agent when blood is oozing from accessible capillaries or venules. In certain kinds of hemorrhage, it can be used to wet pledgets of absorbable gelatin sponge and placed on bleeding tissue or in extraction sockets with or without sutures. It is particularly useful whenever blood is flowing from accessible capillaries and small venules.

General Dosing Information

Table 5.1 lists the general dosing information for specific hemostatics.

Dosage Adjustments

The actual dose for each patient must be individualized according to factors such as his or her size, age and physical status. Reduced doses of vitamin K may be indicated for patients who are taking anticoagulants as opposed to those who have malabsorption problems. The other hemostatic agents should be used as needed.

Special Dental Considerations

Cross-Sensitivity

Patients may experience delayed healing using the gelatin, cellulose and collagen hemostatics. This is more often observed when the surgical site is infected.

Patient Monitoring: Aspects to Watch

Patients receiving vitamin K, especially parenterally, may experience allergic reactions such as rash, urticaria and anaphylaxis.

Adverse Effects and Precautions

The incidence of adverse reactions to hemostatic agents is relatively low. Many reactions are temporary. Idiosyncratic and allergic reactions account for a small minority of adverse responses. See Table 5.2.

Pharmacology

Absorbable Gelatin Sponge

The absorbable gelatin sponge promotes the disruption of platelets and acts as a framework for fibrin, probably because of its phys-

ical effect rather than the result of its alteration of the blood clotting mechanism. It can be placed in dry form or may be moistened with sterile saline or thrombin solution and used in extraction sites.

Oxidized Cellulose

Oxidized cellulose is a chemically modified form of surgical gauze or cotton. Its hemostatic action depends on the formation of an artificial clot by cellulosic acid, which has a marked affinity for hemoglobin.

Oxidized Regenerated Cellulose

Oxidized regenerated cellulose probably serves as a hemostatic by providing a physical effect rather than altering the normal physiological clotting mechanism.

Microfibrillar Collagen Hemostat

This hemostatic agent is used topically to trigger the adhesiveness of platelets and stimulate the release phenomenon to produce aggregation of platelets leading to their disintegration and to release coagulation factors that, together with plasma factors, enable fibrin to form. The physical structure of microfibrillar collagen hemostat adds strength to the clot.

Collagen Absorbable Hemostat

When collagen comes into contact with blood, platelets aggregate and release coagulation factors, which together with plasma factors, cause the formation of fibrin and a clot.

Vitamin K

Two forms of naturally occurring vitamin K have been isolated and prepared synthetically. The naturally occurring forms are designated vitamins K_1 and K_2. Vitamin K_1 is present in most vegetables, particularly in their green leaves. Vitamin K_2 is produced by intestinal bacteria. Menadione has vitamin K activity and is derived from a breakdown of the vitamin K molecule by intestinal bacteria and is sometimes referred to as vitamin K_3. Menadiol sodium diphosphate or vitamin K_4 is a water-soluble derivative that is converted to menadione in the liver.

Table 5.2

Hemostatic Agents: Adverse Effects, Precautions and Contraindications

Agent	Adverse effects	Precautions/contraindications
Absorbable hemostatic agents		
Oxidized cellulose	May lead to a foreign body reaction	Extremely friable and difficult to place Should not be used at fracture sites because it interferes with bone regeneration Should not be used as a surface dressing except for the immediate control of hemorrhage, as cellulosic acid inhibits epithelialization Should not be used in combination with thrombin because the hemostatic action of either alone is greater than that of the combination
Oxidized regenerated cellulose	None of significance to dentistry	Placement in extraction sites may delay healing; it should not be placed in fracture sites because it may interfere with callus formation and may cause cyst formation Encapsulation of fluid and foreign bodies possible
Collagen absorbable hemostat	Incidence of pain has been reported to increase when this material is placed in extraction sockets Allergic reactions can occur in patients with known sensitivity to bovine material	Should not be used in mucous membrane closure because it may interfere with healing due to mechanical interposition Should not be left in infected or contaminated space because of possible delay in healing and increased likelihood of abscess formation Should not be used in patients with a known sensitivity to bovine material Should not be overpacked because collagen absorbable hemostat absorbs water and can expand to impinge on neighboring structures Should not be used in cases where point of hemorrhage is submerged, because collagen must be in direct contact with bleeding site to achieve desired effect
Microfibrillar collagen hemostat	May potentiate abscess formation, hematoma and wound dehiscence	Is not intended to treat systemic coagulation disorders Placement in extraction sites has been reported to increase pain Should not be left in infected or contaminated spaces because of possible adhesion formation, allergic reaction, foreign body reaction Interferes with wound margins
Absorbable gelatin sponge	May form a nidus for infection or abscess formation	Should not be overpacked in extraction sites or surgical defects because it may expand to impinge on neighboring structures

Continued on next page

Table 5.2 (cont.)

Hemostatic Agents: Adverse Effects, Precautions and Contraindications

Agent	Adverse effects	Precautions/contraindications
Systemic agents that modify blood coagulation		
Vitamin K_1 or phytonadione	Parenteral administration can cause transient "flushing sensations" and "peculiar sensations" of taste; also (rarely) dizziness, rapid and weak pulse, profuse sweating, brief hypotension, dyspnea and cyanosis; allergic sensitivity, including an anaphylactoid reaction, have been reported	Should not be injected IV Patient undergoing prothrombin reduction therapy should not receive vitamin K preparations except under a physician's supervision Determine if patient is taking anticoagulants, as the drug can decrease effect of anticoagulant Contraindicated in patients with known sensitivity to the drug
Vitamin K_4 or menadiol sodium diphosphate	Adverse reactions are similar to those produced by phytonadione, but incidence is low	Before administering drug, determine if patient is receiving anticoagulant therapy; a patient undergoing prothrombin reduction therapy should not receive vitamin K preparations except under physician supervision If patient is taking anticoagulants, this agent may decrease their effectiveness
Vitamin K_3 or menadione	Adverse reactions are similar to those produced by phytonadione, but incidence is low	Requires normal flow of bile or administration of bile salts Patient undergoing prothrombin reduction therapy should not receive vitamin K preparations except under physician supervision
Thrombin (topical)		
Thrombin	Allergic reactions can occur in patients with known sensitivity to bovine material	Thrombin must not be injected into blood vessels because it might cause serious or even fatal embolism from extensive intravascular thrombosis; instead, should be applied to surface of bleeding tissue as solution or powder

Vitamins K_1, K_2 or menadione are required for the production of the functional forms of six coagulation proteins: prothrombin, factors VII, IX and X and proteins C and S.

Hypoprothrombinemia may result from inadequately available vitamins K_1 and K_2 because of decreased synthesis by intestinal bacteria, inadequate absorption from the intestinal tract or increased requirement by the liver for normal synthesis of prothrombin. Liver dysfunction may also decrease the production of prothrombin, but the hypoprothrombinemia from hepatic cell injury may not respond to the administration of vitamin K as many coagulation proteins are produced in hepatocytes.

Insufficient vitamin K in ingested foods becomes significant only when the synthesis of the vitamin by intestinal bacteria is markedly reduced by the oral administration of antibacterial agents. Biliary obstructions or intestinal disorders may result in an inadequate rate of absorption of vitamin K.

Phytonadione (vitamin K₁)

Phytonadione (vitamin K₁)

Vitamin K_1 is required for the production of the functional forms of six coagulation proteins: prothrombin, factors VII, IX and X and proteins C and S.

Menadiol sodium diphosphate (vitamin K₄)

Vitamin K_4, because of its water solubility, is absorbed from the intestinal tract even in the absence of bile salts.

Menadione (vitamin K₃)

Menadione is a synthetic water-soluble form of vitamin K, which is sometimes referred to as vitamin K_3. Although it is readily absorbed from the intestine, menadione must be converted to vitamin K_2 by the liver. Therefore, it requires a normal flow of bile into the intestine or the concomitant administration of bile salts.

Thrombin

Thrombin is a sterile protein substance that is an essential component of blood coagulation. It combines with fibrinogen to form fibrin.

Patient Advice

- Let the patient know that a hemostatic has been used, what kind of hemostatic it is and why it was used.
- Advise the patient to let you know if bleeding continues from the surgical site.

Astringents

Astringents cause contraction of tissues. They accomplish this by constricting small blood vessels, extracting water from tissue or precipitating protein.

Table 5.3

Astringents: Dosage Information

Generic name	Brand name(s)	Usual adult dosage	Content/form
Aluminum chloride	Gingi-Aid, Hemodent ★, Hemodettes, Hemogin-L, Rastringent, Styptin, Ultradent	Apply product directly to tissues using a cotton pledget or apply to gingival retraction cords	**Gel:** 20% (Hemodettes) **Solution:** 20% (Hemodent, Styptin), 25% (Gingi-Aid, Rastringent, Ultradent) **Ointment:** 25% (Hemogin-L) **Retraction cords:** Average concentration of 0.915, 3.5 mg/in
Aluminum potassium sulfate	generic	Any concentration, including 100% powder, can be used	**Powder:** 100% Various concentrations, all available and prepared by chemical supply houses
Aluminum sulfate	Gel-Cord	Apply product directly to tissues using a cotton pledget or apply to gingival retraction cords	**Gel:** In unit-dose cartridge **Impregnated retraction cord:** Average concentration of 0.48, 0.85, 1.45 mg/in **Topical solution:** 25%
Ferric sulfate	Astringadent ★, Hemodent-FS, Stasis, ViscoStat	Apply product directly to tissues using a cotton pledget or apply to gingival retraction cords	**Solution:** 13.3% (Astringadent), 15.5 (Hemodent-FS), 20% (ViscoStat—for use in infuser kit), 21% (Stasis)

★ *indicates a product bearing the ADA Seal of Acceptance.*

Table 5.4

Astringents: Adverse Effects

Agent	Adverse effects
Aluminum chloride	Concentrated solutions of aluminum chloride are acidic and may have an irritating and even caustic effect on tissues
Aluminum potassium sulfate	May have an irritating effect
Aluminum sulfate	May have an irritating and even caustic effect
Ferric sulfate	Compound may cause tissue irritation to a greater degree than aluminum compounds

Accepted Indications

Dentists can apply astringents to gingival tissues before taking impressions or placing Class V or root-surface restorations. They can be used alone or in combination with retraction cords. Aluminum and iron salts are the compounds used as astringents in dentistry.

Aluminum Chloride

Aluminum chloride causes contraction or shrinking of tissue, making it useful in retracting gingival tissue. It also reduces secretions and minor hemorrhage.

Aluminum Potassium Sulfate

Aluminum potassium sulfate, or alum, is not widely used even though it is relatively innocuous, because its tissue retraction and hemostatic properties are limited.

Aluminum Sulfate

Aluminum sulfate, as with other aluminum salts, serves as an effective astringent for gingival retraction and hemostatic action.

Ferric Sulfate

Ferric sulfate is an effective and safe astringent and hemostatic for use in gingival retraction. It can also be used in vital pulpotomies.

General Dosing Information

Table 5.3 lists the general dosing and administration information for specific astringents.

Adverse Effects

The incidence of adverse reactions to astringents is relatively low. Most reactions (presented in Table 5.4) are temporary. The adverse effects listed in Table 5.4 apply to all major types of astringents.

Pharmacology

The ability of any astringent to contract or shrink mucous membrane or skin tissue is related to its mode of action involving protein precipitation and water absorption.

Gingival Retraction Cords

Gingival retraction cords can be used alone or in combination with astringents or vasoconstrictors. They are usually made of cotton and are woven in various ways to suit the practitioner's preference. They are also available in a variety of diameters to accommodate the variation in gingival sulcus width and depth.

These cords can be impregnated with astringents or vasoconstrictors either by the manufacturer or at chairside. Aluminum chloride, aluminum sulfate and ferric sulfate are used as the astringents, while racemic epinephrine is used as the vasoconstrictor.

Although epinephrine cord is used by a majority of practitioners rather than an astringent cord for gingival retraction and hemostasis, epinephrine cord is contraindicated in patients with a history of cardiovascular diseases, diabetes and hyperthyroidism and in those taking monoamine oxidase inhibitors, rauwolfias and ganglionic blocking agents.

Some practitioners and educators believe that epinephrine-containing retraction cord and solutions should not be used in dentistry. However, plasma epinephrine concentration increased significantly only after 60 min in a study of healthy subjects without a history of high blood pressure. In spite of the elevated plasma epinephrine levels, the subjects' heart rates, mean arterial pressures and pulse pressure products were not significantly different when the same subjects were exposed to a potassium aluminum sulfate (alum) impregnated cord. The gingival tissues of the subjects were intact, however. Therefore, the patient's medical history, oral health, type of procedure to be done, amount and length of retraction, and exposure of the vascular bed should be considered before deciding to use epinephrine-containing retraction cords. While Table 5.5 provides gingival retraction cord information, Table 5.6 shows the adverse effects, precautions and contraindications of a variety of commercially available retraction cords.

Accepted Indications

Gingival retraction cord is used for all kinds of gingival retraction before taking impressions or placing restorations.

General Dosing Information

Dosage Adjustments

The actual maximum dose for each patient must be individualized depending on factors such as oral health and sensitivity.

Table 5.5

Gingival Retraction Cords: Usage Information*

Generic name	Brand name(s)	Content/form
Retraction cord, plain	Gingi-Plain, Gingi-Plain Z-Twist, Hemodent, Retrax, Sil-trax Plain, Ultrapak	**Gingi-Plain Firm Cord:** #1 (thin); #2 (medium); #3 (thick) **Gingi-Plain Z-Twist Braided Cord:** #00 (very thin); #1 (thin); #2 (medium); #3 (thick) **Hemodent:** #9 (medium thin); #3 (medium heavy) **Retrax Twisted Cord:** #7 (thin); #8 (small); #9 (medium); #10 (large) **Siltrax-Plain Braided Cord:** #7 (thin); #8 (small); #9 (medium); #10 (large) **Ultrapak:** Ultrapak #000 (ultra thin); #00 (very thin); #0 (thin); #1 (medium); #2 (thick); #3 (ultra thick)
Retraction cord with aluminum chloride	Hemodent ★, Retreat	**Hemodent:** #9 (medium thin); #3 (medium heavy), 0.915 mg/in **Retreat:** #1 (thin); #2 (medium); #3 (thick)

★ *indicates a product bearing the ADA Seal of Acceptance.*
A number of retraction cords are available with racemic epinephrine in concentrations ranging from 0.3-1.45 mg/in and varying concentrations of zinc phenylsulfonate.

Continued on next page

Table 5.5 (cont.)
Gingival Retraction Cords: Usage Information*

Generic name	Brand name(s)	Content/form
Retraction cord with aluminum sulfate	Gingi-Aid Z-Twist, Pascord, R-Cord, Sil-Trax AS	**Gingi-Aid Z-Twist Braided Cord:** #00 (very thin); #1 (thin); #2 (medium); #3 (thick); 0.5 mg/in **Pascord Twisted Cord:** #7 (thin), 0.48 mg/in; #8 (small), 0.48 mg/in; #9 (medium), 0.85 mg/in; #10 (large), 1.45 mg/in **R-Cord:** Braided cord with or without epinephrine **Sil-Trax AS Braided Cord:** #7 (thin), 0.48 mg/in; #8 (small), 0.48 mg/in; #9 (medium), 0.85 mg/in; #10 (large), 1.45 mg/in
Retraction cord with potassium aluminum sulfate	GingiBraid, GingiKnit, Gingi-Tract, Sil-Trax, Sulpak, Sultan Ultra, UniBraid	**GingiBraid:** 0 (fine); 1 (small); 2 (medium); 3 (large); also available plain **GingiKnit:** 000 (very fine); 00 (fine); 0 (small); 1 (medium); 2 (large); 3 (extra large) **Gingi-Tract:** Thin, medium, thick **Sil-Trax AS:** #7 (thin); #8 (small); #9 (medium); #10 (large); available with epinephrine **Sulpak:** Braided cord in thin, medium, large **Sultan:** Braided cord in thin, medium, large; available with either aluminum potassium sulfate or racemic epinephrine **UniBraid:** 0 (fine); 1 (small); 2 (medium); 3 (large); also available plain
Retraction cord with epinephrine	Gingi-Pak	#1 (thin); #2 (medium); #3 (thick) 0.5 mg/in
Retraction cord with racemic epinephrine	R-Cord, Racord, Sil-Trax AS, Sil-Trax EPI, Sultan	**Racord Twisted Cord:** #7 (thin), 0.50 mg/in.; #8 (small), 0.50 mg/in.; #9 (medium), 0.85 mg/in.; #10 (large), 1.15 mg/in **Sil-Trax AS:** 0.48-1.45 mg racemic epinephrine/in **Sil-Trax EPI Braided Cord:** #7 (thin), 0.50 mg/in; #8 (small), 0.50 mg/in; #9 (medium), 0.85 mg/in; #10 (large), 1.15 mg/in **Sultan:** 0.108-0.48 mg/in
Retraction cord with zinc chloride	Sultan	0.06-0.218 mg/in

*A number of retraction cords are available with racemic epinephrine in concentrations ranging from 0.3-1.45 mg/in and varying concentrations of zinc phenylsulfonate.

Adverse Effects and Precautions

The incidence of adverse reactions to gingival retraction cords is relatively low. Most reactions are temporary, but gingival tissue destruction may permanently alter gingival architecture, especially after vigorous cord placement.

Pharmacology

Gingival retraction cords work mechanically to widen the gingival sulcus. With the addition of astringents or vasoconstrictors, the gingival tissue is retracted further. The astringents act by constricting blood vessels, extracting water from tissue or precipitating proteins.

Table 5.6

Gingival Retraction Cords: Adverse Effects, Precautions and Contraindications

Type of cord	Adverse effects	Precautions/contraindications
Retraction cord, plain	None of significance to dentistry	None of significance to dentistry
Retraction cord with aluminum chloride	May cause irritation or tissue destruction	Contraindicated in those with a history of allergy
Retraction cord with aluminum sulfate	May cause irritation or tissue destruction	None of significance to dentistry
Retraction cord with potassium aluminum sulfate	May cause irritation or tissue destruction	None of significance to dentistry
Retraction cord with epinephrine	May cause irritation or tissue destruction	Patient's medical history and oral health, type of procedure to be done, amount and length of retraction, and exposure of the vascular bed should be considered before epinephrine-containing retraction cords are used Contraindicated in patients with a history of cardiovascular diseases Contraindicated in patients with a history of diabetes Contraindicated in patients with a history of hyperthyroidism Contraindicated in patients with a history of hypertension Contraindicated in patients with a history of arteriosclerosis Contraindicated in patients taking tricyclic antidepressants Contraindicated in patients taking monoamine oxidase inhibitors Contraindicated in patients taking rauwolfias Contraindicated in patients taking ganglionic blocking agents

Continued on next page

Table 5.6 (cont.)

Gingival Retraction Cords: Oral Adverse Effects, Precautions and Contraindications

Type of cord	Adverse effects	Precautions/contraindications
Retraction cord with racemic epinephrine	May cause irritation or tissue destruction	Patient's medical history and oral health, type of procedure to be done, amount and length of retraction, and exposure of the vascular bed should be considered before epinephrine-containing retraction cords are used
		Contraindicated in patients with a history of cardiovascular diseases
		Contraindicated in patients with a history of diabetes
		Contraindicated in patients with a history of hyperthyroidism
		Contraindicated in patients with a history of hypertension
		Contraindicated in patients with a history of arteriosclerosis
		Contraindicated in patients taking tricyclic antidepressants
		Contraindicated in patients taking monoamine oxidase inhibitors
		Contraindicated in patients taking rauwolfias
		Contraindicated in patients taking ganglionic blocking agents

Suggested Readings

American Medical Association. AMA drug evaluations annual 1992. Chicago: American Medical Association; 1992.

Colman RW, Hirsch J, Marder VJ, Salzman EW, eds. Hemostatics and thrombosis: Basic principles and clinical practice. 3rd ed. Philadelphia: Lippincott; 1994.

Vitamin K. Facts and comparisons 1987; June 1987: 83-84a.

Chapter 6

Corticosteroids

Martha Somerman, D.D.S., Ph.D.

It is imperative that dentists understand the basic principles of corticosteroid therapy. First, dental treatment procedures have to be altered for patients taking steroid medications. Second, steroids are used in clinical dentistry, mainly owing to their anti-inflammatory properties. In dentistry, steroids have been prescribed for treatment of recurrent oral ulcerations and other mucosal lesions such as erosive lichen planus and pemphigus. In most of these situations, topical steroids are used; therefore, adrenal suppression—although possible—is not a likely consequence of therapy. However, dentists also prescribe systemic steroids for severe oral ulcerations and also for facial pain associated with inflammation.

Steroid therapy, especially chronic, inhibits adrenal gland function. The adrenal glands, composed of an inner zone called the adrenal medulla and an outer zone called the adrenal cortex, are multifunctional endocrine organs. The medulla produces epinephrine and norepinephrine, which are catecholamines required for maintaining a variety of physiological functions—control of blood pressure, myocardial contractility and excitability, and regulation of body metabolism. They also enable the body to appropriately respond to stressful situations.

The cortex produces three types of hormones:

- glucocorticoids, which regulate carbohydrate, protein and fat metabolism and are required for suppression of inflammation;

- mineral corticoids, which help to regulate sodium and potassium levels;
- sex hormones, which have a secondary role in sexual maturation.

Secretion of these hormones is carefully regulated through various mechanisms with a hypothalamic-pituitary feedback loop for glucocorticoids.

This chapter focuses on the use of synthetic glucocorticoids for their oral-related anti-inflammatory and immunosuppressive actions. Glucocorticoids are very valuable in treating oral conditions as well as non–oral-related diseases; however, their long-term use (especially systemic) can result in significant detrimental side effects. Dentists should not prescribe corticosteroids for longer than 2 w without re-evaluating the disease state and, when necessary, consulting with the patient's physician. It is important for dentists to recognize the pathological state of patients who have an excessive production of adrenal cortex hormones. An excess secretion can result from a disease, a syndrome or another condition affecting the anterior pituitary gland, the hypothalamus or the adrenal gland itself. In particular, patients with glucocorticoid hypersecretions may have Cushing's syndrome, which is manifested as adiposity of the face (sometimes known as "moon-face") and neck, truncal obesity, muscular wasting and hirsutism. Other symptoms that may or may not be present include hypertension resulting from retention of fluid, decreased collagen production, osteoporosis, an increased susceptibility to infection, increased blood glucose, a decrease in eosinophils and lymphocytes, and reports of bruising easily and poor wound healing.

In contrast, people with adrenal insufficiency experience weakness, weight loss, orthostatic hypotension (postural syncope), nausea and vomiting. With severe insufficiency or adrenal suppression, patients cannot produce steroids in response to stress; in extreme situations this may result in cardiovascular collapse. Chronic loss of adrenal function is called Addison's disease.

Importantly, patients who are prescribed corticosteroids over a long period may manifest some of the symptoms of Cushing's syndrome, such as suppressed adrenal gland function. These patients may physically respond to stressful situations as would people with adrenal insufficiency—by going into adrenal crisis, which may include cardiovascular collapse. Therefore, dentists must carefully evaluate patients who are receiving or have a history of receiving steroid therapy, and they should pursue a consultation with a physician when more detailed information is needed to elicit the duration of time a patient has taken a specific steroid dosage.

Adrenal gland function may be suppressed in patients who have taken as little as 20-30 mg of a corticosteroid (prednisone) per day for 7 to 10 days during the past year. Ordinarily, patients on alternate-day steroid therapy have significantly less adrenal suppression than patients receiving daily therapy. Before beginning dental treatment, dentists must assess patients who take any type or dose of corticosteroid. For example, in the case of a patient taking a high dose of a corticosteroid as part of long-term maintenance therapy, the dentist—in consultation with the patient's physician—should establish appropriate dose levels before beginning dental treatment. In most situations, the dose is usually increased temporarily, with a subsequent decrease back to the patient's maintenance dose after the procedure, as detailed below. (For reference, the normal stress response is equivalent to 60 mg of prednisone per day. Thus, an appropriate dose is often close to 60 mg.) In addition to alteration of steroid medication, severely immunocompromised patients may require prophylactic antibiotic coverage.

General protocol for steroid supplementation
High risk. These are patients receiving daily steroid therapy (dose from 50 to over 60 mg/day of prednisone, or equivalent) each day. No supplementation is required for an oral examination. However, procedures associated with mild to moderate stress require steroid supplementation. Usually, the patient should take a double dose on the day of the procedure and decrease back to the original dose within 2 days. For advanced surgical procedures, the patient should take an optimum dose of steroid (for instance, 60 mg) on the day of surgery. Dosage is then decreased 50% daily from the procedure date until the patient's normal dose is reached.

Also, as steroids have both anti-inflammatory and immunosuppressive activity, patients who are severely compromised are at high risk of developing infections. Therefore, use of antibiotic prophylaxis is recommended for such patients.

Significant risk. In this category are patients who formerly took steroids at doses generally of 20 mg or higher per day and whose steroid therapy lasted 10 days or more within the previous 2 w. These patients usually require 20-40 mg of corticosteroids the day of the procedure, cut to half on day 2, with no steroids on day 3. After 2 w, no replacement therapy is indicated.

Low risk. These patients are receiving alternate-day steroid therapy. There is some question as to whether these patients need supplemental therapy, especially if the dosage was for a short term. However, it is best to perform dental procedures on the off-day of steroid therapy. It is assumed that patients receiving alternate-day steroid therapy will have regained an adequate stress response from the time they change their regimen from every-day to alternate-day therapy within the 2 w preceding dental treatment.

In all situations listed above, dentists who are seeing these types of patients may consult with the patient's physician. As needed, an adrenal corticotropic hormone (ACTH) stimulation test (rarely used) can be used to measure the adrenal glands' ability to respond to orally delivered ACTH.

Accepted Indications

For the most part, corticosteroids provide symptomatic relief, with little effect on controlling disease. Labeled indications for corticosteroids include replacement therapy for adrenal insufficiencies; anti-inflammatory and immunosuppressive action; and treatment of chronic asthma, autoimmune diseases and some hematologic disorders. Among the disorders and diseases treated with corticosteroids are

- endocrine disorders,
- hematologic disorders,
- dermatologic diseases (including their oral manifestations),
- ophthalmic diseases,
- respiratory diseases,
- neoplastic diseases,
- gastrointestinal disorders.

Therapeutically, the most important function of glucocorticoids is their ability to inhibit accumulation of neutrophils and monocytes at sites of inflammation and also their suppression of such cells' phagocytic, bactericidal and antigen-producing activity. On the negative side, these attributes result in compromising the immune system, making such patients highly susceptible to common and uncommon pathogens. This is a major complication of chronic steroid treatment.

Steroids have been used as intra-articular injections to reduce inflammation at local sites. In these cases, the recommendation is to repeat injections no more frequently than q 3 w.

Repeated injections can cause severe joint damage. In general, corticosteroids should not be administered for intra-articular injection in patients with arthroplasty of joint (increased risk of infection); blood-clotting disorders; intra-articular fracture (will delay healing); periarticular infection; osteoporosis; or unstable joints. Furthermore, their use for temporomandibular joint disorders warrants further research.

Systemic Corticosteroids

General Dosing Information

Systemic dosing is typically provided in the form of oral liquid or tablets or intramuscular injection. Concentrations vary depending on the particular indication and size of the joint or other region of treatment, tissue vascularity in the area of injection, and individual patient characteristics (especially disease state) and response to previous or existing concentrations and doses of corticosteroid. As a rule, the lowest effective dose for the shortest duration of time is recommended. If long-term use is planned, frequent monitoring of drug effect is required.

As dentists prescribe mostly topical steroids, Table 6.1 provides information on representative examples of drugs to be used systemically, separated into short-acting, intermediate-acting and long-acting systemic steroids; a more comprehensive table (6.4) for topical corticosteroids appears later in the chapter, and also in Table 24.2, Chapter 24, "Musculoskeletal/Connective Tissue Drugs."

Maximum Recommended Doses

The maximum recommended doses for systemic corticosteroid formulations per procedure or appointment are 5-20 mg of prednisone for maintenance dose and 5-60 mg for continuous or alternate-day therapy, but doses depend on the patient's condition. Dosing schedules and maximum doses are based on the assumption that the dentist has

Table 6.1

Systemic Corticosteroids: Dosing Information

Generic name	Brand name(s)	Usual adult dosage	Maximum adult dosage	Usual child dosage	Pregnancy risk category	Content/form
Short-acting: duration 10-90 min (based on t ½)						
Cortisone	Cortone Acetate, generic; Cortone [CAN]	**Oral:** 25-300 mg/day, single or divided dose **IM:** 20-300 mg/day	300 mg/day	**Oral:** 2.5-10 mg/kg	C	**Tablets:** 5, 10, 25 mg; 5, 25 mg [CAN] **Injection:** 50 mg/mL, in 10-mL vials
Intermediate-acting: duration several h						
Prednisone	Deltasone, Liquid Pred, Meticorten, Prednisone Intensol, Orasone, Prednicen-M, Sterapred; Apo-Prednisone [CAN], Winpred [CAN]	**Oral:** 5-60 mg/day single or divided dose	250 mg/day	**Oral, suspension, syrup or tablet:** 0.05-2 mg/kg/day	C	**Oral suspension, concentrate:** 30% alcohol: 5 mg/mL, in 30-mL vial **Oral suspension:** 5% alcohol: 5 mg/5 mL, in 5- and 500-mL vials **Syrup:** 5 mg/5 mL, 120 mg/240 mL **Tablet:** 1, 2.5, 5, 10, 20, 50 mg
Long-acting: duration ≥ 5 h						
Betamethasone	Celestone; Betnelan [CAN], Celestone [CAN]	**Oral, syrup or tablets:** 600 μg (0.6 mg)-7.2 mg/day in single or divided dose **IM/IV:** 0.6-9 mg/day	9 mg/day	**Oral, syrup or tablets:** 0.0175-0.25 mg/kg/day OR 0.5-7.5 mg/m²/day **IM:** 0.0175-0.125 mg/kg/day OR 0.5-7.5 mg/m²/day	C	**Injection:** 3 mg/mL, in 5-mL vial **Syrup:** 0.06 mg/5 mL, in 118-mL vial **Tablets:** 0.6 mg

[CAN] indicates a drug available only in Canada.

determined (through taking a health history and interviewing the patient) that the patient is in general good health and is not taking any medications that can interact with the corticosteroid agent.

Dosage Adjustments

The actual maximum dose for each patient must be individualized depending on his or her size, age and physical status; other drugs he or she may be taking; and duration of existing corticosteroid therapy (long-term use considerations). Reduced maximum doses may be indicated for pediatric and geriatric patients, patients with serious illness or disability, and patients with medical conditions or who are taking drugs that alter responses to corticosteroids.

Special Dental Considerations

Drug Interactions of Dental Interest

The following drug interactions and related problems involving systemic corticosteroids

Table 6.2

Systemic Corticosteroids: Possible Interactions With Other Agents

Drug taken by patient	Interaction with systemic corticosteroids	Dentist's action
Acetaminophen	Corticosteroid induction of hepatic enzymes may increase formation of hepatotoxic acetaminophen metabolites, thereby increasing risk of hepatotoxicity	Use precaution in patients with history of liver disease
Amphotericin B or carbonic anhydrase inhibitor	*Hypokalemia, edema, heart disease*	Cautious use of steroids in patients taking drugs in first column
Anabolic steroids or androgen	Increased incidence of acne	
Antacids	Possible decrease in absorption of corticosteroids	May require adjustment in steroid dose
Antidiabetic agents	*Steroids may increase blood glucose concentration*	May require adjustments of both steroids and antidiabetic drugs
Salicylates (NSAIDs)	Increased gastrointestinal side effects	Avoid prescribing aspirin-containing products
Digitalis glycosides	Increased risk of arrhythmias due to hypokalemia	Use steroids cautiously
Hepatic enzyme-inducing agents	*Decreased steroid effectiveness owing to increased hepatic microsomal enzymes*	May need to adjust dose of steroids
Some β$_2$ adrenergic agonists	*May cause pulmonary edema*	Discontinue steroid use if signs of edema occur
Potassium- and sodium-altering agents— including vitamin supplements, foods and diuretics	*Could increase or decrease effect of either agent (depends on dose); may result in hypokalemia or increased blood pressure*	Monitor cardiac function and serum potassium; if necessary, adjust sodium and potassium intake and discuss with patient
Vaccines	*Increased risk of developing viral disease*	May require postponement of vaccination

Italics indicate information of major clinical significance.

(Table 6.2) are potentially of clinical significance in dentistry. In addition, estrogen increases biosynthesis of transcortin from the liver; therefore, patients with elevated estrogen levels will have increased concentrations of total plasma cortisol. Also, hypothyroidism may decrease metabolism of glucocorticoids.

Laboratory Value Alterations

- Under stress situations, patients can be tested, as needed, for integrity of the hypothalamic-pituitary-adrenal axis (HPA). The test involves injecting (IM or IV) cosyntropin, a synthetic peptide corresponding to residues 1-24 of human ACTH. There are varying ways to determine activity, but for the rapid stimulation test, cortisol blood levels are determined immediately before injection of 0.25 mg of peptide and then levels of cortisol are measured 30 min later. Levels need to increase more than 20 μg/100 mL to be considered a normal response.
- The dentist also may wish to request tests for CBC, calcium, cholesterol and lipid, glucose, platelet count, potassium and sodium.

Special Patients

Pregnant and nursing women

In animal studies, birth defects have been reported; however, additional studies are required in humans. Steroids cross the placenta, with some suggestions of decreased birth weight and stillbirth. Breast-feeding is not recommended for women taking high doses of steroids; however, only about 1% of the dose is excreted into breast milk.

Pediatric, geriatric and other special patients

Many of these steroids can alter kidney and liver function, which may be particularly damaging to older and younger patients. Therefore, dentists may need to adjust dose levels accordingly.

Steroids should be used with extreme caution in pediatric patients, owing to significant side effects that include retardation of growth.

While receiving steroid therapy, geriatric patients are more likely to develop hypertension, as well as osteoporosis (particularly postmenopausal women).

Risk/benefit of steroid therapy needs to be considered for immunocompromised patients because steroids mask more serious symptoms of their disease.

Patient Monitoring: Aspects to Watch

- Symptoms of blood dyscrasias (such as infection, bleeding and poor healing): for patients with these symptoms, the dentist should request a medical consultation for blood studies and postpone dental treatment until normal values are re-established
- Vital signs, at every appointment: necessary to monitor possible cardiovascular side effects
- Salivary flow: as a factor in caries, periodontal disease and candidiasis
- Dose and duration of steroid therapy: to assess stress tolerance and risk of immunosuppression
- Need for medical consultation: to assess disease control and patient's stress tolerance

Adverse Effects and Precautions

Systemic corticosteroids, especially when taken for long periods, can result in significant adverse effects. Many reactions, such as electrolyte imbalance and immune system impairment, can be life-threatening. Toxic systemic reactions are generally associated with chronic therapy. Idiosyncratic and allergic reactions account for a small minority of adverse responses.

As a rule, side effects are increased with duration and concentration of dose. Therefore, the dentist needs to consider side effects related to intake of other medications (if the patient is taking the steroid for more than 2 w) or for patients with other diseases or disorders such as hypertension, congestive heart failure, blood disorders, diabetes, osteoporosis and immunocompromised situations.

The adverse effects listed in Table 6.3 apply to all major types of systemic corticosteroids. (Precautions and contraindications are usually related to and/or associated with long-term use.) In addition, withdrawal from

Table 6.3

Systemic Corticosteroids: Adverse Effects, Precautions and Contraindications

Body system	Adverse effects	Precautions/contraindications
General	Owing to too-quick withdrawal: flare-up of underlying disease, acute adrenal insufficiency; also (rarely), pseudotumor cerebri	Some effects of withdrawal—fever, myalgia, arthralgia, and malaise—may be difficult to separate from underlying disease
CV	*Hypertension, cardiovascular collapse;* hypertension	*Use cautiously with patients who have heart disease*
CNS	Behavioral disturbances (rare)	Changes in behavioral pattern
Endoc	Growth arrest, hyperglycemia, suppression of HPA	Limit use in small children Use cautiously in patients with diabetes Adrenal crisis under stress
EENT	Cataracts, glaucoma, blurred vision	Patients at risk are children and those with ophthalmic conditions
GI	Increased GI upset, nausea, vomiting, peptic ulcers	Use cautiously with patients who have ulcers
Hema	*Increased susceptibility to infection*	*Use cautiously in immunocompromised patients*
Integ	Acne, poor or delayed wound healing, hirsutism, striae, ecchymoses	Healing after oral surgical procedures should be monitored closely
Metab	Catabolism, fat redistribution	Patients receiving long-term steroid therapy may require protein supplements owing to catabolic effects of steroids
Musc	Fractures, osteoporosis, muscular weakness	Use with patients who have osteoporosis, myasthenia gravis and other musculoskeletal disorders is not recommended
Oral	Dry mouth, poor or delayed wound healing, petechiae, candidiasis	Caries, masked oral infections Surgery or deep scaling may require administration of prophylactic antibiotics because of risk of infection
Renal	Fluid/electrolyte abnormalities	Use cautiously with patients who have renal disease

Italics indicate information of major clinical significance.

steroids may cause significant side effects as well. Importantly, side effects in both situations—that is, withdrawal or long-term use—are potentially life-threatening. Therefore, before systemic steroids are prescribed or withdrawn, the risks and benefits for each patient must be analyzed carefully.

Pharmacology

Systemic and Topical Corticosteroids

Mechanism of action/effect. The effectiveness of steroid hormones is based on their ability to bind to cytosolic receptors in target tissues and subsequently enter the nucleus, where the steroid-receptor complex interacts with nuclear chromatin. This results in a cascade of events including the expression of hormone-specific ribonucleic acids, or RNAs, which in turn increases synthesis of specific proteins that mediate distinct physiological functions. The glucocorticoid cortisol is a normal circulating hormone secreted by the adrenal gland that functions in regulating normal metabolism and providing resistance to stress. In addition, at high levels—whether the result of disease or drug intake—glucocorticoids can have one or more physiological effects. These include

- altering levels of blood cells in the plasma (that is, decreasing eosinophils, basophils, monocytes and lymphocytes and increasing levels of hemoglobin, erythrocytes and polymorphonuclear leukocytes), which decreases circulating levels of cells involved in fighting off infections and results in increased susceptibility to infections;
- reducing the inflammatory response as a result of a decrease in lymphocytes as well as altering lymphocytes' ability to inhibit the enzyme-phospholipase A2, which is required for production of prostaglandins and leukotrienes;
- suppressing the hypothalmic-pituitary-adrenal (HPA) axis, thus inhibiting further synthesis of glucocorticoids.

Therefore, patients taking glucocorticoids warrant special attention as discussed in the introduction to this chapter.

Absorption. Systemically, most glucocorticoids are rapidly and readily absorbed from the GI tract because of their lipophilic character. Also, absorption occurs via synovial and conjunctival spaces.

Topically, absorption through the skin is very slow. However, chronic use in a nasal spray, for example, for use in seasonal rhinitis, can lead to pulmonary epithelial atrophy. Furthermore, excessive or prolonged use of topical steroids can result in sufficient absorption to cause systemic effects.

Both cortisone and prednisone contain a keto group at position II that must be hydroxylated in the liver to become activated. Thus, these drugs should be avoided in patients with abnormal liver function. Also, topical application of position II ketocorticoids is ineffective as a result of inactivity of this form of the steroid.

Distribution. In general, circulating cortisol is bound to plasma proteins: about 80 to 90% bound to transcortin—a cortisol-binding globulin with high affinity—while about 5 to 10% binds loosely to albumin. About 3 to 10% remains in the free (bioactive) form. Transcortin can bind to most synthetic glucocorticoids as well. However, some steroids, such as dexamethasone, do not bind to transcortin and, thus, are almost 100% in free form.

Biotransformation. Inactivation occurs primarily in the liver and also in the kidney, mostly to inactive metabolites. However, cortisone and prednisone are activated only after being metabolized to hydrocortisone and prednisolone, respectively. Fluorinated corticosteroids are metabolized more slowly than the other members of this group.

Elimination. About 30% of inactive metabolite is metabolized further and then excreted in the urine.

Patient Advice

- Emphasize the importance of good oral hygiene to prevent soft-tissue inflammation.

- Caution the patient to prevent injury when using oral hygiene aids; he or she should use a soft toothbrush and have the dentist or hygienist evaluate his or her brushing and flossing techniques.
- Suggest the use of daily home fluoride preparations if chronic dry mouth occurs.
- Suggest the use of sugarless gum, frequent sips of water or artificial saliva substitutes if chronic dry mouth occurs.
- Caution against using mouthrinses with high alcohol content, as they have drying effects on the oral mucosa.

Topical Corticosteroids

Accepted Indications

Topical steroids are indicated for use in dentistry as adjunctive treatment and temporary relief of symptoms associated with nonviral oral inflammation and ulcerative lesions. Such conditions include recurrent aphthous ulcers, desquamative gingivitis and lichen planus. Topical steroids are not recommended for routine gingivitis, where it is more important to establish and remove causative factors and improve oral hygiene.

General Dosing Information

Topical dosing is typically provided in the form of a gel, cream, ointment, lotion or aerosol (see Table 6.4). Concentrations vary depending on the particular indication and region of treatment and on individual patient characteristics such as response to previous or existing concentrations and doses of corticosteroid, as well as size of lesion and, to a lesser extent, patient age and weight. In general, the lowest effective dose and volume of corticosteroids are recommended. For example, areas with thinner skin (for example, facial) require low-potency corticosteroid preparations for long-term therapy. Medium- and high-potency corticosteroids should be used only in more severe situations. In addition, occlusal dressings are available for chronic or severe situations.

Maximum Recommended Doses

Dosing schedules and maximum doses are based on the assumption that the dentist has determined (through taking a health history and interviewing the patient) that the patient is in general good health and is not taking any medications that can interact with the corticosteroid agent. The dose recommended is based on location of lesion and, in many cases, confirmation by biopsy.

Dosage Adjustments

The actual maximum dose for each patient must be individualized depending on the severity of the lesion and the patient's physical status; other drugs he or she may be taking; and duration of existing corticosteroid therapy (long-term use considerations). Reduced maximum doses may be indicated for pediatric and geriatric patients, patients with serious illness or disability and patients with medical conditions or drugs that alter response to corticosteroids.

Laboratory Value Alterations

See the description for systemic corticosteroids.

Cross-Sensitivity

Cross-sensitivity is of more concern with systemic corticosteroids but can be seen with long-term use of topical corticosteroids.

Special Patients

Cross-sensitivity is of more concern with systemic corticosteroids but can be seen with long-term use of topical corticosteroids.

Pregnant and nursing women

Extensive use of topical corticosteroids is not recommended for pregnant patients or patients planning to become pregnant.

The concentration of topical corticosteroids in breast milk is not known.

Pediatric, geriatric, and other special patients

Pediatric patients have thinner skin and may absorb topical corticosteroids more quickly than older patients. HPA suppression, Cushing's syndrome and intracranial hypertension have been documented in children

Table 6.4

Topical Corticosteroids: Dosing Information

Generic name*	Brand name(s)	Usual adult dosage	Usual child dosage	Pregnancy risk category	Content/form
Betamethasone (medium to high potency)	Benisone, Beta-Val, Diprosone, Valisone	Apply once/day-tid to affected area after meals and at bedtime	Not established, but use least amount that yields effect	C	**Cream:** 0.05%–0.1% in 5-, 15-, 45-g tubes **Ointment:** 0.05%–0.1% in 5-, 15-, 45-g tubes
Clobetasol (high potency)	Temovate	**Topical, ointment:** Apply to affected area after meals and at bedtime	Not established, but use least amount that yields effect	C	**Ointment:** 0.05% in 1-oz tubes
Dexamethasone (low potency)	Decadron	**Topical, elixir:** Rinse with 1 tsp for 2 min qid; do not swallow **Topical, cream:** Apply to affected area after meals and at bedtime	Not established, but use least amount that yields effect	C	**Elixir:** 0.5 mg/5 mL in 5-, 20-, 100-, 237-, 240-, 500-mL bottles **Cream:** 0.1% in 15- and 30-g tubes
Fluocinonide (high potency)	Lidex	**Topical, ointment:** Apply to affected area after meals and at bedtime	Not established, but use least amount that yields effect	C	**Ointment:** 0.05% in 1-oz tubes
Hydrocortisone (cortisol) (low potency)	Alphaderm HC, Anusol-HC, Hytone, Orabase-HCA ; Protocream-HC	Apply to affected area after meals and at bedtime	Not established, but use least amount that yields effect	C	**Cream:** 0.5%–2.5% in 1-, 2-oz tubes and 5-, 30-g tubes **Lotion:** 0.5%–2.5% in 1-, 2-oz tubes **Ointment:** 0.5%–2.5% in 1-oz tubes

Continued on next page

Table 6.4 (cont.)

Topical Corticosteroids: Dosing Information

Generic name*	Brand name(s)	Usual adult dosage	Usual child dosage	Pregnancy risk category	Content/form
Hydrocortisone with iodoquinolone (low potency)	Vytone	**For patients susceptible to candidiasis—topical, cream and ointment:** Apply once/day-tid to affected area after meals and at bedtime	Not established, but use least amount that yields effect	C	**Cream:** 1% hydrocortisone, 1% iodoquinolone
Triamcinolone acetonide (medium potency)	Aristocort A, Kenalog in Orabase, Oralone, generic; Oracort [CAN]	**Topical, cream:** Apply to affected area bid-tid after meals and at bedtime **Topical, oral suspension:** 5 mL qid after meals and at bedtime; do not swallow	Not established, but use least amount that yields effect	C	**Cream:** 0.025%, 0.1%, 0.5% in 5-g tubes **Oral suspension:** 0.1%, 0.2 % in 200-mL bottles
Triamcinolone acetonide with nystatin (medium potency)	Mytrex, nystatin/triamcinolone acetonide; triamcinolone acetonide	**For patients susceptible to candidiasis—topical, cream and ointment:** Apply to affected area after meals and at bedtime	Not established, but use least amount that yields effect	C	**Cream:** 0.025%–0.1%; 100,000 units nystatin/1 mg triamcinolone acetonide/g

[CAN] indicates drugs available only in Canada.

* Several other topical corticosteroids are available that vary in their potency (which is indicated in parentheses). Among the most commonly used are alclometasone (Aclovate) (low), amcinonide (Cyclocort) (medium to high), desoximetasone (Topicort) (high), fluocinolone (Fluonid, Synalar) (medium), flurandrenolide (Cordran; Drenison [CAN]) (medium).

using topical corticosteroids; therefore, low-potency (unfluorinated) topical steroids should be used with children.

There are no appropriate studies that provide information on the effects of topical steroids when used by older people. However, geriatric patients may have alterations in skin/mucosa requiring altered and, in many cases, lower doses.

Patient Monitoring: Aspects to Watch

See the description for systemic corticosteroids. Corticosteroids can mask underlying infection and lead to misdiagnosis.

Adverse Effects and Precautions

Topical corticosteroids have fewer side effects than those given by the systemic route. However, there is some systemic absorption through the oral mucosa. The absorption of topical agents increases with potency and prolonged use. Very rarely, adverse effects usually seen with systemic corticosteroid use are noted with topical steroid use. Idiosyncratic and allergic reactions—burning, itching, irritation, dryness, allergic contact dermatitis, hyperesthesia, skin atrophy (local infection), telangiectasia—account for a minority of adverse responses.

Pharmacology

See the description for systemic corticosteroids.

Patient Advice

- Good oral hygiene is important in preventing soft-tissue inflammation.
- The patient should use a topical corticosteroid after brushing and eating and at bedtime for optimal effect.
- Use on oral herpetic ulcerations is contraindicated.

- The patient should apply the agent with a cotton-tipped applicator by pressing, not rubbing, the paste on the lesion.
- When a topical corticosteroid is used to treat oral lesions, a tissue response should be noted within 7-14 days. If not, the patient should return for oral evaluation. If corticosteroids are used chronically, the patient should return for frequent recall visits.
- If irritation, infection or sensitization occurs at site, the patient should discontinue use and return for evaluation.
- The patient should avoid exposing the affected area to sunlight; burns may occur.
- These agents are for external use only.
- The patient should prevent the topical steroid from coming in contact with his or her eyes.
- The patient should not bandage or wrap the affected area unless directed to do so.
- The patient should report adverse reactions.
- The patient should avoid taking anything by mouth for ½ h and 1 h after topical use in mouth (as a mouthrinse or an ointment).

Suggested Readings

Effect of corticosteroids for fetal maturation on perinatal outcomes. NIH consensus statement. 1994:12(2):1-24.

MacKay S, Eisendrath S. Adverse reaction to dental corticosteroids. Gen Dent 1992;40:136-8.

Rodu B, Mattingly G. Oral mucosal ulcers: diagnosis and management. JADA 1992;123:83-6.

Rosenberg SW, Arm RN, eds. Clinician's guide to treatment of common oral conditions. 4th ed. Baltimore: American Academy of Oral Medicine; 1997.

Vincent SD, Lilly GE, Baker KA. Clinical, historic and therapeutic features of cictricial pemphigoid. A literature review and open therapeutic trial with corticosteroids. Oral Surg Oral Med Oral Pathol 1993;76:453-9.

Chapter 7

Antibiotics

Clay Walker, Ph.D.

The term "antibiotic" was initially used to refer to any compound produced by a microorganism that inhibited another microorganism. Through common usage, this definition has evolved to include any natural, semisynthetic or, in some cases, totally manmade antimicrobial agent that inhibits bacterial growth. An antibiotic can be classified as either bactericidal or bacteriostatic. Bactericidal drugs, such as penicillins, directly kill an infecting organism; bacteriostatic drugs, such as tetracyclines and erythromycin, inhibit the proliferation of bacteria by interfering with an essential metabolic process but are eliminated by the host's immune defense system.

In general, there is no advantage in selecting a bactericidal rather than a bacteriostatic antibiotic for the treatment of healthy people. However, if the patient is immunocompromised either by concurrent treatment (such as cancer chemotherapy or drugs associated with a bone-marrow transplant) or by a pre-existing disease (such as HIV infection), a bactericidal antibiotic would be indicated.

For an antimicrobial agent to be useful in the treatment of pathogenic microorganisms, the following criteria should be met:
- the microorganism must be susceptible to the agent;
- the agent must be capable of penetrating to the site of the infection;
- adequate concentrations of the agent must be achieved and maintained at the site of the infection;
- the agent should be low in toxicity to the host but should exhibit selective toxicity to the microorganisms;
- the agent should not readily promote resistance or create a serious imbalance in the normal flora of the host.

This chapter focuses on the compounds that are clinically applicable for treating dental-related microbial infections and diseases; it also describes agents that dental patients may be receiving as concurrent therapy for medical conditions. It cannot provide comprehensive coverage of all available antimicrobial agents, nor can it cover every potential adverse effect that may have been directly or indirectly associated with the use of different antimicrobial agents.

The chapter is organized as follows:
- penicillins and cephalosporins;
- macrolides;
- tetracyclines;
- clindamycin;
- metronidazole;
- quinolones;
- sulfonamides.

Penicillins and Cephalosporins

Antibiotics belonging to these two classes are referred to as "β-lactam antibiotics" due to the presence of the β-lactam ring common to all drugs in these classes. These drugs are considered bactericidal because they directly result in the death of bacteria by inhibiting specific bacterial enzymes required for the assembly of the bacterial cell wall. Many of the β-lactam antibiotics are rendered inactive by the bacterial production of β-lactamase, an enzyme that hydrolyzes the β-lactam ring and renders the antibiotic inactive. The bacterial production of β-lactamase is the primary reason that treatment with penicillins or cephalosporins can fail.

The cephalosporins and the closely related cephamycins are normally listed together as a single related group and are similar to the penicillins in structure and action. Although penicillins are usually superior for treating dental-related infections, the cephalosporins/cephamycins are included in this chapter because they are frequently used in medical practice and may be encountered in patients seeking dental treatment.

Dosage information for oral administration only is provided in Table 7.2. These are the dosages more frequently recommended for the treatment of dental-related infections. Higher and more frequent oral dosages may be indicated for severe or life-threatening infections. Other semisynthetic penicillins (azlocillin, mezlocillin, piperacillin, ticarcillin, methicillin) as well as most of the cephalosporins/cephamycins (cephalothin, cephapirin, cefazolin, cefamandole, cefoxitin, cefonicid, cefotaxime, ceftizoxime, ceftazidime, cefoperazone) are available only for intramuscular or intravenous injection owing to poor oral absorption and instability in the presence of gastric acids. These are generally reserved for the treatment of severe infections and diseases that require hospitalization.

Accepted Indications

Table 7.1 lists penicillins and cephalosporins and common indications for their use.

General Dosing Information

See Table 7.2 for dosage information.

Table 7.1

Penicillins and Cephalosporins: Characteristics and Common Indications for Use

Generic name	Characteristics	Common indications for use
Penicillins		
Amoxicillin	Similar to ampicillin but yields higher serum levels More rapidly and completely absorbed from stomach than ampicillin Penetrates gingival crevicular fluid well but is hydrolyzed rapidly if significant levels of β-lactamases are present	Has same uses as ampicillin Designed specifically for oral administration
Amoxicillin/clavulanic acid	Has same properties as amoxicillin but is resistant to wide range of β-lactamases Penetrates gingival crevicular fluid well Resistant to most β-lactamases produced by oral bacteria	Broad-spectrum antibiotic with excellent activity against many β-lactamase-producing oral and nonoral bacteria
Ampicillin	Provides broad-spectrum activity against both gram-negative and gram-positive bacteria Stable to stomach acids and readily absorbed from the stomach Susceptible to β-lactamases	Broad-spectrum penicillin for use against a variety of bacteria that do not produce β-lactamase (for example, *Escherichia coli*, as well as *Neisseria, Haemophilus* and *Proteus* species)

Continued on next page

Table 7.1 (cont.)

Penicillins and Cephalosporins: Characteristics and Common Indications for Use

Generic name	Characteristics	Common indications for use
Penicillins (cont.)		
Carbenicillin indanyl	Stable to gastric acids Relatively resistant to certain β-lactamases produced by gram-negative bacteria	Indicated in the treatment of penicillin-resistant *Proteus* and *Pseudomonas* species
Cloxacillin	Relatively resistant to β-lactamases produced by *Staphylococcus aureus* but not to other bacterial β-lactamases	Use is generally limited to treatment of infections involving β-lactamase-producing staphylococcal microorganisms such as *Staphylococcus aureus*
Dicloxacillin	Same as for cloxacillin	Same as for cloxacillin
Nafcillin	Relatively stable to β-lactamase produced by *Staphylococcus aureus* Inactivated to varying degree by gastric acids Irregular absorption following oral dosage	Primarily used for treatment of infections due to *Staphylococcus aureus*
Oxacillin	Same as for cloxacillin	Same as for cloxacillin
Penicillin G benzathine suspension	Active against most gram-positive but not gram-negative bacteria Unstable to gastric acid Susceptible to β-lactamases Poor and unpredictable absorption after an oral dose, so usually given IM	Drug of choice for wide variety of serious infections, such as pneumococci, meningococcal meningitis, gonorrhea, syphilis, hemolytic streptococci, actinomycosis
Phenoxymethyl-penicillin (Penicillin V)	Activity primarily limited to gram-positive bacteria Stable to stomach acids Susceptive to β-lactamases Readily absorbed from the stomach	Use is limited to treatment of minor infections such as ulcerative gingivostomatitis, and the prophylaxis and continued treatment of streptococcal infections
Cephalosporins		
Cefaclor Cefadroxil Cefixime Cefuroxime Cephalexin Cephradine	All can be given orally Primarily excreted through the kidneys	Primary use is the treatment of urinary tract infections Most dental-related infections can be better treated with a penicillin

Table 7.2

Penicillins and Cephalosporins: Oral Dosage Information

Generic name	Brand name(s)	Usual adult dosage	Maximum adult dosage	Maximum child dosage	Pregnancy risk category	Content/form	Oral dosage suggestions
		Penicillins					
Amoxicillin	Amoxil, Polymox, Trimox	250 or 500 mg tid	4 g/day	**Weight < 20 kg:** 20-40 mg/kg in divided doses tid	B	**Tablets:** 125, 500 mg **Oral suspension:** 125, 250 mg/5 mL	Given without regard to meals
Amoxicillin/ clavulanic acid	Augmentin	250 or 500 mg tid	4.5 g/day	**Weight < 20 kg:** 20-40 mg/kg in divided doses tid	B	**Tablets:** 250, 500 mg **Oral suspension:** 125, 250 mg/5 mL	Given without regard to meals
Ampicillin	Amcill, Omnipen, Polycillin, Principen	250 or 500 mg qid	4 g/day	**Weight < 20 kg:** 100-200 mg/kg in divided doses qid	B	**Capsules:** 50, 500 mg **Oral suspension:** 125, 500 mg/5 mL	Given 1-2 h before meal
Bacampicillin	Spectrobid	400 or 800 mg bid	3.2 g/day	25-50 mg/kg in 2 divided doses	Not listed	**Tablets:** 400 mg **Oral suspension:** 125 mg/5 mL	Given without regard to meals
Carbenicillin	Geocillin	500 or 1,000 mg qid	**Solution:** 4 g/day solution **Tablets:** Not listed	Not recommended for children	Not listed	**Tablets:** 500 mg **Pediatric solution:** not available	Given without regard to meals
Cloxacillin	Cloxapen, Tegopen	250 or 500 mg qid	6 g/day	**Weight < 20 kg:** 50-100 mg/kg in 4 divided doses qid	B	**Capsules:** 250, 500 mg **Oral suspension:** 125 mg/5 mL	Given 1-2 h before meal

Continued on next page

Table 7.2 (cont.)

Penicillins and Cephalosporins: Oral Dosage Information

Generic name	Brand name(s)	Usual adult dosage	Maximum adult dosage	Maximum child dosage	Pregnancy risk category	Content/form	Oral dosage suggestions
Penicillins (cont.)							
Dicloxacillin	Dynapen, Dycill, Pathocil	250 or 500 mg qid	6 g/day	**Weight < 40 kg:** 25 mg/kg as 4 divided doses qid	B	**Capsules:** 25, 250, 500 mg **Oral suspension:** 62.5 mg/5 mL	Given 12 h before meal
Nafcillin	Unipen	250 or 500 mg qid	6 g/day	100-200 mg/kg in divided doses given q 4-6 h	Not listed	**Capsules and tablets:** 100, 250, 500 mg	Given 1 h before or 2 h after meal
Oxacillin	Bactocill, Prostaphlin	500-1,000 mg qid	6 g/day	**Weight < 20 kg:** 50-100 mg/kg administered in a single dose	B	**Capsules:** 50 or 500 mg **Oral suspension:** 250 mg/5 mL	Given 1 h before or 2 h after meal
Penicillin G benzathine suspension*	Penicillin-G, Benzylpenicillin	200,000-800,000 units qid	2,000,000 units/day (1,248 mg/day)	50,000-100,000 units/kg as 2 divided doses	B	**Tablets:** 200,000-800,000 units each	Given 1 h before or 2 h after meal
Phenoxymethyl-penicillin (Penicillin V-potassium)	Betapen-K, Pen-Vee K, Phenoxymethyl-penicillin, V-Cillin K, Veetids	250 or 500 mg qid	7.2 g/day	**Weight < 20 kg:** 50-100 mg/kg in 4 divided doses qid	B	**Tablets:** 125, 250, 500 mg **Oral suspension:** 125, 250 mg/5 mL	Given 1 h before or 2 h after meal
Cephalosporins							
Cefaclor	Ceclor	250 mg tid	4 g/day	**Weight < 20 kg:** 20 mg/kg in divided doses tid	B	**Capsules:** 250, 500 mg **Oral suspension:** 125, 375 mg/5 mL	Given without regard to meals

Cefadroxil	Duricef, Ultracef	500 mg bid or 1,000 mg/day	4 g/day	**Weight < 40 kg:** 30 mg/kg in divided doses bid	B	**Capsules:** 500 mg **Oral suspension:** 125, 500 mg/5 mL	Given without regard to meals
Cefixime	Suprax	200 mg bid or 400 mg q day	Not available	**Weight < 40 kg:** 8 mg/kg in single dose or divided doses bid	B	**Tablets:** 200, 400 mg **Oral suspension:** 100 mg/5 mL	Given without regard to meals
Cefuroxime	Ceftin	250 mg bid	Not available	**Age < 12 y:** 125 mg bid for child under 12 years of age	B	**Tablets:** 125, 250, 500 mg **Oral suspension:** Not available	Given without regard to meals
Cephalexin	Biocef, Cefanex, Keftab, Keflex	250 mg qid or 500 mg bid	4 g/day	**Weight < 40 kg:** 25-50 mg/kg in divided doses bid	B	**Tablets:** 250, 500 mg **Oral suspension:** 125, 250 mg/5mL oral suspension	Given without regard to meals
Cephradine	Anspor, Velosef	250 or 500 mg qid	4 g/day	**Weight < 40 kg:** 25-50 mg/kg in divided doses bid	B	**Capsules:** 250, 500 mg **Oral suspension:** 125, 250 mg/5mL	Given without regard to meals

* Also available as salt of potassium or sodium or in combination with procaine (parenteral only).

Dosage Adjustments

Under normal circumstances, penicillins and cephalosporins are rapidly eliminated from the body primarily through the kidneys but, in a small part, in the bile and by other routes. In the case of patients with reduced renal function, dosages should be adjusted downward relative to creatinine clearance rates in consultation with the patient's physician. In patients undergoing peritoneal dialysis, an alternative antibiotic should be considered because most penicillins and cephalosporins are effectively removed from the bloodstream by hemodialysis.

Special Dental Considerations

Drug Interactions of Dental Interest

Probenecid, when used concurrently with penicillins and cephalosporins, may decrease renal tubular secretion of these drugs; this may result in increased and prolonged antibiotic blood levels.

The concurrent use of allopurinol with ampicillin, amoxicillin or amoxicillin/clavulanic acid substantially increases the incidence of rashes in patients receiving both drugs relative to that in patients receiving the antibiotic alone.

Amoxicillin/clavulanic acid should not be coadministered with the antiabuse drug disulfiram.

Laboratory Value Alterations

- High urine concentrations of a penicillin or cephalosporin may result in false-positive reactions when the urine is tested for the presence of glucose using certain commercially available test kits.

Cross-Sensitivity

Before initiating therapy with any penicillin or cephalosporin, careful inquiry should be made concerning previous hypersensitivity reactions to any penicillin, cephalosporin, or other allergens. Serious and occasionally fatal hypersensitivity (anaphylactoid) reactions have been reported in patients receiving penicillin or cephalosporin therapy. These reactions are more apt to occur in people with a history of penicillin and/or cephalosporin hypersensitivity and/or a history of sensitivity to multiple allergens. Penicillins and cephalosporins should be used with caution in patients who have a history of significant allergies and/or asthma. Because of the similarity in the structure of the penicillins and cephalosporins, patients allergic to one class may manifest cross-reactivity to members of the other class. Cross-reactivity to cephalosporins may occur in as many as 20% of the patients who are allergic to penicillins.

Special Patients

Pregnant and nursing women

Penicillins and cephalosporins are secreted in human breast milk, and caution should be exercised when a drug from either group is administered to nursing women. Clinical experience with the penicillins and cephalosporins during pregnancy has not shown any positive evidence of adverse effects on the fetus. However, there have been no adequate and well-controlled studies in pregnant women that show conclusively that harmful effects of these drugs on the fetus can be ruled out. Therefore, penicillins and cephalosporins should be used during pregnancy only if clearly needed.

Patient Monitoring: Aspects to Watch

- Patients with a history or suspected history of hypersensitivity to a penicillin or cephalosporin: if given any antibiotic in this class, should be observed for any difficulty in breathing for a minimum of 1 h before being released

Adverse Effects and Precautions

Adverse effects, precautions and contraindications related to penicillins and cephalosporins are listed in Table 7.3.

Table 7.3

Penicillins and Cephalosporins: Adverse Effects, Precautions and Contraindications

Body system	Adverse effects	Precautions/contraindications
General	Hypersensitivity	Up to 10% of all patients may have some sensitivity or allergy
		Mild reactions are often limited to rash or skin lesions of head and neck, but may include facial swelling
		More severe reactions may involve swelling and tenderness of joints
		Hypersensitivity reactions occur more frequently in patients with infectious mononucleosis after they have been treated with ampicillin or amoxicillin
	Superinfection	Superinfection, or overgrowth by resistant bacteria or *Candida*, can occur after prolonged use or high dosage
	Direct toxicity	Rare; most likely to occur in patients who have impaired renal function or in elderly people
CNS	Varied	Reversible hyperactivity, agitation, anxiety, insomnia, confusion and/or dizziness have been reported
GI	Gastric upset	Can range from mild to severe and can include nausea, vomiting, diarrhea, gastritis, stomatitis and enterocolitis; more common with amoxicillin/clavulanic acid and the cephalosporins than with other penicillins
Resp	Anaphylactic or anaphylactoid reactions	Can cause death in highly sensitized subjects; reactions occur after administration by injection more often than by oral route

Pharmacology

Penicillins

Because penicillin absorption after oral administration is influenced by the presence of food in the stomach, more predictable blood levels can be obtained if it is given on an empty stomach. Alternatively, predictable blood levels are also seen when penicillin is given parenterally.

Once absorbed, penicillin is widely distributed throughout the body, including the saliva and gingival crevicular fluid. It does not pass the blood-brain barrier in normal patients, but during meningitis it does pass through and may be clinically effective. Penicillin is rapidly eliminated from plasma by the kidneys, crosses the placenta and has been found in cord blood and amniotic fluid.

Penicillins are excreted in breast milk

in low concentrations. Although significant problems in humans have not been documented, risk-benefit must be considered, as penicillin use by nursing mothers may lead to sensitization, diarrhea and candidiasis.

Cephalosporins

The cephalosporins pass into most body fluids and tissues in adequate levels to allow their use in the treatment of most infections. They can also pass through the placenta and occur in small amounts in the milk of lactating mothers. Most cephalosporins are excreted unchanged in the urine.

Patient Advice

- In case of the development of any adverse effect (rash; nausea; vomiting; diarrhea; swelling of lips, tongue or face; fever and so forth), the patient should be advised to stop taking the medication and promptly inform the dentist.

Macrolides

The macrolide group of antibiotics contains approximately 40 different compounds, but only a limited few have clinical use. Erythromycin has generally been the most effective and is widely used as an alternative to penicillins for the treatment and prevention of infections caused by gram-positive microorganisms. Clarithromycin, a semisynthetic macrolide antibiotic, is similar to erythromycin, but has a broader spectrum of activity. Both antibiotics have good activity against most gram-positive bacteria associated with the mouth. Unlike erythromycin, clarithromycin has relatively good activity against a number of gram-negative bacteria.

In recent years, a novel class of antibiotics called the azalides has surfaced. These new macrolide derivatives appear superior to erythromycin and clarithromycin in that they offer better pharmacokinetic properties, excellent tissue distribution, longer therapeutic half-life and activity against many gram-negative and gram-positive bacteria. Of the azalides, azithromycin has received extensive clinical use.

Accepted Indications

Erythromycin, clarithromycin and azithromycin are indicated in the treatment of mild-to-moderate infections involving the upper and lower respiratory tract and for uncomplicated skin and skin structure infections due to susceptible strains of *Staphylococcus aureus, Streptococcus pyogenes,* or *Streptococcus agalactiae* (see Table 7.4). These drugs are indicated as an alternate in patients with hypersensitivity to penicillins. Azithromycin is not indicated for use in individuals under 16 years of age or in the treatment of patients with pneumonia who are judged to be inappropriate for outpatient oral therapy.

General Dosing Information

See Table 7.5 for dosage information.

Dosage Adjustments

Erythromycin and azithromycin are principally eliminated from the body via the liver. Therefore, dosages and/or the dosage interval should be adjusted when these drugs are administered to a patient with impaired hepatic function. Clarithromycin is eliminated via the liver and kidney and may be administered without dosage adjustment in patients with hepatic impairment and normal renal function. However, in the presence of severe renal impairment with or without coexisting hepatic impairment, decreased dosage or prolonged dosage intervals may be appropriate.

Special Dental Considerations

Drug Interactions of Dental Interest

Concomitant use of erythromycin with certain other drugs, such as theophylline, oral anticoagulants or digoxin, can result in

Table 7.4

Macrolides: Characteristics and Common Indications for Use

Generic name	Characteristics	Common indications for use
Azithromycin	Broad spectrum of activity for both gram-positive and gram-negative bacteria Given once daily	Indicated in the treatment of patients aged ≤ 16 y who have mild-to-moderate infections
Clarithromycin	Active against gram-positive and many gram-negative bacteria	Treatment of mild-to-moderate respiratory infections and uncomplicated skin infections
Erythromycin base	Active against gram-positive bacteria, particularly gram-positive cocci Provides only limited activity against gram-negative bacteria Yields irregular and unpredictable serum levels Given during a fasting state	Treatment of upper and lower respiratory tract, skin and soft tissue infections of mild-to-moderate severity Alternative to penicillin G and other penicillins for treatment of gram-positive coccoid infections in patients with hypersensitivity to penicillins
Erythromycin ethylsuccinate	Activity same as for erythromycin base	Uses same as for erythromycin base
Erythromycin stearate	Activity same as for erythromycin base Less subject to gastric acids than erythromycin base Yields more predictable serum levels	Uses same as for erythromycin base

elevated serum levels for these drugs and may, in the case of theophylline, lead to toxicity. The use of erythromycin in patients receiving carbamazepine, cyclosporine, hexobarbital or phenytoin may result in elevated serum levels of erythromycin. The concurrent use of erythromycin and ergotamine or dihydroergotamine has been associated with acute ergot toxicity in some patients. Erythromycin has been reported to decrease the clearance rate of triazolam and may increase the pharmacological effect of this drug. Although the above effects have not been reported in clinical trials with azithromycin or clarithromycin, specific drug-to-drug interaction studies have not been performed. Therefore, caution should be exercised when either azithromycin or clarithromycin is used concomitantly with any of the above drugs.

Aluminum- and magnesium-containing antacids reduce the peak serum levels obtained with azithromycin.

Concurrent use with ampicillin, gentamicin and cefamanadole can antagonize the action of these drugs. Concurrent use with clindamycin is contraindicated because of similar modes of action.

Laboratory Value Alterations

• There are no reported laboratory test

Table 7.5

Macrolides: Oral Dosage Information

Generic name	Brand name(s)	Usual adult dosage	Maximum adult dosage	Maximum child dosage	Pregnancy risk category	Content/form	Oral dosage suggestions
Azithromycin	Zithromax	500 mg initial loading dose, followed by single dose of 250 mg/day	Not listed	Age < 16 y: Safety not clearly established for children	B	**Capsules:** 250 mg	Given 1 h before or 2 h after meal
Clarithromycin	Biaxin	250 or 500 mg bid	Not listed	Age < 12 y: Safety not established	C	**Tablets:** 250, 500 mg	May be given without regard to meals
Erythromycin base	E-Mycin, Ery-Tab, Erythromycin Base Filmtab	250 mg qid	4 g/day	30-50 mg/kg in divided doses qid	B	**Tablets:** 250, 500 mg	Given 1 h before or 2 h after meal
Erythromycin ethylsuccinate	E.E.S., Pediamycin, Eryped, Erythro	400 mg qid	4 g/day	30-50 mg/kg in divided doses qid	B	**Tablets:** 400 mg **Oral suspension:** 200, 400 mg/ 5 mL	May be given without regard to meals
Erythromycin stearate	Erypar, Erythrocin, Erythrocot	250 mg qid	4 g/day	30-50 mg/kg in divided doses qid	B	**Tablets:** 250, 500 mg	Given 1 h before or 2 h after meal

alterations for azithromycin or clarithromycin.

- Erythromycin interferes with the fluorometric determination of urinary catecholamines.

Cross-Sensitivity

Erythromycin, azithromycin or clarithromycin are contraindicated in patients with known hypersensitivity to any of the macrolide antibiotics.

Special Patients

Pregnant and nursing women

Clarithromycin should not be used in pregnant women except in clinical circumstances in which no alternative therapy is appropriate. If pregnancy occurs while taking the drug, the patient should be advised of the potential hazard to the fetus. Although no evidence of impaired fertility or harm to the fetus has been found with either erythromycin or azithromycin, these drugs should be used during pregnancy only if needed.

Erythromycin is secreted in human breast milk and should be used with caution in nursing mothers. As it is not known if either clarithromycin or azithromycin are secreted in human breast milk, the same cautions should be applied to these drugs as well.

Pediatric, geriatric and other special patients

The safety of clarithromycin has not been established for children aged < 12 y, and the safety of azithromycin has not been established for children and youths aged < 16 y.

Dosage adjustment does not appear to be necessary in elderly patients who have normal renal and hepatic function.

Adverse Effects and Precautions

Serious adverse effects are rarely encountered with these drugs. The majority of the side-effects associated with erythromycin, azithromycin and clarithromycin have been of a mild and transient nature. The most frequently reported events have been diarrhea, nausea, abnormal taste, dyspepsia, abdominal pain/discomfort and headache (see Table 7.6).

Pharmacology

The macrolides inhibit bacterial protein synthesis by binding reversibly to the 50S ribosomal subunits of sensitive bacteria. Erythromycin base is incompletely absorbed from the upper part of the small intestine. The drug is inactivated by gastric acid and is thus administered as protected tablets or capsules that dissolve in the duodenum. Food in the stomach delays the drug's ultimate absorption. The esters of erythromycin, erythromycin stearate and ethylsuccinate provide greater stability and facilitate absorption. Both clarithromycin and azithromycin are better absorbed than erythromycin and yield higher serum levels.

Table 7.6

Macrolides: Adverse Effects, Precautions and Contraindications

Body system	Adverse effects	Precautions/contraindications
General	Shifts in oral flora and possible colonization by exogenous organisms may occur during oral therapy Allergic reactions are rare, but can be manifested as skin rashes Epigastric distress most common side effect	Erythromycin, azithromycin and clarithromycin cross the placenta, and erythromycin and azithromycin should be given during pregnancy with caution; clarithromycin should not be given during pregnancy due to potential adverse effects to fetus Erythromycin, and most likely azithromycin and clarithromycin, are secreted in human breast milk and should be given to nursing mothers with caution Azithromycin is not approved for youths under 16 years and clarithromycin is not approved for children under 12 years
CV	Heart palpitations, chest pain (both extremely rare)	Use with caution in patients with history of cardiac arrhythmias; consider alternate antibiotic
CNS	Dizziness, headache, vertigo (extremely rare)	Transient hearing loss has been associated with large doses of erythromycin in patients with renal impairment
GI	Nausea, vomiting, abdominal pain and diarrhea (all relatively common but rarely severe)	Dose-related, more common in children and young adults
GU	Vaginitis (extremely rare)	More common in patients with history of antibiotic-associated vaginitis
HB	Hepatotoxicity Nephritis (extremely rare)	Caution should be exercised if administrated to patients with impaired hepatic function Cholestatic hepatitis may occur with erythromycin estolate but rarely with other forms

The macrolides diffuse readily into intracellular fluids, and antibacterial activity can be achieved at essentially all body sites with the exception of the brain and cerebrospinal fluid.

Patient Advice

- Any of these drugs may cause gastric discomfort and may result in diarrhea, abdominal cramping, nausea, unpleasant taste and/or headache.
- Clarithromycin may have adverse effects on fetal development and should not be taken by pregnant patients; use of this drug should be immediately stopped if pregnancy occurs.

Tetracyclines

The tetracyclines, which include tetracycline, doxycycline and minocycline, all have essentially the same spectrum of activity. They are considered to be bacteriostatic at normal dosages and inhibit bacterial protein synthesis in sensitive bacteria by binding to the 30S ribosomal subunits and preventing the addition of amino acids to the growing peptide chain. At high concentrations, the tetracyclines are bactericidal for bacterial cells and may inhibit protein synthesis in mammalian cells.

The advantage of using either doxycycline or minocycline, rather than tetracycline, is that the former two antibiotics are absorbed better after oral administration. This greater absorption results in higher serum levels and a lesser need for frequent dosing. Unfortunately, resistance to one tetracycline often indicates resistance to all tetracyclines.

Accepted Indications

The tetracyclines are broad-spectrum antibiotics and as such are frequently indicated in the treatment of gram-positive and gram-negative bacterial infections of the head and neck as well as other regions of the body (see Table 7.7). Dental applications include the adjunctive treatment of refractory periodontitis

and juvenile periodontitis, dental abscesses, soft tissue abscesses, and as an alternative when penicillins are contraindicated or when β-lactamase-producing microorganisms are involved. Due to bacterial resistance, the tetracyclines are not indicated in the treatment of streptococcal or staphylococcal infections.

Resistance to tetracycline-HCl has become so widespread that this drug is rarely used in clinical medicine. However, the drug still appears to be beneficial in the treatment of certain dental infections, including periodontitis, that do not respond favorably to conventional periodontal therapy.

General Dosing Information

See Table 7.8 for dosage information.

Dosage Adjustments

Because tetracyclines have been shown to depress plasma prothrombin activity, patients receiving anticoagulant therapy may require downward adjustment of the anticoagulant dosage.

If renal impairment exists, the recommended doses for any tetracycline may lead to excessive systemic accumulation of the antibiotic and, possibly, liver toxicity. The antianabolic action of the tetracyclines may cause an increase in blood urea nitrogen. In patients with significant renal insufficiency, this may lead to azotemia, hyperphosphatemia and acidosis. Total dosages of any tetracycline should therefore be decreased in patients with renal impairment by reduction of recommended individual doses and/or by extending the time between doses.

Special Dental Considerations

Drug Interactions of Dental Interest

As described above, the tetracyclines may depress plasma prothrombin activity and should be used with caution in patients receiving anticoagulant therapy.

The concurrent use of tetracycline and methoxyflurane has been reported to result in fatal renal toxicity.

Because bacteriostatic antibiotics such as the tetracyclines may interfere with the bactericidal action of penicillins and cephalosporins, it is not advisable to administer these antibiotics concomitantly.

Concurrent use of tetracyclines with oral contraceptives may render the contraceptives less effective.

Divalent cations bind the tetracyclines to different degrees. Therefore, bismuth subsalicylate and antacids containing aluminum, calcium or magnesium interfere with the absorption of these antibiotics and should not be ingested at the same time as a tetracycline.

Laboratory Value Alterations
- False elevations of urinary catecholamine levels may occur due to interference with the fluorescence test.

Cross-Sensitivity
A hypersensitivity or allergic reaction to one tetracycline is indicative of hypersensitivity to all other tetracyclines.

Special Patients
Pregnant and nursing women
All tetracyclines cross the placenta and form a stable calcium complex in bone-forming tissue. This can have toxic effects on the developing fetus and result in the retardation of skeletal development. Evidence of embryotoxicity has also been noted. Therefore, tetracyclines should not be administered to pregnant women or to women who intend to become pregnant.

Tetracyclines are secreted in breast milk and should not be administered to nursing mothers because the antibiotics are deposited in growing bone plates and the developing teeth.

Pediatric, geriatric and other special patients
Tetracycline drugs should not be used in children aged ≤ 8 y because these drugs may cause permanent discoloration of the teeth.

In brief, tetracyclines should not be administered for dental purposes to any children 8 years or younger, to pregnant or nursing women or to women taking oral

Table 7.7
Tetracyclines: Characteristics and Common Indications for Use

Generic name	Characteristics	Common indications for use
Doxycycline hyclate	Has the same characteristics as tetracycline except that it is absorbed more completely following oral administration and yields higher serum levels	Uses same as for tetracycline (below)
Minocycline hydrochloride	Has the same characteristics as tetracycline except that it is absorbed more completely following oral administration and yields higher serum levels More lipophilic than doxycycline and provides better tissue penetration	Uses same as for tetracycline (below)
Tetracycline hydrochloride	Broad-spectrum antibiotic with activity against gram-positive and gram-negative bacteria, mycoplasmas, rickettsial and chlamydial infections	Adjunctive treatment of adult periodontitis and juvenile periodontitis Treatment of acute necrotizing ulcerative gingivitis and dental abscesses Alternative to penicillins for treatment of actinomycosis and other oral infections

Table 7.8

Tetracyclines: Oral Dosage Information

Generic name	Brand name(s)	Usual adult dosage	Maximum adult dosage	Maximum child dosage	Pregnancy risk category	Content/form	Oral dosage suggestions
Doxycycline hyclate	Doryx, Doxycin, Doxylin, Monodox, Vibramycin, Vibra-tabs	100 mg bid on 1st day, followed by 100 mg/day as either single dose or 50 mg bid	300 mg/day	**Age > 8 y:** 4 mg/kg divided into equal doses bid on 1st day, followed by 2 mg/kg as single dose or divided into equal doses bid	D	**Capsules:** 50, 100 mg **Oral suspension:** 25 or 50 mg/5 mL	Given 1 h before or 2 h after meal
Minocycline hydrochloride	Dynacin, Minocin	200 mg loading dose, followed by 100 mg bid	350 mg on 1st day, then 200 mg/day	**Age > 8 y:** 4 mg/kg initially followed by 2 mg/kg bid	D	**Capsules:** 50, 100 mg **Oral suspension:** 50 mg/5 mL	Given 1 h before or 2 h after meal
Tetracycline hydrochloride	Achromycin, Achromycin V, Sumycin	250 mg qid	4 g/day	**Age > 8 y:** 25-50 mg/kg in equal doses bid	D	**Capsules:** 250, 500 mg **Oral suspension:** 125 mg/5 mL	Given 1 h before or 2 h after meal

contraceptives. An alternative antibiotic should be used in place of a tetracycline.

Adverse Effects and Precautions

The adverse effects of and precautions and contraindications related to the tetracyclines are listed in Table 7.9.

Pharmacology

The tetracyclines are readily absorbed from the gastrointestinal tract following oral administration. Most of the absorption takes place in the stomach and upper small intestine and is greater in the fasting state. The tetracyclines are distributed throughout the body and readily penetrate soft tissues, the CNS and the brain. The drugs readily cross the placenta and enter the fetal circulation and amniotic fluid. Relatively high concentrations are also present in breast milk. The drugs are stored in the reticuloendothelial cells of the liver, spleen and bone marrow, and in the bone, dentin and enamel of unerupted teeth.

Excretion is via the urine and feces; the primary route is the kidneys. However, renal clearance of minocycline is much lower than tetracycline and persists in the body long after

Table 7.9
Tetracyclines: Adverse Effects, Precautions and Contraindications

Body system	Adverse effects	Precautions/contraindications
General	Benign intracranial hypertension	Manifested as headache and blurred vision
CNS	Dizziness, vertigo and tinnitus may occur with minocycline	Avoid operating vehicles or hazardous machinery
GI	Nausea, heartburn, epigastric pain, vomiting and diarrhea relatively common with oral administration Superinfection or overgrowth of intestinal flora by tetracycline-resistant organisms	Avoid taking medication immediately before bedtime to help alleviate symptoms of epigastric distress and heartburn
HB	Mild leukopenia	Should not be used when patients are taking anticoagulants such as coumarin, heparin and protoamine because of depressed plasma prothrombin; use with these anticoagulants could require downward adjustment of the anticoagulant
Integ	Maculopapular and erythematous rashes Photosensitivity	Avoid direct sunlight if possible Stop dosage if skin erythema occurs Use of sunscreen may be recommended
Oral	Deposits in the calcifying areas of the bones and teeth and permanent discoloration when administered to children aged < 8 y Superinfection or overgrowth of oral flora by tetracycline-resistant organisms	Do not administer to children aged < 8 y, during pregnancy or to nursing mothers Minocycline may produce a grayish pigmentation in gingiva and may discolor permanent, erupted teeth
Renal	Increase in blood urea nitrogen	Adjusted dosages required if renal impairment exists

administration is stopped. Doxycycline is not eliminated by the same pathways as are the other tetracyclines and does not accumulate significantly in the blood of patients with renal failure.

Patient Advice

- Photosensitivity manifested by an exaggerated sunburn may occur in patients taking tetracyclines. Patients apt to be exposed to direct light or ultraviolet light should be advised that this reaction can occur and that the dosage should be discontinued at the first evidence of skin erythema. This reaction is relatively rare with minocycline.
- Patients who experience central nervous system symptoms should be cautioned against driving vehicles or operating hazardous machinery while taking minocyclines.
- Concurrent use of tetracyclines may render oral contraceptives less effective.
- If patients are taking calcium-containing products, iron or antacids, they should not be given tetracyclines, with the exception of doxycycline.

Clindamycin

Clindamycin is the single member of this antibiotic family that is clinically used. Although not structurally related to erythromycin, it shares the same mode of action in that it binds to the 50S ribosomal subunits and inhibits bacterial protein synthesis in sensitive organisms. Clindamycin is relatively active against gram-positive and gram-negative anaerobic bacteria, including most of those associated with the mouth. Essentially, all gram-negative aerobic bacteria are resistant.

Accepted Indications

Clindamycin is generally reserved for the treatment of serious infections of the respiratory tract, skin and soft tissue, female genital tract, intra-abdominal infections and abscesses, and septicemia involving gram-positive and/or gram-negative anaerobes, streptococci, staphylococci, and mixed infections involving anaerobes and facultative gram-positive bacteria. See Table 7.10.

General Dosing Information

See Table 7.11 for dosage information.

Dosage Adjustments

In patients with severe renal and/or hepatic impairment, clindamycin should be administered only for very severe infections, with the dosages and dosage intervals adjusted accordingly.

Special Dental Considerations

Drug Interactions of Dental Interest

Clindamycin has been shown to have neuromuscular blocking properties that may enhance the action of other neuromuscular blocking agents and should be used with caution in patients receiving such agents.

Table 7.10

Clindamycin: Characteristics and Common Indications for Use

Generic name	Characteristics	Common indications for use
Clindamycin hydrochloride	Active against most gram-positive bacteria including many staphylococcal and streptococcal species Excellent activity against both gram-positive and gram-negative anaerobic bacteria	Treatment of severe infections caused by anaerobic bacteria Adjunct to treatment of adult refractory periodontitis

Table 7.11
Clindamycin: Oral Dosage Information

Generic name	Brand name(s)	Usual adult dosage	Maximum adult dosage	Maximum child dosage	Pregnancy risk category	Content/form	Oral dosage suggestions
Clindamycin hydrochloride	Cleocin HCl, Cleocin Pediatric	150-300 mg qid	1.8 g/24 h	8-12 mg/kg/day in 3-4 equally divided doses	B	**Capsules:** 75, 150, 300 mg **Oral suspension:** 75 mg/5 mL	Given without regard to meals

Cross-Sensitivity

There are no cross-sensitivities reported between clindamycin and any other antibiotic group. However, the 75- and 150-mg capsules of clindamycin-HCl contain FD&C Yellow no. 5 (tartrazine), which may cause allergic reactions in some patients with hypersensitivity to aspirin.

Special Patients

Pregnant and nursing women

Clindamycin is secreted in breast milk in sufficient concentrations to cause disturbances of the intestinal flora of infants and should not be administered to nursing mothers unless warranted by severe clinical circumstances. Jaundice and abnormalities in liver function tests also may occur.

The safety of clindamycin for use during pregnancy has not been established.

Pediatric, geriatric and other special patients

Clindamycin should not be administered to older patients who have an associated severe illness that may render them more susceptible to diarrhea.

The drug should be administered with caution to any patient with a history of gastrointestinal disease, particularly colitis, or to a patient with severe renal disease and/or severe hepatic disease.

Adverse Effects and Precautions

Any broad-spectrum antibiotic therapy may result in the disturbance of the normal intestinal flora and lead to colonization by the opportunistic pathogen *Clostridium difficile*.

This may result in a severe form of colitis, referred to as "pseudomembraneous colitis," which can be fatal. The disease may begin during therapy or it may be delayed for several weeks after the cessation of therapy. Although the disease can occur following therapy with a number of antibiotics, its incidence has been higher after the use of the intravenous form of clindamycin (clindamycin phosphate). However, it has been reported to occur after the use of oral clindamycin hydrochloride as well. Therefore, the drug should always be used with caution and reserved for severe infections that are not amenable to other therapy.

Pharmacology

Clindamycin is nearly completely absorbed from the stomach after oral administration and the absorption is not appreciably influenced by the presence of food. The drug is widely distributed to many fluids and tissues, including bone. However, significant concentrations are not obtained in the cerebrospinal fluid even if the meninges are inflamed. The drug readily crosses the placental barrier and enters the fetal circulation. Clindamycin concentrates in the polymorphonuclear leukocytes and alveolar macrophages and in soft tissue abscesses.

The drug is excreted in the urine and the feces. Antimicrobial activity may persist in the colonic contents for up to 1 w after therapy is stopped, and the growth of sensitive microorganisms in the colon may be suppressed for up to 2 w.

Table 7.12
Clindamycin: Adverse Effects, Precautions and Contraindications

Body system	Adverse effects	Precautions/contraindications
General	Generalized mild-to-moderate skin rashes due to hypersensitivity to clindamycin (appear in up to 10% of patients) Hypersensitivity reactions to tartrazine, yellow dye present in some clindamycin capsules (can occur in patients who are allergic to aspirin)	Should be discontinued if hypersensitivity reaction occurs Should be used with caution in patients with aspirin hypersensitivity
GI	Diarrhea, abdominal pain, esophagitis and stomach irritation are relatively common Pseudomembranous colitis has been associated with parenteral administration of clindamycin but rarely with oral administration (incidence of PMC varies from 0.01%-10.00% and appears more frequently in elderly people and patients with previous history of colitis)	Oral dosages should be taken with food and a full glass of water to help prevent stomach irritation Drug should be discontinued if diarrhea persists and patient immediately referred to a physician
HB	Jaundice and abnormalities in liver function tests have occurred	Use with caution in patients with history of liver disorders; for long-term therapy, monitor liver function tests

Patient Advice

- Dosage should be stopped in the case of persistent diarrhea or severe abdominal pain, or if blood appears in the stool.
- Dosage should be stopped in the event of a skin rash, as this may indicate hypersensitivity to the drug.

Metronidazole

Metronidazole was initially introduced in the 1960s as a treatment for trichomonal vaginitis. The observation that the drug also had a beneficial effect on acute ulcerative gingivitis led to studies culminating in its use in the treatment of anaerobic bacterial infections. Indeed, the drug is still used in the treatment of infections caused by anaerobic protozoa. However, its primary use is in the treatment of obligate anaerobic bacteria associated with the mouth, the intestinal tract and the female genital tract.

Metronidazole has been used with considerable success as an adjunct to the treatment of periodontitis; this probably is related to its high activity against the gram-negative anaerobic bacilli that are often associated with the disease. The concurrent oral administration of metronidazole with either amoxicillin or amoxicillin/clavulanic acid has been used with some success in the treatment of both juvenile and adult forms of periodontitis. The combination of metronidazole and amoxicillin has been reported to be particularly effective in the treatment of *Actinobacillus actinomycetemcomitans*-associated periodontitis.

Metronidazole has been used in combination with both amoxicillin and amoxicillin/clavulanic acid for the adjunctive treatment of juvenile periodontitis in those in their late teens and young adults and in the treatment of refractory periodontitis that has not responded favorably to other forms of periodontal therapy. The dosages used for these combination therapies have usually consisted of 250 mg of metronidazole and 250 mg of amoxicillin or amoxicillin/clavulanic acid given concurrently at 8-h intervals (tid) for a period of 7 to 10 days.

Note: The combined use of metronidazole with amoxicillin or amoxicillin/clavulanic acid has not been approved by the Food and Drug Administration in this country.

Accepted Indications

Metronidazole is generally reserved for the treatment of serious infections of the lower respiratory tract, skin and soft tissue, female genital tract, intra-abdominal infections and abscesses, bones and joints, and bacterial septicemia involving obligate gram-positive anaerobic cocci, gram-negative anaerobic bacilli and *Clostridium* species.

The drug is indicated in the treatment of symptomatic and asymptomatic trichomoniasis in both females and males and in the treatment of amebic dysentery.

Metronidazole is indicated in the treatment of antibiotic-associated colitis and in pseudomembraneous colitis due to infection by *Clostridium difficile* (see Table 7.13).

General Dosing Information

See Table 7.14 for dosage information.

Dosage Adjustments

Patients with severe hepatic disease or impairment metabolize metronidazole slowly, with a resultant accumulation in the plasma. For such patients, the drug should be given with caution and the dosages adjusted downward from those normally given. However, for patients receiving renal dialysis, adjustment is not necessary because metronidazole is rapidly removed by dialysis.

In elderly patients, the pharmacokinetics of the drug may be altered and monitoring of serum levels may be necessary to adjust the dosage.

Table 7.13
Metronidazole: Characteristics and Common Indications for Use

Generic name	Characteristics	Common indications for use
Metronidazole	Antibacterial activity against all anaerobic cocci and both gram-negative bacilli and gram-positive spore-forming bacilli Nonsporulating gram-positive bacilli are often resistant as are most facultative bacteria	Indicated in treatment of trichomoniasis, amebiasis and giardiasis as well as a variety of infections caused by obligate anaerobic bacteria Indicated in treatment of obligate anaerobic bacterial infections associated with mouth, intestinal tract and female genital tract Has been used as adjunct in treatment of periodontitis

Table 7.14
Metronidazole: Oral Dosage Information

Generic name	Brand name(s)	Maximum adult dosage	Usual adult dosage	Maximum child dosage	Pregnancy risk category	Content/form	Oral dosage suggestions
Metronidazole	Flagyl, Protostat	4 g/day	250 mg tid-qid	Not recommended for children	B	Tablets: 250, 500 mg Oral suspension: Not available	Given without regard to meals

Special Dental Considerations

Drug Interactions of Dental Interest

Metronidazole has been reported to potentiate the anticoagulant effect of warfarin and other oral coumarin anticoagulants, resulting in a prolongation of prothrombin time.

The simultaneous administration of drugs that induce microsomal liver enzymes or enzyme activity—such as phenytoin, phenobarbital, or cimetidine—may affect the clearance rate of metronidazole.

In patients stabilized on relatively high doses of lithium, short-term metronidazole therapy has been associated with the elevation of serum lithium and, in some cases, with signs of lithium toxicity.

Abdominal cramping, nausea, vomiting, headache and flushing may occur if alcoholic beverages are consumed during the period of metronidazole administration.

Metronidazole should not be given to patients who are presently taking or have taken in the past 2 w the antiabuse drug disulfiram, since psychotic reactions have been reported when the two drugs are taken concurrently.

Laboratory Value Alterations

- Metronidazole may interfere with certain types of determination of serum chemistry values, and values of 0 may be obtained for aspartate transaminase (AST), serum glutamic-oxaloacetic transaminase (SGOT), alanine amino transferase (ALT), serum glutamate pyruvate transaminase (SGPT), lactic dehydrogenase (LDH), triglycerides and/or hexokinase glucose.

Cross-Sensitivity

Metronidazole is contraindicated in patients with a history of hypersensitivity to metronidazole or any other nitroimidazole derivative.

Special Patients

Pregnant and nursing women

Because of the potential for tumorigenicity in animal studies and because metronidazole passes the placental barrier and is secreted in breast milk, the drug should not be given to either pregnant women or nursing mothers.

Pediatric, geriatric and other special patients

As the pharmacokinetics of metronidazole may be altered in elderly patients, the drug should be given with caution and only when an alternative antibiotic is not available.

The safety and effectiveness of metronidazole has not been established in children except for the treatment of amebiasis.

Patients with Crohn's disease should not be treated with metronidazole, as the drug may potentiate the tendency for the formation of gastrointestinal and certain extraintestinal cancers.

Patient Monitoring: Aspects to Watch

- In elderly patients or patients with severe hepatic disease or impairment: drug serum levels (to avoid toxicity)

Adverse Effects and Precautions

Several serious adverse reactions have been associated with the use of metronidazole (see Table 7.15). The most serious have been convulsive seizures and peripheral neuropathy, the latter being characterized by numbness or paresthesia of an extremity. Patients should be specifically warned about these reactions and told to stop taking the drug if any neurological symptoms should occur.

The most common adverse effects involve the gastrointestinal tract. Nausea has been reported in approximately 12% of the patients receiving the drug. This may be accompanied by headache, anorexia and, occasionally, vomiting, diarrhea, epigastric distress and abdominal cramping.

Pharmacology

Metronidazole is usually completely and promptly absorbed after oral administration and achieves therapeutic levels in the serum about 1 h after the first dosage. The drug is readily distributed throughout the body and penetrates well into body tissues and fluids, including vaginal secretions, saliva, breast

Table 7.15

Metronidazole: Adverse Effects, Precautions and Contraindications

Body system	Adverse effects	Precautions/contraindications
General	Nasal congestion, fever, decrease of libido, fleeting joint pains	None of significance to dentistry
CNS	Convulsive seizures, peripheral neuropathy, dizziness, vertigo, ataxia, confusion, irritability, depression, weakness and insomnia	Dosage should be stopped immediately if any neurological symptoms occur
GI	Nausea possibly accompanied by headache, anorexia, vomiting, diarrhea and abdominal cramps (experienced by approximately 12% of patients)	Symptoms of nausea are common and may be lessened if medication is taken at meals
GU	Dysuria, cystitis, polyuria, incontinence and sense of pelvic pressure Urine may be darkened	Use with caution in patients with history of kidney disorders
Oral	Sharp, unpleasant metallic taste is not uncommon Furry tongue, glossitis and stomatis may occur and are associated with sudden overgrowth of *Candida* Dryness of mouth	Unpleasant taste may be lessened somewhat if medication is taken with food

milk and cerebrospinal fluid. In pregnancy, the drug passes the placental barrier and enters the fetal circulation.

The liver is the same site for the metabolism of metronidazole and accounts for more than 50% of the systemic clearance. However, unchanged metronidazole and its metabolites are excreted in various proportions in the urine.

Patient Advice

- Patients should be informed of the adverse effects that have been associated with taking metronidazole. Approximately 12% of patients will probably experience nausea with or without an accompanying headache and possibly other gastrointestinal symptoms. A sharp, unpleasant, metallic taste may also occur.
- The use of alcoholic beverages while taking the drug or within a day of cessation of the drug may result in abdominal distress, nausea, vomiting and/or headache.

- As convulsive seizures and peripheral neuropathy have occurred in patients treated with metronidazole, patients should be instructed to immediately stop taking the drug and contact the dentist if any neurological symptoms such as dizziness, vertigo, ataxia, confusion, depression, weakness or insommia occur.

Quinolones

The quinolones are a group of 1,8-naphthyridine derivatives that are not chemically related to any other antibacterial agents. These are synthetically produced drugs and therefore are not true antibiotics, because they are not the by-product of microorganisms. Nalidixic acid, which was introduced into clinical use in 1964, is the prototype of the quinolone drugs. A number of other drugs, chemically similar to nalidixic acid but with an improved antibacterial spectrum, have been synthesized. These can be divided into the older quinolones, such as nalidixic acid, which have limited antibacterial activity, and the newer second-generation quinolones. The latter have a much broader spectrum of activity and only recently have become clinically available.

Ciprofloxacin, a fluorinated quinolone carboxylic derivative, is an example of the newer drugs and is currently the most frequently used quinolone. This antimicrobial agent has excellent activity against a wide range of gram-negative organisms, including many that are resistant to third-generation cephalosporins, broad-spectrum penicillins and the newer semisynthetic aminoglycosides. It also produces good activity against gram-positive bacteria and is particularly useful for managing mixed infections. However, most anaerobic bacteria, including those of the mouth, are resistant to the drug. It is very likely that a number of patients coming for dental treatment will be taking ciprofloxacin; fortunately, this drug reportedly does not cross-react with most antibiotics. In fact, it has been reported to have an additive effect with antibiotics such as the β-lactams, aminoglycosides, clindamycin and metronidazole.

Accepted Indications

Ciprofloxacin is indicated in the treatment of infections caused by aerobic or facultative gram-negative rods or by *Staphylococcus aureus*, *Staphylococcus epidermidis*, *Streptococcus pyogenes* or *Streptococcus faecalis* that involve the lower respiratory tract, the skin and skin structures, the bones and joints and the urinary tract. The drug is also indicated in the treatment of infectious diarrhea caused by enterotoxigenic strains of *Escherichia coli*, or by *Campylobacter jejuni* or *Shigella* species. The drug is not indicated in the treatment of infections caused by obligate anaerobic bacteria. See Table 7.16.

General Dosing Information

See Table 7.17 for dosage information.

Dosage Adjustments

In patients who have impaired renal clearance and are not undergoing renal dialysis, dosage intervals should be adjusted based on serum creatinine levels. For patients who are undergoing renal dialysis, dosages of 250-500 mg should be given either q day or should be based on serum creatinine levels.

For patients with changing renal function or for patients with both renal and hepatic insufficiency, adjusted dosages should be based on serum concentrations of ciprofloxacin.

Special Dental Considerations

Drug Interactions of Dental Interest

Concurrent administration of ciprofloxacin with theophylline may lead to elevated serum concentrations of theophylline and substantially increase the risk of theophylline-associated adverse reactions. Serious and fatal reactions have occurred in patients receiving these two drugs together.

Table 7.16

Ciprofloxacin: Characteristics and Common Indications for Use

Generic name	Characteristics	Common indications for use
Ciprofloxacin	Bactericidal Broad spectrum of activity against both gram-positive and gram-negative bacteria Inactive against most anaerobic bacteria	Indicated in treatment of infections of the lower respiratory tract, skin, bone and joints, and urinary tract and for the treatment of infectious diarrhea

Ciprofloxacin has been shown to interfere with the metabolism of caffeine. This may lead to reduced clearance of caffeine and the prolongation of its effects, particularly in people sensitive to caffeine.

Concurrent administration with antacids containing magnesium, aluminum or calcium or with divalent and trivalent cations such as iron may substantially interfere with the absorption of ciprofloxacin. To a lesser extent, this effect is observed with multivitamins containing zinc.

Ciprofloxacin has been reported to enhance the effects of the anticoagulant warfarin and its derivatives. If it is necessary to administer these drugs concomitantly, prothrombin time should be monitored.

In patients receiving cyclosporine, ciprofloxacin may result in transient elevations of serum creatinine.

Due to the risk of seizures and convulsions, ciprofloxacin should be used with extreme caution in patients with known or suspected CNS disorders, such as severe cerebral arteriosclerosis, epilepsy or other factors that predispose people to seizures.

Cross-Sensitivity

A history of hypersensitivity to ciprofloxacin or to any other quinolone is a contraindication to its use.

Special Patients

Pregnant and nursing women

The safety and effectiveness of ciprofloxacin in pregnant or lactating women has not been established. The drug should be used during pregnancy only if the potential benefit justifies the potential risk to the fetus.

Ciprofloxacin is excreted in human milk. Due to the potential for serious adverse reactions in nursing infants, nursing should be discontinued if it is necessary to administer ciprofloxacin to the mother.

Pediatric, geriatric and other special patients

The safety and effectiveness of ciprofloxacin in children and adolescents aged < 18 y has not been established.

Patient Monitoring: Aspects to Watch

Serum creatinine levels should be monitored in patients receiving ciprofloxacin who have severe renal impairment.

Due to the potential for serious adverse reactions, serum levels of theophylline should be monitored closely if it is necessary to administer ciprofloxacin to patients receiving theophylline.

Adverse Effects and Precautions

Adverse effects that were thought to be probably or possibly related to ciprofloxacin therapy have been reported in 16% of the patients treated. The most frequent reported adverse effects, in order of occurrence, have been nausea, diarrhea, vomiting, abdominal pain/discomfort, headache, restlessness and rash (see Table 7.18). Each of these has been reported in 1% to 5% of patients receiving the drug.

Table 7.17

Ciprofloxacin: Oral Dosage Information

Generic name	Brand name(s)	Usual adult dosage	Maximum adult dosage	Maximum child dosage	Pregnancy risk category	Content/form	Oral dosage suggestions
Ciprofloxacin	Cipro	250 or 500 mg bid	1.5 g/day	Age < 18 y: Safety and effectiveness not established	C	**Tablets:** 250, 500, 750 mg **Oral suspension:** Not available	Given without regard to meals

Table 7.18

Ciprofloxacin: Adverse Effects, Precautions and Contraindications

Body system	Adverse effects	Precautions/contraindications
General	Photosensitivity, flushing, fever, edema of face, neck, lips, or hands (these occur in about 1% of patients) Allergic reactions ranging from urticaria to anaphylactic reactions have been reported but are rare	Stop therapy if signs of allergic reactions observed Patients allergic to one quinolone may be allergic to others
CV	Palpitation, atrial flutter, hypertension, angina pectoris, myocardial infarction (relatively rare)	None of significance to dentistry
CNS	Dizziness, lightheadedness, insomnia, hallucinations, manic reaction, irritability, convulsive seizures, depression, drowsiness, weakness and malaise (incidence relatively high in patients receiving theophylline and ciprofloxacin concurrently)	Caution advised in prescribing for patients with CNS disorders
EENT	Blurred vision, disturbed vision, decreased visual acuity, diplopia, tinnitus, hearing loss (effects may be CNS-related; incidence higher in patients receiving theophylline concomitantly)	Avoid concomitant usage with theophylline
GI	Nausea (most common side effect and may occur in 5% of patients; effect may be lessened by taking medication with food); also diarrhea, vomiting, abdominal discomfort, dysphagia, gastrointestinal bleeding	Use of drug may have to be discontinued if GI problems persist
GU	Urine retention, vaginitis	None of significance to dentistry
Musc	Joint or back pain, joint stiffness, neck or chest pain, flare-up of gout (first two are reported in about 1% of patients)	Use of drug may have to be discontinued in patients with gout
Oral	Painful oral mucosa and oral candidiasis; bad taste in mouth (more likely to occur with high or prolonged dosage)	Patient should be monitored for signs of oral candidiasis
Renal	Nephritis (reported in about 1% of patients), renal failure	Reduced dose recommended in patients with renal impairment
Resp	Epistaxis, laryngeal or pulmonary edema, dyspnea, bronchospasm (all relatively rare)	Use of drug may have to be discontinued if respiratory problems persist

Pharmacology

Ciprofloxacin is rapidly absorbed from the stomach after oral administration. Serum concentrations increase proportionately with dosage, and maximum serum concentrations are obtained 1-2 h after oral administration. After absorption, the drug is widely distributed throughout the body. Tissue concentrations often exceed serum concentrations in both men and women, particularly in the genital tissue. The drug is present in antibacterial concentrations in saliva, nasal and bronchial secretions, sputum, breast milk, skin blister fluid, lymph, peritoneal fluid and prostatic secretions. Ciprofloxacin is also present in lung, skin, fat, muscle, cartilage and bone. The drug diffuses across the placenta to enter the fetal circulation.

When ciprofloxacin is given concomitantly with food, there is delay in its absorption with a corresponding delay in peak serum levels; however, overall absorption is not substantially affected.

Concomitant administration of ciprofloxacin with theophylline decreases the clearance of theophylline and results in an increased risk of a patient's developing CNS or other adverse reactions.

In patients with reduced renal function, the half-life of the drug is slightly prolonged and dosage adjustments may be required.

Patient Advice

- Patients should be advised that ciprofloxacin can be taken with or without a meal. The preferred time of dosing is 2 h after a meal. Patients should be advised to drink fluids liberally and not to take antacids containing magnesium, aluminum, or calcium, products containing iron or multivitamins containing zinc.
- Patients should be advised that moderate to severe photosensitivity may occur and be manifested as exaggerated sunburn; excessive sunlight should be avoided.
- The drug may cause dizziness and light-headedness; therefore, patients should know how they react to the drug before they operate an automobile or machinery or engage in activities requiring mental alertness or coordination.
- There is a possibility of caffeine accumulation when coffee, tea or other caffeine-containing products are consumed while taking the drug.

Sulfonamides

The sulfonamides, or "sulfa drugs," are antimetabolites that competitively inhibit the synthesis of folic acid and folic acid derivatives in bacterial cells. Folic acid derivatives are essential for the synthesis of DNA precursors in both mammalian and bacterial cells. Unlike mammalian cells, bacterial cells are unable to absorb folic acid across the cell membrane and must synthesize it within the cell.

The sulfonamides competitively compete with para-aminobenzoic acid (PABA), which is required by bacteria in the metabolic pathway for the synthesis of folic acid. When a sulfonamide is substituted in place of PABA, the pathway cannot proceed any further and the bacterium is unable to synthesize the purine moieties needed for DNA synthesis. However, because inhibition by sulfonamides is competitive, the continued inhibition of growth depends on high concentrations of the drug. If the drug concentration falls below the competitive level, the synthesis of folic acid continues.

Most bacteria readily develop or acquire resistance to the sulfonamides through genetic transfer. This has been partially overcome by the use of a drug combination consisting of trimethoprim (also a competitive inhibitor of folic acid synthesis, but at a different point in the metabolic pathway) and sulfamethoxazole, a sulfonamide. The combination has been given the name "co-trimoxazole." Trimethoprim acts synergistically with sulfamethoxazole because both drugs inhibit sequential steps in the folic acid pathway. Although each of the drugs is bacteriostatic when used alone, the combination appears to be bactericidal. Use of co-trimoxazole is limited primarily to the treatment of urinary infections, chronic bronchitis and acute otitis media infections in children, and as a prophylaxis for traveler's diarrhea. Dental infections are usually better treated with a more appropriate antibiotic.

Accepted Indications

Sulfonamides are indicated in the treatment of urinary tract infections due to *Escherichia coli*, *Klebsiella*, *Enterobacter* or *Proteus* species.

They are used in the treatment of acute otitis media in children aged > 2 y or of chronic bronchitis in adults caused by susceptible strains of *Streptococcus pneumoniae* or *Haemophilus influenzae*. However, these drugs are not indicated for prophylactic or prolonged administration for patients with otitis media at any age.

Sulfonamides can be useful in the treatment of *Shigella* enteritis when antimicrobial therapy is indicated.

Finally, these agents frequently are used prophylactically for people traveling to countries in which the water and food may be contaminated with fecal organisms such *Escherichia coli*, *Klebsiella* or *Enterobacter*. See Table 7.19.

General Dosing Information

See Table 7.20 for recommended dosages.

Dosage Adjustments

Trimethoprim and sulfamethoxazole should be given with caution to patients with impaired renal or hepatic function, to those with possible folate deficiency (for example, elderly people, chronic alcoholics, patients receiving anticonvulsant therapy or patients with malabsorption syndrome or in malnutrition states), and to those with severe allergy or bronchial asthma. In such patients, lower dosages or a prolonged interval between doses may be indicated.

Special Dental Considerations

Drug Interactions of Dental Interest

Trimethoprim and sulfamethoxazole may prolong the prothrombin time in patients receiving the anticoagulant warfarin or its derivatives. The drug combination may inhibit the hepatic metabolism of phenytoin and result in excessive phenytoin serum levels.

In patients receiving thiazide diuretics, particularly elderly patients, an increased incidence of thrombocytopenia with purpura has been reported when trimethoprim and sulfamethoxazole are given concomitantly with the diuretic.

Laboratory Value Alterations

- The trimethoprim component may interfere with serum methotrexate assay when a bacterial dihydrofolate reductase is used as the binding protein.

Cross-Sensitivity

Trimethoprim and sulfamethoxazole use is contraindicated in patients with hypersensitivity to trimethoprim or any sulfonamide.

Table 7.19

Trimethoprim and Sulfamethoxazole: Characteristics and Common Indications for Use

Generic name	Characteristics	Common indications for use
Trimethoprim and sulfamethoxazole	Spectrum of activity limited to gram-negative aerobic or facultative bacteria and to a few streptococcal species; little activity against most gram-positive bacteria or anaerobic bacteria	Preventive prophylaxis for traveler's diarrhea Treatment of acute otitis media in children, chronic bronchitis in adults, urinary tract infections and *Shigella*-associated enteritis

Special Patients

Pregnant and nursing women

A trimethoprim-and-sulfamethoxazole combination is not indicated for use in either pregnant or lactating women. Sulfonamides, including the sulfamethoxazole component, pass the placenta and enter the fetal circulation. Sulfa drugs are also excreted in breast milk.

Pediatric, geriatric and other special patients

There may be an increased risk of severe adverse reactions in elderly patients, particularly in the presence of complicating conditions—for example, impaired kidney and/or liver function—or when the patients are concomitantly using other drugs (see Drug Interactions). Severe skin reactions, generalized bone marrow depression or a specific decrease in platelets are frequently reported adverse effects in elderly patients.

Trimethoprim and sulfamethoxazole should not be given to infants aged < 2 mo except in unusual clinical circumstances in which another antimicrobial agent cannot be used.

Trimethoprim and sulfamethoxazole should not be given to patients receiving a thiazide diuretic because an increased incidence of thrombocytopenia has been reported when the two drugs are given concomitantly.

Patient Monitoring: Aspects to Watch

Hypersensitivity to sulfa drugs is relatively common and is usually manifested as rash and urticaria.

Adverse Effects and Precautions

The adverse effects associated with the sulfonamides are numerous and varied (Table 7.21), with an overall incidence of about 5%. The most common adverse reactions are gastrointestinal disturbances, which may include nausea, vomiting and/or anorexia, and allergic skin reactions such as rash and urticaria.

Table 7.20
Trimethoprim and Sulfamethoxazole: Oral Dosage Information

Generic name	Brand name(s)	Usual adult dosage	Maximum adult dosage	Maximum child dosage	Pregnancy risk category	Content/ form	Oral dosage suggestions
Trimethoprim and sulfamethoxazole	Bactrim, Septra	**Oral suspension:** 20 mL bid **Tablets, double-strength:** 1 tablet bid **Tablets, regular:** 2 tablets bid	Not listed	8 mg/kg trimethoprim and 40 mg/kg sulfamethoxazole given in 2 equal doses bid	C	**Tablets, double-strength:** 160 mg trimethoprim/ 800 mg sulfamethoxazole **Tablets, regular:** 80 mg trimethoprim/ 400 mg sulfamethoxazole **Oral suspension:** 40 mg trimethoprim/ 200 mg sulfamethoxazole/5 mL	Given without regard to meals

Table 7.21

Trimethoprim and Sulfamethoxazole: Adverse Effects, Precautions and Contraindications

Body system	Adverse effects	Precautions/contraindications
General	Hypersensitivity manifested as skin rash most common, anaphylactic reactions, serum sicknesslike syndrome, photosensitivity, allergic myocarditis Weakness, fatigue, insomnia	Dosage should be immediately stopped if skin rash develops
CNS	Convulsions, ataxia, vertigo, tinnitus, headache, depression, nervousness, apathy, hallucinations	If convulsions occur, use of drug should be discontinued; use of drug may have to be discontinued if other CNS symptoms persist
GI	Nausea, vomiting, anorexia, glossitis, stomatitis (all relatively common) Diarrhea (rare)	Medical attention is necessary if GI symptoms persist
Hema	Agranulocytosis, thrombocytopenia, leukopenia, neutropenia, eosinophilia	Not recommended for patients with hepatic impairment If blood dyscrasia is suspected, appropriate laboratory tests should be ordered
Musc	Arthralgia, myalgia	
Renal		Not recommended for patients with renal impairment

Pharmacology

The trimethoprim-and-sulfamethoxazole combination is rapidly absorbed after oral administration with peak serum levels for the individual components occurring 1 to 4 h after dosage. The trimethoprim component is widely distributed, is concentrated in the tissues and readily enters cerebrospinal fluid and sputum. The sulfamethoxazole component is widely distributed through the body fluids and crosses the placenta to enter the fetal circulation. Both components are secreted in human breast milk.

About 60% of trimethoprim and 25% to 50% of sulfamethoxazole are excreted in the urine within 24 h of dosage.

Patient Advice

• Trimethoprim and sulfamethoxazole should be discontinued at the first appearance of skin rash or any sign of an adverse reaction. Clinical signs of a rash, sore throat, fever, cough, shortness of breath, pallor, purpura or jaundice may be early indications of serious reactions.

Suggested Readings

Mandell GL, Sande MA. Antimicrobial agents: Penicillins, cephalosporins, and other β-lactam antibiotics. In: Goodman and Gilman's the pharmacological basis of therapeutics. 8th ed. New York: Pergamon Press; 1990:1065-97.

Mandell GL, Sande MA. Antimicrobial agents: Tetracyclines, chloramphenicol, erythromycin, and miscellaneous antibacterial agents. In: Goodman and Gilman's the pharmacological basis of therapeutics. 8th ed. New York: Pergamon Press; 1990:1117-45.

Mandell GL, Sande MA. Antimicrobial agents: Sulfonamides, trimethoprim-sulfamethoxazole, quinolones, and agents for urinary tract infections. In: Goodman and Gilman's the pharmacological basis of therapeutics. 8th ed. New York: Pergamon Press; 1990:1047-64.

Physicians' desk reference. 51st ed. Montvale, N.J.: Medical Economics; 1997.

Walker CB. Antimicrobial agents and chemotherapy. In: Slots J, Taubman M, eds. Contemporary oral microbiology and immunology. St. Louis: Mosby; 1992:242-64.

Walker CB. Selected antimicrobial agents: Mechanisms of action, side effects, and drug interactions. In: Slots J, Rams T, eds. Periodontology 2000. Vol. 10: Systemic and topical antimicrobial therapy in periodontics. Copenhagen: Munksgaard; 1996:12-28.

Chapter 8

Antifungal and Antiviral Agents

Martha Somerman, D.D.S., Ph.D.

Antifungal Agents

Fungal infections occur less frequently than bacterial and viral infections; they are encountered in the mouth, an area that favors the growth of certain fungal strains. This is especially true for immunocompromised patients, for patients whose tissues are subjected to poorly fitting prostheses or nonremovable prostheses that have accumulated plaque, for patients with xerostomia, and for patients taking antibiotics who have an increased risk of developing oral and vaginal yeast infections. *Candida* infections of the mouth frequently go undiagnosed in hospitalized patients as well as in patients who require supervised care. The result may be oral pain of such severity that food intake is negatively affected—a significant concern for all patients, and especially those who cannot communicate their pain, such as ailing nursing home residents.

Once a fungal infection of the mouth has been established, it is important that precautions are taken to prevent recurring fungal infection. These would include disposal of previously used toothbrushes and other contaminated oral hygiene devices and a careful cleaning of dentures by the patient and/or dental staff. Appropriate brushing requires sonication to remove hard deposits and rinsing with a disinfectant. To treat the fungal infection itself, antifungal agents are required. This chapter is limited to two principal categories of antifungal drugs, polyenes and azoles, as these are pertinent to dentistry. In addition, some antifungal agents are now being used in combination with corticosteroids. For example, the combination of the polyene, nystatin and triamcinolone (Mycolog II, Mytrex) has been recommended for use in treating angular cheilitis and has been shown to be effective during the first few days of treatment. However, if inflammation persists, U.S. Pharmacopeia medical experts recommend the use of nystatin alone or other topical antifungal agents alone. In addition, some dentists report that antifungal vaginal creams—such as miconazole (Monistat 7), nystatin vaginal suppositories, clotrimazole (Mycelex-G)—have proven effective in cases in which other topical antifungal agents have not been beneficial.

Dosing information on antifungal drugs is provided in Table 8.1.

Accepted Indications

Drug Categories
Azoles
Systemic antifungals are used to treat serious, chronic extensive mucocutaneous candidiasis caused by *Candida* species. Many of the azoles are used to treat orapharyngeal candidiasis. They are also used for other fungal infections, such as aspergillosis, blastomycosis, chromomycosis, coccidioidomycosis, cryptococcosis and histoplasmosis.

Polyenes
Polyenes are used for local treatment of fungal

infections of the mouth caused by *Candida albicans* and other *Candida* species.

Fungal Infections

Candidiasis
Candidiasis is the most frequent fungal infection affecting the mouth. In general, when there is no systemic problem, candidiasis responds to topical therapy.

Actinomycosis
Actinomycosis is caused by an organism with both fungal and bacterial properties, with the most common sites being cervicofacial.

Histoplasmosis
Histoplasmosis is a deep fungal infection that may affect the mouth. A biopsy is required, as it can be clinically confused with epidermoid carcinoma.

Others
Other fungal infections that are seen in the mouth include aspergillosis, blastomycosis and coccidioidomycosis.

General Dosing Information
General dosing information is provided in Table 8.1. Dosing depends on severity of the fungal infection; therefore, selection of topical forms for less complicated infections and systemic forms for greater severity is typical.

Maximum Recommended Doses
With many fungal infections, lesions tend to recur after treatment when use of the drug is discontinued. This situation may require use of the agent 48 h after symptoms disappear and, in certain cases, long-term therapy— with caution, however, because of the potential for development of resistant strains. Furthermore, because resistant strains of candidal organisms have been reported to be associated more often with systemic therapy, systemic use of antifungal agents for oral infections should be considered cautiously. Resistant strains may render a drug ineffective against life-threatening candidal infections such as those that occur in immunocompromised patients.

Dosage Adjustments
No detailed information is available on age-related changes in patients taking antifungal drugs. However, elderly patients are more likely to have hepatic- and renal-associated problems requiring adjustment in dose of drug and/or dosing time.

Special Dental Considerations

General Considerations
- Examine oral mucous membranes for signs of fungal infection.
- Examine for evidence of oral *Candida* infection.
- A culture may be required to confirm the fungal organism.
- Long-term therapy may be needed to clear the infection.
- To prevent reinoculation of *Candida* infection, patients should dispose of their toothbrushes or other contaminated oral hygiene devices used during the period of infection. Patients who wear full dentures should soak their appliances nightly in an antifungal solution while their oral fungal infection is being treated.
- Determine if medication controls the disease.
- Place patients on a schedule of frequent recall visits to evaluate their healing response.
- Assess patients' salivary flow as a factor in caries, periodontal disease and candidiasis.
- Caution patients about the use of broad-spectrum antibiotics, which can alter the gastrointestinal flora and result in candidiasis.

Drug Interactions of Dental Interest
Azoles
- Absorption of the antifungal drugs itraconazole and ketoconazole can be altered by drugs such as antacids, anticholinergics/antispasmotics, histamine H_2-antagonist, omeprazole and sucralfate. Therefore, advise patients to take the above medications at least 2 h after taking the antifungal agent.
- Use of antidiabetic agents in conjunction

Table 8.1

Antifungal Agents: Dosage Information

Generic name	Brand name(s)	Usual adult dosage	Usual child dosage	Pregnancy risk category	Content/form
			Azoles		
Clotrimazole	Gyne-Lotrimin, Lotrimin, Mycelex, Mycelex Troche; Canesten [CAN], Myclo [CAN], Neo-Zol [CAN]	**Topical cream, lotion:** Rub into affected area bid for 1-8 w **Oral troches:** Dissolve 10-mg troches in mouth 5 times a day for 14 days, 3-5 10-mg tablets q day for 14 days or apply ointment to the affected area qid for 14 days	**Age < 5 y—oral:** Oral suspension rather than tablets (same as adult dose) **Infants:** Not established	**Cream, lotion:** B **Oral suspension:** Not available **Tablets:** C	**Cream, lotion:** 10 mg/g **Oral suspension:** 10 mg/mL **Tablets:** 10 mg
Fluconazole	Diflucan	**Tablets:** 200 mg immediately, then 100 mg daily for 7-14 days **Oral suspension:** 200-400 mg/day	Not established	C	**Oral suspension:** 10 mg/mL, 40 mg/mL **Tablets:** 50, 100, 200 mg; 50, 100 mg [CAN]
Itraconazole	Sporanox	**Tablets:** 200-400 mg/day	Not established	C	**Tablets:** 100 mg; 100 mg [CAN]
Ketoconazole	Nizoral; Akorazol [CAN]	**Tablets:** 200-400 mg q day **Cream:** Rub gently onto affected area q day or bid and/or bedtime	**Age > 2 y—oral:** 5-10 mg/kg/day **Age > 2 y—topical:** Same as adult **Infants:** Not established	**Cream:** C **Tablets:** C	**Cream:** 2% in 15-g tubes **Tablets:** 200 mg
			Polyenes		
Amphotericin B	Fungizone	**Oral suspension:** 1 mL (100 mg) of liquid, swish and swallow qid for 2 w	1 mL (100 mg) of liquid, swish and swallow qid for 2 w	**Cream, lotion, ointment:** B **Oral suspension:** C	**Cream, lotion, ointment:** 3% **Oral suspension:** 100 mg/mL in bottles of 24 mL (to be swished and swallowed or to be used IV for severe infections)

Nystatin	Mycostatin, Nilstat, Nystex, O-V Statin, PMS Nystatin; Nadostine [CAN], Nyaderm [CAN]	In general, treatment should continue 48 h after symptoms disappear to prevent relapse **Tablets/troches:** 200,000-400,000 units 4-5 times/day, dissolved slowly and completely in mouth; patients who have difficulty dissolving tablets may need to use oral suspension form **Oral suspension:** swish and swallow 400,000-600,000 units qid **Cream/ointment:** Cover the area of infection bid-tid, after meals and at bedtime	In general, treatment should continue 48 h after symptoms disappear to prevent relapse **Tablets/troches:** 200,000-400,000 units 4-5 times/day, dissolved slowly and completely in mouth; do not use in children aged under 5 y, but use oral suspension instead **Oral suspension:** Swish and swallow 400,000-600,000 units qid; dose is lower in newborns and infants, 100,000-200,000 units four times/day **Cream/ointment:** Cover the area of infection bid-tid	**Tablets:** B **Oral suspension:** C	**Tablets:** 500,000 units **Troches/pastilles:** 200,000 units **Oral suspension:** 100,000 units/mL; available in 5 mL, 60 mL, and 480 mL **Cream/ointment:** 100,000 units/g in 15-g and 60-g tubes
Nystatin with triamcinolone acetonide	Mycolog II, Mytrex	In general, treatment should continue 48 h after symptoms disappear to prevent relapse **Cream/ointment:** cover the area of infection bid-tid, after meals and at bedtime	In general, treatment should continue 48 h after symptoms disappear to prevent relapse **Cream/ointment:** cover the area of infection bid-tid	C	**Cream:** Nystatin 100,000 units and triamcinolone acetonide 0.1% in 1.5-g, 15-g, 30-g, 60-g, 120-g tubes **Ointment:** Nystatin 100,000 units and triamcinolone acetonide 0.1% in 15-g, 30-g, 60-g, 120-g tubes

[CAN] indicates a drug available only in Canada.

with the antifungal agents fluconazole and itraconazole may result in altered blood glucose.

- Anticoagulant effects, such as increased prothrombin time, may occur in patients taking warfarin in conjunction with antifungal agents.
- Concurrent use of antihistamines (such as terfenadine) with the azoles itraconazole and ketoconazole has led to cardiac arrhythmias and death.
- Concurrent use of alcohol or hepatoxicity medications may result in increased liver damage; therefore, patients who are taking medications over the long term or who have a history of liver disease should be monitored carefully, and such patients should not drink alcohol.
- A disulfiram-like reaction can result from concurrent ingestion of alcohol and ketoconazole; therefore, advise patients to avoid alcoholic beverages.
- Concurrent use of antifungal agents and cyclosporine and phenytoin may inhibit the metabolism of the latter, resulting in toxic levels of cyclosporine and phenytoin; therefore, both of these medications need to be monitored closely.
- The antifungal agent itraconazole may increase serum digoxin concentrations; therefore, digoxin concentration must be monitored to avoid toxicity.

Polyenes

Amphotericin B. Increased toxicity has been reported with the following agents: cyclosporine and aminoglycosides (nephrotoxicity); corticosteroids (hypokalemia).

Special Patients

Pregnant and nursing women

Most antifungal agents are classified as B or C in the pregnancy risk category; however, controlled studies are not available, so caution should be taken in prescribing such medications to pregnant women. As some antifungal agents do enter breast milk, the dentist should recommend precautions for those who are nursing. However, nystatin has not been shown to enter breast milk.

Pediatric, geriatric and other special patients

Many antifungal agents can alter kidney and liver function, which may be severely damaging to older and younger patients. Therefore, dentists may need to adjust dose levels accordingly.

Adverse Effects and Precautions

Table 8.2 lists the adverse effects and precautions related to antifungal agents.

Pharmacology

The mechanism by which the polyenes amphotericin B and nystatin inhibit fungal growth is essentially the same. The agents bind to sterols on the cell membranes of target fungi, resulting in defective membranes and allowing for leakage of intracellular components. The result is cell lysis.

In contrast, azole antifungal agents interfere with cytochrome P-450 activity, necessary for the demethylation of 14-α methylsterol to ergosterol. Ergosterol is the major sterol associated with fungal cell membranes. Thus, lack of this sterol results in loss of membrane function. Also, in *Candida albicans,* azoles inhibit transformation of blastospores into invasive mycelial form. The effect of azoles may be fungistatic or fungicidal depending on concentration.

Patient Advice

The following general advice can be given to all patients who have a fungal infection.

- Long-term therapy may be needed to clear the infection and/or prevent relapse.
- Patients should complete the entire course of their medication.
- Patients should not use commercial mouthwashes for mouth infections unless they are prescribed by the dentist.
- Patients should soak full or partial dentures in a suitable antifungal solution on a nightly basis while treating oral lesions.

Table 8.2

Antifungal Agents: Adverse Effects, Precautions and Contraindications

Agent	Adverse effects	Precautions/contraindications
Azoles		
Clotrimazole	**GI:** Nausea and vomiting *HB: Abnormal liver function tests* **Integ:** Rash, urticaria, stinging, burning, peeling, blistering	Should not be used for treatment of systemic fungal infection Sugar content of lozenge preparations warrant use of other options in caries-prone patients Contraindicated in patients with hypersensitivity
Fluconazole	**GI:** Nausea, vomiting, diarrhea, cramping, flatus **HB:** Hepatotoxicity, hepatitis, jaundice **Integ:** Skin rash, exfoliative skin disorders such as Stevens-Johnson syndrome (rare), photosensitivity **Renal:** Renal disease	Renal dysfunction Hepatic dysfunction Contraindicated in patients with hypersensitivity
Itraconazole	**CV:** Hypertension, edema, hypokalemia, malaise **CNS:** Headache, dizziness, anorexia, fatigue, fever **GI:** Nausea, vomiting, diarrhea, abdominal pain, hepatitis, hepatic dysfunction **GU:** Impotence **HB:** Hepatotoxicity **Integ:** Rash, pruritus	Liver dysfunction and rare cases of serious adverse cardiovascular events, including death, have been reported when terfenadine (Seldane) is given in conjunction with itraconazole Contraindicated in patients who also are taking terfenadine Contraindicated in patients with hypersensitivity
Ketoconazole	**CNS:** Headache, dizziness, lethargy, anxiety, insomnia, dreams, paresthesia **Endoc:** Gynecomastia, depressed adrenocortical function **GI:** Nausea, vomiting, anorexia, diarrhea, cramps, abdominal pain, constipation, flatulence, GI bleeding **GU:** Impotence **HB:** Hepatotoxicity **Integ:** Pruritus (cream and oral), severe irritation and stinging (cream), fever, chills, photophobia, rash, dermatitis, purpura, urticaria	Renal disease Hepatic disease (periodic liver function tests are recommended) Drug-induced achlorhydria Rare cases of serious adverse cardiovascular events, including death, have been reported when terfenadine is given in conjunction with ketoconazole Contraindicated in patients who are taking terfenadine Contraindicated in patients with hypersensitivity

Italics indicate information of major clinical significance.

Continued on next page

Table 8.2 (cont.)

Antifungal Agents: Adverse Effects, Precautions and Contraindications

Agent	Adverse effects	Precautions/contraindications
Polyenes		
Amphotericin B	**CV:** Hypotension, hypertension **CNS:** *Fever, chills,* delirium, convulsions **Endoc:** *Hypokalemia, hypomagnesemia* **GI:** *GI disturbance* **GU:** Urinary retention **Hema:** *Phlebitis, anemia,* leukocytosis, leukopenia **HB:** Acute liver failure **Integ:** Hypersensitivity, burning, itching, redness at site **Renal:** *Nephrotoxicity*	Contraindicated in patients with sensitivity to amphotericin B
Nystatin	**GI:** *Nausea, vomiting, anorexia, diarrhea, abdominal pain* **Integ:** Hypersensitivity reaction, rash, urticaria (rare) **Oral:** Bad taste with oral suspension and lozenges	Sugar content of some lozenge preparations may warrant use of other options in caries-prone patients Contraindicated in patients with hypersensitivity to nystatin
Nystatin with triamcinolone acetonide	**Integ:** Dryness, acne, allergic dermatitis, skin maceration and atrophy, burning, irritation	Avoid use of occlusive dressings Contraindicated in patients with hypersensitivity to nystatin or triamcinolone

Italics indicate information of major clinical significance.

- If an oral infection has occurred, patients should soak their full or partial dentures in an antifungal solution overnight until lesions are absent; prolonged infections may require fabrication of a new prosthesis.
- To prevent reinoculation of *Candida* infections, patients should dispose of any toothbrushes or other contaminated oral hygiene devices they used during the period of infection.
- Patients should be told that good oral hygiene is important in preventing gingival inflammation.
- Patients should avoid mouthrinses with high alcohol content because of their drying effects.
- If patients experience chronic dry mouth, they may need to use home fluoride preparations on a daily basis. They also can use sugarless gum, frequent sips of water or artificial saliva substitutes if they are experiencing chronic dry mouth.
- Patients should be cautioned to be careful to prevent injury when using oral hygiene aids.

Suggested Readings

Hansten PD, Horn JR. Terfenadine drug interactions. Drug Interactions Newsletter (August Special Issue) 1992; 586-8.

Rosenberg SW, Arm RN, eds. Clinician's guide to treatment of common oral conditions. 4th ed. Baltimore: American Academy of Oral Medicine; 1997.

United States Pharmacopeial Convention Inc. Drug information for the health care professional. Vol. I. 15th ed. Rockville, Md.: United States Pharmacopeial Convention Inc.; 1995.

Wynn RL. Erythromycin and ketoconazole (Nizoral) associated with terfenadine (Seldane)-induced ventricular arrhythmias. Gen Dent 1993;41:27-9.

Antiviral Agents

Viral infections can and do occur in the mouth. Signs of viral infection include malaise, anorexia, fever, myalgia, crops of vesicle formation and coated tongue. Ruptured vesicles usually produce pain. General treatment of viral infections is often palliative, aimed at making the patient comfortable and providing adequate liquids to prevent dehydration. Usually, lesions resolve in 10 to 14 days.

Viral infections encountered in dental practice include hepatitis; hand-foot-and-mouth disease (group A coxsackievirus); primary herpes simplex infection (such as gingiva stomatitis) and recurrent herpes simplex infection (such as herpes labialis); herpangina; herpes zoster; varicella; and human immunodeficiency (HIV). The above conditions are not necessarily conditions for which the dentist will be prescribing, but the dentist must be aware of them and of their recommended treatment. For example, hepatitis B vaccine is currently recommended for all individuals, and therefore the dentist should inquire while taking a patient's medical history whether he or she has been vaccinated. In addition, some of the diagnostic characteristics of these viruses are seen in the mouth.

Use of antiviral agents is often limited to immunocompromised patients, and doses should be as low as possible.

Most viral-associated lesions of the mouth and elsewhere are preceded by a viral prodrome of local tingling, malaise, anorexia and/or fever. Smears may be warranted to determine if lesions are viral. The major type of viral lesion of the mouth is vesiculobullous in nature and can be noted as small vesicular lesions. Group A coxsackievirus lesions—most frequently noted in children in the summer and fall—are often noted on the palate; in addition, the virus may cause parotitis and also herpangina. Treatment of group A coxsackievirus is palliative.

How viruses develop. Viruses are composed of single- or double-stranded nucleic acids, either DNA or RNA. Viruses, as obligate intracellular parasites, lack both a cell wall and a cell membrane and are not involved in metabolic activities independent of the host. However, within the host, they transmit genetic information and also replicate. Invasion by a virus does not necessarily result in cell destruction. Destruction of the host depends on release of virus from the cell, ability of the virus to influence cell metabolism, and release of toxins by the virus. Several results are possible, including cytolysis, metabolic dysfunction, cell transformation or no pathological effects. Host defense mechanisms are critical for fighting viral infections. Any disease state or drug therapy that compromises the host response can result in fatal viral infection.

The requirement that the host supply metabolic activity for viral reproduction results in difficulties in developing antiviral drugs selective enough to inhibit viral reproduction without causing damage to the host. Nonetheless, drugs have been developed with selective activity against viral reactions. Antimicrobial agents are not effective against viruses. Discussed below are antiviral agents that dental professionals will most frequently encounter and prescribe.

Resistance to antiviral agents. Similarly to other antimicrobial agents, viral resistance to antiviral agents has become an increasing problem. There are many reasons for resistance and depending on the specific drug, there can be multiple mechanisms for resistance. For example, it is believed that with acyclovir, resistant herpes simplex viruses have been developed due to alterations in either the viral thymidine kinase or the viral DNA polymerase (for example, deficient kinase). At the clinical level, significant mucocutaneous infections have been noted in AIDS patients associated with acyclovir-resistant strains of herpes virus simplex.

Aphthous ulcers. Distinction should be made between commonly occurring intraoral ulcers (such as aphthae) that do not have a viral etiology and those associated with intraoral herpes. While aphthae are not of viral etiology, it is important to mention a drug recently approved by the FDA for their treatment: amlexanox (brand name Aphthasol). This is the only drug the FDA has approved for treatment of aphthae.

Accepted Indications

Because of substantial toxicity and side effects, antiviral agents usually are reserved for immunocompromised patients with mucocutaneous HSV-associated lesions. There are some suggestions that topical acyclovir may be used for recurrent herpes labialis for all patients. This is based on the fact that there is often an initial tingling (prodrome period) before onset of the lesion, as well as on the belief that its use at this time can decrease pain and duration of symptoms. Other treatment may include anesthetic agents, nutritional supplements and antipyretics, as needed.

General Dosing Information

General dosing information is provided in Table 8.3.

For aphthous ulcers, amlexanox, available in a 5% paste, should be applied directly to aphthae qid after brushing and after meals. Side effects are rare, but local irritation is occasionally reported. Systemic absorption is negligible.

Dosage Adjustments

Antiviral agents have significant side effects and toxicity. Thus, the lowest possible dose, where a benefit can be seen, should be used.

Table 8.3

Antiviral Agents: Dosage Information

Generic name	Brand name(s)	Usual adult dosage	Usual child dosage	Pregnancy risk category	Content/form
Acyclovir	Zovirax; Avirax [CAN]	**For herpes simplex—oral:** 200 mg q 4 h **For herpes simplex— topical:** ½-in ribbon of ointment for a 4-in-sq surface q 3 h	**Age ≤ 2 y, for herpes simplex:** Not established; consult physician	C	**Capsules:** 200 mg; 200 mg [CAN] **Tablets:** 400, 800 mg; 200, 400, 800 mg [CAN] **Oral suspension:** 40 mg/mL; 40 mg/mL [CAN] **Ointment:** 5% (50 mg/g) in 3-, 15-g tubes; 5% (50 mg/g) in 3-, 15-g tubes [CAN]
Penciclovir	Denavir	**Topical:** Apply to affected area at onset of symptoms q 2 h for 4 days	Not established	B	**Ointment:** 10 mg/g in 2-g tubes

[CAN] indicates a drug available only in Canada.

Special Dental Considerations

Drug Interactions of Dental Interest

As acyclovir is a nephrotoxic medication, it may increase nephrotoxicity. Probenecid and other nephrotoxic agents may increase levels of acyclovir and, thus, toxicity.

Cross-Sensitivity

Patients taking antiviral agents may have a sensitivity to nephrotoxic and hepatotoxic drugs.

Special Patients

Pregnant and nursing women

Antiviral agents are contraindicated for pregnant and nursing women (unless the benefit justifies the risk to the fetus).

Acyclovir does pass into breast milk, but no toxicity has been reported.

Pediatric, geriatric and other special patients

Both renal and hepatic toxicity are associated with antiviral agents. Thus, precautions must be taken in patients at risk of renal and/or hepatic dysfunction—not uncommon in older people and children.

Adverse Effects and Precautions

Table 8.4 lists adverse effects and precautions for antiviral agents.

Patient Monitoring: Aspects to Watch

- Recurrent and persistent oral lesions: These may be an indication of more serious disease; careful diagnosis may warrant biopsy and evaluation for HSV, AIDS and carcinoma

Table 8.4

Antiviral Agents: Adverse Effects, Precautions and Contraindications

Body system	Adverse effects	Precautions/contraindications
Systemic acyclovir		
General	None significant to dentistry	Contraindicated in patients with hypersensitivity to acyclovir
CNS	Neuropsychiatric toxicity (may be more common in immunocompromised and geriatric patients) Light-headedness, dizziness	Contraindicated in patients who have neurologic abnormalities or abnormal neurologic reactions to cytotoxic medications
GI	GI disturbances; anorexia	None significant to dentistry
HB	None significant to dentistry	Patients with serious hepatic abnormalities, because of difficulties with biotransformation
Musc	Tremors	None significant to dentistry
Oral	Taste disturbances	None significant to dentistry
Renal	*Acute renal insufficiency due to precipitation of acyclovir in renal tubes has been reported*	Maintain adequate hydration to prevent precipitation of acyclovir in the renal tubules Adults with chronic renal impairment require reduced dose Patients who have serious electrolyte abnormalities

Italics indicate information of major clinical significance.

Continued on next page

Table 8.4 (cont.)

Antiviral Agents: Adverse Effects, Precautions and Contraindications

Body system	Adverse effects	Precautions/contraindications
Topical acyclovir and penciclovir		
General	Hypersensitivity at the local site Mild pain, burning, stinging	Contraindicated in patients with hypersensitivity to acyclovir and/or penciclovir Effects of penciclovir have not been established in immunocompromised patients Avoid contact with eye
Oral	Taste disturbances	None significant to dentistry

Pharmacology

Nucleoside antiviral agents act by being phosphorylated by the host cell or virus for antiviral activity, usually to the triphosphate form (as with acyclovir and penciclovir). Once activated, the antiviral phosphorylated form intereferes with the viral DNA polymerase, inhibiting viral DNA replication.

Patient Advice

- For topical use, patients should apply agent using a finger cot or some type of protective covering.

- Patients should avoid using mouthrinses that have a high alcohol content.
- Patients should dispose of toothbrushes used during period of infection.

Suggested Readings

Boyd MR, Kern ER, Safrin S. Penciclovir: a review of its spectrum of activity, selectivity and cross-resistance pattern. Antiviral Chem Chemother 1993;4(Supplement 1):3-11.

Erlick KS, Mills J, Chatis P, et al. Acyclovir-resistant herpes simplex virus infections in patients with acquired immunodeficiency syndrome. N Engl J Med 1989;320:293-6.

Field AK, Biron KK. "The end of innocence" revisited: resistance of herpesviruses to antiviral drugs. Clin Microbiol Rev 1994;7:1-13.

Chapter 9.

Topical Antiseptics

Chris H. Miller, Ph.D.; B. Ellen Byrne, R.Ph., D.D.S., Ph.D.

An antiseptic is a broad-spectrum antimicrobial chemical solution that is applied topically to body surfaces to reduce the microbial flora in preparation for surgery or at an injection site. In contrast, antibiotics (see Chapter 7) are organic chemical substances originally produced by microorganisms and used systemically or topically to treat infectious diseases in humans, animals and plants. Disinfectants (see Chapter 28) are antimicrobial chemical solutions used on inanimate surfaces. Sterilants are agents that, when used properly, can kill all microbes. Germicides (see Chapter 28) are agents that can kill at least some microbes; sporocides, fungicides, virucides, bacteriocides and tuberculocides are agents that can kill specific types of microbes.

The antimicrobial activity of antiseptics usually is weaker than that of disinfectants and sterilants because less harsh, or weaker, chemicals usually must be applied to body surfaces to avoid irritating the tissues. However, the antimicrobial activity of antiseptics can be lethal to the microbes on the body surfaces (the word "bactericidal" contains the stem "-cidal," derived from the Latin root meaning "destroy"), or the activity may merely inhibit the growth of microbes (the word "bacteriostatic" contains the stem "-static," derived from the Latin root meaning "inhibit"). The specific activity depends on the nature of the antiseptic chemical and the microbes involved.

In general, antiseptics have a broad spectrum of activity in killing a wide variety of microbes. However, they are not considered to be sterilants, although they may kill all the microbes on a particular surface at a given time. Some antiseptics have substantivity, also known as residual, long-lasting or persistent activity. These agents adhere to tissue surfaces and may remain active for a period of a few hours after their application.

In dentistry, antiseptics are grouped into three classes: handwashing agents, skin and mucosal antiseptics and root canal and cavity preparations.

Handwashing Agents

There are two types of microbial flora on the skin: resident flora and transient flora. The resident flora, also referred to as the "colonizing flora," consist of microbes that colonize the skin; in other words, they attach to, multiply on and are considered permanent residents of the skin. Prominent members of the resident flora include *Staphylococcus epidermidis* and several species of *Corynebacterium*, *Acinetobacter*, *Propionibacterium* and *Peptococcus*. Members of the resident flora are not readily removed from the skin by mechanical friction.

The transient flora, also referred to as the "contaminating flora," comprise microbes that are not consistently found on the skin and that, after being acquired, exist for a relatively short time (usually until the next handwashing). They are acquired by contact with contaminated surfaces and can include any known microbe. Because members of the transient flora do not colonize the skin, they are readily removed by mechanical friction, such as that in handwashing. This is fortunate, because the transient flora are those most involved in spreading diseases by contaminating people's hands.

Accepted Indications

Handwashing with a detergent solution facilitates the suspension of most of the transient microbes and a few of the resident microbes from the surface of the skin; subsequent rinsing removes the microbes from the hands. Thus, both mechanical friction and rinsing are crucial for effective handwashing. The addition of an antimicrobial agent to the handwashing detergent adds another important component to the process, that of destroying most of the remaining transient microbes and even some, but not all, of the resident flora.

Handwashing products include

- antimicrobial soap, which contains an ingredient with in vitro and in vivo activity against skin flora;
- healthcare personnel handwash, a broad-spectrum, antimicrobial preparation that reduces the number of transient flora on intact skin to a baseline level (it is fast-acting, nonirritating and designed for frequent use);
- surgical hand scrub, a broad-spectrum, fast-acting, persistent and nonirritating preparation that contains an antimicrobial ingredient designed to significantly reduce the number of microorganisms on intact skin.

The antimicrobial agents in handwashing agents include chlorhexidine gluconate, *para*-chloro-*meta*-xylenol, iodophors (which contain iodine) and triclosan (Table 9.1).

Chlorhexidine gluconate. Chlorhexidine gluconate, or CHG, is a fairly broad-spectrum antimicrobial agent that is intermediate in its speed of action. It has a high affinity for skin, and it continues to be effective for at least 6 h. There have been relatively few reports of adverse reactions (Table 9.2) to chlorhexidine, although a few allergic reactions have been noted.

Iodophors. Iodophors are complexes of iodine and an organic carrier that increase the solubility of iodine and provide a reservoir of iodine. An example is the complex of iodine with polyvinylpyrrolidone (povidone-iodine). With iodophors, the presence of free iodine (the antimicrobial component) is increased during dilution; the recommended levels for free iodine in antiseptics are 1 to 2 mg per L (1-2 parts per million). Iodophors have an intermediate speed of action and a low level of persistence. Table 9.1 lists some iodophor products, their forms and their uses.

Para-chloro-meta-xylenol. *Para*-chloro-*meta*-xylenol also is known as PCMX or chloroxylenol. It is intermediate in its speed of action and exhibits some persistence in its activity. The incidence of adverse reactions to PCMX is low. Preparations with lower concentrations of PCMX are more appropriate for routine handwashing than as surgical scrubs. Some PCMX products are shown in Table 9.1.

Triclosan/irgasan. Triclosan, or irgasan, is 2,4,4'-trichloro-2'-hydroxydiphenolchlorophenol. Its speed of action is intermediate and it does have some persistence on the skin. At lower concentrations, it is bacteriostatic. This antiseptic agent is the common active ingredient in household liquid antibacterial soaps, deodorant soaps and underarm deodorants and is present in similar concentrations in products marketed to healthcare professionals. These preparations, some of which are listed in Table 9.1, are more appropriate for routine handwashing than as surgical scrubs.

General Usage Information

See Table 9.1.

Adverse Effects and Precautions

See Table 9.2.

Table 9.1

Handwashing Agents: Usage Information

Generic name	Brand name(s)	Content/form	Actions/uses
4% chlorhexidine gluconate solution	BrianCare Antimicrobial Skin Cleanser ★ Dencide Antimicrobial Solution, Dyna-Hex 4% Antimicrobial Skin Cleanser ★ Excell Antimicrobial Skin Cleanser, Hibiclens Antimicrobial Skin Cleanser ★ Luroscrub Antimicrobial Skin Cleanser ★ Maxiclens ★ Novoclens Topical Solution ★ Scrub-Stat IV Antimicrobial Solution ★	4% chlorhexidine gluconate, 4% isopropyl alcohol	Very effective against gram-positive bacteria, moderately effective against gram-negative bacteria, bacteriostatic only against mycobacteria According to laboratory studies, can eliminate infectivity of lipophilic viruses such as HIV, influenza and herpes simplex but is not very effective against hydrophilic viruses such as poliovirus and some enteric viruses
2% chlorhexidine gluconate solution	Chlorostat Antimicrobial Skin Cleanser ★ Cida-Stat Antimicrobial Solution ★ Dyna-Hex 2% Antimicrobial Skin Cleanser ★	2% chlorhexidine gluconate, 4% isopropyl alcohol	Not as effective as the 4% solution but has similar spectrum of activity
Iodophors	Betadine Surgical Scrub (1% available iodine), Sana Scrub Surgical Scrub (0.75% available iodine)	0.75%, 1% available iodine	Very effective against gram-positive bacteria and moderately effective against gram-negative bacteria, the tubercle bacillus, fungi and many viruses
Para-chloro-*meta*-xylenol (PCMX) (chloroxylenol)	DermAseptic (3% PCMX), PCMX Scrub (3% PCMX), Lurosep Antimicrobial Lotion Soap (0.5% PCMX), Vironex (0.5% PCMX with Nonoxynol-9)	0.5%, 3% PCMX, 0.5% PCMX with Nonoxynol-9	Although some studies have shown CHG and iodophors to be more active than PCMX against skin flora, PCMX is a fairly broad-spectrum antimicrobial agent that is moderately effective against gram-positive bacteria and somewhat effective against gram-negative bacteria, the tubercle bacillus and some fungi and viruses
Triclosan or irgasan	Dial Liquid Antimicrobial Soap (0.2% triclosan), Lysol I.C. Antimicrobial Soap (0.3% triclosan), Septisol Solution (0.25% irgasan)	0.2%, 0.3% triclosan, 0.25% irgasan	Moderately effective against gram-positive bacteria and most gram-negative bacteria, but it may be less effective against *Pseudomonas aeruginosa*; somewhat effective against the tubercle bacillus; level of its effectiveness against viruses is unknown

★ *indicates a product bearing the ADA Seal of Acceptance.*
The products listed here might not include all of those that are available. Also, the listing of a product does not denote its superiority to any other product that is either listed or not listed, nor does it guarantee its availability or quality.

Table 9.2

Handwashing Agents: Adverse Effects, Precautions and Contraindications

Body system	Adverse effects	Precautions/contraindications
General	Allergic reaction in sensitive persons (may occur with any product)	Avoid contact with agent if sensitive
EENT	Eye damage (with chlorhexidine gluconate)* Damage to the middle ear (with chlorhexidine gluconate)*	Avoid placing chlorhexidine gluconate in eyes and ears
Endoc	Induction of hyperthyroidism in infants by iodine	Do not use iodophors on infants
Integ	Skin irritation (with iodophor products)	Rinse off iodophors after handwashing

*Chlorhexidine is nontoxic on the skin but may cause damage if placed directly into the eye or ear.

Suggested Readings

Aly R, Maibach HI. Comparative antibacterial efficacy of a 2-minute surgical scrub with chlorhexidine gluconate, povidone-iodine, and chloroxylenol sponge brushes. Am J Infect Control 1988;16:173-7.

Denton GW. Chlorhexidine. In: Block SS, ed. Disinfection, sterilization, and preservation. Philadelphia: Lea and Febiger; 1991:274-89.

Gottardi W. Iodine and iodine compound. In: Block SS, ed. Disinfection, sterilization, and preservation. Philadelphia: Lea and Febiger; 1991:152-66.

Larson E, Mayur K, Laughon BA. Influence of two handwashing frequencies on reduction of colonizing flora with three handwashing agents used by health care personnel. Am J Infect Control 1989;17:83-8.

Larson E, Talbot GH. An approach for selection of health care personnel handwashing agents. Infect Control 1986;7:419-24.

Skin and Mucosal Antiseptics

In dentistry, antiseptics may be used on the skin or the oral mucosa to reduce the microbial load before injections, incisions, or other invasive procedures. Such agents should be fast-acting and nonirritating. Both alcohols and iodine preparations used separately or in combination have been shown to reduce the microbial load on body surfaces.

Alcohols. Isopropyl (2-propanol, isopropanol) and ethyl (ethanol) alcohols are used as skin antiseptics, but because of the burning or stinging sensations they cause, they are not recommended for use on mucosal tissues. Although there are some differences in the antiseptic activity of ethyl and isopropyl alcohols, their concentration is more important in determining their overall effectiveness. Because some water must be present to enhance the denaturation of microbial proteins (which is the mechanism of antimicrobial action), effective concentrations range from 60% to 90% aqueous solutions. Usually, however, to reduce chances of skin irritation and drying, an amount of alcohol no higher than 70% by weight is used.

Iodophors. As mentioned above, presurgical preparation of the skin may involve an alcohol treatment followed by application of an iodophor. The antimicrobial activity of iodophor preparations involves the binding of iodine to amino acids, thus causing changes in protein structure and functioning. Iodine binds to the S-H group of cysteine, which interferes with the bridging of peptides during protein synthesis. Also under alkaline conditions, iodine can bind to the N-H group of several amino acids interfering with peptide bond formation. Iodine solutions stain and may irritate the skin, whereas iodophors have reduced staining properties and are less irritating.

Accepted Indications

See Table 9.3.

General Usage Information

See Table 9.3.

Adverse Effects and Precautions

See Table 9.4.

Suggested Readings

Brenman HS, Randell E. Local degerming with povi-done-iodine. II. Prior to gingivectomy. J Periodontol 1974;45: 870-2.

Groschel DHM, Pruett TL. Surgical antisepsis. In: Block SS, ed. Disinfection, sterilization, and preservation. Philadelphia: Lea and Febiger; 1991:642-54.

Larson EI, Morton HE. Alcohols. In: Block SS, ed. Disinfection, sterilization, and preservation. Philadelphia: Lea and Febiger; 1991:191-203.

Randell E, Brenman HS. Local degerming with

Table 9.3

Skin and Mucosal Antiseptics: Usage Information

Generic name	Brand name(s)	Content/form	Actions/uses
Ethyl alcohol	(generic)	70% ethyl alcohol	Very effective; gives rapid protection against most vegetative gram-positive and gram-negative bacteria; has good activity against the tubercle bacillus, most fungi and many viruses
Iodophors	Betadine Solution (1% available iodine), Sana Prep Solution (0.75% available iodine)	0.75%, 1% available iodine	May be applied to oral mucosa to reduce bacteremias during treatment of patients who are at increased risk of developing endocarditis (as indicated by American Heart Association) or who may be somehow immuno-compromised and have a neutropenia; antiseptic mouthrinses containing chlorhexidine or phenolic compounds also may be used in these instances (see Chapter 11); aqueous iodine preparations or a tincture of iodine (iodine in alcohol) also may be used for skin antisepsis
Isopropyl alcohol	(generic)	70% isopropyl alcohol	Alcohols are very effective and give rapid protection against most vegetative gram-positive and gram-negative bacteria; has good activity against the tubercle bacillus, most fungi and many viruses

The products listed here might not include all of those that are available. Also, the listing of a product does not denote its superiority to any other product that is either listed or not listed, nor does it guarantee its availability or quality.

Table 9.4

Skin and Mucosal Antiseptics: Adverse Effects, Precautions and Contraindications

Body system	Adverse effects	Precautions/contraindications
General	Defatting of skin and enhanced exposure of bacteria in hair follicles (alcohols) Painful stinging and burning when applied directly to mucosa and wounds (alcohols) Possible irritation (iodophors) Possible induction of hyperthyroidism in infants by iodine	Do not use alcohols or alcohol-based products on mucous membranes Do not use iodophors on infants

povidone-iodine. Part I. Prior to dental prophylaxis. J Periodontol 1974;45:866-9.

Zinner DD, Jablon JM, Saslaw MS. Bacteriocidal properties of povidone-iodine and its effectiveness as an oral antiseptic. Oral Surg 1961;14:1377-82.

Root Canal Medications/ Dressings

Irrigants. Irrigants are used during root canal therapy to flush debris from the canal, lubricate the canal, disinfect the canal, and act as a tissue or debris solvent. The three preparations most commonly used as irrigants are sodium hypochlorite, ethylenediamine-tetra-acetic acid and hydrogen peroxide.

Intracanal medications. The primary purpose of intracanal medications is to reduce microflora in the root canal after canal debridement while producing a minimal effect on normal host tissue. A secondary reason is to reduce postinstrumentation pain. The medications most commonly used for this purpose are calcium hydroxide, phenolic compounds, and the aldehyde formocresol (formaldehyde 48.5%, cresol 48.5%).

Accepted Indications

Irrigants
Sodium hypochlorite (NaOCl)
See Table 9.5.

Ethylenediamine-tetra-acetic acid (EDTA)
EDTA is a chelator, an organic substance that removes metal ions such as calcium by binding them chemically. This action aids in removal of calcified tissue. See Table 9.5.

Hydrogen peroxide 3% (H_2O_2)
Hydrogen peroxide should not be sealed into a canal because of the danger of forcing infected material beyond the apex. In pulp canals, hydrogen peroxide should be used carefully to avoid emphysema of the adjacent soft tissue. See Table 9.5.

Intracanal medications
Calcium hydroxide
See Table 9.5.

Phenolic compounds
Phenolic compounds such as camphorated parachlorophenol, which are considered protoplasmic poisons, are potent antimicrobial agents. They are capable of destroying tissue cells by binding cell membrane lipids and proteins. See Table 9.5.

Eugenol
Eugenol, which is an antiseptic and anodyne, is the essential chemical in clove oil and has similar uses. It is used in protective packs after excision of gingival tissues and is found in some temporary cements. Eugenol can also be used as an antiseptic in root canal therapy and for temporary relief of toothache.

Aldehydes
Formocresol is used routinely in pulpotomy procedures in primary teeth and as a temporary intracanal medicament.

Zinc oxide and zinc oxide-eugenol preparations
Zinc oxide is slightly antiseptic and weakly astringent and is used in combination with eugenol in many dental preparations. Some preparations use oils other than eugenol. Zinc oxide-eugenol preparations are used as therapeutic bases, temporary fillings, inlay and crown cements, periodontal surgical dressings and root canal sealers. The therapeutic value of zinc oxide-eugenol preparations is based on their compatibility with both hard and soft tissues of the mouth as well as their analgesic and topical local anesthetic effects. Zinc oxide-eugenol cements are recognized particularly for their sedative effect on pulpal tissue, especially in the restoration of teeth with deep carious lesions. Additionally, zinc oxide-eugenol cements are mildly antiseptic and provide a good marginal seal and good thermal insulation.

Zinc oxide-eugenol mixtures set into a hardened mass when mixed; the setting process involves both chemical and physical processes. Dressings containing zinc oxide and eugenol can be applied to the gingiva after surgical periodontal procedures. These dressings usually contain other ingredients such as tannic acid, rosin and oils such as mineral, peanut or vegetable oils. In some zinc oxide preparations, eugenol is completely replaced by other oils. These products are marketed as two components that must be combined and mixed to a paste or a putty-like consistency before being applied as a dressing to the tissue. One component is generally a powder consisting of zinc oxide, rosin, tannic acid, binders and soluble salts; the other component is a liquid consisting of eugenol, other oils or both.

General Usage Information

See Table 9.5.

Adverse Effects and Precautions

See Table 9.6.

Suggested Readings

Ingle JI, Bakland LF. Endodontics. 4th ed. Baltimore: Williams & Wilkins; 1994.

Walton RE, Torabinejad M. Principles and practice of endodontics. 2nd ed. Philadelphia: WB Saunders; 1996.

Table 9.5

Root Canal Medications and Dressings: Usage Information

Generic name	Brand name(s)	Content/form	Actions/uses
Aldehydes			
Formocresol	Buckley's Formo Cresol ★	**Liquid:** 35% cresol, 19% formaldehyde, 17.5% glycerine, 28.5% water	Vital pulp therapy in primary teeth
	Formo Cresol ★	**Liquid:** 48.5% cresol, 48.5% formaldehyde, 3% glycerine	Vital pulp therapy in primary teeth
Intracanal medications			
Calcium hydroxide (Ca[OH]₂)	Calcium hydroxide powder (generic) ★	Calcium hydroxide, USP, powder	Used to create an environment for healing pulpal and periapical tissues, to produce antimicrobial effects, to aid in elimination of apical seepage, to induce formation of calcified tissue, and to prevent inflammatory resorption after trauma
	Pulpdent Temp Canal	Calcium hydroxide in aqueous methylcellulose	Used to create an environment for healing pulpal and periapical tissues, to produce antimicrobial effects, to aid in elimination of apical seepage, to induce formation of calcified tissue, and to prevent inflammatory resorption after trauma

★ indicates a product bearing the ADA Seal of Acceptance.
The products listed here might not include all of those that are available. Also, the listing of a product does not denote its superiority to any other product that is either listed or not listed, nor does it guarantee its availability or quality.

Continued on next page

Table 9.5 (cont.)

Root Canal Medications and Dressings: Usage Information

Generic name	Brand name(s)	Content/form	Actions/uses
Irrigants			
Ethylenediamine-tetra-acetic acid (EDTA)	EDTA (generic)	17% in aqueous solution, pH 8.0	In combination with sodium hypochlorite, EDTA removes smear layer; alone, aids in removal of calcified tissue by chelating metal ions
	EDTAC	EDTA with Centrimide	In combination with sodium hypochlorite, EDTA removes smear layer; alone, aids in removal of calcified tissue by chelating metal ions
	File-EZE	EDTA in an aqueous solution	In combination with sodium hypochlorite, EDTA removes smear layer; alone, aids in removal of calcified tissue by chelating metal ions
	RC Prep ★	Urea peroxide 10%, EDTA 15% in a special water soluble base	In combination with sodium hypochlorite, EDTA removes smear layer; alone, aids in removal of calcified tissue by chelating metal ions
	REDTA	EDTA 17% in an aqueous solution, pH of 8.0	In combination with sodium hypochlorite, EDTA removes smear layer; alone, aids in removal of calcified tissue by chelating metal ions
Hydrogen peroxide 3% (H_2O_2)	generic	Aqueous solution	Oxidizing power of hydrogen peroxide kills certain anaerobic bacteria in cultures; in contact with tissues, its germicidal power is very limited because it is readily decomposed by organic matter and antimicrobial effect lasts only as long as oxygen is being released; can be used to cleanse and treat infected pulp canals
Sodium hydrochlorite (NaOCl)	Chlorox	5.25% sodium hypochlorite	Has a solvent action on pulp tissue and organic debris, is used for irrigation of root canals, and is useful for cleaning dentures; aqueous solutions of 2.5% and 5% sodium hypochlorite are reported to be equally effective in dissolving pulpal debris when used as root canal irrigants

★ indicates a product bearing the ADA Seal of Acceptance.
The products listed here might not include all of those that are available. Also, the
listing of a product does not denote its superiority to any other product that is either
listed or not listed, nor does it guarantee its availability or quality.

Continued on next page

Table 9.5 (cont.)

Root Canal Medications and Dressings: Usage Information

Generic name	Brand name(s)	Content/form	Actions/uses
		Irrigants (cont.)	
	Hypogen	5.25% sodium hypochlorite	Has a solvent action on pulp tissue and organic debris, is used for irrigation of root canals, and is useful for cleaning dentures; aqueous solutions of 2.5% and 5% sodium hypochlorite are reported to be equally effective in dissolving pulpal debris when used as root canal irrigants
		Miscellaneous preparations	
Zinc oxides	COE-Pak ★	**Paste 1:** 45% zinc oxide, 37% magnesium oxide, 11% peanut oil, 6% mineral oil, 1% chloroxylenol, chlorothymol and coumarin, 0.02% Toluidine-Red pigment **Paste 2:** 43% polymerized rosin, 24% coconut fatty acid, 10% ethyl alcohol, 9% petroleum jelly, 4% gum elemi, 4% lanolin, 3% ethyl cellulose, 1.5% chlorothymol, 1% carnauba, 0.2% zinc acetate, 0.1% spearmint oil	Periodontal dressing
	Perio-Care Periodontal Dressing ★	**Paste:** 38.5% magnesium oxide, 29.8% vegetable oils, 19.2% zinc oxide, 12.5% calcium hydroxide, 0.2% coloring **Gel:** 63.2% resins, 29.8% fatty acids, 3.5% ethyl cellulose, 3.5% lanolin	Periodontal dressing
	Perio-Putty	**Base:** 3.1% polyvinylpyrrolidone-iodine complex, 9% polymer, 5% benzocaine, 82.9% fillers **Catalyst:** 19.9% zinc oxide, 10.3% magnesium oxide, 12.3% mineral and vegetable oils, 58% inert fillers **Skin lubricant:** 95% silicone oils, 5% inert fillers	Periodontal dressing with skin lubricant

★ indicates a product bearing the ADA Seal of Acceptance.
The products listed here might not include all of those that are available. Also, the listing of a product does not denote its superiority to any other product that is either listed or not listed, nor does it guarantee its availability or quality.

Continued on next page

Table 9.5 (cont.)

Root Canal Medications and Dressings: Usage Information

Generic name	Brand name(s)	Content/form	Actions/uses
Miscellaneous preparations (cont.)			
	Zinc Oxide, U.S.P. ★	Zinc oxide powder	Periodontal dressing
	Zone Periodontal Pack	**Base:** 3.1% polyvinylpyrrolidone-iodine complex, 38.3% rosin, 2% chlorobutanol, 10% mineral oil, 9.3% isopropyl myristate, 37.3% propylene glycol monoisostearate	Periodontal dressing
Zinc oxide-eugenol	Kirkland Periodontal Pack ★	**Powder:** 40% zinc oxide, 40% rosin, 20% tannic acid **Liquid:** 46.5% eugenol, 46.5% peanut oil, 7.5% rosin	Periodontal dressing
	Peridres	**Powder:** 49% rosin, 46% zinc oxide, 3% tannic acid, 3% kaolin **Liquid:** 98% eugenol, 2% thymol	Periodontal dressing
Phenolic compounds			
Parachlorophenol (PCP)	Cresanol Root Canal Dressing	**Liquid:** 25% parachlorophenol, 25% metacresyl acetate, 50% camphor	Intracanal medicament
	M.C.P. Root Canal Dressing ★	**Liquid:** 25% metacresyl-acetate, 25% parachlorophenol, 50% camphor	Intracanal medicament
	Parachlorophenol Liquefied	**Liquid:** 98% parachlorophenol, 2% glycerin	Intracanal medicament
Camphorated parachlorophenol (CPC)	Camphorated Parachlorophenol, U.S.P. ★	**Liquid:** 35% parachlorophenol and 65% camphor	Intracanal medicament
Eugenol	Eugenol U.S.P. ★	**Liquid:** 100% eugenol	Anodyne/oral tissues, teeth

★ *indicates a product bearing the ADA Seal of Acceptance.*
The products listed here might not include all of those that are available. Also, the listing of a product does not denote its superiority to any other product that is either listed or not listed, nor does it guarantee its availability or quality.

Table 9.6

Root Canal Medications: Adverse Effects, Precautions and Contraindications

Body system	Adverse effects	Precautions/contraindications
General	Sodium hypochlorite is caustic and not suitable for application to wounds or areas of infection in soft tissues	Minimize soft-tissue contact
	Hydrogen peroxide should be used carefully to avoid emphysema of adjacent soft tissue	
	Phenolic compounds can destroy tissue cells by binding cell membrane lipids and proteins	
	Combined action of cresol, a protein-coagulating phenolic compound, and formaldehyde, an alkylating agent, make formocresol extremely cytotoxic and capable of causing widespread necrosis of vital tissue in the mouth or elsewhere	

Chapter 10

Agents Affecting Salivation

John Yagiela, D.D.S., Ph.D.

Anticholinergic Drugs

Saliva plays a vital role in protecting the health of soft and hard tissues of the mouth and in such functions as taste, mastication and deglutition. Excessive salivation, however, can complicate the performance of dental procedures such as the taking of impressions and the placement of restorations.

A number of anticholinergic drugs—otherwise referred to as cholinergic antagonists, antimuscarinic agents or parasympatholytics—are effective antisialogogues and are used by dentists and physicians for treating inappropriate salivary secretions and for reducing normal salivation to facilitate the performance of intraoral procedures. Because none of these agents is selective in its action, they all have a tendency to produce side effects, and this must be considered before proceeding with antisialogogue therapy. The anticholinergic drugs included in this chapter are limited to agents that have been approved for use to control salivation or that are used in dentistry for that purpose.

Accepted Indications

The control of salivation for dental procedures is a generally recognized but not officially accepted indication for these drugs. Atropine, glycopyrrolate, methantheline, propantheline and scopolamine are the most commonly used agents. These drugs also have several medical indications. For example, parenteral atropine has been approved

- for the control of bradycardia and first-degree heart block associated with excessive vagal activity or administration of succinylcholine;
- to inhibit salivation and respiratory tract secretions during general anesthesia;
- to minimize the muscarinic side effects of cholinesterase inhibitors used to reverse the action of neuromuscular blocking drugs.

Parenteral glycopyrrolate has been approved for the same purposes, except for the prophylaxis of succinylcholine-induced bradyarrhythmias. It also is indicated before general anesthesia to reduce secretion of gastric acid and to minimize the danger of pulmonary aspiration. Parenteral scopolamine has been approved for the control of secretions during general anesthesia and as a preanesthetic sedative and anesthetic adjunct in conjunction with opioid analgesics.

Anticholinergic drugs also have been approved for the management of peptic ulcers and various gastrointestinal, biliary and genitourinary disorders. For most drugs and conditions, these indications are considered obsolete. Selected anticholinergic drugs also are used to treat parkinsonism and as mydriatics and cycloplegics in ophthalmology. Atropine is a recognized antidote for the muscarinic toxicity of mushrooms, parasympathomimetic agonists and anticholinesterase drugs, insecticides and nerve gases.

General Dosing Information

Low doses of the anticholinergic drugs described in this chapter for blocking excessive salivary secretion, properly adjusted for route of administration, are relatively selective in effect. Larger doses, such as those required to treat vagally induced bradyarrhythmias, uniformly produce side effects, including pronounced dryness of the mouth. General dosing guidelines for the control of salivation and uses associated with general anesthesia are provided in Table 10.1.

Maximum Recommended Doses

Maximum recommended doses have not been established for single administrations of anticholinergics beyond the usual doses indicated in Table 10.1.

Dosage Adjustments

Within the recommended range, the dose of an anticholinergic drug may be adjusted according to need. For control of salivation, a low dose may be adequate when only moderation of salivation is required, whereas a larger dose may be necessary if secretions are preventing the successful accomplishment of a procedure, such as an impression. Reduced doses should be considered for infants, geriatric patients and those with medical conditions that alter their responses to anticholinergic drugs.

Special Dental Considerations

Drug Interactions of Dental Interest

Drug interactions and related problems involving anticholinergic antisialogogues listed in Table 10.2 are potentially of clinical significance in dentistry. Cross-sensitivities are provided in Table 10.3.

Laboratory Value Alterations

- Gastric acid secretion tests are impaired by anticholinergic drugs because they decrease stimulation of gastric acids.
- Radionuclide gastric emptying tests are impaired by anticholinergic drugs because of delayed gastric emptying.
- Phenolsulfonphthalein excretion tests are impaired by atropine because the two agents compete for the same transport mechanism.

- Serum uric acid is decreased in patients with hyperuricemia or gout who are receiving glycopyrrolate.

Cross-Sensitivity

Table 10.3 lists potential cross-sensitivities between anticholinergic agents and other drugs.

Special Patients

Pregnant and nursing women

Atropine and scopolamine cross the placenta. Although there is no evidence of teratogenic effects, intravenous atropine can cause tachycardia in the fetus, and parenteral scopolamine given during labor may adversely affect the neonate by depressing the CNS and reducing vitamin K-dependent clotting factors. Glycopyrrolate, methantheline and propantheline are quaternary ammonium compounds, and it is unlikely that they reach the fetal circulation in large amounts.

All anticholinergic drugs may inhibit lactation. In addition, atropine and scopolamine are distributed into breast milk. Although single doses to control salivation have not been associated with any health problem, it may be advisable for nursing mothers to collect sufficient milk to cover the 8-h period after taking an anticholinergic drug.

Pediatric, geriatric and other special patients

Pediatric patients. Infants and small children are especially sensitive to the toxic effects of anticholinergic drugs, even when the dose is corrected for body size. Because of their high metabolic rate, children generate relatively large amounts of heat and must dissipate that heat in a warm environment by sweating. Blockade of acetylcholine-mediated perspiration by these agents can quickly lead to grossly elevated temperatures. Flushing of the skin is an important early visual cue that steps must be taken to improve heat loss. Young children may also be especially sensitive to the CNS effects of atropine and scopolamine.

Geriatric patients. Geriatric patients are particularly susceptible to the parasympatholytic effects of anticholinergic drugs on

Table 10.1

Anticholinergic Drugs: Dosage Information

Generic name	Brand name(s)	Usual adult dosage	Usual child dosage	Pregnancy risk category	Content/form
Atropine sulfate	Sal-Tropine ★	**To control salivation—oral:** 0.3–1.2 mg **In anesthesia:** 2 mg orally or 0.2–0.6 mg IM ½–1 h before induction for prophylaxis of excessive secretions, 0.4–1 mg IV (up to 2 mg total) for arrhythmia, 0.3–1.2 mg for use with anticholinesterase in reversal of neuromuscular blockade	**To control salivation—oral:** 0.01 mg/kg up to 0.4 mg **In anesthesia—IV:** 0.01–0.03 mg/kg IV for arrhythmia, 0.01–0.02 mg/kg for use with anticholinesterase in reversal of neuromuscular blockade	C	**Injection, 0.05 mg/mL:** in 5-mL syringes **Injection, 0.1 mg/mL:** in 5-, 10-mL syringes **Injection, 0.3 mg/mL:** in 1-, 30-mL vials **Injection, 0.4 mg/mL:** in 1-mL ampules and 1-, 10-, 30-mL vials **Injection, 0.5 mg/mL:** in 1-, 30-mL vials and 5-mL syringes **Injection, 0.8 mg/mL:** in 0.5-, 1-mL ampules and 0.5-mL syringes **Injection, 1 mg/mL:** in 1-mL ampules and 10-mL syringes **Tablets:** 0.4 mg **Tablets, soluble:** 0.4, 0.6 mg

		Usual Adult Dosage	Usual Pediatric Dosage		Available Forms
Glycopyrrolate	Robinul, Robinul Forte	**To control salivation—oral:** 1-2 mg. **In anesthesia:** 4.4 µg/kg IM ½-1 h before induction for prophylaxis of excessive secretions (including gastric), 0.1 mg IV q 2-3 min for arrhythmia, 0.2 mg/1 mg neostigmine or 5 mg pyridostigmine for reversal of neuromuscular blockade	**To control salivation:** Not established. **In anesthesia:** 4.4-8.8 µg/kg IM ½-1 h before induction for prophylaxis of excessive secretions (including gastric), 4.4 µg/kg q 2-3 min up to 0.1 mg for arrhythmias; 0.2 mg/1 mg neostigmine or 5 mg pyridostigmine for reversal of neuromuscular blockade	B	**Injection, 0.2 mg/mL:** in 1-, 2-, 5-, 20-mL vials. **Tablets:** 1, 2 mg
Methantheline bromide	Banthine	**To control salivation—oral:** 50-100 mg	**To control salivation:** 12.5-50 mg	C	**Tablets:** 50 mg
Propantheline bromide	Pro-Banthine	**To control salivation—oral:** 15-30 mg	**To control salivation:** 0.375 mg/kg up to adult dose	C	**Tablets:** 7.5, 15 mg
Scopolamine butylbromide [CAN]	Buscopan [CAN]	**To control salivation—oral:** 10-20 mg	Not established	C	**Injection, 20 mg/mL:** in 1-mL ampules. **Suppositories:** 10 mg. **Tablets:** 10 mg
Scopolamine hydrobromide	(generic)	**To control salivation—oral:** 0.3-0.6 mg * **In anesthesia—IM:** 0.2-0.6 mg (for prophylaxis of excessive secretions). **As an anesthetic adjunct—IV, IM, SC:** 0.32-0.65 mg	**To control salivation:** Not established. **Age 4-7 mo, in anesthesia—IM:** 0.1 mg (for prophylaxis of excessive secretions). **Age 7 mo-3 y, in anesthesia—IM:** 0.15 mg (for prophylaxis of excessive secretions). **Age 3-8 y, in anesthesia—IM:** 0.2 mg (for prophylaxis of excessive secretions). **Age 8-12 y, in anesthesia—IM:** 0.3 mg (for prophylaxis of excessive secretions)	C	**Injection, 0.3 mg/mL:** in 1-mL vials. **Injection, 0.4 mg/mL:** in 0.5-mL ampules and 1-mL vials. **Injection, 0.86 mg/mL:** in 0.5-mL vials. **Injection, 1 mg/mL:** in 1-mL vials

★ indicates a drug that has the ADA Seal of Acceptance.
[CAN] indicates a drug that is available only in Canada.
* Requires oral ingestion of solution designed for injection, usually with flavoring agent to improve taste.

Table 10.2

Anticholinergic Drugs: Possible Interactions With Other Drugs

Drug taken by patient	Interaction with anticholinergic drugs	Dentist's action
Antacids or absorbent antidiarrheal drugs	*May impair absorption of anticholinergic drug*	Avoid administration of an anticholinergic drug within 2-3 h of ingestion of the interacting drug
Antimyasthenics	Muscarinic effects are blocked by anticholinergic drugs, possibly obscuring early signs of an antimyasthenic overdose	Use cautiously
CNS depressants	Summation of CNS depression with scopolamine; hallucination and behavioral disturbances have been reported with parenteral lorazepam and scopolamine	Use cautiously
Drugs with anticholinergic side effects: antiparkinsonism drugs, antipsychotic agents, carbamazepine, digoxin, dronabinol, orphenadrine, procainamide, quinidine, sedative antihistamines, tricyclic antidepressants	*Additive anticholinergic effects*	Use cautiously
Ketoconazole	*Absorption may be impaired by increased gastric pH caused by anticholinergic drugs*	Have the patient take ketoconazole at least 2 h before the anticholinergic drug
Metoclopramide	Effect of hastening gastric emptying may be blocked by anticholinergic drugs	Use cautiously
Opioid analgesics	Summation of constipating effects	Use cautiously
Potassium chloride	*Delayed absorption may increase gastrointestinal toxicity of potassium chloride*	Avoid concurrent use

Italics indicate information of major clinical significance.

Table 10.3

Anticholinergic Drugs: Potential Cross-Sensitivity With Other Drugs

A person with a sensitivity to	May also have a sensitivity to
Any belladonna alkaloid	Atropine or scopolamine
Methantheline	Propantheline (and vice versa)

visceral smooth muscle. Although single doses, as used in dentistry for control of salivation, are generally well tolerated by elderly people, large doses of atropine and scopolamine have been associated with excessive depressant and excitatory CNS reactions. Repeated doses can cause constipation and, especially in men, urinary retention. Xerostomia, increased dental caries and fungal infections are dental concerns associated with chronic use in elderly patients. In addition, patients aged > 40 y are at increased risk of an acute attack of previously undiagnosed angle-closure glaucoma.

Patients with medical problems. Patients with certain medical problems are especially susceptible to the adverse effects of anticholinergic drugs. These include patients with obstructive or paralytic gastrointestinal and urinary tract disorders, cardiac disease and angle-closure glaucoma. Specific recommendations regarding these patients are listed in Table 10.4.

Patient Monitoring: Aspects to Watch
- Cardiovascular status (arterial blood pressure, heart rate, electrocardiogram) with parenteral anticholinergic drugs

Adverse Effects and Precautions
The adverse effects of the anticholinergic drugs are the predictable consequences of the inhibition of various physiological actions of acetylcholine. Single oral doses of agents

Table 10.4
Anticholinergic Drugs: Adverse Effects, Precautions and Contraindications

Body system	Adverse effects	Precautions/contraindications
General	Skin rash, urticaria Decreased sweating, hyperthermia *(mainly in small children)*	Monitor temperature in patients with fever *Contraindicated in patients with history of drug sensitivity to the anticholinergic drug considered for use*
CV	*Tachycardia,* hypertension Orthostatic hypotension (with large doses of quaternary ammonium derivatives)	*Avoid large doses or parenteral administration in patients with cardiac disease, tachycardia or acute hypovolemia* Use cautiously in patients with Down's syndrome, hyperthyroidism, hypertension or pregnancy toxemia
CNS	CNS depression, drowsiness, dizziness, tiredness, anterograde amnesia, confusion with *scopolamine* or atropine CNS excitation, headache, hallucination, seizures with *scopolamine* or atropine	Children with brain damage are more likely to develop CNS effects
EENT	*Mydriasis, cycloplegia, blurred vision and increased intraocular pressure, especially with scopolamine or atropine*	Use cautiously with patients who have open-angle glaucoma Increased mydriatic effect is likely in patients with Down's syndrome *Contraindicated in patients with history of angle-closure glaucoma*

Italics indicate information of major clinical significance.

Continued on next page

Table 10.4 (cont.)

Anticholinergic Drugs: Adverse Effects, Precautions and Contraindications

Body system	Adverse effects	Precautions/contraindications
GI	Constipation, obstruction, gastric reflux, nausea and vomiting *(mainly with chronic use)*	*Patients with obstructive or paralytic GI disease, intestinal atony, hiatal hernia, reflux esophagitis or ulcerative colitis are at risk of exacerbating their existing disorder* Patients with reflux esophagitis or obstructive GI disease have an increased risk of emesis during anesthesia when an anticholinergic drug is used preoperatively
GU	Urinary retention *(mainly with chronic use)*	*History of obstructive or paralytic uropathy, prostatic hypertrophy or urinary retention increases risk of urinary retention* Renal function impairment may prolong anticholinergic effects
HB		Hepatic function impairment may prolong anticholinergic effects
Musc	Muscle weakness (large doses of quaternary ammonium derivatives)	*Myasthenia gravis increases risk of muscle weakness*
Oral	*Xerostomia*, difficulty in swallowing Increased incidence/severity of dental caries, periodontal disease and candidiasis *(with chronic use)*	Patients with xerostomia are likely to experience increased inhibition of salivation
Resp	Dryness of respiratory tree Decreased ventilation from muscle weakness (large doses of quaternary ammonium derivatives)	Pulmonary problems from obstruction of bronchial passages by thickened secretions are more likely with patients—especially young children and bedridden patients—who have chronic pulmonary disease *Myasthenia gravis increases risk of impaired ventilation*

Italics indicate information of major clinical significance.

used to control salivation are usually well tolerated, but large parenteral doses invariably induce a host of side effects. Although these effects may be unpleasant, they are virtually never life-threatening except in small children and medically compromised patients. The adverse effects and precautions and contraindications listed in Table 10.4 apply to all routes of administration.

Pharmacology

Anticholinergic drugs competitively block the effects of acetylcholine and cholinergic drugs at muscarinic receptor sites. Muscarinic receptors mediate tissue responses to parasympathetic nervous system stimulation and cholinergic-induced sweating and vasodilation. Tertiary amines, such as atropine and especially scopolamine, may produce

CNS effects because of their ability to cross the blood-brain barrier. Quaternary amines, such as glycopyrrolate, methantheline and propantheline, are largely excluded from the brain and do not act directly on the CNS. The existence of muscarinic receptor subtypes (designated M_1 through M_5) also accounts for some of the differences in peripheral effects among the anticholinergic drugs because of different relative affinities of the drugs for these subtypes. It has been determined that the M_3 receptor supports serous salivary gland secretion and the M_2 receptor is responsible for parasympathomimetic cardiac effects. In tissues where acetylcholine release at muscarinic receptors is chronically active, anticholinergic drugs will exert pronounced antimuscarinic effects. If acetylcholine or other cholinergic drugs are absent, anticholinergic drugs will elicit little or no observable effect.

Atropine and scopolamine, two naturally occurring belladonna alkaloids, are well absorbed from the gastrointestinal tract; however, absorption is less complete with the synthetic quaternary ammonium drugs. Atropine is partially metabolized in the liver and excreted in the urine as both the parent compound and metabolite. A similar fate presumably occurs with the other anticholinergic agents. Table 10.5 lists the time to effect and duration of effect of anticholinergic drugs used orally for control of salivation.

Patient Advice

- Patients should be aware of the potential common side effects, such as dryness of the mouth, nose and throat; difficulty in swallowing; and inhibition of sweating.
- Parents should be warned of the potential for hyperthermia in small children, especially when the children are overdressed, physically active or in a warm environment.
- Because of the possibility of psychomotor impairment after use of scopolamine, driving or other tasks requiring alertness and coordination should be avoided or performed with added caution, as appropriate, on the day of treatment. It is also desirable to avoid the use of alcohol or other CNS depressants during this time.

Suggested Readings

Brown JH, Taylor P. Muscarinic receptor agonists and antagonists. In: Hardman JG, Limbird LE, eds. Goodman & Gilman's the pharmacological basis of therapeutics. 9th ed. New York: McGraw-Hill; 1996:141-60.

Mandel ID. The role of saliva in maintaining oral homeostasis. JADA 1989;119:298-304.

Table 10.5

Anticholinergic Drugs*: Pharmacokinetic Parameters

Drug	Time of onset (min)	Duration of effect (h)	Amine structure
Atropine	60 to 120	4 to 6	Tertiary
Scopolamine	30 to 60	4 to 6	Tertiary
Glycopyrrolate	30 to 45	6 to 8	Quaternary
Methantheline	30 to 45	6	Quaternary
Propantheline	30 to 45	6	Quaternary

*Drugs administered orally for control of salivation.

Cholinergic Drug: Pilocarpine

In contrast to the anticholinergic agents, cholinergic drugs produce effects that mimic those of acetylcholine, the natural ligand for cholinergic receptors. Additional terms used to identify cholinergic drugs include cholinergic agonists, cholinomimetics, parasympathomimetics and muscarinic agonists. Pilocarpine, a naturally occurring cholinergic agonist, is the only drug currently approved for the treatment of xerostomia. Diseases or conditions that cause xerostomia commonly result in opportunistic infection, increased caries and difficulty in speaking and in maintaining normal dietary intake. Although pilocarpine has been used as a sialogogue for nearly a century to treat such diverse conditions as Sjögren's syndrome and postradiation xerostomia, it was approved for the latter purpose by the U.S. Food and Drug Administration only in 1994, after being developed under the provisions of the Orphan Drug Act of 1983.

Successful stimulation of salivary secretion by pilocarpine requires the presence of intact salivary gland tissue and nerve supply. In the case of radiation therapy, this requirement may be met by residual active tissue in the irradiated field or healthy tissue outside the field.

Accepted Indications

Pilocarpine has been approved for the relief of xerostomia caused by radiation therapy of the head and neck. In its topical forms, pilocarpine has also been approved for treating various types of glaucoma and producing pupillary constriction (miosis) after surgery or ocular examination.

General Dosing Information

As shown in Table 10.6, the usual adult daily dose of pilocarpine is 5 mg tid. A dose of 10 mg tid may be tried in refractory cases; however, the incidence of dose-related side effects increases at this dosage, and as a general rule, the dentist should use the lowest effective dose that is tolerated by the patient. Pilocarpine has not been tested in children.

Special Dental Considerations

Drug Interactions of Dental Interest
Table 10.7 lists possible drug interactions and related problems involving pilocarpine that are potentially of clinical significance in dentistry.

Cross-Sensitivity
Patients sensitive to other forms of pilocarpine dosage (that is, ophthalmic) should be considered sensitive to oral pilocarpine.

Special Patients
Pregnant and nursing women
There are no data regarding the influence of pilocarpine on reproduction and fetal development. Pilocarpine has been designated as FDA pregnancy category C. It has not been determined if pilocarpine is distributed into breast milk, and there are no reports of related problems in humans.

Table 10.6

Pilocarpine: Dosage Information

Generic name	Brand name(s)	Usual adult dosage	Usual child dosage	Pregnancy risk category	Content/form
Pilocarpine hydrochloride	Salagen	5 mg tid **In refractory cases:** 10 mg tid	Not established	C	Tablets: 5 mg

Pediatric, geriatric and other special patients
Pilocarpine has not been tested for, nor is it indicated for, use in children.

There appears to be no special concern regarding pilocarpine and the geriatric population, although elderly people are more likely to have specific medical problems, such as angle-closure glaucoma, pulmonary disease or cardiovascular disease, that may complicate pilocarpine therapy.

Adverse Effects and Precautions

Most of the adverse effects observed with pilocarpine (Table 10.8) are dose-dependent extensions of the drug's ability to stimulate cholinergic muscarinic receptors. Hypertension may be an important exception to this generalization. Excessive secretions (sweating, bronchial secretions, rhinitis) are the most common side effects associated with oral pilocarpine.

Pharmacology

Pilocarpine stimulates muscarinic receptors to elicit most of its effects. Muscarinic receptors are linked to specific G proteins that mediate intracellular signaling in response to drug-receptor binding. For the M_3 receptor involved in salivary secretion, stimulation of its G protein causes the intracellular formation of inositol 1,4,5-trisphosphate and diacylglycerol, which promote secretion and smooth muscle contraction. Anomalous hypertensive responses to pilocarpine may be due to ganglionic or adrenal medullary stimulation. Pilocarpine, which is a tertiary amine, gains access to the CNS and can produce excitatory reactions.

Pilocarpine is readily absorbed from the gastrointestinal tract. Peak drug effects occur within 1 h and last 3-5 h. Pilocarpine is partially metabolized, possibly in the plasma or at neuronal synapses, and is then excreted in the urine.

Patient Advice

- Because adverse effects are dose-dependent, patients should be cautioned to take the medication as directed.
- If dizziness, lightheadedness or blurred vision occurs, patients should refrain from driving or other tasks requiring alertness, coordination and visual acuity until the problem is resolved.

Table 10.7

Pilocarpine: Possible Interactions With Other Drugs

Drug taken by patient	Interaction	Dentist's action
Drugs with anticholinergic activity: anticholinergics, antiparkinson drugs, antipsychotic agents, carbamazepine, digoxin, dronabinol, orphenadrine, procainamide, quinidine, sedative antihistamines, tricyclic antidepressants	*Antagonistic drug effects*	Use cautiously when the anticholinergic effect of the interacting drug is not the goal of therapy; otherwise consult with a physician to optimize drug treatment
Drugs with cholinergic activity: cholinergic antiglaucoma drugs, antimyasthenic agents, bethanechol	Summation of drug effects	Use cautiously
β-adrenergic blocking drugs	*Summation of drug effects on cardiac automaticity and conduction*	Use cautiously

Italics indicate information of major clinical significance.

Table 10.8
Pilocarpine: Adverse Effects, Precautions and Contraindications

Body system	Adverse effects	Precautions/contraindications
General	Sweating, chills, flushing	*Contraindicated in patients with history of drug sensitivity to pilocarpine*
CNS	Confusion, headache	Psychiatric disorders increase risk of CNS disturbances
CV	Bradycardia, *tachycardia*, atrioventricular heart block *Hypertension*, transient hypotension	*Patients with cardiovascular disease have increased risk of cardiovascular instability*
EENT	Increased intraocular pressure, blurred vision, eye pain, lacrimation	*Patients with angle-closure glaucoma or acute iritis have an increased risk of acute attack of glaucoma* History of or predisposition for retinal detachment may increase risk of detachment
GI	Nausea and vomiting, diarrhea	
GU	Frequent urination	Use in patients with nephrolithiasis may lead to renal colic
HB		Patients with cholelithiasis have increased risk of acute biliary disorder
Musc	Tremors	
Resp	Bronchoconstriction, increased mucous secretions, wheezing, pulmonary edema Rhinitis, nose bleed	*History of asthma, chronic bronchitis or chronic obstructive pulmonary disease increases risk of respiratory distress*

Italics indicate information of major clinical significance.

Suggested Readings

Fox, PC, Atkinson JC, Macynski AA, et al. Pilocarpine treatment of salivary gland hypofunction and dry mouth (xerostomia). Arch Intern Med 1991;151:1149-52.

Johnson JT, Ferretti GA, Nethery WJ, et al. Oral pilocarpine for post-irradiation xerostomia in patients with head and neck cancer. N Engl J Med 1993;329:390-5.

Wynn RL. Oral pilocarpine (Salagen)—a recently approved salivary stimulant. Gen Dent 1996;44:26,29-31.

Saliva Substitutes

When salivary function is absent or minimal, cholinergic drug therapy with pilocarpine or related agents is ineffective. Replacement of missing saliva is a natural therapeutic alternative. Water is most commonly used by patients afflicted with chronic xerostomia because of its unique advantages of availability and low cost. Water is a poor substitute for saliva, however, because it lacks necessary ions, buffering capacity and lubricating mucins. Saliva substitutes, or artificial salivas, are designed to more closely match the chemical and physical characteristics of saliva. These preparations often contain complex mixtures of salts, with cellulose derivatives or animal mucins added to increase viscosity (often a viscosity greater than that of natural saliva, in an attempt to improve retention within the mouth). Flavoring agents, usually sorbitol or xylitol, are generally added to improve taste, and parabens are sometimes included to inhibit bacterial growth. A deficiency of all artificial salivas to date is their complete lack of anti-infective proteins, such as immunoglobulin A, histatins and lysozyme.

Accepted Indications

Saliva substitutes are indicated for the symptomatic relief of dry mouth and dry throat in patients with xerostomia.

General Dosing Information

Saliva substitutes are meant to be taken ad libitum throughout the day, usually in the form of sprays, to keep the oral mucosa moist. There are no specific dosing guidelines, nor are there specific recommendations for special patients. Table 10.9 lists, by manufacturer's brand name, the ingredients of each commercially available preparation.

Special Dental Considerations

Patients with severe xerostomia who use a saliva substitute containing sorbitol on a regular basis may be at increased risk of caries associated with a very limited fermentation of sorbitol. A proper professionally designed topical fluoride treatment program undertaken to protect the teeth of the patient with xerostomia from caries should also overcome any problem posed by sorbitol.

Table 10.9

Saliva Substitutes: Product Information

Brand name(s)	Content/form
Entertainer's Secret	**Solution:** sodium carboxymethylcellulose, dibasic sodium phosphate, potassium chloride, parabens, aloe vera gel, glycerin in 60-mL spray
Moi-Stir, Moi-Stir Swabsticks	**Solution:** sodium carboxymethylcellulose, dibasic sodium phosphate, calcium, magnesium, potassium and sodium chlorides, parabens, sorbitol in 120-mL pump spray and 3-stick packets
Mouthkote	**Solution:** mucoprotective factor, yerba santa, saccharin, sorbitol, xylitol in 60- and 240-mL spray
Optimoist	**Solution:** hydroxyethyl cellulose, acesulfame potassium, calcium phosphate monobasic, citric acid, sodium benzoate, sodium hydroxide, sodium monofluorophosphate in 60- and 355-mL spray
Saliva Substitute★	**Solution:** sodium carboxymethylcellulose, sorbitol in 5- and 120-mL vials
Salivart★	**Solution:** sodium carboxymethylcellulose, dibasic potassium phosphate, calcium, magnesium, potassium and sodium chlorides, sorbitol, nitrogen propellant in 25- and 75-mL spray cans
Salix	**Lozenges:** hydroxypropyl methylcellulose, carboxymethylcellulose, dicalcium phosphate, malic acid, hydrogenated cottonseed oil, sodium citrate, citric acid, silicon dioxide, sorbitol
Xero-Lube★	**Solution:** hydroxyethylcellulose, dibasic and monobasic potassium phosphates, calcium, magnesium and potassium chlorides, sodium fluoride, methylparaben, flavor, xylitol in 6-oz spray

★ indicates a product bearing the ADA Seal of Acceptance.

There are no known drug interactions involving saliva substitutes, nor any need for patient monitoring pertaining to these products. Laboratory tests are likewise unaffected.

Cross-Sensitivity

Saliva substitutes containing parabens pose a risk of cross-sensitivity in patients allergic to parabens, para-aminobenzoic acid or its derivatives, such as ester local anesthetics. Some products contain other ingredients that pose additional risks of allergic cross-reactions.

Adverse Effects and Precautions

Aside from the allergic potential of parabens or other components of selected preparations and the possibility of increased caries incidence with sorbitol, there are few potential adverse effects or precautions associated with saliva substitutes. Microbial contamination is a possibility with multiple dose formulations, but this risk is partially offset by the inclusion of paraben preservatives.

Pharmacology

Saliva substitutes are physically active agents. When used regularly, they help minimize the sequelae of xerostomia by keeping the oral mucosa moist and lubricated. Surface abrasion is reduced, and patients are more able to perform the everyday activities of speaking,

eating and sleeping. Long-term compliance, however, is a problem with these products because of their perceived inconvenience and relatively high cost.

Because saliva substitutes are quickly swallowed and their activity is of limited duration, they must be administered repeatedly. The components of the ingested solution undoubtedly undergo gastrointestinal absorption; however, there is no information on the pharmacokinetics of the currently available saliva substitutes.

Patient Advice

- Patients should be informed of the necessity of the continual use of saliva substitutes.
- Patients with chronic xerostomia should be educated on the need for regular professional care and for a high degree of compliance with the dental professional's recommendations for minimizing caries and soft-tissue pathology.

Suggested Readings

Jacob RF. Management of xerostomia in the irradiated patient. Clin Plast Surg 1993;20:507-16.

Levine MJ. Development of artificial salivas. Crit Rev Oral Biol Med 1993;4:279-86.

Levine MJ, Aguirre A, Hatton MN, Tabak LA. Artificial salivas: present and future. J Dent Res 1987;66(Special Issue):693-8.

Chapter 11.

Mouthrinses and Dentifrices

Angelo J. Mariotti, D.D.S., Ph.D.

Mouthrinses

As the first major component of the alimentary canal, the mouth contains unique anatomical and physiological characteristics that affect the therapeutic outcome of topically applied agents. Therefore, the pharmacokinetics (that is, the activity involving processes such as the rate and extent of absorption, distribution and elimination of drugs from the body over time) of rinses in the mouth depend on how drugs are administered, when they are administered, the type of drug and the drug formulation.

Mouthrinses or mouthwashes fall into two categories:
- a vehicle for therapeutic agents to treat disease states;
- liquids with a pleasant taste and odor used primarily for cosmetic purposes (that is, to overcome mouth odors).

The three principal uses of mouthrinses are reduction of plaque formation on teeth and oral mucosa, prevention or remineralization of carious lesions and control of halitosis.

Each type of mouthrinse has its own associated traits.

Chlorhexidine rinses are available by prescription only, while all others are available over the counter. Mouthrinses containing chlorhexidine are the only products that have received FDA approval for efficacy in reducing plaque and gingival inflammation.

Fluoride rinses will substantially reduce carious lesions, but these agents have little or no effect in reducing supragingival plaque.

Oxygenating compounds should not be considered for frequent and extended use, as damage to oral tissues can result. In solutions containing carbamide peroxide, 33.5% of carbamide peroxide is converted to hydrogen peroxide, which in turn has the potential to damage oral tissues in doses exceeding 3% hydrogen peroxide. A solution of 10% carbamide peroxide releases approximately 3% hydrogen peroxide when introduced into the mouth.

Since the introduction of the first prebrushing rinse, the marketing of similar generic products has proliferated. Although some studies have reported plaque reductions in patients using these agents, a large number of studies found no advantage of using prebrushing rinses in reducing plaque levels. Thus, the recommendation of prebrushing rinses is questionable.

As for cosmetic mouthrinses to freshen breath, dentists should keep in mind that the reasons for halitosis are complex. The impact of mouthrinses in disguising malodor is transitory and ineffective. To effectively diagnose and treat the cause of halitosis, the dentist must perform a thorough examination.

Although mouthrinses containing chlorine dioxide are sold in the United States, adequate controlled trials of their efficacy for plaque and halitosis reduction are not available.

Accepted Indications

Mouthrinses are used in dentistry for a variety of reasons: to freshen breath, to prevent or control tooth decay, to reduce plaque formation on teeth and gums, to prevent or reduce gingivitis or to produce a combination of these effects.

General Dosing Information

The usual adult dosage (and often the geriatric dosage) for mouthrinses (Table 11.1) is 10-20 mL for therapeutic rinses; it is not established for cosmetic and prebrushing rinses and so can be dictated by individual choice. For oxygenating agents, dosage regimens are more restrictive, in terms of frequency and duration of usage. Duration of rinsing varies by type used. Safety and efficacy typically have not been established for mouthrinse use by pediatric patients.

Maximum Recommended Doses

Maximum recommended doses for mouthrinses are typically what can be held in the mouth comfortably (10-20 mL). The exception is an oxygenating agent of 1.5% hydrogen peroxide (Peroxyl), which is used in smaller quantities. Depending on whether the formulations are purchased over the counter (with directions on packaging) or prescribed (with directions on the label), additional mouthrinse should be taken only after sufficient time has been allowed for the therapeutic effect of the previous dose to need augmentation.

Dosage Adjustments

The actual maximum dose for each patient must be individualized depending on factors such as his or her size, age and physical status; ability to effectively rinse and expectorate; oral health; and sensitivity. Mouthrinses are not often prescribed for pediatric patients and as patients often swallow some of the product, reduced maximum doses may be indicated for geriatric patients, patients with serious illness or disability, and patients with medical conditions or who are taking drugs that alter oral responses to mouthrinses.

Special Dental Considerations

Drug Interactions of Dental Interest

The following drug interactions and related problems involving mouthrinses are potentially of clinical significance in dentistry. Concurrent use of agents that contain either calcium hydroxide or aluminum hydroxide may form a complex with the fluoride ions and reduce a rinse's effectiveness in the mouth. Concomitant use of chlorhexidine and stannous fluoride mouthrinses may reduce the efficacy of each agent.

Cross-Sensitivity

Some patients can develop allergic reactions (skin rash, hives, swelling of face, and so forth) to rinses. If this occurs, treatment should be discontinued immediately.

Special Patients

Problems with oral rinses containing fluorides in humans who are pregnant or breast feeding have not been documented with normal daily use.

Patient Monitoring: Aspects to Watch

- Extrinsic staining and increased calculus buildup: possible in some instances (see Table 11.2)
- Patients in recovery from alcoholism: caution should be used in prescribing mouthrinses containing alcohol to these patients
- Rinsing with water or drinking anything after using the mouthrinse: should be avoided for for at least 30 min to prevent clearance of the drug from the mouth and reduction in effectiveness of the mouthrinse

Adverse Effects and Precautions

The incidence of adverse reactions to mouthrinses is relatively low. Many reactions (burning, taste alterations, tooth staining) are temporary. Idiosyncratic and allergic reactions account for a small minority of adverse

Table 11.1

Mouthrinses: Dosage and Usage Information

Generic name/active ingredient	Brand name(s)	Usual adult dosage*	Usual child dosage†	Indications	Content
Anesthetic mouthrinse	Chloraseptic Mouthwash	10 mL prn (no more often than q 3 h)	Not indicated for children	Topical anesthesia	1.4% phenol, 12.5% alcohol
Chlorhexidine ‡	Peridex ★, PerioGard	15 mL swished for 30 s and expectorated; use bid	Not established	Antibacterial	**Peridex ★:** 0.12% chlorhexidine, 11.6% alcohol **PerioGard:** 0.12% chlorhexidine, 11.6% alcohol
Cosmetic mouthrinses	Cepacol, Lavoris Crystal Fresh, Lavoris Mint, Lavoris Original Cinnamon, Lavoris Original, Lavoris Peppermint, Listermint Mint, Oxyfresh Natural Mouthrinse, Platinum, Rembrandt Mouth Refreshing Rinse, Retardex Oral Rinse, Scope Mouthwash and Gargle, Scope Mouthwash and Gargle with Baking Soda, Signal Mouthwash, Therasol Mouthwash	Amount, duration and frequency of mouthrinse used depends on individual choice	Use of mouthrinses is not recommended for children	Masking of odors in mouth	**Cepacol:** 14.5% alcohol, miscellaneous ingredients **Lavoris Crystal Fresh, Original, Peppermint:** alcohol, citric acid, sodium hydroxide, zinc oxide, miscellaneous ingredients **Lavoris Mint, Cinnamon:** alcohol, aromatic oils, zinc chloride and/or zinc oxide **Listermint Mint (alcohol-free):** zinc chloride, sodium benzoate, sodium lauryl sulfate, miscellaneous ingredients **Oxyfresh Natural Mouthrinse (alcohol-free):** oxygene (contains chlorine dioxide), miscellaneous ingredients **Platinum:** monofluorophosphate, tetrapotassium pyrophosphate, miscellaneous ingredients **Rembrandt Mouth Refreshing Rinse (alcohol-free):** sodium benzoate, methyl paraben, miscellaneous ingredients *Continued on next page*

Continued on next page

★ indicates a product bearing the ADA Seal of Acceptance.

* Geriatric dosage is same as usual adult dosage.

† Pediatric safety and efficacy have not been established except with fluoride rinses in children aged 6 y and older.

‡ Pregnancy risk category B. Pregnancy risk categories have not been established for other products in this table.

Table 11.1 (cont.)

Mouthrinses: Dosage and Usage Information

Generic name/ active ingredient	Brand name(s)	Usual adult dosage*	Usual child dosage†	Indications	Content
Cosmetic mouthrinses (*cont.*)					**Retardex Oral Rinse (alcohol-free)** Ciosysii (contains chlorine dioxide), miscellaneous ingredients **Scope Mouthwash and Gargle:** 18.9% alcohol, sodium benzoate, cetylpyrionium chloride, benzoic acid, domiphen bromide, miscellaneous ingredients **Scope Mouthwash and Gargle with Baking Soda:** 9.9% alcohol, cetylpyridinium chloride, domiphen bromide, miscellaneous ingredients **Signal Mouthwash:** 14.5% alcohol, sodium lauryl sulfate, miscellaneous ingredients **Therasol Mouthwash:** 8% alcohol, 0.3% C31G (alkyl dimethyl amine oxide and alkyl dimethyl glycine), miscellaneous ingredients
Fluorides	Act Fluoride Anti-Cavity Dental Rinse; Reach Act for Kids Fluoride Anti-Cavity Treatment ★; Dentinbloc Dentin Desensitizer; Fluorigard Anti-Cavity Dental Rinse ★; Phos-Flur Daily Oral Rinse ★; Point-Two Dental Rinse; PreviDent Dental Rinse ★; Reach Fluoride Dental Rinse; NaFrinse Acidulated Oral Rinse ★; Oral-B Anti-Cavity Dental Rinse ★; Pro-Dentx 0.2% Neutral Sodium Fluoride Rinse ★	10 mL of sodium fluoride swished for 60 s and expectorated q day; patient should not eat or drink for 30 min after rinsing	**Age < 6 y:** Not recommended **Age ≥ 6 y:** Children can rinse with 10 mL of 0.05% sodium fluoride for 60 s and expectorate q day and should not eat or drink for 30 min after rinsing	Prevention or remineralization of carious lesions	**Act Fluoride Anti-Cavity Dental Rinse:** 0.05% sodium fluoride, 7% alcohol **Dentinbloc Dentin Desensitizer:** 1.09% sodium fluoride, 0.4% stannous fluoride, 0.14% hydrogen fluoride **Fluorigard Anti-Cavity Dental Rinse ★;** **Phos-Flur Daily Oral Rinse ★:** 0.02% fluoride **Point-Two Dental Rinse:** 0.2% sodium fluoride, 6% alcohol **PreviDent Dental Rinse ★:** 0.2% sodium fluoride, 6% alcohol **Reach Act for Kids Fluoride Anti-Cavity Treatment ★:** 0.05% sodium fluoride

Category	Products	Active ingredients	Clinical uses	Pediatric dosage†	Usual adult dosage*
Fluorides (cont.)		**Reach Fluoride Dental Rinse; NaFrinse Acidulated Oral Rinse ★; Oral-B Anti-Cavity Dental Rinse ★:** 0.05% sodium fluoride **Pro-Dentx 0.2% Neutral Sodium Fluoride Rinse ★**			
Oxygenating agents	Gly-Oxide, Orajel Rinse, Perimax Hygenic Perio Rinse, Peroxyl Mouthrinse	**Gly-Oxide:** 10% carbamide peroxide **Orajel Rinse:** 4% alcohol, 1.5% hydrogen peroxide **Perimax Hygenic Perio Rinse:** 1.5% hydrogen peroxide **Peroxyl Mouthrinse:** 1.5% hydrogen peroxide, 6% alcohol	Cleansing suppurating wounds and inflamed mucous membranes	Not established	Regimens used for rinses containing oxygenating agents will vary depending on formulation: e.g., recommendation for Gly-Oxide is that several drops be applied to affected areas, followed by a 2-3-min rinsing; the recommendation for Peroxyl Mouthrinse is that 10 mL of it be used, followed by a 60-s rinsing
Phenolic compounds	Listerine ★ §	**Listerine ★****: 0.092% eucalyptol, 0.062% thymol, 0.06% methyl salicylate, 0.042% menthol, ranging from 21.6 (**Cool Mint, Fresh Burst**) to 26.9% (**Original**) alcohol	Antibacterial	Not established	20 mL swished full strength for 30 s and expectorated bid or prn dentist
Prebrushing rinses	Advanced Formula Plax	**Advanced Formula Plax:** principal ingredients by volume include water, glycerin, 8.5% alcohol, tetrasodium pyrophosphate, benzoic acid, sodium lauryl sulfate, sodium benzoate	Impairing attachment of plaque to tooth and therefore aiding in mechanical removal of plaque	Not established	Efficacy has not been established for adult or geriatric population

Continued on next page

★ indicates a product bearing the ADA Seal of Acceptance.
* Geriatric dosage is same as usual adult dosage.
† Pediatric safety and efficacy have not been established except with fluoride rinses in children aged 6 y and older.
§ Although Listerine was the first antiseptic oral rinse formulated, today there are a significant number of generic compounds with similar antibacterial properties. See footnote on page 204 for examples.

Table 11.1 (cont.)

Mouthrinses: Dosage and Usage Information

Generic name/ active ingredient	Brand name(s)	Usual adult dosage*	Usual child dosage†	Indications	Content
Sanguinarine	Viadent Oral Rinse	Swish 10 mL for 60 s and expectorate prn dentist	Not established	Antibacterial	0.03% sanguinaria extract, 10% alcohol

★ indicates a product bearing the ADA Seal of Acceptance.

* Geriatric dosage is same as usual adult dosage.

† Pediatric safety and efficacy have not been established except with fluoride rinses in children aged 6 y and older.

Phenolic Compounds: *Various phenolic compound mouthrinses are available generically as store brands. The following generic products carry the ADA Seal of Acceptance: Albertson's Antiseptic Mouth Rinse; Ames Blue Mint Antiseptic Mouth Rinse; Arbor Antiseptic Mouth Rinse; Arbor Antiseptic Mouth Rinse, blue mint; Bi-Mart Blue Mint Antiseptic Mouth Rinse; Brite-Life Antiseptic Mouth Rinse; Brooks Antiseptic Mouth Rinse; Brooks Blue Mint Antiseptic Mouth Rinse; Chateau Antiseptic Mouth Rinse; Cool Mint Listerine Antiseptic; CVS Antiseptic Mouth Rinse, Blue Mint; Diamond Products Original Flavor Antiseptic Mouth Rinse; Discount Drug Mart Food Fair Blue Mint Antiseptic Mouth Rinse; Dominick's Antiseptic Mouth Rinse; Drug Emporium Antiseptic Mouth Rinse; Drug Emporium Blue Mint Antiseptic Mouth Rinse; Drug Guild Antiseptic Mouth Rinse; Eckerd Antiseptic Mouth Rinse; Equate Antiseptic Mouth Rinse; Fame Antiseptic Blue Mint Mouth Rinse; Family Pharmacy Antiseptic Mouth Rinse; FDC Antiseptic Mouth Rinse; Food Lion Antiseptic Mouth Rinse; Fred Myer Antiseptic Mouth Rinse; Fred's Antiseptic Mouth Rinse; Fred's Blue Mint Antiseptic Mouth Rinse; FreshBurst Listerine Antiseptic; Full Value Antiseptic Mouth Rinse; Full Value Blue Mint Antiseptic Mouth Rinse; Furr's Antiseptic Mouth Rinse; Giant Eagle Blue Mint Antiseptic Mouth Rinse; Giant Eagle Antiseptic Mouth Rinse; Goldline Antiseptic Mouth Rinse; Good Neighbor Pharmacy Antiseptic Mouth Rinse; Good Neighbor Pharmacy Blue Mint Antiseptic Mouth Rinse; Good Sense Blue Mint Antiseptic Mouth Rinse; Good Sense Antiseptic Mouth Rinse; Hannaford Antiseptic Mouth Rinse; Happy Harry's Antiseptic Mouth Rinse; Harmon Antiseptic Mouth Rinse; Harmon Blue Mint Antiseptic Mouth Rinse; Harris Teeter Antiseptic Mouth Rinse; Health Mart Antiseptic Mouth Rinse, blue mint; Hills Antiseptic Mouth Rinse; Hills Blue Mint Antiseptic Mouth Rinse; Homebest Antiseptic Mouth Rinse; Homebest Blue Mint Antiseptic Mouth Rinse; Hy-Vee Antiseptic Mouth Rinse; Hy-Vee Blue Mint Antiseptic Mouth Rinse; K&B Antiseptic Mouth Rinse; K&B Blue Mint Antiseptic Mouth Rinse; Kroger Antiseptic Mouth Rinse; Kroger Blue Mint Antiseptic Mouth Rinse; Leader Antiseptic Mouth Rinse; Legend Antiseptic Mouth Rinse; Longs Antiseptic Mouth Rinse; Longs Blue Mint Antiseptic Mouth Rinse; Marquee Antiseptic Mouth Rinse; May's Antiseptic Mouth Rinse; May's Blue Mint Antiseptic Mouth Rinse; Medalist Antiseptic Mouth Rinse; Meijer Antiseptic Mouth Rinse; Meijer Blue Mint Antiseptic Mouth Rinse; Money Supply Antiseptic Mouth Rinse; Navarro Antiseptic Mouth Rinse; Navarro Blue Mint Antiseptic Mouth Rinse; Oral Pure Antiseptic Mouth Rinse; Oral Pure Blue Mint Antiseptic Mouth Rinse; Osco Antiseptic Mouth Rinse; Osco Blue Mint Antiseptic Mouth Rinse; Our Family Antiseptic Mouth Rinse; Our Family Blue Mint Antiseptic Mouth Rinse; Perfect Choice Blue Mint Antiseptic Mouth Rinse; Perrigo Antiseptic Mouth Rinse; Perrigo Blue Mint Mouth Rinse; Phar-Mor Antiseptic Mouth Rinse; Phar-Mor Antiseptic Mouth Rinse, blue mint; Price Chopper Antiseptic Mouth Rinse; Price Chopper Blue Mint Antiseptic Mouth Rinse; Publix Antiseptic Mouth Rinse; Publix Blue Mint Antiseptic Mouth Rinse; Quality Choice Blue Mint Antiseptic Mouth Rinse; Raley's Antiseptic Mouth Rinse; Safeway Antiseptic Mouth Rinse; Sav-On Antiseptic Mouth Rinse; Sav-On Blue Mint Antiseptic Mouth Rinse; Schnucks Antiseptic Mouth Rinse; Shaw's Antiseptic Mouth Rinse; Shurfine Antiseptic Mouth Rinse; Smith's Antiseptic Mouth Rinse; Smith's Blue Mint Antiseptic Mouth Rinse; Smitty's Antiseptic Mouth Rinse; Spartan Antiseptic Mouth Rinse; Spartan Blue Mint Antiseptic Mouth Rinse; Stater Bros. Markets Antiseptic Mouth Rinse; Stater Bros. Markets Blue Mint Antiseptic Mouth Rinse; Super G Antiseptic Mouth Rinse; Swan Antiseptic Mouth Rinse; Target Antiseptic Mouth Rinse; Target Blue Mint Antiseptic Mouth Rinse; The Pharm Blue Mint Antiseptic Mouth Rinse; The Pharm Antiseptic Mouth Rinse; Top Care Antiseptic Mouth Rinse; Ultra Fresh Antiseptic Mouth Rinse; Ultra Fresh Blue Mint Antiseptic Mouth Rinse; Valu-Rite Antiseptic Mouth Rinse; Venture Antiseptic Mouth Rinse; Venture Blue Mint Antiseptic Mouth Rinse; Vi-Jon Antiseptic Mouth Rinse; Walgreens Antiseptic Mouth Rinse; Walgreens Fresh Mint Antiseptic Mouth Rinse; Wegmans Antiseptic Mouth Rinse; Wegmans Blue Mint Antiseptic Mouth Rinse; Weis Quality Antiseptic Mouth Rinse; Weis Quality Blue Mint Antiseptic Mouth Rinse; Western Family Antiseptic Mouth Rinse; Western Family Blue Mint Antiseptic Mouth Rinse*

Table 11.2

Mouthrinses: Adverse Effects, Precautions, and Contraindications

Generic name	Adverse effects	Precautions/contraindications
Chlorhexidine	Allergic reaction (skin rash, hives, swelling of face), alteration of taste, staining of teeth, staining of restorations, discoloration of tongue, increase in calculus formation, parotid duct obstruction, parotitis, desquamation of oral mucosa, irritation to lips or tongue, oral sensitivity	Permanent staining of margins of restorations or composite restorations Should not be used as sole treatment of gingivitis Contraindicated in patients with sensitivity to chlorhexidine
Cosmetic mouthrinses	Alcohol content in these mouthrinses can have a drying effect on the oral mucosa, particularly in people who have low salivary flow; however, the flowing agents in them may stimulate salivary flow	Should be used cautiously in young children and in people who have low salivary flow due to age or drugs Contraindicated in patients with allergic reactions Contraindicated in patients with oral ulcerations Contraindicated in patients with oral desquamative diseases
Fluorides	Ulcerations of oral mucosa, fluorosis, osteosclerosis, diarrhea, bloody vomit, nausea, stomach cramps, black tarry stools, drowsiness, faintness, stomach cramps or pain, unusual excitement if swallowed	Chronic systemic overdose may induce fluorosis and changes in bone Contraindicated in patients with dental fluorosis Contraindicated in patients who exhibit fluoride toxicity from systemic ingestion Contraindicated in patients who have severe renal insufficiency
Oxygenating agents	Chemical burns of oral mucosa, decalcification of teeth, black hairy tongue	Should not be used for extended periods of time because of possible side effects mentioned at left Contraindicated for treatment of periodontitis or gingivitis
Phenolic compounds	Burning sensation, bitter taste, drying out of mucous membranes	Should not be used as sole treatment of gingivitis Contraindicated in patients with oral ulcerations or desquamative diseases Contraindicated in children (because of high alcohol content)
Prebrushing rinses	None reported	Negligible effects on plaque make these agents of little use in the treatment of carious lesions or periodontal diseases, including gingivitis
Sanguinarine	Allergic reaction (skin rash, hives, swelling of face), burning sensation, bitter taste	Should not be used as sole treatment of gingivitis Contraindicated in patients with sensitivity to sanguinaria extract

responses. The adverse effects listed in Table 11.2 apply to all major types of mouthrinses.

Pharmacology

Chlorhexidine

Chlorhexidine is a bisbiguanide with broad-spectrum antibacterial activity. It is a symmetrical, cationic molecule that binds strongly to hydroxylapatite, the organic pellicle of the tooth, oral mucosa, salivary proteins and bacteria. As a result of the binding of chlorhexidine to oral structures, the drug exhibits substantivity (for example, 30% of the drug is retained after rinsing with subsequent slow release over time). Chlorhexidine is poorly absorbed from the gastrointestinal tract, and whatever is absorbed is excreted primarily in the feces. Depending on the dose, chlorhexidine can be bacteriostatic or bactericidal. Bacteriostasis results from interference with bacterial cell wall transport systems. Bactericidal concentrations concentrate in and disrupt the cell wall, which leads to leakage of intra-cellular proteins.

Cosmetic Mouthrinses

Mouthrinses used to mask oral odor pose several problems. Breath odors can result for a myriad of reasons, including poor oral hygiene, oral or systemic disease, types of food eaten and bacterial flora in the alimentary canal and on the tongue. Furthermore, the duration of action of mouthrinses in masking halitosis is quite variable, but these agents generally have short durations of action because of poor substantivity.

Fluorides

Fluoride has been shown to dramatically reduce carious lesions in both children and adults. Fluoride ion is assimilated into the apatite crystal of enamel and stabilizes the crystal, making teeth more resistant to decay. Fluoride has also been shown to help remineralize incipient carious lesions. The germicidal activity of these agents is negligible.

Oxygenating Agents

Oxygenating agents release oxygen as an active intermediate, loosening debris in inaccessible areas. Oxygenating agents also have been reported to induce damage in bacterial cells by altering membrane permeability. The germicidal activity of these agents is negligible. The substantivity of oxygenating agents is poor.

Phenolic Compounds

Antibacterial activity is created by a combination of essential oils (eucalyptol [0.092%], thymol [0.062%], methyl salicylate [0.06%] and menthol [0.042%]) in an alcohol-based (21.6 to 26.9%) vehicle. Essential oils have been implicated in inhibiting bacterial enzymes and reducing pathogenicity of plaque. The substantivity of phenolics is poor.

Prebrushing Rinses

The exact mechanism that prebrushing rinses use to "loosen" plaque is not known and is questionable. However, it has been suggested that surface active agents (for example, sodium lauryl sulfate, sodium benzoate) make plaque soluble and therefore easier to remove.

Sanguinarine

Sanguinarine is a benzophenanthridinealkaloid extract from the root of *Sanguinaria canadensis* and has broad-spectrum antibacterial activity. Sanguinarine has been reported to bind to reactive sulfhydryls, which causes the cell to be less enzymatically active.

Note: Although alcohol can denature bacterial cell walls, it serves as a vehicle in most mouthrinses.

Patient Advice

- The effectiveness of any mouthrinse is tied to the use of the agent as prescribed by the dentist. This means the proper dose, duration of time in the mouth and frequency of rinsing must be carefully followed. If a patient misses a dose, he or she should apply the mouthrinse as soon as possible; however, doubling the dose will offer no benefit.

- To receive the greatest antiplaque or anti-caries benefit, the patient should rinse before retiring to bed.
- After using a mouthrinse, the patient should not rinse with water or drink anything for at least 30 min. Immediately drinking or rinsing with water will increase clearance of the drug from the mouth and will reduce the effectiveness of the mouthrinse. Furthermore, changes in taste sensation may occur by rinsing the mouth with water immediately after using a mouthrinse.
- Keep these mouthrinses out of the reach of young children, as ingestion of 4 or more oz of rinses containing alcohol can cause alcohol intoxication.

Suggested Readings

Ciancio SG. Chemical agents: plaque control, calculus reduction and treatment of dentinal hypersensitivity. Periodontology 2000 1995;8:75-86.

Dawes C. Clearance of substances from the oral cavity—implications for oral health. In: Edgar WM, O'Mullane DM, eds. Saliva and oral health. 2nd ed. London: British Dental Association; 1996:67-80.

Fine DH. Chemical agents to prevent and regulate plaque development. Periodontology 2000 1995;8:87-107.

Mariotti A, Hefti A. Drugs for the control of supragingival plaque. In: Stitzel CR, Craig RE, eds. Modern pharmacology. 5th ed. Boston: Little, Brown; 1997:533-40.

Dentifrices

Oral hygiene is a critical aspect of all dental therapy. Proper oral hygiene reduces the buildup of dental plaque on tooth surfaces and reduces the incidence of dental caries as well as various types of periodontal diseases. Dentifrices—which help remove dental plaque by enhancing the mechanical scrubbing and cleaning power of a toothbrush — are pastes, gels or powders used with a toothbrush to aid in the cleaning of accessible tooth surfaces. Dentifrices typically contain abrasives (to remove debris and residual stain), foaming agents (a preference of consumers), humectants (to prevent loss of water from preparation), thickening agents or binders (to stabilize dentifrice formulations and prevent separation of liquid and solid phases), flavoring (a preference of consumers) and therapeutic agents.

Depending on the dentifrice, the principal therapeutic outcomes can include reduction of caries incidence by assimilation of the fluoride ion into the apatite crystal of enamel (as a result of sodium fluoride, stannous fluoride, sodium monofluorophospate); reduction of tooth hypersensitivity by blocking dentin tubules and thereby reducing fluid exchange (as a result of strontium chloride, sodium citrate, potassium nitrate); cosmetic whitening of teeth by peroxides (as a result of hydrogen peroxide) and/or abrasives; reduction of calculus by chelation of divalent cations in saliva (as a result of pyrophosphates or zinc citrate); and reduction of plaque formation by reducing enzymatic activity of microorganisms and by an antibacterial effect (as a result of triclosan).

Most dentifrices marketed to the public can be broadly classified as agents for

- caries prevention,
- reduction of tooth sensitivity,
- cosmetics,
- reduction of calculus formation,
- plaque formation reduction,
- gingivitis reduction.

Triclosan (2,4,4,'-Trichloro-2'-hydroxdiphenyl ether) is a new antiplaque/antigingivitis agent available in dentifrices. The addition of a copolymer, vinylmethyl-ether maleic acid (Gantrez), has been shown to improve the effectiveness of triclosan by enhancing its retention (substantivity) by hard and soft surfaces. This formula (Colgate Total) has been approved by the Food and Drug Administration for sale in the United States and is ADA-accepted. Claims allowed are for the reduction of plaque, gingivitis, calculus and caries. Studies as early as 1973 showed that this chemical agent had a broad-spectrum antimicrobial effect against a wide range of gram-positive and gram-negative bacteria found in the mouth. The minimal concentration of triclosan for oral pathogens is 0.3 mg/mL. Triclosan's antibacterial activity is not affected by anionic agents, such as lauryl sulfate, which are essential to dentifrice and mouthwash formulations—a fact that broadens its range of use. In doses lower than 0.5%, taste perception is minimally affected; however, at concentrations of greater than 0.5%, undesirable effects on taste occur.

Accepted Indications

Dentifrices are used in dentistry for cosmetic purposes and to provide caries prevention, tooth sensitivity reduction, calculus reduction, plaque reduction, and gingivitis reduction or a combination of all these effects. The agent triclosan is used in dentifrices for caries prevention and plaque, calculus and gingivitis reduction.

General Dosing Information

Depending on the patient's age and the dentifrice used (see Table 11.3), the usual adult dosage is approximately 1.5 mg of fluoride.

Dosage Adjustments

The actual maximum dose for each patient must be individualized depending on factors such as his or her size, age and physical status; ability to effectively rinse and expectorate; oral health; and sensitivity. Highly fluoridated dentifrices are not often prescribed for young pediatric patients, and reduced maximum doses may be indicated for certain patients, such as those with physical or mental disabilities.

A list of caries prevention dentrifices with the active ingredient fluoride follows.

Aim Baking Soda Gel with Fluoride

Aim Regular Strength Gel with Fluoride

Aim Extra Strength Toothpaste ★

Aquafresh for Kids Toothpaste ★

Aquafresh Triple Protection Toothpaste ★

Arbor Fluoride Toothpaste ★

Arm and Hammer Dental Care Gel with Fluoride

Brooks Sodium Fluoride Toothpaste ★

Chateau Fluoride Toothpaste ★

Close-Up Fluoride Toothpaste

Close-Up Fluoride Gel

Colgate Cavity Protection Gel with Baking Soda ★

Colgate Cavity Protection Toothpaste with Baking Soda ★

Colgate Cavity Protection Toothpaste/Great Regular Flavor ★

Colgate Cavity Protection Toothpaste/Winterfresh Gel ★

Colgate Junior Cavity Protection ★

Colgate Junior Gel ★

Colgate Total ★

Crest Cavity Protection Gel ★

Crest Cavity Protection Gel with Baking Soda ★

Crest Cavity Protection Toothpaste ★

Crest Cavity Protection Toothpaste with Baking Soda ★

Crest Kids SparkleFun Cavity Protection Gel ★

Drug Emporium Fluoride Toothpaste ★

Enamelon

Equate Fluoride Toothpaste ★

Finast Fluoride Toothpaste ★

Food Lion Fluoride Toothpaste ★

Fred's Fluoride Toothpaste ★

Giant Eagle Fluoride Toothpaste ★

Gleem Toothpaste

Good Sense Fluoride Toothpaste ★

Grand Union Fluoride Toothpaste ★

Hannaford Fluoride Toothpaste ★

Homebest Fluoride Toothpaste ★

Hy-Vee Sodium Fluoride Toothpaste ★

Interplak Toothpaste with Fluoride

Kroger Fluoride Toothpaste ★

Leader Sodium Fluoride Toothpaste ★

Longs Fluoride Toothpaste ★

Meijer Fluoride Toothpaste ★

Mentadent Fluoride Toothpaste w/Baking Soda:Peroxide ★

Mouth Kote Toothpaste

Oral-B Sesame Street Fluoride Toothpaste ★

Osco Fluoride Toothpaste ★

Pepsodent Baking Soda Gel

Pepsodent Fluoride Toothpaste

Perrigo Fluoride Toothpaste ★

Price Chopper Fluoride Toothpaste ★

Quality Choice Mint Flavor Toothpaste ★

Raley's Fluoride Toothpaste ★

Sav-On Fluoride Toothpaste ★

Shane Fluoride Toothpaste ★

Shaw's Fluoride Toothpaste ★

Sheffield's Fluoride Toothpaste ★

Shoprite Fluoride Toothpaste ★

Swan Sodium Fluoride Toothpaste ★

Tom's Natural Baking Soda Toothpaste with Fluoride

Tom's Natural Toothpaste for Children with Fluoride

Tom's Natural Toothpaste with Calcium and Fluoride ★

Tom's Natural Toothpaste with Propolis and Myrrh

Top Care Sodium Fluoride Toothpaste

Topol Smoker's Fluoride Gel ★

Topol Smoker's Toothpaste with Fluoride ★

Ultra Brite Gel

Ultra Brite Toothpaste

Ultra Fresh Fluoride Toothpaste ★

Valu-Rite Fluoride Toothpaste ★

Walgreens Sodium Fluoride Toothpaste ★

Wegmans Fluoride Toothpaste ★

Weis Quality Fluoride Toothpaste ★

★ indicates a product bearing the ADA Seal of Acceptance.
* Fluoride from either sodium fluoride or monofluorophosphate.

Table 11.3

Sensitivity Reduction, Cosmetic and Calculus Prevention Dentifrices

Product	Therapeutic/active ingredient
Prevention of dentinal sensitivity*	
Aquafresh Sensitive Teeth Toothpaste	5% potassium nitrate, 0.15% sodium fluoride
Crest Sensitivity Protection Fluoride Toothpaste ★	5% potassium nitrate, 0.15% sodium fluoride
Fresh Mint Sensodyne Toothpaste ★	Fluoride
Oral-B Sensitive with Fluoride Paste	5% potassium nitrate, 0.14% sodium fluoride
Protect Sensitive Teeth Gel Toothpaste ★	5% potassium nitrate, 0.15% sodium fluoride
Rembrandt Whitening Toothpaste for Sensitive Teeth	5% potassium nitrate, 0.76% sodium monofluorophosphate, citroxain
Sensodyne Toothpaste for Sensitive Teeth and Cavity Protection with Baking Soda	5% potassium nitrate, 0.15% sodium fluoride
Sensodyne Cool Gel Toothpaste for Sensitive Teeth and Cavity Prevention Desensitizing Dentifrice	5% potassium nitrate, 0.15% sodium fluoride
Cosmetic*	
Caffree Anti-Stain Fluoride Toothpaste	Fluoride
Colgate Platinum Tooth Whitener Toothpaste	2% tetrasodium phosphate, 10% aluminum oxide, 0.76% sodium monofluorophosphate
Pearl Drops Baking Soda Whitening Toothpaste	Fluoride
Pearl Drops Extrastrength Whitening Toothpaste with Fluoride	Fluoride
Pearl Drops Whitening Gel	Fluoride
Pearl Drops Whitening Toothpolish with Fluoride	Fluoride
Rembrandt Whitening Toothpaste	44% dicalcium phosphate dihydrate, 0.76% sodium monofluorophosphate (1,000 ppm), citroxain
Prevention of calculus*	
Aquafresh Whitening Toothpaste	Sodium fluoride
Aim Anti Tartar Gel Formula with Fluoride	Zinc citrate, 0.76% sodium monofluorophosphate
Aquafresh Tartar Control Toothpaste ★	Tetrapotassium pyrophosphate, tetrasodium pyrophosphate, 0.221% sodium fluoride

Continued on next page

Table 11.3 (cont.)

Sensitivity Reduction, Cosmetic and Calculus Prevention Dentifrices

Product	Therapeutic/active ingredient
Prevention of calculus* (cont.)	
Close-Up Tartar Control Gel	Zinc citrate, 0.76% sodium monofluorophosphate
Colgate Tartar Control Formula Gel Micro Cleaning Formula ★	Tetrasodium pyrophosphate, 0.15% sodium fluoride
Colgate Tartar Control Formula Toothpaste Micro Cleaning Formula ★	Tetrasodium pyrophosphate, 0.15% sodium fluoride
Colgate Total ★	0.30% triclosan, 0.15% sodium fluoride
Crest Multi-Care	Tetrasodium pyrophosphate, 0.15% sodium fluoride
Crest Tartar Protection Fluoride Gel ★	Tetrapotassium pyrophosphate, disodium pyrophosphate, tetrasodium pyrophosphate, 0.15% sodium fluoride
Crest Tartar Protection Fluoride Toothpaste ★	Tetrapotassium pyrophosphate, disodium pyrophosphate, tetrasodium pyrophosphate, 0.15% sodium fluoride (1,100 ppm)
Prevent Tartar Prevention Toothpaste with Fluoride	Zinc chloride, 0.76% monofluorophosphate
Prevention of plaque*	
Colgate Total ★	0.30% triclosan, 0.15% sodium fluoride
Viadent Fluoride Gel	Sanguinaria, 0.76% sodium monofluorophosphate
Viadent Fluoride Paste	Sanguinaria, 0.76% sodium monofluorophosphate
Prevention of gingivitis*	
Colgate Total ★	0.30% triclosan, 0.15% sodium fluoride
Crest Gum Care	Stannous fluoride, 0.15% sodium fluoride

★ *indicates a product bearing the ADA Seal of Acceptance.*
* *These dentifrices also possess caries-preventive properties.*

Special Dental Considerations

Drug Interactions of Dental Interest

The following drug interactions and related problems involving dentifrices are potentially of clinical significance in dentistry.

Many of the ingredients of dentifrices, as well as products containing stannous fluoride, interact with chlorhexidine and should not be used concomitantly but, rather, used at least 30 min apart. Use of a chlorhexidine rinse followed by a fluoride dentifrice may reduce the efficacy of each agent.

Cross-Sensitivity

Some patients can develop allergic reactions (skin rash, hives, desquamation) to dentfrices and should discontinue use of the product immediately.

Special Patients

Patients with physical or mental disabilities may have difficulty clearing dentifrice from the mouth. These patients should receive additional help from caretakers.

Patient Monitoring: Aspects to Watch

See Table 11.4.

Adverse Effects and Precautions

The incidence of adverse reactions to dentifrices is relatively low. Many reactions (burning or taste alterations) are temporary. Idiosyncratic and allergic reactions account for a small minority of adverse responses. The adverse effects listed in Table 11.4 apply to all major types of dentifrices. Some patients cannot use tartar-control products because of the

Table 11.4

Dentifrices: Adverse Effects, Precautions and Contraindications

Dentifrice type	Adverse effects	Precautions/contraindications
Calculus-reducing formulas	Development of dentinal hypersensitivity and tissue irritation, but incidence is low	None of significance
Fluoride formulas	Fluorosis	Precautions include telling the caregivers of pediatric patients to make sure a pea-sized amount is used on toothbrush so that amount of fluoride ingested is minimized
Gingivitis-reducing formulas	None of significance	Products containing stannous fluoride may produce reversible staining of teeth
Plaque-reducing formulas	Allergic reaction, burning sensation, bitter taste	None of significance
Sensitive-teeth formulas	Allergic reactions (most products contain parabens, to which some patients may be allergic)	Differential diagnosis is important to rule out other reasons for sensitivity—for example, cracked tooth or caries
Whitening formulas	Burning sensation, drying out of mucous membranes, taste alteration, gingival abrasion, enamel erosion	Not all discolorations of enamel (for example, enamel mottling, tetracycline staining, aging-extrinsic enamel) are responsive to extrinsic bleaching via dentifrices

development of dentinal hypersensitivity or soft tissue irritation. For information on desensitizing agents, see Chapter 13.

Pharmacology

Calculus-Reducing Formulas

The precise mechanism of supragingival calculus formation is not known; however, it is assumed that most calculus-reducing formulas reduce crystal growth on tooth surfaces. One way in which crystal growth on enamel is retarded is by the chelation of cations by the active ingredient found in dentifrices.

Fluoride Formulas

Fluoride has been shown to dramatically reduce carious lesions in both children and adults. Fluoride ion is assimilated into the apatite crystal of enamel and stabilizes the crystal, making it more resistant to decay. Fluoride has also been shown to remineralize carious lesions.

Gingivitis- and Plaque-Reducing Formulas

Sanguinarine has been reported to bind to reactive sulfhydryls, causing reduced enzymatic activity in the bacterial cell. Another antibacterial agent that has recently been introduced into dentifrices has been triclosan. Triclosan is both a bisphenol and a nonionic germicide that is effective against gram-positive and gram-negative bacteria and is on the U.S. market. A number of studies have shown this agent reduces plaque and gingivitis by approximately 25-30%. A dentifrice containing stannous fluoride has been shown to reduce gingivitis by 20%, but the mechanism of action is unclear.

Sensitive-Teeth Formulas

Several mechanisms of action have been proposed for these agents, including retention of fluid exchange following occlusion of dentin tubules by ions as well as potassium-induced depolarization of the dentinal nerve, thereby reducing nerve activity.

Whitening Formulas

Whitening of teeth can occur by two mechanisms. One method is mechanical, in which an abrasive is used to remove debris from the tooth. The other method involves the use of peroxides, which react with water to form free oxygen radicals that help to whiten the teeth, or a combination of mechanical and chemical actions.

Patient Advice

- The effectiveness of any dentifrice lies in use of the agent as prescribed by the doctor. For antiplaque or anticaries dentifrices, the greatest benefit will be obtained if the patient brushes before bedtime.

Suggested Readings

Chikte UM, Rudolph MJ, Reinach SG. Anti-calculus effects of dentifrice containing pyrophosphate compared with control. Clin Prev Dent 1992;14(4):29-33.

Ismail AI. Fluoride supplements: current effectiveness, side effects, and recommendations. Community Dent Oral Epidemiol 1994;22(3):164-72.

McGuire S. A review of the impact of fluoride on adult caries. J Clin Dent 1993;4(1):11-23.

Riordan PJ. Fluoride supplements in caries prevention: a literature review and proposal for a new dosage schedule. J Public Health Dent 1993;53(3):174-89.

Rolla G, Ellingsen JE. Clinical effects and possible mechanisms of action of stannous fluoride. Int Dent J 1994;44(1) (Supplement):99-105.

Rolla G, Ogaard B, Cruz R de A. Clinical effect and mechanism of cariostatic action of fluoride-containing toothpastes: a review. Int Dent J 1991;41(3):171-4.

Stephen KW. Fluoride toothpastes, rinses, and tablets. Adv Dent Res 1994;8(2):185-9.

Stookey GK, DePaola PF, Featherstone JD, et al. A critical review of the relative anticaries efficacy of sodium fluoride and sodium monofluorophosphate dentifrices. Caries Res 1993;27(4):337-60.

US Department of Health and Human Services. Public Health Service report on fluoride benefits and risks. Washington, D.C.: US Government Printing Office, 1991;HHS publication no. (CDC)91-801. (MMWR Morb Mortal Wkly Rep; Recommendations and Reports series No. RR-7; no. 40).

Chapter 12

Systemic and Topical Fluorides

Kenneth H. Burrell, D.D.S., S.M.

With today's array of available systemic and topical fluoride products, it is not surprising that confusion abounds concerning their proper use. Factors that should be taken into account when considering a fluoride regimen are the age of the patient, the patient's caries rate and other caries-producing factors.

Age of the patient. Patients aged < 6 y are at risk of developing enamel fluorosis from excessive amounts of fluoride in the water supply, inappropriate and injudicious use of fluoride supplements and regular, inadvertent ingestion of fluoride-containing over-the-counter products. Ingestion of fluoride in food products also contributes to a child's total daily fluoride intake.

Improper use of fluoride supplements by itself can cause fluorosis. With the exception of unnecessarily or incorrectly prescribed fluoride supplements, no other factors alone are thought to contribute to dental fluorosis. Patients should follow instructions on the labels of over-the-counter fluoride-containing products so that they can avoid unintended fluoride ingestion.

The patient's caries rate. Patients without caries or with no apparent risk of caries may require nothing more than the 0.7 to 1.2 parts per million fluoride in the municipal water supply or an appropriate fluoride-supplement dosage schedule, along with the daily use of a fluoride-containing dentifrice and semiannual postprophylaxis fluoride applications. Patients with low caries rates or a slight risk may require the additional use of a 0.05% sodium fluoride over-the-counter

mouthrinse or a 0.4% stannous fluoride gel. Patients with moderate-to-high caries rates and moderate-to-severe risk of caries may also require the daily use of neutral or acidulated 1.1% sodium fluoride gel.

Other caries-producing factors. A patient's existing fluoride regimen is an important part of his or her dental history, but, of course, it is not the only consideration when trying to determine treatment for caries. The patient's oral hygiene regimen, diet and medical history, and whether or not pit and fissure sealants have been placed on newly erupted teeth, must also be taken into account. Twice-daily brushing and once-daily interdental cleaning, usually with floss, should be adequate for most patients, provided these procedures are done properly and thoroughly. A well-balanced diet with a minimum amount of snacking also should reduce the risks of dental caries. Important events in a patient's medical history can change that regimen, however. Diminished salivary flow, or xerostomia, can be caused by medications, head and neck irradiation for cancer treatments and some diseases, such as Sjögren's syndrome. Xerostomia can increase the caries rate dramatically so that a patient's diet, oral hygiene and fluoride use may require modification after its onset.

Clinical judgment is important for successful treatment. Correct diagnosis as a result of careful history-taking, meticulous examination and competent interpretation of diagnostic tests can increase the likelihood of successful prevention or treatment outcome.

Systemic Fluorides

Accepted Indications

Fluoride in water supplies and fluoride supplements are considered to be long-term caries preventives by making fluoride available systemically while tooth enamel is forming. When fluoride levels in drinking water are below 0.6 ppm, a fluoride supplement should be considered (see Table 12.1). An analysis of the home drinking water may not be adequate, however. The patient's parents or guardians may need to be questioned about the child's usual source of drinking water. Many bottled waters do not contain optimal amounts of fluoride. Day care centers may have fluoridated drinking water that is at levels adequate to preclude prescribing a fluoride supplement.

General Dosing Information

Fluoride in drinking water concentrated at between 0.7 and 1.2 ppm offers the maximum reduction in dental caries with the minimal amount of enamel mottling, or fluorosis.

The calculations for the optimal range of fluoride in drinking water have also been used to determine dosage for fluoride supplements and are used for children aged between 6 mo and 16 y when the fluoride in drinking water is below 0.6 ppm. Table 12.1 shows the recommended fluoride supplement dosage schedule.

Systemic dosing of fluoride supplements is typically prescribed in the form of either drops, tablets or dual-use topical/systemic swish-and-swallow solutions.

General dosage forms include tablets and lozenges available in 0.25 mg, 0.50 mg and 1 mg. Fluoride drops are available in various concentrations, which affects the number of drops per dose. Thus, it is important to specify the concentration of the drops prescribed. A combination fluoride supplement/mouthrinse is also available, with each 5 mL (one teaspoonful) containing 1 mg of fluoride from 2.20 mg of sodium fluoride and orthophosphoric acid.

Fluoridated salt. Salt fluoridation is not used in the United States but is used in some countries, such as Mexico and Switzerland, where water fluoridation is not possible. Fluoride has been shown to be effective at a concentration of 200-250 mg/kg of table salt.

Table 12.1

Systemic Fluoride Supplements: Recommended Dosage Schedule of the American Dental Association, the American Academy of Pediatric Dentistry and the American Academy of Pediatrics

| Age | Fluoride ion level in drinking water (ppm)* | | |
	< 0.3 ppm	0.3-0.6 ppm	> 0.6 ppm
Birth-6 mo	None	None	None
6 mo-3 y	0.25 mg/day†	None	None
3-6 y	0.50 mg/day	0.25 mg/day	None
6-16 y	1.0 mg/day	0.50 mg/day	None

1.0 ppm = 1 mg/liter.
† 2.2 mg sodium fluoride contains 1 mg fluoride ion.

Fluoridated milk. A small number of studies have been conducted to determine the caries-inhibiting effects of fluoride in cow's milk. Although reductions in caries related to fluoridated milk have shown promise, more studies are required. There is concern that the effectiveness of fluorides in milk products may be reduced because fluoride combines with calcium to form calcium fluoride, which is poorly absorbed in the stomach. Fluoridated milk products are not available in the United States.

Fluoridated chewing gum. In several European countries, chewing gum is used as an adjunctive vehicle for delivering fluoride topically to teeth. The concentration of fluoride in these gums is approximately 0.25 mg of fluoride per stick of gum. Use of fluoridated chewing gums results in a salivary fluoride concentration similar to that achieved by using other fluoride sources such as dentifrices or mouthrinses. In addition, fluoride gums have the added advantage of simultaneously stimulating salivary flow and raising salivary and plaque pH. Such effects may be particularly advantageous to xerostomatic patients. However, there are, to date, no definitive clinical studies on the anticaries protective effect of these gums, and further studies are required before any conclusions regarding their efficacy can be reached.

Maximum Recommended Doses

No more than 120 mg of fluoride should be dispensed to a patient at one time. One tablet of the prescribed dose should be taken per day with water or juice. Taking fluoride supplements with milk and other dairy products is not recommended because they can combine with the calcium to become poorly absorbed calcium fluoride. The tablet strength is determined by the concentration of fluoride in the patient's source of drinking water

and the age of the child. Tables 12.1 and 12.2 show the maximum recommended dose is 1 mg per day.

Dosage Adjustments

The actual maximum dose for each patient must be individualized depending on the patient's size, age and physical status; other drugs he or she may be taking; and tolerance of prior or existing doses administered for fluoride therapy. Reduced doses may be indicated for patients based on changes in their water supply's fluoride content, which may result from relocation or any adverse side effects experienced.

Special Dental Considerations

Drug Interactions of Dental Interest
Calcium-containing products and food interfere with the absorption of systemic fluoride.

Cross-Sensitivity
Allergic rash and other idiosyncratic reactions have rarely been reported. Gastric distress, headache and weakness have been reported in cases of excessive ingestion.

Special Patients
Fluoride supplements are not recommended for patients other than children living in areas with fluoride levels such as those described in Table 12.1.

Patient Monitoring: Aspects to Watch
Fluoride supplements can cause fluorosis if used in areas where drinking water contains fluoride levels greater than the levels outlined in Table 12.1.

Adverse Effects and Precautions
No adverse reactions or undesirable side effects have been reported when fluoride supplements have been taken as directed. Excessive use may result in dental fluorosis, especially in areas where the fluoride level in

Table 12.2

Systemic Fluorides: Dosage Information

Generic name	Brand name(s)	Usual child dosage*	Maximum child dosage
Sodium fluoride, tablets and lozenges—0.25 mg fluoride	**Tablets:** Fluor-A-Day ★, Fluoritab ★, Luride Lozi-Tabs ★, Luride SF Lozi-Tabs ★ **Lozenges:** Fluor-A-Day ★	1 tablet or lozenge per day taken with water or juice dissolved in mouth or chewed	Prescribe no more than 480 tablets or lozenges
Sodium fluoride, tablets and lozenges—0.5 mg fluoride	**Tablets:** Fluor-A-Day ★, Fluoritab ★, Luride Lozi-Tabs ★ **Lozenges:** Fluor-A-Day ★	1 tablet or lozenge per day taken with water or juice dissolved in mouth or chewed	Prescribe no more than 240 tablets or lozenges
Sodium fluoride, tablets and lozenges—1 mg fluoride	**Tablets:** Fluor-A-Day ★, Fluoritab ★, Luride Lozi-Tabs ★ **Lozenges:** Fluor-A-Day ★	1 tablet or lozenge per day taken with water or juice and dissolved in mouth or chewed	Prescribe no more than 120 tablets or lozenges
Sodium fluoride, drops—0.5 mg/mL fluoride	**Drops:** Luride ★, Pediaflor	½ dropperful = 0.25 mg 1 dropperful = 0.5 mg 2 droppersful = 1 mg	Prescribe no more than 200 mL
Sodium fluoride, drops—2 mg/mL fluoride	**Drops:** Karidium ★	2 drops = 0.25 mg 4 drops = 0.5 mg 8 drops = 1 mg	Prescribe no more than 30 mL
Sodium fluoride, drops—2.5 mg/mL fluoride	**Drops:** Fluor-A-Day ★	2 drops = 0.25 mg 4 drops = 0.5 mg 8 drops = 1 mg	Prescribe no more than 30 mL
Sodium fluoride, drops—5 mg/mL fluoride	**Drops:** Fluoritab ★	1 drop = 0.25 mg 2 drops = 0.5 mg 4 drops = 1 mg	Prescribe no more than 23 mL
Sodium fluoride, rinse—0.2 mg/mL fluoride	**Rinses:** Phos-Flur ★	1 mg fluoride/teaspoonful (0.2 mg fluoride/mL) swished for 1 min then swallowed	Prescribe no more than 500 mL

★ *indicates a product bearing the ADA Seal of Acceptance.*
* *These supplements are for children only. There is no dose for adult or geriatric patients.*

drinking water is high. Therefore, fluoride supplements are not recommended where the water content of fluoride is at or above 0.6 ppm.

In children, acute ingestion of 10-20 mg of sodium fluoride can cause excessive salivation and gastrointestinal disturbances. Ingestion of 500 mg can be fatal. Oral or intravenous fluids containing calcium, or both, may be indicated.

Precautions. If the fluoride level is unknown, the drinking water must be tested for fluoride content before supplements are prescribed. For testing information, ask the local or state health department. Determining a proper dosage schedule can be a complex task if a patient has exposure to a number of different water supplies. Once a proper schedule is established, however, the effectiveness of the schedule requires the patient's long-term compliance.

Contraindications. The fluoride dosage schedule was designed to take into account the widespread use of fluorides that can contribute to the increased frequency and severity of fluorosis. Fluoride supplements are contraindicated for children drinking water with fluoride concentrations at or above 0.6 ppm.

Pharmacology

Systemic and Topical Fluorides

Mechanism of action/effect. After early studies showed that fluoride reduced the solubility of powdered enamel and dentin, investigators began trying to determine how fluoride works to reduce dental caries. However, the mechanism or mechanisms of action are still incompletely understood. Nevertheless, fluoride is thought to work in many ways. It has been speculated that a combination of actions work to reduce the severity and frequency of dental caries, which is the result of excessive demineralization in the demineralization-remineralization process. This excessive demineralization occurs after repeated acid attacks that result when bacterial plaque metabolizes sugars ingested during meals and snacks. Clinical manifestations of dental caries become evident when demineralization predominates over time and upsets the demineralization-remineralization equilibrium. Fluoride reduces the demineralization of enamel and dentin by reducing the acid production of bacterial plaque and decreasing the solubility of apatite crystals. When fluoride is exposed to apatite crystals, it readily becomes incorporated to reduce the dissolution of apatite during acid attacks. The presence of fluoride, therefore, inhibits demineralization and helps to maintain the equilibrium between demineralization and remineralization during acid attacks.

Absorption. Fluoride is absorbed in the gastrointestinal tract, 90% of it in the stomach. Calcium, iron or magnesium ions may delay absorption.

Distribution. After absorption, 50% of fluoride is deposited in bone and teeth.

Elimination. The major route of excretion is the kidneys. Fluoride is also excreted by the sweat glands, the gastrointestinal tract and in breast milk.

Patient Advice

- Patients and their guardians should be advised to take systemic fluorides as directed.
- Patients or their guardians should notify the prescriber when their water supply has changed as the result of a move or a change in schools or by the addition of fluoride to the water supply.
- These products should be kept from children's reach; they are often formulated to have a pleasant taste and children therefore are more likely to consume them if they are easily accessible.

Topical Fluorides

Accepted Indications

Topical preparations are used in the prevention and treatment of dental caries.

Concentrations of 1,500 ppm or below are sold as over-the-counter preparations for the prevention of dental caries. Preparations that are prescribed for topical home use generally consist of higher concentrations of fluoride and are indicated for both treatment and prevention. Patients who are either at high risk of developing dental caries or who experience high caries rates are candidates for daily use of these products. However, high-concentration preparations that are usually applied annually or after dental prophylaxis in children are applied to prevent caries.

Some kinds of fluoride compounds at certain concentrations can be used to reduce dentinal hypersensitivity. Sodium fluoride (151,000 ppm fluoride ion), in equal amounts of kaolin and glycerin, has been shown to be effective for this purpose when professionally applied and burnished into affected areas using orangewood sticks. A water-free 0.4% (1,000 ppm fluoride ion) stannous fluoride gel has also been demonstrated to reduce dentinal hypersensitivity when patients use it daily at home.

There is evidence that a 0.4% stannous fluoride toothpaste has been shown to reduce gingivitis with daily use.

General Dosing Information

Topical dosing is typically provided in the form of liquid solutions, gels, foams, varnishes, pastes, rinses and dentifrices. Concentrations can vary depending on oral health and sensitivity, the particular indication involved, region of treatment, response to previous or existing concentrations and doses of fluoride as well as individual patient characteristics such as age, weight, physical status, and ability to effectively rinse and expectorate. See Table 12.3.

Doses of topically applied solutions, gels, foams and varnishes are typically applied with a cotton swab, a toothbrush, a carrier or as a rinse. To control the dosing of high fluoride concentrations so that excessive amounts of fluoride are not in the mouth and to control salivary contamination, cotton rolls, a saliva ejector or high vacuum suction can be used. Because varnishes are applied to adhere to teeth for prolonged periods, all residual fluoride is swallowed. Between 0.3-0.5 mL of varnish is used per patient so that about 5-11 mg is ingested. This amount is consistent with ingestion calculations for other professionally applied fluoride preparations.

When it comes to fluoride dentifrices, more frequent brushing may be required, but this depends on the patient's caries risk. A 0.4% stannous fluoride gel might be considered as an alternative to brushing with a dentifrice, however. In this way, the patient can receive the benefit of the same fluoride exposure as with the dentifrice without a dentifrice's cleansing properties, which may not be necessary. Also, the cleansing properties of a dentifrice may not be desirable if topical application of fluoride is required more than twice a day.

Maximum Recommended Doses

The maximum recommended doses for topical fluoride formulations per procedure or appointment are 5 mL of acidulated phosphate fluoride solution, gel or foam, 1.23% fluoride ion; 5 mL of 2% neutral sodium fluoride solution or gel; 0.3-0.5 mL of fluoride-containing varnish, 5% sodium fluoride (2.26% fluoride ion); 0.2-0.4 mL 1.1% neutral and acidulated sodium fluoride gel drops; a pea-sized amount (about 0.25 g) 1,000-1,500 ppm fluoride toothpaste for children aged < 6 y; and 10 mL of 0.05% sodium fluoride mouthrinse for children aged > 6 y. Mouthrinses are not recommended for children aged < 6 y.

Dosage Adjustments

The actual maximum dose for each patient can be individualized depending on the patient's age and physical status, ability to effectively rinse and expectorate and oral health and sensitivity.

Table 12.3

Topical Fluorides: Dosage Information

Generic name/ active ingredient	Brand name(s)	Usual adult dosage*	Maximum adult dosage
Professionally applied fluoride products			
Acidulated phosphate fluoride solutions, gels and foams (1.23% fluoride ion)	**Foams:** Laclede ★ **Gels:** Care-4 ★, Fluorident ★, FluoroCare Time Saver, FluoroCare Thixo-Set ★, Perfect Choice ★, Pro-Dentx ★, Protect ★, Topex	5 mL of solution or gel with 12,300 ppm fluoride ion after dental prophylaxis per fluoride carrier	10 mL
2% neutral sodium fluoride solutions, gels or foams (0.90% fluoride ion)	FluoroCare Neutral, Topex Neutral pH, Neutra-Foam	5 mL of solution, gel or foam with 9,040 ppm fluoride ion after dental prophylaxis per fluoride carrier	10 mL
Fluoride-containing varnishes, 5% sodium fluoride (2.26% fluoride ion)	Duraflor, Duraphat	0.3-0.5 mL of varnish containing 22,600 ppm fluoride ion after dental prophylaxis	0.5 mL
Fluoride prophylaxis pastes (0.40% - 2% fluoride ion)	Glitter, Masnasil, Teledyne Water Pik Prophylaxis Paste, Butler Fluoride Prophylaxis Paste, Unipro Prophy Paste, Prophy Gems, Radant, Topex, Ziroxide, Zircon F	Use amount sufficient to polish the teeth (4,000-20,000 ppm fluoride ion)	Use no more than the amount required to polish the teeth
Prescription fluorides			
1.1% neutral or acidulated sodium fluoride gel (0.50% fluoride ion)	Karigel-N ★, Luride Lozi-Tabs, PreviDent Gel, Theraflur ★	4-8 drops on inner surface of each custom-made tray per day (5,000 ppm fluoride ion)	Maximum amount prescribed is one 24-mL plastic squeeze bottle; maximum adult dose is 16 drops/day
0.2% neutral sodium fluoride rinses (0.09% fluoride ion)	NaFrinse ★, PreviDent ★	Recommended for use by children (920 ppm fluoride ion solution)	
0.044% sodium fluoride and acidulated phosphate fluoride rinses (0.02% fluoride ion)	Phos-Flur ★	10 mL once daily after brushing (200 ppm fluoride ion solution)	Same as usual adult dosage

★ indicates a product bearing the ADA Seal of Acceptance.
[CAN] indicates a product available only in Canada.
* Geriatric dosage is same as adult dosage.

Continued on next page

Table 12.3 (cont.)

Topical Fluorides: Dosage Information

Generic name/ active ingredient	Brand name(s)	Usual adult dosage*	Maximum adult dosage
Over-the-counter fluorides			
Fluoride-containing dentifrices (0.12-0.15% and 0.21% fluoride ion)	Aquafresh Tartar Control Toothpaste ★, Colgate Tartar Control Baking Soda and Peroxide Toothpaste ★, Colgate Tartar Control Gel with Micro Cleaning Crystals ★, Colgate Tartar Control Toothpaste with Micro Cleaning Crystals ★, Colgate Total ★, Crest Sensitivity Protection Fluoride Toothpaste ★, Crest Tartar Protection Fluoride Gel ★, Crest Tartar Protection Fluoride Toothpaste ★, Fresh Mint Sensodyne Fluoride Toothpaste ★, Mentadent Fluoride Toothpaste with Baking Soda and Peroxide ★, Protect Sensitive Teeth Gel Toothpaste ★; Sensodyne-SC Toothpaste [CAN]	Amount sufficient to cover toothbrush bristles: ≈ 1 g per day (1,000-1,500 ppm fluoride ion)	Twice a day or more as recommended
0.4% stannous fluoride gels (0.15% fluoride ion)	Activus ★, Alpha-Dent ★, Easy-Gel, Florentine II ★, Gel-Kam ★, Gel-Tin ★, Perfect Choice ★, Plak Smacker ★, Pro-Dentx ★, Schein Home Care ★, Super-Dent ★	Amount sufficient to cover toothbrush bristles: ≈ 1 g per day (1,000 ppm fluoride ion)	Once a day or more as recommended
0.05% sodium fluoride rinses (0.02% fluoride ion)	Fluorigard ★, NaFrinse Acidulated ★, NaFrinse Neutral ★, Oral-B Rinse Therapy ★, Reach Act, Reach Act for Kids ★	10 mL of solution with 230 ppm fluoride ion	Rinse for 1 min, once daily

★ indicates a product bearing the ADA Seal of Acceptance.
[CAN] indicates a product available only in Canada.
* Geriatric dosage is same as adult dosage.

Special Dental Considerations

Cross-Sensitivity

Although allergies to fluoride probably do not exist, patients may be allergic to some of the ingredients in the various formulations. Some of the 1.23% acidulated phosphate fluoride solutions and gels and some dentifrices contain tartrazines used as color additives. They can cause allergic reactions, especially in patients with hypersensitivity to aspirin.

Adverse Effects and Precautions

Excessive ingestion of fluoride products can produce acute and chronic effects. Ingestion of quantities of fluoride as low as 1 mg per day have been shown to produce mild fluorosis in a small percentage of the population if the ingestion takes place during tooth crown development. The severity and frequency of fluorosis can increase in a population if the recommended dose is exceeded and if the quantity of daily fluoride ingestion increases. Chronic fluoride toxicity, or skeletal fluorosis, may occur after years of daily ingestion of 20-80 mg of fluoride; however, such heavy doses are far in excess of the average intake in the United States. There is no evidence that skeletal changes are produced by ingestion of therapeutic doses of fluoride, however.

Accidental ingestion of high concentrations of fluoride (> 1,500 ppm) can cause gastrointestinal disturbances such as excessive salivation, nausea, vomiting, abdominal pain and diarrhea. Central nervous system disturbances that have been observed include irritability, paresthesia, tetany and convulsions. Respiratory and cardiac failure have also been observed. See Table 12.4.

Dentifrices should not exceed 260 mg of fluoride ion. It is thought that the quantity of fluoride in dentifrice can exceed the 120-mg limit the American Dental Association has established for other fluoride-containing products

Table 12.4

Topical Fluorides: Adverse Effects, Precautions and Contraindications

Type	Adverse effects	Precautions/contraindications
Professionally applied fluoride products		
Acidulated phosphate fluoride solutions, gels and foams (1.23% fluoride ion)	**CNS:** Inadvertent ingestion can produce headaches and weakness; more severe instances of excessive ingestion can cause CNS problems such as irritability, paresthesia, tetany, convulsions, respiratory failure and cardiac failure; fluoride has direct toxic action on nerve tissue **Hema:** Excessive amounts of fluoride can also cause electrolyte disturbances leading to hypocalcemia and hyperkalemia; hypoglycemia is a result of failure of enzyme systems **Musc:** Fluoride has a direct toxic action on muscle and nerve tissue	Some preparations may contain tartrazines (FDC Yellow No. 5), which are used as color additives; tartrazine-containing products are contraindicated in patients allergic to the compound; tartrazine can cause allergic reactions, including bronchial asthma; allergic response is rare, but is frequently observed in patients who also experience hypersensitivity to aspirin

Continued on next page

Table 12.4 (cont.)

Topical Fluorides: Adverse Effects, Precautions and Contraindications

Type	Adverse effects	Precautions/contraindications
Professionally applied fluoride products		
2% neutral sodium fluoride solutions or gels	**CV:** Excessive amounts of fluoride can produce cardiac failure **CNS:** Excessive amounts of fluoride can produce irritability, paresthesia, tetany, convulsions; fluoride has direct toxic action on nerve tissue **GI:** Excessive amounts of fluoride can produce GI disturbances such as excess salivation, nausea, abdominal pain, vomiting and diarrhea **Hema:** Excessive amounts of fluoride can cause electrolyte disturbances leading to hypocalcemia and hyperkalemia. Hypoglycemia is a result of enzyme systems failure **Musc:** Fluoride has direct toxic action on muscle tissue **Resp:** Excessive amounts of fluoride can produce respiratory failure	Not to be used with other professionally applied topical fluoride preparations
Fluoride-containing varnishes, 5% sodium fluoride (2.26% fluoride ion)	**CNS:** Inadvertent ingestion can produce headaches and weakness; more severe instances of excessive ingestion can cause CNS problems such as irritability, paresthesia, tetany, convulsions, respiratory failure and cardiac failure; fluoride has direct toxic action on nerve tissue **Hema:** Excessive amounts of fluoride can also cause electrolyte disturbances leading to hypocalcemia and hyperkalemia; hypoglycemia is a result of failure of enzyme systems **Musc:** Fluoride has a direct toxic action on muscle and nerve tissue	Not to be used in conjunction with other high-concentration topical fluoride solutions when varnish is applied to all tooth surfaces
Fluoride prophylaxis pastes, 4,000-20,000 ppm fluoride	**Oral:** Excessive polishing may remove more fluoride from the enamel surface than fluoride prophylaxis paste can replace	Should be thoroughly rinsed from mouth on completion of prophylaxis
Prescription fluorides		
1.1% neutral or acidulated phosphate fluoride gel-drops (5,000 ppm fluoride ion)	**Oral:** Patients with mucositis may report irritation to the acidulated preparation	Repeated use of acidulated fluoride has been shown to etch glass filler particles in composite restorations and porcelain crowns, facings and laminates As with all fluoride products, children aged < 6 y should be supervised to prevent their swallowing the product, which can lead to fluorosis, nausea and vomiting

Continued on next page

Table 12.4 (cont.)

Topical Fluorides: Adverse Effects, Precautions and Contraindications

Type	Adverse effects	Precautions/contraindications
Prescription fluorides (cont.)		
0.2% neutral sodium fluoride rinse (920 ppm fluoride ion solution)	**General:** Allergic reaction could result from flavoring agent **GI:** Nausea and vomiting may result from inadvertent swallowing **Oral:** Irritation of oral tissues, especially in children with mucositis, may result from alcohol that might be part of the formulation	Should not be used in children aged < 6 y because they cannot rinse without significant swallowing and this product is not for systemic use Should not be swallowed by children of any age and should be kept from their reach
Over-the-counter fluorides		
Dentifrice with 0.12-0.15% and 0.24% fluoride ion (1,000-1,500 ppm fluoride ion)	**General:** Allergic reactions thought to be caused by flavoring agents in some formulations (mint-flavored products have been reported to cause these reactions; however, as a variety of flavoring agents is available, patient should be advised to change to another flavor until a suitable product is found)	To prevent fluorosis, supervise children aged < 6 y so that swallowing does not occur Accidental ingestion of a single dose, which contains 1-2 mg of fluoride ion, is not harmful Intentional ingestion of large amounts of fluoride toothpaste can cause gastric irritation, nausea and vomiting No single container should exceed 260 mg of fluoride ion (it is thought that quantity of fluoride in dentifrice can exceed the 120-mg limit ADA has established for other fluoride-containing products because dentifrices contain humectants and detergents that induce vomiting)
0.4% stannous fluoride gels (1,000 ppm fluoride ion)	**General:** Allergic reactions thought to be caused by flavoring agents in some formulations (mint-flavored products have been reported to cause these reactions; however, as a variety of flavoring agents is available, patient should be advised to change to another flavor until a suitable product is found)	Children aged < 6 y should be supervised to prevent swallowing and fluorosis; accidental ingestion of a single dose (1- to 2-mg ribbon of gel) is not harmful Intentional ingestion of large amounts of gel can cause gastric irritation, nausea and vomiting No single container should exceed 120 mg of fluoride
0.5% sodium fluoride mouthrinses (230 ppm fluoride ion)	**General:** Allergic reactions thought to be caused by flavoring agents in some formulations (mint-flavored products have been reported to cause these reactions; however, as a variety of flavoring agents is available, patient should be advised to change to another flavor until a suitable product is found)	Children aged < 6 y generally should not use this product because of their inability to rinse without swallowing; otherwise, accidental ingestion of a single dose is not harmful Intentional ingestion of several doses can cause gastric irritation, nausea and vomiting Some of these products contain alcohol to promote solubility of flavoring agents; these products should be kept out of children's reach and in childproof caps/packaging

because dentifrices contain humectants and detergents that act to induce vomiting.

Pharmacology

See the discussion earlier in this chapter.

Patient Advice

Although the gel form of 2% neutral sodium fluoride may be more easily applied, clinical evidence of its effectiveness has not been demonstrated. The original application schedule was 4 times per year and was for children at the specific ages of 3, 7, 10, and 13 y. Currently the caries-inhibiting properties of this solution are considered to be equivalent to the APF gels and solutions, which contain a higher concentration of fluoride (12,300 ppm).

Suggested Readings

Levy SM. Review of fluoride exposures and ingestion. Community Dent Oral Epidemiol 1994;22(3):173-80.

Newbrun E. Current regulations and recommendations concerning water fluoridation, fluoride supplements, and topical fluoride agents. J Dent Res 1992;71(5):1255-65.

Ripa LW. A critique of topical fluoride methods (dentifrices, mouthrinses, operator-, and self-applied gels) in an era of decreased caries and increased fluorosis prevalence. J Public Health Dent 1991;51(1):23-41.

Ripa LW. Review of the anticaries effectiveness of professionally applied and self-applied topical fluoride gels. J Public Health Dent 1989;49(5):297-309.

Whitford GM, Allmann DW, Shaked AR. Topical fluoride: effects on physiologic and biochemical process. J Dent Res 1987;66(5):1072-8.

Chapter 13

Desensitizing Agents

Martha Somerman, D.D.S., Ph.D.

Dentin hypersensitivity is characterized by a sharp pain produced in response to mild stimuli that usually disappears with removal of the stimulus. Root sensitivity is a significant problem for many patients and may be a result of, or associated with, scaling and root planing, periodontal surgery, gingival recession, toothbrush abrasion, attrition, erosion, trauma or chronic periodontal disease. It is important to rule out active pathology (for example, root fracture or root surface decay) before providing treatment for root sensitivity. In many situations, root sensitivity decreases with time, but when it does not, it results in extreme discomfort or an inability to eat or drink certain foods, inability to function outdoors in cold weather and, at times, poor oral hygiene that can result in periodontal-related problems. Unfortunately, ideal OTC and professional desensitizing agents with predictable outcomes have not been developed.

Densensitizing agents can be separated into two types: agents applied to the tooth by a practitioner and agents that are for home use. Table 13.1 provides information about currently available products for use in the clinical setting. A major concern with products for home use is the abrasiveness of the paste; however, all ADA-accepted toothpastes have safe levels of abrasive materials.

In-Office Products

Accepted Indications

In-office desensitizing agents are used to provide relief from thermal and tactile sensitivity on exposed root surfaces when pathological causes for pain have been ruled out. Agents containing fluoride also provide an anticaries function.

General Usage Information

Usage and Administration for Adults and Children

See Tables 13.1 and 13.2 for information on usage and administration. As with any agents, if pain persists or worsens, the situation should be re-evaluated. Overuse can be detrimental to tooth structure. Therefore, continued sensitivity, after ruling out other symptoms, can be treated by changing the product versus increasing the dose. Use of increased amounts, beyond those shown in Table 13.1, has not been reported to be effective in decreasing sensitivity.

Special Dental Considerations

- Fluorides interact with calcium-containing products—for example, to form calcium fluoride, which is poorly absorbed.
- Also, certain agents—for example, chlorhexidine—may decrease fluoride's ability to bind to root surfaces. Thus, after using fluoride agents, the patient should not rinse or eat for 1 h.
- Some agents are acidic and thus may cause sensitivity in patients with mucositis.
- Some acidic compounds—for example, oxalate—may cause dulling of porcelain ceramics and decreased effectiveness of bonding cements. Therefore, pumicing the root surface before the use of some desensitizing agents is recommended.

Table 13.1

Desensitizing Fluorides, Oxalates, Varnishes, Sealants and Bonding Agents: Usage Information

Generic name	Brand name(s)	Usage and administration for adults	Usage and administration for children	Content/form	Features/uses
Fluorides					
0.40% stannous fluoride, 1.09% sodium fluoride, 0.14% hydrogen fluoride (eqivalent to 0.717% fluoride and 0.303% Sn)	Dentinbloc Dentin Desensitizer, Pro-Dentx Office Fluorides, Pro-Dentx Comfort Dentin Densensitizer, Gel-Kam ★	Dry dentin surface (isolation not necessary); dispense 10-12 drops into plastic dappen dish; apply saturated cotton pellets to sensitive area for 1 full min; use light pressure and do not burnish; have patient expectorate after application; to overcome pain threshold, sequential 1-min treatments may be required Do not apply with wooden stick	Caution must be taken in use of fluorides as desensitizing agents in children due to possibility of fluorosis and altered bone density **Age < 12 y:** Not intended for this age group	Available in boxes of 50-unit dose treatments (0.75 g/unit)	Has been shown to form particles that block dentin tubules, thereby providing temporary relief from pain associated with root-surface sensitivity
3.9% strontium chloride, 0.42% sodium fluoride	Desensitizer, Health-Dent Desensitizer, Hema-Glu Desensitizer	Dry dentin surface (isolation not necessary); dispense 10-12 drops into plastic dappen dish; apply saturated cotton pellets to sensitive area for 1 full min; use light pressure and do not burnish; have patient expectorate after application; to overcome pain threshold, sequential 1-min treatments may be required Do not apply with wooden stick	Caution must be taken in use of fluorides as desensitizing agents in children due to possibility of fluorosis and altered bone density **Age < 12 y:** Not intended for this age group	**Gel:** 10 mL, 60 mL **Solution:** 10 mL	Has been shown to form particles that block dentin tubules, thereby providing temporary relief from pain associated with root-surface sensitivity
3.28% stannous fluoride	Stani-Max Pro	Dilute 1:1 with water, preferably distilled water, to provide a 1.64% SnF rinse Use in office irrigation or rinse Recommended rinse after scaling and root planing	Caution must be taken in use of fluorides as desensitizing agents in children due to possibility of fluorosis and altered bone density **Age < 12 y:** Not intended for this age group	**Glycerin-based liquid:** 16-oz bottles	Has been shown to form particles that block dentin tubules, thereby providing temporary relief from pain associated with root-surface sensitivity

★ indicates a product bearing the ADA Seal of Acceptance.

Continued on next page

Table 13.1 (cont.)

Desensitizing Fluorides, Oxalates, Varnishes, Sealants and Bonding Agents: Usage Information

Generic name	Brand name(s)	Usage and administration for adults	Usage and administration for children	Content/form	Features/uses
			Fluorides (cont.)		
1.1% neutral sodium fluoride	NiteWhite NSF	Apply in a tray and wear as directed for 5 min/day	Caution must be taken in use of fluorides as desensitizing agents in children due to possibility of fluorosis and altered bone density **Age <12 y:** Not intended for this age group	Gel (content not available)	Has been shown to form particles that block dentin tubules, thereby providing temporary relief from pain associated with root-surface sensitivity
			Oxalates		
Potassium oxalate	Protect	Dry dentin surface (isolation not necessary); dispense 10-12 drops into plastic dappen dish; apply saturated cotton pellets to sensitive area for 1 full min; use light pressure and do not burnish; have patient expectorate after application; to overcome pain threshold, sequential 1-min treatments may be required Do not apply with wooden stick	Not recommended	½-oz bottle, 24 ampules/box	Used for chairside treatment of dentinal hypersensitivity; acidic reagents remove smear layer and demineralize root surface (and may also leave crystals of calcium oxalate on the root surface), which may decrease effectiveness of bond cements and adhesives' interaction with the root surface; therefore, surfaces treated with an oxalate should be pumiced before a bonding agent is used

Agent	Product	Application		Packaging	Uses
Ferric oxalate (6% ferric oxalate)	Sensodyne Sealant	Dry dentin surface (isolation not necessary); dispense 10-12 drops into plastic dappen dish; apply saturated cotton pellets to sensitive area for 1 full min; use light pressure and do not burnish; have patient expectorate after application; to overcome pain threshold, sequential 1-min treatments may be required Do not apply with wooden stick	Not recommended	Available in ½-oz (15 mL) bottles with dispenser	Used for chairside treatment of dentinal hypersensitivity; acidic reagents remove smear layer and demineralize root surface (and may also leave crystals of calcium oxalate on the root surface), which may decrease effectiveness of bond cements and adhesives' interaction with the root surface; therefore, surfaces treated with an oxalate should be pumiced before a bonding agent is used
Aluminum oxalate	Dentin Conditioners	Dry dentin surface (isolation not necessary); dispense 10-12 drops into plastic dappen dish; apply saturated cotton pellets to sensitive area for 1 full min; use light pressure and do not burnish; have patient expectorate after application; to overcome pain threshold, sequential 1-min treatments may be required Do not apply with wooden stick	Not recommended	3 mL/5mL bottle with dispenser	Used for chairside treatment of dentinal hypersensitivity; acidic reagents remove smear layer and demineralize root surface (and may also leave crystals of calcium oxalate on the root surface), which may decrease effectiveness of bond cements and adhesives' interaction with the root surface; therefore, surfaces treated with an oxalate should be pumiced before a bonding agent is used
Varnishes, sealants and bonding agents					
Varnishes: Sodium fluoride	Duraphat, Duraflor	Apply chairside according to manufacturer's recommendations	Not recommended	50 mg/mL, 10-mL tube	**Varnishes:** Used for chairside treatment of dentinal hypersensitivity; varnishes occlude dentinal tubules

Continued on next page

Table 13.1 (cont.)

Desensitizing Fluorides, Oxalates, Varnishes, Sealants and Bonding Agents: Usage Information

Generic name	Brand name(s)	Usage and administration for adults	Usage and administration for children	Content/form	Features/uses
Varnishes, sealants and bonding agents (cont.)					
Sealants: Active ingredient not listed	Barrier Dental Sealant, Pain-Free Desensitizer	Apply chairside according to manufacturer's recommendations	Not recommended	2 component bottles of 5 mL each	**Sealants:** Used for chairside treatment of dentinal hypersensitivity; appear to close dentinal tubules and protect pulp and reduce sensitivity to temperature extremes; compatible with all restorative materials, dental cements, and cavity liners
Bonding agents: Methacrylate polymer	All-Bond DS Desensitizer, Micro prime, Confi-Dental, Gluma Desensitizer	Apply chairside according to manufacturer's recommendations	Not recommended	**Gluma Densensitizer, Confi-Dental:** available in small dispenser bottle **Micro prime:** 5-mL bottle **All-Bond DS Desensitizer:** Kit contains two primers, cleanser, mixing well, brush handle and brush tips	**Bonding agents:** Used for chairside treatment of dentinal hypersensitivity; bonding agents seal dentinal tubules and reduce fluid shifting

Special Patients

Pregnant and nursing women

There is no evidence that desensitizing agents are harmful to pregnant women or during breast feeding. While a minimal amount does cross the placental barrier if these agents are ingested and traces also are found in breast milk, no contraindications are reported when these agents are used as recommended.

Pediatric, geriatric and other special patients

In children, ingestion of high levels of fluoride will cause fluorosis of teeth and osseous changes. In older patients, there is no evidence suggesting a need to modify existing procedures.

Patient Monitoring: Aspects to Watch

- Persistent or increased pain: may require re-evaluation of differential diagnosis as well as consideration of alternative agents, therapies or both

Adverse Effects and Precautions

Fluorides

Fluoride preparations should be kept out of reach of children. On rare occasions, adverse reactions to fluorides, including skin rash, GI upset and headaches, may be noted. Such reactions are reversible upon discontinuing use. Fluoride should not be swallowed.

Patients with gingival sensitivity may be sensitive to the acidity of certain fluoride solutions.

Acidic fluoride solutions may cause dulling of porcelain and ceramic restorations.

Oxalates

Acids may decrease the effectiveness of bonding cements; thus, teeth treated with oxalates should be pumiced before application of bonding agents.

Varnishes, Sealants and Bonding Agents

No adverse effects or precautions have been reported.

Pharmacology

The general principle guiding the development of desensitizing agents is that the number of dental tubules exposed to the mouth correlates with sensitivity; thus, many of the agents are designed to occlude tubules. The most popular theory is that sensitivity in this situation results from the movement of fluid through the exposed tubules, which results in activation of the nerves within the pulp, subsequently registered as pain.

Another strategy, based on the "hydrodynamic theory," includes the development of agents that can depolarize nerves directly. Another theory of dentin hypersensitivity is that of the "dentinal receptor mechanism," which proposes that odontoblasts play a more receptive role; however, agents that induce pain normally fail to evoke pain when applied to exposed dentin. Yet a third theory is that certain polypeptides present within the pulp can modulate nerve impulses within the pulp. Thus, therapies have been directed at agents or procedures or both that can depolarize nerves directly.

Patient Advice

- Patients should be aware that, in general, several factors must be carefully considered in treatment of tooth sensitivity: severity of the problem, physical findings and past treatment. Proper diagnosis is required before initiation of treatment, whether in office or at home.
- Patients must realize that use of a desensitizing agent may not prove effective over a short time (for example, less than 2 w).

Suggested Readings

Curro FA, ed. Tooth hypersensitivity. Dent Clin North Am 1990;July:34(3).

Jackson RJ. Dentifrices for the treatment of dentine hypersensitivity. In: Embery G, Rolla G, eds. Clinical and biological aspects of dentifrices. New York: Oxford University Press; 1992;337-44.

Pashley EL, Tao L, Pashley DH. Effects of oxalate on dentin bonding. Am J Dent 1993;3:116-8.

Richardson DW, Tao L, Pashley DH. Bond strengths of luting cements to potassium oxalate-treated dentin. J Prosthet Dent 1990;63:418-22.

Silverman G, German E, Hanna CB, et al. Assessing the efficacy of three dentifrices in the treatment of dentinal hypersensitivity. JADA 1997;127:191-201.

Home Use Products

Accepted Indications

Densensitizing toothpaste agents are used to provide relief from thermal and tactile sensitivity on exposed root surfaces when pathological causes for pain have been ruled out. In addition, these toothpastes contain fluoride to prevent caries.

General Usage Information

Usage and Administration

See Table 13.2 for general usage information on desensitizing toothpastes.

Special Dental Considerations

Following are special dental considerations for home use desensitizing agents, which are the same as or very similar to those for in-office products listed earlier in this chapter.

Drug Interactions of Dental Interest

- There is some suggestion of interaction of fluorides with calcium-containing products—for example, formation of calcium fluoride, which is poorly absorbed.
- Certain agents—for example, chlorhexidine—may decrease fluoride's ability to bind to the root surface. Thus, after using fluoride agents, the patient should not rinse or eat for 1 h.
- Some agents are acidic and thus may cause sensitivity in patients with mucositis.
- Some acidic compounds—for example, oxalate—may cause dulling of porcelain ceramics and decreased effectiveness of bonding cements. Therefore, pumicing the root surface before use of some desensitizing agents is recommended.

Special Patients

There is no evidence that desensitizing agents are harmful to pregnant women or during breast feeding. In children, high levels of fluoride will cause fluorosis of teeth and osseous changes. In older patients, no alteration of dose is required.

Patient Monitoring: Aspects to Watch

- Persistent or increased pain: may require re-evaluation of differential diagnosis and consideration of alternative agents, therapies or both

Adverse Effects and Precautions

No adverse effects are reported beyond those related to high-dose fluoride. Precautions include the underlying possibility of an undiagnosed serious dental problem that may need prompt dental care. Products should not be used more than 4 w unless recommended by the dentist. Keep out of reach of children. All patients, and especially those with severe dental erosion, should brush properly and lightly with any dentifrice to avoid further removal of tooth structure.

Pharmacology

The general principle guiding development of desensitizing agents, including toothpastes, is that the number of dental tubules exposed to the mouth correlates with sensitivity; thus, most agents are designed to occlude tubules. The most popular theory is that sensitivity in this situation is due to the movement of fluid through the exposed tubules, which results in activation of the nerves within the pulp and subsequently is registered as pain.

Patient Advice

- Patients should be aware that, in general, several factors must be carefully considered in treatment of tooth sensitivity: severity of the problem, physical findings and past treatment. Proper diagnosis is required before initiation of treatment, whether in office or at home.

Table 13.2

Desensitizing Toothpastes: Usage Information

Generic name	Brand name(s)	Usage and administration for adults	Usage and administration for children	Content/form	Features/uses
Sodium fluoride, 5% potassium nitrate	Aquafresh Sensitive Teeth, Crest Sensitivity Protection ★, Oral-B Sensitive, Protect Sensitive Teeth ★, Sensodyne Cool Gel, Sensodyne Tartar Control, Desensitize Plus, Arm & Hammer Dentacare	Apply toothpaste onto soft-bristle toothbrush; brush teeth thoroughly for at least 1 min tid (morning and evening) or as recommended by a dentist or physician; make sure to brush all sensitive areas of the teeth	**Age < 12 y:** Dentist or physician should be consulted before children use this product. **Age < 6 y:** Children should be supervised when using this product; keep out of reach of children	**Tubes:** 1-, 6-oz	Fluoride products are used for prevention of cavities, and added compounds are considered to decrease dentinal hypersensitivity; if pain persists more than 4 w, patient should be re-evaluated to determine cause of sensitivity
Sodium monofluorophosphate, 5% potassium nitrate	Den-Mat Sensitive, Sensodyne Fresh Mint ★, Sensodyne Original, Rembrandt Whitening Sensitive	Apply toothpaste onto soft-bristle toothbrush; brush teeth thoroughly for at least 1 min tid (morning and evening) or as recommended by a dentist or physician; make sure to brush all sensitive areas of the teeth	**Age < 12 y:** Dentist or physician should be consulted before children use this product. **Age < 6 y:** Children should be supervised when using this product; keep out of reach of children	**Tubes:** 1-, 6-oz	Fluoride products are used for prevention of cavities, and added compounds are considered to decrease dentinal hypersensitivity; if pain persists more than 4 w, patient should be re-evaluated to determine cause of sensitivity
10% strontium chloride	Sensodyne-SC [CAN]	Apply toothpaste onto soft-bristle toothbrush; brush teeth thoroughly for at least 1 min tid (morning and evening) or as recommended by a dentist or physician; make sure to brush all sensitive areas of the teeth	**Age < 12 y:** Dentist or physician should be consulted before children use this product. **Age < 6 y:** Children should be supervised when using this product; keep out of reach of children	**Tubes:** 1-, 6-oz	Fluoride products are used for prevention of cavities, and added compounds are considered to decrease dentinal hypersensitivity; if pain persists more than 4 w, patient should be re-evaluated to determine cause of sensitivity

★ indicates a product bearing the ADA Seal of Acceptance.
[CAN] indicates a product available only in Canada.

- Patients must realize that use of a desensitizing agent will not prove effective over a short time unless the product is used for at least 2 w.

Suggested Readings

Curry FA, ed. Tooth hypersensitivity. Dent Clin North Am 1990;July:34(3).

Gilliam DG, Newman HN, Bulman JS, Davies EH. Dentifrice abrasivity and dental hypersensitivity. Results 12 weeks following cessation of 8 weeks' supervised use. J Periodontol 1992;63:7-12.

Kuroiwa M, Kodaka T, Kuroiwa M, Abe M. Dentin hypersensitivity. Occlusion of dentinal tubules by brushing with and without an abrasive dentifrice. J Periodontol 1994;65:291-6.

Ochardson R, Gangarosa LP Sr, Holland GR, Pashley DH. Towards a standard code of practice for evaluating the effectiveness of treatments for hypersensitive dentine. Arch Oral Biol 1994;39:1215-45.

Chapter 14.

Bleaching Agents

B. Ellen Byrne, R.Ph., D.D.S., Ph.D.

Tooth bleaching agents can be classified as to whether they are used for external or internal bleaching and whether the procedure is performed in the office by a dentist or at home by a patient. For tooth bleaching, hydrogen peroxide (H_2O_2) is used alone at levels of 30% or at 10% to 22% levels in a stable gel of carbamide peroxide (urea peroxide) that breaks down to form hydrogen peroxide (3.35% H_2O_2 from 10% carbamide peroxide), urea, ammonia and carbon dioxide. The Food and Drug Administration has not approved peroxide solutions for use as a home bleach, however.

Internal bleaching. Internal bleaching produces reliable results when used to eliminate intrinsic stains in dentin caused by blood breakdown products or endodontics or for stains in receded pulp chambers. However, bleaching should be confined to the dentin; bleaching the cementum, which provides an attachment for the periodontal ligament, has been associated with external root resorption. External root resorption below the gingival attachment is associated with internal bleaching on nonvital teeth that have sustained trauma, poorly sealed canal spaces or heating during the bleaching procedure. It is felt that the bleaching agent diffuses through the dentinal tubules and initiates an inflammatory resorptive response in the cervical area. Unfortunately, external cervical resorption is not seen for approximately 5 to 6 y after internal bleaching. The use of heat is not essential and should be avoided.

Internal bleaching is always an in-office procedure. There are two common approaches

to internal bleaching: the "office bleach" (a one-time application) and the "walking bleach" (sealed inside the tooth for 2 to 3 days). The office bleaching agent is a mixture of Superoxol (30% hydrogen peroxide) and perborate, to which heat is applied by the use of a hot instrument, such as a ball burnisher or an electric heat-producing instrument, for 2 to 5 min to accelerate the bleaching process. Heat has also been associated with external root resorption. Walking bleach seals the Superoxol and perborate mixture inside the tooth for 2 to 3 days. The sodium perborate, a stable white powder, soluble in water, decomposes into sodium metaborate and hydrogen peroxide, thus releasing nascent oxygen. The sodium perborate, which is mixed with the hydrogen peroxide, also releases oxygen. This combination is thought to be synergistic and very effective in bleaching. This technique is called "walking bleach" because the bleaching process actually occurs between dental appointments, during which time the bleaching agents are sealed in the pulp chamber.

External bleaching. External bleaching is indicated for teeth that are discolored from aging, fluorosis or staining due to the effects of tetracycline. External bleaching can be applied by the dentist or staff or can be applied by the patient in home-use bleaching. When dentist-administered and home-use bleaching are used together, it is called "dual bleaching."

Dentist-applied external bleaching can be done with periodic repetitions of an office-bleaching agent using Superoxol, or 30% H_2O_2.

An etching gel containing phosphoric acid applied to selected dark areas increases the penetration of the bleach. Light is used to produce heat, which accelerates the bleaching process. External bleaching may need additional treatment every 1 or 2 y to touch up relapses. Severely stained teeth may require more frequent retreatment.

Home bleaching, supervised by the dentist, is done by the patient at home using a custom-made plastic carrier that holds the bleach against the patient's teeth. After the desired result is achieved, overnight use on a periodic basis (1 to 4 times/mo) can maintain the lightening that has been achieved.

External bleaching is seldom permanent, lasting approximately 1 to 4 y, after which teeth gradually return to their original color. Usually the younger the patient, the longer the bleaching will last. The more difficult it is to bleach a tooth, the more likely it is to discolor again. Bluish-gray stains seem to reappear more quickly than yellow stains. Because reoccurrence of staining is unpredictable, promises about longevity should not be made. Internal bleaching usually lasts longer than external bleaching.

Accepted Indications

Types of tooth discoloration, causes and response to bleaching are provided in Table 14.1. Information on in-office bleaching techniques is provided in Table 14.2; information on dentist-supervised home bleaching is provided in Table 14.3. Brown, blue-gray and gray stains are usually caused by caries, porphyria, fluorosis, dentinogenesis imperfecta and erythroblastosis fetalis. They need microabrasion and restorative care and should not be bleached.

Table 14.1

Types of Tooth Discoloration

Color	Etiology	Ease or difficulty of bleaching
White	Fluorosis	Degree of difficulty depends on extent of fluorosis
Blue-gray	Dentinogenesis imperfecta, erythroblastosis fetalis, tetracycline	Deeply stained blue-gray discolorations, especially those associated with tetracycline, are more difficult to treat than yellow teeth
Gray	Silver oxide from root canal sealers	Dark stains from root canal sealers seldom bleachable, should be treated restoratively
Yellow	Fluorosis, physiological changes due to aging, obliteration of the pulp chamber	Mild uniform yellow discoloration associated with aging or mild uniform fluorosis are easiest to treat
Brown	Fluorosis, caries, porphyria, tetracycline, dentinogenesis imperfecta	Stains that are deeper in color are more difficult to treat
Black	Mercury stain (amalgam), caries, fluorosis	Very dark or black stains from silver-containing root canal sealers or from mercury are seldom bleachable, should be treated restoratively
Pink	Internal resorption	Bleaching is not indicated; treatment consists of endodontics and calcium hydroxide treatment

Table 14.2
Professionally Applied Bleaching Agents: Usage Information

Generic name	Brand name(s)	Indications	Usual adult dosage
Internal bleaching			
30% hydrogen peroxide	Superoxol with sodium perborate ★	Yellow or black stains from endodontics or tetracycline; intrinsic stains when teeth have darkened from blood breakdown products, or in receded pulp chambers	Sealed into pulp chamber for up to 7 days
External bleaching			
30% hydrogen peroxide	Starbrite Gel In-Office Gel ★, Superoxol with sodium perborate ★	Light yellow stains associated with aging or mild fluorosis	Heat applied for 2-5 min; can be used with or without phosphoric acid

★ *indicates a product bearing the ADA Seal of Acceptance.*

Table 14.3
Dentist-Dispensed Home Bleaching Agents: Usage Information*

Generic name	Brand name(s)	Indications	Usual adult dosage
10% carbamide peroxide	Colgate Platinum Tooth Whitener ★	Yellow or brown stains from aging, fluorosis or tetracycline	1 or 2 treatments q day for ½-1 h duration, for 2 w
	Opalescence Whitening Gel ★	Yellow or brown stains from aging, fluorosis or tetracycline	1-2 h q day or night OR every second or third night, depending on patient's needs
	Rembrandt Lighten Bleaching Gel ★	Yellow or brown stains from aging, fluorosis or tetracycline	1 or 2 treatments q day for 1-2 h duration, for a maximum of 4 w

★ *indicates a product bearing the ADA Seal of Acceptance.*
As this book was going to press, NiteWhite received the ADA Seal of Acceptance

General Usage Information

Maximum Recommended Amounts
Average treatment time is generally 2-6 w. More difficult cases require extended treatment and may result in teeth that look chalky. In some patients, stains relapse when treatment is discontinued.

Usage Adjustments
Adult
When having bleaching done at the dental office, some patients, especially those with severe erosion, abrasion or recession, may find the combination of heat and peroxide uncomfortable. These patients are not good candidates for office bleaching. For at-home bleaching, the recommended wearing time varies greatly; the wearing times are determined by the clinical study designs and vary considerably between products. The daily dosage is between ½ h and 10 h for one or two treatments per day.

Special Dental Considerations

Drug Interactions of Dental Interest

Possible interactions between substances such as therapeutics and bleaching agents are provided in Table 14.4.

Special Patients

Pregnant and nursing women

The long-term effects of using in-office or home bleaching agents on the teeth of pregnant women have not been studied; therefore, women who are pregnant or who have a reasonable expectation that they could become pregnant should not undergo treatment. Pregnancy risk category has not been determined.

Pediatric, geriatric and other special patients

Bleaching agents are not indicated for use in children. The gel should be kept away from children.

Patient Monitoring: Aspects to Watch

Long-term use can alter normal oral flora and can contribute to lingual papillary hypertrophy (hairy tongue) and *Candida albicans*.

Adverse Effects and Precautions

See Table 14.5 for adverse effects, precautions and contraindications for in-office and home use of bleaching agents.

Pharmacology

The mechanism of tooth bleaching is not fully understood; however, it is felt that the unstable peroxide breaks down to highly unstable free radicals. These free radicals chemically break larger pigmented organic molecules in the enamel matrix into smaller less pigmented constituents. Higher concentrations, such as 30% hydrogen peroxide, remove the enamel matrix, thereby creating microscopic voids that scatter light and increase the appearance of whiteness until remineralization occurs and the color partly relapses. When the morphology of unbleached teeth is compared to teeth that have been treated with lower concentrations of peroxide, such as carbamide peroxide 10%, the latter seem not to be affected; therefore, different bleaching materials and concentrations may have different modes of action.

The addition of carbopol, a carboxypolymethylene polymer, prolongs the release of hydrogen peroxide from carbamide peroxide. Carbopol, a water-soluble resin used in many household products such as shampoo and

Table 14.4

Bleaching Agents: Possible Interactions With Other Substances

Substance used by patient	Interaction with bleaching agent	Dentist's actions
Alcohol	May possibly result in additive carcinogenicity because peroxides have mutagenic potential and may boost the effects of known carcinogens	Advise patients to avoid these products
Coffee	May compromise treatment results	Advise patients to avoid these products
Tea	May compromise treatment results	Advise patients to avoid these products
Heavy use of tobacco	May compromise treatment results; may possibly result in additive carcinogenicity because peroxides have mutagenic potential and may boost the effects of known carcinogens	Advise patients to avoid these products

Table 14.5

Bleaching Agents: Adverse Effects, Precautions and Contraindications

Body system	Adverse effects	Precautions/contraindications
General	Prolonged use of 30% H_2O_2 can destroy cells, and for cells that are not destroyed, prolonged use may potentiate the carcinogenic effects of carcinogens	Patients should not smoke or use other potential carcinogens during treatment
Oral	Due to acidic nature of some of these products, patients can experience transient dentin sensitivity that goes away when the bleaching is discontinued High concentrations of H_2O_2, or Superoxol, used in office bleaching may produce what appear to be tissue burns—white areas on the gingiva that are caused by oxygen gas bubbles and are not true burns, although discomfort can feel like a burn	Patients with root sensitivity may not want to have treatment because treatment can aggravate sensitivity In cases of tissue burns (see description at left), rinse affected area for 1-5 min

toothpaste, is used as a thickening agent. It does not break down, nor does it increase the breakdown of the bleaching agent. The carbopol binds to the peroxide and triples or quadruples the active release time of peroxide. Products without carbopol are more fluid and bleach more slowly due to the reduced activity time and greater loss of bleach from the tray.

Patient Advice

The following advice pertains to patients who are using home bleaching agents:

- The more treatments per day, the faster the bleaching; however, this concentrated use of bleaching agents can also increase sensitivity.

- The patient should not wear the appliance while eating.
- Users should discontinue treatment with the bleaching agent if the teeth, gums or bite become uncomfortable.
- The dentist should check the patient's mouth every 1-6 w to ensure that no damage has been done to the teeth, gums or dental restorations.

Suggested Readings

Albers HF. Lightening natural teeth. ADEPT Report 1991;2(1):1-24.

Harrington GW, Natkin F. External resorption associated with bleaching of pulpless teeth. J. Endod 1979;5:344-8.

Haywood VB, Leonard RH, Nelson CF, Brunson WD. Effectiveness, side effects and long-term status of night-guard vital bleaching. JADA 1994;125(9):1219-26.

Chapter 15

Drugs for Medical Emergencies in the Dental Office

Stanley F. Malamed, D.D.S.

Medical emergencies can and do occur in dental offices. Surveys have demonstrated that it is likely that at least one potentially life-threatening emergency situation will develop during a dentist's practice lifetime. (See Chapter 16 for a discussion of how to manage emergency situations.)

Each professional staff member in every dental office should be trained to recognize and manage any emergency situation that might arise.

Although certain categories of emergency drugs are suggested for the dental office emergency kit, it must be emphasized that administering emergency drugs will always be secondary to providing basic life support during an emergency. Indeed, during all emergency situations, health care professionals should strictly adhere to the P, A, B, C, D emergency management protocol:

P = position;

A = airway;

B = breathing;

C = circulation;

D = definitive treatment (which might include administration of drugs).

Because dentists' levels of training in emergency management can vary significantly, it is impossible to recommend any one list of emergency drugs or any one proprietary emergency drug kit that meets the needs and abilities of all dentists. For this reason, dentists should develop their own emergency drug and equipment kits, based on their level of expertise in managing emergencies.

Although no state dental boards have established specific recommendations as to which emergency drugs and equipment a dentist must have available, state boards of dental examiners do mandate that certain drugs and items of emergency equipment be available in offices where dentists employ intramuscular or intravenous parenteral sedation or general anesthesia. Specialty groups, such as the American Dental Society of Anesthesiology, the American Association of Oral and Maxillofacial Surgeons and the Academy of Pediatric Dentistry, have instituted guidelines for the use of sedation and general anesthesia, which dictate the emergency drugs that must be readily available. The following drug categories are mandated by many state boards of dental examiners for doctors who have been permitted to use parenteral conscious sedation, deep sedation or general anesthesia:

• vasopressor;
• corticosteroid;
• bronchodilator;
• muscle relaxant;
• narcotic antagonist;
• benzodiazepine antagonist;
• antihistamine (histamine-blocker);
• anticholinergic;
• cardiac medications: epinephrine, antiarrhythmic, vasodilator;
• antihypertensive.

Dentists should not include in the emergency kit any drug or item of emergency equipment they are not trained to use. For example, dentists who are not well-trained in tracheal intubation should not include a laryngoscope and endotracheal tubes in their emergency kits; likewise, dentists who are not proficient in venipuncture should not have an anticonvulsant drug, such as diazepam, in their kits because anticonvulsant drugs must be administered intravenously. Also, dentists should not use anticonvulsants if they are unable to ventilate a patient who is unconscious and apneic, as is likely to occur when anticonvulsant drugs are administered to terminate a seizure.

Table 15.1 lists four levels of drugs and medical equipment that can help the dentist design an emergency kit that will be suitable for the level of emergency preparedness of his or her dental office:

- Level 1 drugs are those deemed most important or critical;
- Level 2 drugs are less critical but can be included in the emergency drug kits of dentists trained to use them;
- Level 3 drugs are those employed for advanced cardiac life support;
- Level 4 includes antidotal drugs that are used to reverse the clinical actions of previously administered medications.

Accepted Indications

Table 15.2 describes the emergency clinical indications for injectable and noninjectable drugs.

General Dosing Information

Table 15.2 provides the dosing information for injectable and noninjectable drugs.

Special Dental Considerations

Drug Interactions of Dental Interest

Table 15.3 lists the possible interactions of injectable and noninjectable emergency drugs with other drugs.

Adverse Effects and Precautions

Table 15.4 lists the adverse effects and precautions related to injectable and noninjectable emergency drugs with other drugs.

Table 15.1

Levels and Types of Injectable and Noninjectable Drugs and Equipment for Emergencies in Dental Offices

Injectable drugs	Noninjectable drugs	Equipment
Level 1 (basic critical drugs)		
Endogenous catecholamine: Epinephrine (1:1,000)	**Oxygen**	**Oxygen delivery system** including positive-pressure/demand valve, bag, valve, mask device, pocket mask; **high-volume suction and aspirator tips or tonsillar suction; syringes; tourniquets; Magill intubation; forceps**
Histamine blocker: Diphenhydramine, chlorpheniramine	**Vasodilator:** Nitroglycerin	
	Bronchodilator: Albuterol	
	Antihypoglycemic: Orange juice, regular (not diet) soft drinks	
Level 2 (noncritical drugs)		
Anticonvulsant: Diazepam	**Anticholinergic:** Atropine	**Cricothyrotomy device:** oropharyngeal or nasopharyngeal airways, or both
Analgesic: Morphine sulfate	**Respiratory stimulant:** Aromatic ammonia, spirits of ammonia	**Laryngoscope and endotracheal tubes**
Vasopressor: Methoxamine		**Equipment for intravenous infusion:** infusion solution such as 5% dextrose and water (D5W); intravenous tubing; catheters, winged infusion sets, or both
Antihypoglycemic: Glucagon HCl, 50% dextrose		
Corticosteroid: Anti-inflammatory hydrocortisone, sodium succinate		
Antihypertensive: Antianginal, ß-adrenergic blocking agents such as esmolol, labetalol		

Level 3 (advanced cardiac life support drugs)

Endogenous catecholamine: Epinephrine (1:10,000, for IV administration)

Anticholinergic, antidysrhythmic: Atropine

Antiarrhythmic: Lidocaine

Antiarrhythmic: Procainamide

Antiarrhythmic: Bretylium tosylate

Antiarrhythmic: Verapamil

Alkalinizing agent: Sodium bicarbonate

Analgesic: Morphine sulfate

Calcium salt: Calcium chloride

Level 4 (antidotal drugs)

Narcotic antagonist: Naloxone (example)

Benzodiazepine antagonist: Flumazenil (example)

Table 15.2

Injectable and Noninjectable Emergency Drugs: Dosage Information

Generic name	Brand name(s)	Maximum adult dosage (mg/kg)	Maximum child dosage (mg/kg)	Pregnancy risk category	Content/form	Indications
			Level 1 (basic critical drugs)			
Endogenous catecholamine (sterile solution): Epinephrine 1:1,000	Ana-Guard, Epi-Pen Auto-Injector	**To manage allergic reaction—IM or SC:** 0.2-1.0 mL (mg); small dose should be administered initially and increased, if necessary **Note:** When epinephrine is administered IM, buttocks should be avoided and mid-deltoid or vastus lateralis muscles should be used instead **To manage asthma and certain allergic reactions, such as angioedema, urticaria, serum sickness and anaphylaxis—SC:** 0.2-1.0 mL (mg); small dose should be administered initially and increased, if necessary; preferred route of administration is SC **For cardiac resuscitation—IV:** 0.5 mL (0.5 mg) diluted to 10 mL with sodium chloride injection **Note:** External cardiac compression should be continued after IV administration in patients who have had cardiac arrest to ensure distribution of the epinephrine to coronary circulation **Note:** Drug should be administered only when physical and electromechanical attempts at resuscitation have failed	**For asthmatic pediatric patients—SC:** 0.01 mg/kg or 0.3 mg/m² to a maximum of 0.5 mg; dose should be repeated every 4 h, if needed **To manage asthma and certain allergic reactions, such as angioedema, urticaria, serum sickness and anaphylaxis—SC:** 0.01 mg/kg or 0.3 mg/m² body surface to a maximum of 0.5 mg; dose should be repeated every 4 h, if needed; preferred route of administration is SC	C	**Note:** When diluted, can be administered IV; each mL contains 1 mg of epinephrine hydrochloride dissolved in water for injection, with sodium chloride added for isotonicity **Syringe:** IM 0.15 mg/0.3 mL Epi-Pen Jr. Autoinjector; IM 0.3 mg/0.3 mL Epi-Pen Autoinjector; IM, IV, SC 1.0 mg/mL Ana-Guard **Vial—IM, IV, SC:** 0.1 mg/mL in 3- and 10-mL vials; 1.0 mg/mL in 3- and 10-mL vials	For relief of respiratory distress due to bronchospasm To provide rapid relief of hypersensitivity reactions from drugs and other allergens, anaphylaxis, anaphylactic shock

Histamine blocker: Diphenhydramine	Benadryl	**IV or deep IM:** 10-50 mg; 100 mg, if required, to a maximum daily dose of 400 mg **Overdosage:** Overdosage can be manifested by CNS symptoms ranging from depression to excitation; stimulation is particularly likely in children; atropine-like signs and symptoms—dry mouth; fixed, dilated pupils; flushing; gastrointestinal symptoms—also can develop	**IV or deep IM:** 5 mg/kg/24 h or 150 mg/m²/24 h	B	**IV, IM:** 10 mg/mL, 50 mg/mL	For allergic reactions, allergies, anaphylactic reactions, angioedema; mild, uncomplicated skin manifestation of urticaria and angioedema **Age ≥ 60 y:** More likely to cause dizziness, sedation and hypotension
Histamine blocker: Chlorpheniramine	Chlor-Trimeton, Chlor-Pro 10, generic	**IM or IV:** 4 mg tid-qid up to 40 mg/day **Overdosage:** Overdosage can be manifested by CNS symptoms ranging from depression to excitation; stimulation is particularly likely in children; atropine-like signs and symptoms—dry mouth; fixed, dilated pupils; flushing; gastrointestinal symptoms—also can develop	**IM or IV:** 2 mg tid-qid	C	**Chlorpheniramine—IV, IM:** 10 mg/mL Chlor-Trimeton	For allergic reactions, allergies, anaphylactic reactions, angioedema; mild, uncomplicated skin manifestation of urticaria and angioedema **Age ≥ 60 y:** More likely to cause dizziness, sedation and hypotension
Oxygen		**Inhalation:** Administered at a flow rate, calculated in L/min, that is adequate to alleviate the presenting signs and symptoms	**Inhalation:** Administered at a flow rate, calculated in L/min, that is adequate to alleviate the presenting signs and symptoms		In compressed gas cylinders in a variety of sizes; portability of the oxygen cylinder is a desirable characteristic; a minimum supply for emergency use is one E-cylinder	Any emergency situation in which respiratory distress is evident

Continued on next page

Table 15.2 (cont.)

Injectable and Noninjectable Emergency Drugs: Dosage Information

Generic name	Brand name(s)	Maximum adult dosage (mg/kg)	Maximum child dosage	Pregnancy risk category	Content/form	Indications
			Level 1 (basic critical drugs) (cont.)			
Vasodilators, antianginals, antihypertensives, CV drugs: Nitroglycerin	Nitrostat, Nitrolingual Spray	**Oral—sublingual tablets:** One tablet (0.15-0.6 mg) should be dissolved under tongue or in buccal pouch at first sign of an acute anginal attack; dose may be repeated every 5 min until relief is obtained; if pain persists after administration of 3 tablets in a 15-min period, a physician should be notified **Oral—lingual aerosol spray:** At onset of an anginal attack, 1 (0.4-0.8 mg) or 2 metered doses should be sprayed onto or under the tongue; no more than 3 metered doses are recommended during a 15-min period; if chest pain persists, prompt medical attention is recommended **Overdosage:** Severe hypotension and reflex tachycardia, which can be managed by elevating the patient's legs and temporarily terminating administration of the drugs, can occur	Not established	C	**Sublingual tablets:** 0.15, 0.3, 0.4, 0.6 mg **Translingual spray:** Nitrolingual, 0.4, 0.8 mg/dose **Vaporoles:** amyl nitrite (yellow), 0.3 mL	For the prophylaxis, treatment and management of patients with angina pectoris

	Adult dosage	Child dosage	How supplied	Comments
Bronchodilator: Albuterol — Ventolin, Proventil	2 inhalations repeated every 4-6 h; for some patients, 1 inhalation q 4 h may be adequate; neither more frequent administrations nor a larger number of inhalations are recommended; if a previously effective dosage regimen fails to provide the usual relief, medical advice should be sought immediately, as this is a sign of seriously worsening asthma and requires reassessment of therapy	**Age < 14 y:** Not established **Age ≥ 14 y:** 2 inhalations repeated every 4-6 h; for some patients, 1 inhalation q 4 h may be adequate; neither more frequent administrations nor a larger number of inhalations are recommended; if a previously effective dosage regimen fails to provide the usual relief, medical advice should be sought immediately, as this is a sign of seriously worsening asthma and requires reassessment of therapy	**Inhalation aerosol:** 0.09 mg/inhalation, 200 inhalations	For relief of bronchospasm in patients aged ≥ 4 y who have reversible obstructive airway disease; for prevention of exercise-induced bronchospasm in patients aged ≥ 4 y
Antihypoglycemics (orange juice, nondiet soft drinks)	Orange juice or regular (not diet) cola beverages are administered in 4-oz increments every 5-10 min until patient has returned to normal level of consciousness	Orange juice or regular (not diet) cola beverages are administered in 4-oz increments every 5-10 min until patient has returned to normal level of consciousness	**Liquids:** Available in 12-oz cans	For hypoglycemia in the conscious patient
Level 2 (noncritical drugs)				
Anticonvulsant: Diazepam — D-Val, Valium	Should be individualized (titrated) for maximum beneficial effect **IM:** 2-20 mg, depending on indication and its severity; should be administered slowly, at least 1 min for each mL (5 mg) **Patients with status epilepticus and severe recurrent convulsive seizures —IM:** 5-10 mg initially and repeated, if necessary, at 10- to 15-min intervals	**Older children—IV:** 2-20 mg, depending on indication and its severity **Patients with status epilepticus and severe recurrent convulsive seizures—IV:** maximum of 30 mg	Not established **Solution for injection—IV:** 5 mg/mL	A useful adjunct in treating status epilepticus and severe recurrent convulsive seizures

Continued on next page

Table 15.2 (cont.)

Injectable and Noninjectable Emergency Drugs: Dosage Information

Generic name	Brand name(s)	Maximum adult dosage (mg/kg)	Maximum child dosage	Pregnancy risk category	Content/form	Indications
			Level 2 (noncritical drugs) (cont.)			
Analgesic: Morphine sulfate	Astramorph PF, Duramorph, generic; Epimorph [CAN], Morphine Forte [CAN], Morphine Extra-Forte [CAN], Morphine H.P. [CAN]	**IV:** small incremental doses of 2-5 mg every 5-30 min until desired effect is achieved **Overdosage:** Is characterized by respiratory depression with or without concomitant CNS depression; because respiratory arrest can result either through direct depression of respiratory center or as result of hypoxia, dentist's first action should be ensuring adequate respiratory exchange through provision of patent airway and institution of assisted or controlled ventilation **Note:** Naloxone, the narcotic antagonist, is a specific antidote; usually given in 0.4-mg doses; should be administered IV simultaneously with respiratory resuscitation; naloxone injection and resuscitative equipment should be immediately available for administration in case of life-threatening or intolerable side effects **Note:** Low doses of IV-administered morphine have little effect on CV stability; high doses are excitatory, resulting from sympathetic hyperactivity and increase in circulating catecholamines **Note:** CNS excitation, resulting in convulsions, can accompany high doses of morphine administered IV **Note:** Dysphoric reactions and toxic psychoses have also been reported	In dentistry, not used with children	C	**Solution for injection—IM, IV, SC:** 2, 4, 5, 8, 10, 15 mg/mL	To manage pain that is not responsive to nonnarcotic analgesics; for treatment of pain and anxiety associated with acute myocardial infarction

Vasopressor, sympathomimetic agent: Methoxamine	Vasoxyl	**To correct fall in blood pressure—IM:** 10-15 mg; amount depends on degree of fall **To correct fall in systolic pressure to 60 mm/Hg or less—IV:** 3-5 mg; this dose can be accompanied by 10-15 mg IM for more prolonged effect **Whenever an emergency exists—IV:** 3-5 mg; this dose can be accompanied by 10-15 mg IM for more prolonged effect **Overdosage:** Can be manifested as undesirable elevation in blood pressure and/or bradycardia	Not established	C	20 mg in 1-mL ampules	For the support or maintenance of blood pressure
Antihypoglycemic: Glucagon hydrochloride	Glucagon; generic	1 mg by subcutaneous, IM or IV injection; patient usually awakens within 15 min; if response is delayed, there is no contraindication to administration of 1-2 additional doses of glucagon; however, in view of deleterious effects of cerebral hypoglycemia and depending on duration and depth of coma, use of parenteral glucose must be considered; IV glucose must be given if patient fails to respond to glucagon **Note:** Should not be administered at concentrations greater than 1 mg/mL **Note:** Is generally well-tolerated and no cases of overdosage of glucagon have been reported; if overdosage were to occur, it would not be expected to cause consequential toxicity, but would be expected to be associated with nausea, vomiting, gastric hypotonicity and diarrhea	**Weight > 20 kg—IM, IV, SC:** 1 mg **Weight < 20 kg—IM, IV, SC:** 0.5 mg or dose equivalent to 20-30 µg/kg; patient usually awakens within 15 min; if response is delayed, there is no contraindication to the administration of 1-2 additional doses of glucagon; however, in view of deleterious effects of cerebral hypoglycemia and depending on duration and depth of coma, use of parenteral glucose must be considered; IV glucose must be given if patient fails to respond to glucagon **Note:** Supplementary carbohydrates should be given as soon as possible, especially to children or adolescent patients	B	**Solution for injection—IM, IV, SC:** 10 mg/mL	For the management of severe hypoglycemic reactions **Note:** Patients with Type I diabetes do not have as great a response to blood glucose levels as do stable Type II diabetes patients

Continued on next page

[CAN] indicates a drug available only in Canada.

Table 15.2 (cont.)

Injectable and Noninjectable Emergency Drugs: Dosage Information

Generic name	Brand name(s)	Maximum adult dosage	Maximum child dosage (mg/kg)	Pregnancy risk category	Content/form	Indications
			Level 2 (noncritical drugs) (cont.)			
Antihypoglycemic: Dextrose 50%	generic	IV: 20-50 mL at a rate of 10 mL/min; most patients regain consciousness rapidly (5-10 min); additional 50 mL may be needed in some patients; supplementary carbohydrates should be given as soon as possible. **Note:** Is generally well-tolerated	0.5-1 g/kg/dose; D50W is diluted 1:1, producing D25W to avoid hypertonicity. **Note:** Supplementary carbohydrates should be given as soon as possible, especially to children or adolescent patients	C	50-mL glass ampules	For the management of severe hypoglycemic reactions (patients with Type I diabetes do not have as great a response to blood glucose levels as do stable Type II diabetes patients)
Anti-inflammatory adrenal corticosteroid: Hydrocortisone sodium succinate	A-hydroCort, Solu-Cortef, generic	Should be administered IV in emergency situations, but can also be administered IM; usual starting dose is 100 mg administered IV over 30 s	Not established	C	**Solution for injection—IM, IV:** 100 mg in 1-mL vials, 250 mg in 2-mL vials, 500 mg in 4-mL vials, 1 g in 8-mL vials. **Act-O-Vial System:** 100 mg, diluted to 50 mg/mL	For treating primary or secondary adrenocortical insufficiency as well as acute adrenocortical insufficiency; also for treatment of shock that proves unresponsive to conventional therapy if adrenocortical insufficiency exists or is suspected; to control severe or incapacitating allergic conditions intractable to adequate trials of conventional treatment in bronchial asthma and drug hypersensitivity reactions

| Anti-hypertensive, antianginal, β-adrenergic blocking agent: Esmolol | Brevibloc | **Injection:** Should be diluted to 10-mg/mL infusion by addition of two 2.5-g ampules to a 500-mL container of a compatible IV solution

For intra- or postoperative tachycardia or hypertension: Not always advisable to slowly titrate dose of esmolol to a therapeutic effect; for immediate control of tachycardia, hypertension or both, give 80-mg (approximately 1 mg/kg) bolus dose over 30 s, then 150-μg/kg/min infusion, if necessary; adjust infusion rate, as necessary, up to 300 μg/kg/min to maintain desired heart rate/blood pressure

For intra- or postoperative tachycardia or hypertension, alternative method: Loading dose infusion of 500 μg/kg/min for 1 min, then 4-min maintenance infusion of 50 μg/kg/min; if adequate therapeutic effect is not noted within 5 min, repeat same loading dose and follow with maintenance infusion increased to 100 μg/kg/min

(continued on next page) | Not established | C | **Solution for injection—IV:** 2.5 g/10 mL, 100 mg/10 mL | For treatment of tachycardia and hypertension that occur intraoperatively and postoperatively during surgery or emergence from anesthesia |

Continued on next page

Table 15.2 (cont.)

Injectable and Noninjectable Emergency Drugs: Dosage Information

Generic name	Brand name(s)	Maximum adult dosage (mg/kg)	Maximum child dosage	Pregnancy risk category	Content/form	Indications
		Level 2 (noncritical drugs) (cont.)				
Anti-hypertensive, antianginal, β-adrenergic blocking agent: Esmolol (cont.)		**Note:** Can be mixed with these IV solutions: 5% dextrose (D5) and water, D5 in lactated Ringer's, D5 in Ringer's, D5 and 0.45% sodium chloride, D5 and 0.9% sodium chloride, lactated Ringer's, 0.45% sodium chloride, 0.9% sodium chloride; is *not* compatible with sodium bicarbonate injection **Overdosage:** Acute toxicity, secondary to massive accidental overdosage of esmolol, has occurred due to errors in dilution; result has been hypotension, bradycardia, drowsiness and loss of consciousness; patient should be placed in a supine position and legs should be raised to improve blood supply to brain; effects have resolved within 10 min, in some cases, with administration of a vasopressor agent **Note:** Bradycardia can be treated with atropine; bronchospasm with a ß2-agonist or a theophylline derivative or both; symptomatic hypotension can be managed with IV fluids, vasopressor agents or both				

| Anti-hypertensive, antianginal, β-adrenergic blocking agent: Labetalol | Normodyne, Trandate (labetalol) | **Labetalol:** Intended for IV use in hospitalized patients

Overdosage: Acute toxicity, secondary to massive accidental overdosage of labetalol, has occurred, and result has been hypotension, bradycardia, drowsiness and loss of consciousness; patient should be placed in a supine position and legs should be raised to improve blood supply to brain; effects have resolved within 10 min, in some cases, with administration of a vasopressor agent

Note: Bradycardia can be treated with atropine; bronchospasm with a β₂-agonist or a theophylline derivative or both; symptomatic hypotension can be managed with IV fluids, vasopressor agents or both | Not established | C | **Solution for injection—IV:** 5 mg/mL in 4-, 8-, 20-, and 40-mL vials | For control of blood pressure in patients with severe hypertension |

Continued on next page

Table 15.2 (cont.)

Injectable and Noninjectable Emergency Drugs: Dosage Information

Generic name	Brand name(s)	Maximum adult dosage (mg/kg)	Maximum child dosage	Pregnancy risk category	Content/form	Indications
		Level 2 (noncritical drugs) (cont.)				
Anticholinergic, antiarrhythmic Atropine	Sal-Tropine, generic	**Injection—IM, IV, SC:** 0.5 mg (range, 0.4-0.6 mg) **As an antisialagogue before induction of anesthesia—IM:** 0.5 mg (range, 0.4-0.6 mg) **For bradyarrhythmias—IV:** 0.4-1 mg q 1-2 h, as needed; larger doses up to maximum of 2 mg may be required **Overdosage—IV, slow:** Physostigmine 1-4 mg rapidly abolishes delirium and coma caused by large doses of atropine (see Table 15.4 for adverse reactions) **Note:** Fatal dose level of atropine is not known; doses of 200 mg have been used, and doses as high as 1,000 mg have been given to adults	**Injection—IV:** 0.01-0.33 mg/kg **Overdosage—IV, slow:** Physostigmine 0.5-1 mg rapidly abolishes delirium and coma caused by large doses of atropine (see Table 15.4 for adverse reactions) **Note:** In children, doses of 10 mg or less may be fatal; with a dose as low as 0.5 mg, undesirable minimal symptoms or responses of overdosage may occur, and these increase in severity and extent with larger doses of the drug (excitement, hallucinations, delirium and coma with dose of 10 mg or more)	C	**Solution for injection—IM, IV, SC:** 0.1, 0.4, 0.5, 1 mg/mL and 0.4 mg/0.5 mL ampules	As an antisialagogue for preanesthetic medication; to restore cardiac rate and arterial pressure when vagal stimulation causes a sudden decrease in pulse rate and cardiac action; to lessen the degree of atrioventricular heart block when increased vagal tone is a major factor in conduction defect (as in some cases due to digitalis); to overcome severe bradycardia and syncope owing to hyperactive carotid sinus reflex
Respiratory stimulants	Aromatic ammonia, spirits of ammonia	**Inhalation:** Vaporole containing ammonia is crushed between the user's fingers and held beneath patient's nose, thus permitting patient to inhale the ammonia	Though rarely indicated in children, dosage and method of administration same as for adults	Not available	**Vaporoles:** 0.3 mL	Respiratory depression not induced by opioid analgesics; vasodepressor syncope

		Level 3 (advanced life-support drugs)				

Drug	Trade name	Adult dosage	Pediatric dosage	Category	Preparation	Use
Endogenous catecholamine: Epinephrine (1:10,000)	Adrenalin	**IV or endotracheally:** 0.5-1.0 mg; higher range of doses should be used and repeated at least every 5 min	**IV or endotracheally:** 0.01 mg/kg (0.1 mL/kg of the 1:10,000 solution)	C	**Solution:** 1 mg epinephrine/10 mL of solution in syringes	For patients who have suffered cardiac arrest
Anticholinergic, antiarrhythmic: Atropine	Sal-Tropine, generic	**Injection, IM, IV, SC:** 0.5 mg (range 0.4-0.6 mg) **As an antisialagogue before induction of anesthesia—IM:** 0.5 mg (range 0.4-0.6 mg) **For bradyarrhythmias—IV:** 0.4-1.0 mg q 1-2 h, as needed; larger doses up to maximum of 2 mg may be required **Overdosage—IV, slow:** Physostigmine 1-4 mg rapidly abolishes delirium and coma caused by large doses of atropine (see Table 15.4 for adverse reactions) **Note:** Fatal dose level of atropine is not known; doses of 200 mg have been used, and doses as high as 1,000 mg have been given to adults	Intravenous doses in children range from 0.01 to 0.33 mg per kg of body weight **Overdosage—IV, slow:** Physostigmine 0.5-1 mg rapidly abolishes delirium and coma caused by large doses of atropine (see Table 15.4 for adverse reactions) **Note:** In children, doses of 10 mg or less may be fatal; with a dose as low as 0.5 mg, undesirable minimal symptoms or responses of overdosage may occur, and these increase in severity and extent with larger doses of the drug (excitement, hallucinations, delirium and coma with dose of 10 mg or more)	C	**Solution for injection—IM, IV, SC:** 0.1 mg/mL, 0.4 mg/mL, 0.5 mg/mL, and 1.0 mg/mL in ampules and vials; 0.4 mg/0.5 mL in ampules	As an antisialagogue for preanesthetic medication; to restore cardiac rate and arterial pressure when vagal stimulation causes a sudden decrease in pulse rate and cardiac action; to lessen degree of atrio-ventricular heart block when increased vagal tone is a major factor in conduction defect (as in some cases due to digitalis); to overcome severe bradycardia and syncope due to hyperactive carotid sinus reflex

Continued on next page

Table 15.2 (cont.)

Injectable and Noninjectable Emergency Drugs: Dosage Information

Generic name	Brand name(s)	Maximum adult dosage (mg/kg)	Maximum child dosage	Pregnancy risk category	Content/form	Indications
Level 3 (advanced life-support drugs) (cont.)						
Antiarrhythmic: Lidocaine	Xylocaine, generic	**Injection:** Bolus of 1 mg/kg, with additional bolus injections of 0.5 mg/kg repeated q 8-10 min, if needed, to total dose of 3 mg/kg; dosage should be reduced for debilitated and/or elderly patients, commensurate with their age and physical status **Overdosage:** Signs and symptoms of an overdose are described in Table 15.4; should convulsions or signs of respiratory depression and arrest develop, airway patency and adequacy of ventilation must be ensured immediately; when convulsions persist despite ventilation with oxygen, small increments of anticonvulsants, such as diazepam, may be administered IV	**Injection:** Bolus of 1 mg/kg, with additional bolus injections of 0.5 mg/kg repeated q 8-10 min, if needed, to total dose of 3 mg/kg; dosage should be reduced for children, commensurate with their age and physical status	B	**Solution for injection:** 1%, 2%, 5% in vials and syringes	For the acute management of ventricular arrhythmias such as those occurring in relation to acute myocardial infarction; drug of choice for suppression of ventricular tachycardia and ventricular fibrillation, as well as ventricular premature complexes in critically ill patients

| Antiarrhythmic: Procainamide | Pronestyl | **For ventricular tachycardia or premature ventricular complexes—IV:** 100 mg initially, then 50 mg q 5 min until one of the following has been observed: (1) the dysrhythmia has been suppressed, (2) hypotension has ensued, (3) the QRS complex has been widened by 50% of its original width or (4) total of 1 g has been administered

Overdosage: After IV administration, transiently high plasma levels of procainamide can induce hypotension, affecting systolic pressure more than diastolic pressure, especially in hypertensive patients; such high plasma levels can also produce CNS depression, tremor and even respiratory depression; management of overdosage includes general positioning-, airway-, breathing- and circulation-supportive measures (P, A, B, C), close observation, monitoring of vital signs and, possibly, intravenous pressor agents and mechanical cardiorespiratory support | Not established | C | **Solution for injection:** 100 mg/mL in 10-mL syringes and vials; 500 mg/mL in 2-mL vials | Useful in suppressing premature ventricular complexes and recurrent ventricular tachycardia that cannot be controlled by lidocaine; rarely used to treat ventricular fibrillation because it takes so long to reach adequate blood levels even after intravenous administration; can also be used to convert supraventricular arrhythmias |

Table 15.2 (cont.)

Injectable and Noninjectable Emergency Drugs: Dosage Information

Generic name	Brand name(s)	Maximum adult dosage (mg/kg)	Maximum child dosage	Pregnancy risk category	Content/form	Indications
		Level 3 (advanced life-support drugs) (cont.)				
Antiarrhythmic agent: Bretylium tosylate	Bretylol, generic	**Injection—IM, IV:** Used clinically only for treatment of life-threatening ventricular arrhythmias under constant electrocardiographic monitoring; meant for short-term use only; patients should be kept supine during course of bretylium therapy or be closely observed for postural hypotension **For immediate management of life-threatening ventricular arrhythmias such as ventricular fibrillation or hemodynamically unstable ventricular tachycardia—IV, rapid:** 5 mg/kg; other usual cardiopulmonary resuscitative procedures, including electrical conversion, should be employed before and after injection in accordance with good medical practice; if ventricular fibrillation persists, the dosage can be increased to 10 mg/kg and repeated as necessary **Overdosage:** In the presence of life-threatening arrhythmias, underdosing with bretylium probably presents a greater risk to patients than potential overdosage	5 mg/kg; may be increased to 10 mg/kg	C	**Solution for injection:** 50 mg/mL in 10-mL vials; 1 mg/mL generic	For prophylaxis and therapy of ventricular fibrillation; for treatment of life-threatening ventricular arrhythmias (such as ventricular tachycardia) that have failed to respond to adequate doses of a first-line antiarrhythmic such as lidocaine

Antiarrhythmic: Verapamil	Calan, Iseptin, generic	**Injection—IV:** Bolus of 0.075-0.150 mg/kg (maximum 10 mg) over 1 min; peak therapeutic effects occur within 3-5 min of bolus injection **If initial response is inadequate:** Repeated doses of 0.15 mg/kg (maximum 10 mg) q 30 min after first dose **Overdosage:** Treat all verapamil overdoses as serious and maintain observation for at least 48 h under continuous hospital care	**Age 1-15 y:** Initially, 0.1-0.3 mg/kg (usual single dose 2.5 mg), not to exceed 5 mg; for repeat dose 30 min after initial dose, do not exceed 10 mg as a single dose	C	**Solution for injection:** 2.5 mg/mL in 2-mL ampules	For management of paroxysmal supraventricular tachycardia that does not require cardioversion
Alkalinyzing agent: Sodium bicarbonate	generic	1 mEq/kg initially; maximum of 50% of this dose can be given for subsequent doses, which should not be given more frequently than every 10 min	1 mEq/kg/dose	C	**Injectable solution:** 4.2%, 5%, 7.5% and 8.4% in 5-, 10-, 50- and 500-mL vials	Because of absence of proven efficacy and numerous adverse effects, for use (if at all) only after application of more definitive and better substantiated interventions: prompt defibrillation, effective chest compression, endotracheal intubation and hyperventilation with 100% oxygen, and use of such drugs as epinephrine and lidocaine (these interventions take 10 min; thereafter, sodium bicarbonate therapy, although not recommended, can be considered in specific clinical circumstances, such as documented pre-existing metabolic acidosis with or without hyperkalemia)

Continued on next page

Table 15.2 (cont.)

Injectable and Noninjectable Emergency Drugs: Dosage Information

Generic name	Brand name(s)	Maximum adult dosage (mg/kg)	Maximum child dosage (mg/kg)	Pregnancy risk category	Content/form	Indications
Level 3 (advanced life-support drugs) (cont.)						
Analgesic: Morphine sulfate	Astramorph PF, Duramorph, generic; Epimorph [CAN], Morphine Forte [CAN], Morphine Extra-Forte [CAN], Morphine H.P. [CAN]	**Injection—IM, IV, SC:** Small incremental doses of 2-5 mg q 5-30 min until desired effect is achieved **Overdosage:** Is characterized by respiratory depression with or without concomitant CNS depression; because respiratory arrest can result either through direct depression of respiratory center or as result of hypoxia, dentist's first action should be ensuring adequate respiratory exchange through provision of patent airway and institution of assisted or controlled ventilation **Note:** Naloxone, the narcotic antagonist, is a specific antidote; usually given in 0.4-mg doses; should be administered IV simultaneously with respiratory resuscitation; naloxone injection and resuscitative equipment should be immediately available for administration in case of life-threatening or intolerable side effects **Note:** Low doses of IV-administered morphine have little effect on CV stability; high doses are excitatory, resulting from sympathetic hyperactivity and increase in circulating catecholamines **Note:** CNS excitation, resulting in convulsions, can accompany high doses of morphine administered IV **Note:** Dysphoric reactions and toxic psychoses have also been reported	**Analgesic—IV, very slow:** 50-100 µg/kg	C	**Solution for injection:** 2, 4, 5, 8, 10, 15 mg/mL	To manage pain that is not responsive to nonnarcotic analgesics; for the treatment of pain and anxiety associated with acute myocardial infarction

| Calcium salt:
Calcium
chloride | generic | **Injection—IV, slow:** 2-4 mg/kg of a 10%
solution and repeated at 10-min intervals if
considered necessary

Overdosage: Too rapid administration can
lower blood pressure and produce cardiac
syncope | **Injection:** 5-7 mg/kg; first dose
should be infused slowly (no faster
than 1 mL/min) and repeated once
after 10 min, if required | C | **Solution in prefilled
syringes or ampules:**
10 mL of 10%
solution of calcium
chloride with 13.6
mEq of calcium
(1 mL = 100 mg) | Only for treatment of
acute hyperkalemia,
hypocalcemia or calcium
channel blocker toxicity |

Continued on next page

Table 15.2 (cont.)

Injectable and Noninjectable Emergency Drugs: Dosage Information

Generic name	Brand name(s)	Maximum adult dosage (mg/kg)	Maximum child dosage	Pregnancy risk category	Content/form	Indications
			Level 4 (antidotal drugs)			
Narcotic antagonist: Naloxone	Narcan ★, generic	**For reversal of respiratory depression—IV:** 0.1-0.2 mg IV q 2-3 min to desired degree of reversal (adequate ventilation and alertness without significant pain or discomfort); repeat doses may be required within 1-2 h, depending on amount, type (short- or long-acting) and time since last administration of narcotic; supplemental IM doses of naloxone have been shown to produce a longer lasting effect **Note:** Can be injected IM, IV or SC, but most rapid onset of action follows IV use; IV route is recommended in emergency situations **Note:** Larger than necessary dosage of naloxone can result in significant reversal of analgesia and increase in blood pressure; in addition, too rapid a reversal can induce nausea, vomiting, sweating and circulatory stress **Note:** Because duration of action of some narcotics can exceed that of naloxone, patient should be kept under continued observation and repeated doses of naloxone should be administered, if necessary	**For reversal of respiratory depression—IV:** Increments of 0.005 to 0.010 mg q 2- to 3-min to desired degree of reversal	B	**Solution for injection:** 0.02 mg/mL in 2-mL vials; 0.4 mg/mL in 1-, 2- and 10-mL vials; 1.0 mg/mL in 1-, 2-, 5- and 10-mL vials	For complete or partial reversal of narcotic depression (including respiratory depression) induced by opioids, including natural and synthetic narcotics, propoxyphene, methadone and the narcotic-antagonist analgesics nalbuphine, pentazocine and butorphanol; also indicated for suspected acute opioid overdosage

		Note: For partial reversal of narcotic depression after use of narcotics during surgery, smaller doses of naloxone are usually adequate; dose should be titrated according to patient's response Overdosage: In humans, no clinical experience with overdosage of naloxone				
Benzodiazepine antagonist: Flumazenil	Romazicon	For reversal of conscious sedation or in general anesthesia—IV only: Initially, 0.2 mg (2 mL) administered over 15 s; if desired level of consciousness has not been obtained after waiting an additional 45 s, further dose of 0.2 mg can be injected and repeated at 60-s intervals, where necessary, up to additional 4 doses to maximum total dose of 1 mg (10 mL); dose should be individualized according to patient's response; most patients respond to doses of 0.6-1 mg Resedation: Repeated doses can be administered at 20-min intervals, as needed Repeat treatment: No more than 1 mg (administered at 0.2 mg/min) should be administered at any one time; no more than 3 mg should be given in any 1-h period Overdosage: Large IV doses of flumazenil administered to healthy normal volunteers in absence of a benzodiazepine agonist produced no serious adverse reactions, severe signs or symptoms or clinically significant laboratory test abnormalities; reversal with an excessively high dose of flumazenil can produce anxiety, agitation, increased muscle tone, hyperesthesia and possible convulsions	Same as adult dosage	C	Solution for injection: 0.1 mg/mL in 5-mL and 10-mL multiple-use vials	For complete or partial reversal of sedative effects of benzodiazepines in cases in which general anesthesia has been induced and/or maintained with benzodiazepines or sedation has been produced with benzodiazepines for diagnostic and therapeutic procedures, and for management of an overdose of benzodiazepine

★ indicates a drug bearing the ADA Seal of Acceptance.

Table 15.3

Injectable and Noninjectable Emergency Drugs: Possible Interactions With Other Drugs

Drug taken by patient	Interaction with emergency injectable and noninjectable drugs	Dentist's action
Level 1 (basic, noncritical drugs)		
Histamine blockers: Diphenhydramine, chlorpheniramine	Histamine blockers have additive effects with alcohol and other central nervous system depressants such as sedatives, hypnotics and tranquilizers	In the case of an emergency, there is no situation in which a drug-to-drug interaction would be of concern
Bronchodilator: Albuterol	Other sympathomimetic aerosol inhalers should not be used concomitantly with albuterol so as to minimize the risk of deleterious CV events Albuterol should be administered with extreme caution to patients receiving monoamine oxidase (MAO) inhibitors or tricyclic antidepressants because the action of albuterol on the CV system can be potentiated.	See note above
Level 2 (noncritical drugs)		
Anticonvulsant: Diazepam	If combined with other psychotropic or anticonvulsant drugs—such as phenothiazines, opioids, barbiturates, monoamine oxidase inhibitors and other antidepressants—CNS and respiratory depressant actions of diazepam can be potentiated	In the case of an emergency, there is no situation in which a drug-to-drug interaction would be of concern
Analgesic: Morphine	Depressant effects of morphine are potentiated by either concomitant administration or the presence of other central nervous system depressants such as alcohol, sedatives, histamine-blockers or psychotropic drugs such as monoamine oxidase inhibitors, phenothiazines, butyrophenones and tricyclic antidepressants	See note above
Vasopressor, sympathomimetic agent: Methoxamine	The pressor effect of methoxamine can be markedly potentiated when administered in conjunction with monoamine oxidase inhibitors, tricyclic antidepressants, vasopressin or ergot alkaloids such as ergotamine, ergonovine or methylergonovine	See note above
Level 3 (advanced cardiac life support drugs)		
Injectable antiarrhythmic: Lidocaine	Lidocaine HCl should be used with caution in patients with digitalis toxicity that is accompanied by atrioventricular block; concomitant use of beta-blocking agents or cimetidine can reduce hepatic blood flow and thereby reduce lidocaine clearance	In the case of an emergency, there is no situation in which a drug-to-drug interaction would be of concern
Injectable antiarrhythmic: Procainamide	If other antiarrhythmic drugs are being administered, additive effects can occur with administration of procainamide, so a reduction in dosage may be necessary	See note above
Antiarrhythmic agent: Bretylium tosylate	The pressor effects of catecholamines, such as dopamine or norepinephrine, are enhanced by bretylium	See note above

Continued on next page

Table 15.3 (cont.)

Injectable and Noninjectable Emergency Drugs: Possible Interactions With Other Drugs

Drug taken by patient	Interaction with emergency injectable and noninjectable drugs	Dentist's action
Level 3 (advanced cardiac life support drugs) (cont.)		
Antiarrhythmic agent: Verapamil	Concomitant therapy with β-adrenergic blockers and verapamil can result in additive negative effects on heart rate, atrioventricular conduction or cardiac contractility or both Concomitant administration of verapamil with oral antihypertensive agents will usually have an additive effect on lowering blood pressure; patients receiving this combination should be monitored appropriately	In the case of an emergency, there is no situation in which a drug-to-drug interaction would be of concern
Calcium chloride: Calcium salt	Calcium increases ventricular irritability and can precipitate digitalis toxicity in those who are taking digitalis	See note above
Level 4 (antidotal drugs)		
Benzodiazepine antagonist: Flumazenil	Interaction with CNS depressants other than benzodiazepines has not been specifically studied; however, no deleterious interactions were seen when flumazenil was administered after narcotics, inhalational anesthetics, muscle relaxants and muscle relaxant antagonists administered in conjunction with sedation or anesthesia	In the case of an emergency, there is no situation in which a drug-to-drug interaction would be of concern

Table 15.4

Injectable and Noninjectable Emergency Drugs: Adverse Reactions, Precautions and Contraindications

Type of drug	Adverse reactions	Precautions/contraindications
		Level 1 (basic, critical drugs)
Epinephrine 1:1,000	**General:** Transient and minor side effects of anxiety, headache, fear and palpitations may be noted with therapeutic doses, most often in patients with hyperthyroidism	Should be protected from exposure to light; solution should not be used if it is pinkish or darker than light yellow or if it contains a precipitate
		Is preferred treatment for life-threatening allergic reactions even though it contains a sodium bisulfite, a product that in other drugs can cause allergic-type reactions, including anaphylaxis or life-threatening or less severe asthmatic episodes, in certain susceptible patients; because alternatives to using epinephrine in life-threatening situations may not be acceptable, presence of sulfite in this product should not deter dentist from administering it for treatment of serious allergic or other life-threatening situations
Histamine blockers: Diphenhydramine, chlorpheniramine	**CNS:** Sedation, dizziness, sleepiness and disturbed coordination **GI:** Epigastric distress **Resp:** Thickening of bronchial secretions	Can diminish mental alertness in children; in young children, in particular, can produce excitation
Oxygen	None	Not indicated for patients experiencing hyperventilation
Vasodilators, antianginals, antihypertensives, CV drugs: Nitroglycerin	**General:** The most frequent (2%) adverse reaction associated with administration of nitroglycerin is headache; other adverse reactions that occur in less than 1% of patients receiving nitroglycerin include tachycardia, nausea, vomiting, apprehension, restlessness, muscle twitching, retrosternal discomfort, palpitations, dizziness and abdominal pain	Should be used with caution in patients with severe hepatic or renal disease
		Excessive hypotension, especially for prolonged periods, should be avoided because of potentially deleterious effects on brain, heart, liver, and kidneys from poor perfusion and attendant risk of ischemia, thrombosis and altered function of these organs; paradoxical bradycardia and increased angina pectoris can accompany nitroglycerin-induced hypotension
		Contraindicated in patients with hypersensitivity to nitroglycerin or other organic nitrates, hypotension or uncorrected hypovolemia, increased intracranial pressure and inadequate cerebral circulation

Drug	Adverse reactions	Precautions/Notes
Bronchodilator: Albuterol	**CNS:** Tremor (< 15%), dizziness (< 5%), nervousness (< 10%) **CV:** Adverse reactions to albuterol are similar to those of other sympathomimetic amines, although incidence of some CV events is less with albuterol than with isoproterenol; palpitations (10% albuterol; 15% isoproterenol), tachycardia (10% for both), increased blood pressure (< 5% for both) **GI:** Nausea (< 15%), heartburn (< 5%)	Albuterol should be used with caution in patients with CV disorders, especially coronary insufficiency, cardiac arrhythmias and hypertension; in patients with convulsive disorders, hyperthyroidism, or diabetes mellitus and in patients who are unusually responsive to sympathomimetic amines Contraindicated in patients with a history of hypersensitivity to any of its components As with other inhaled β-adrenergic agonists, albuterol inhalation aerosol can produce paradoxical bronchospasm that can be life-threatening; fatalities have been reported in association with excessive administration of inhaled sympathomimetic drugs; though the precise cause of death is not known, cardiac arrest following the development of severe acute asthmatic crisis and subsequent hypoxia is suspected
Antihypoglycemics (orange juice, nondiet soft drinks)	None of significance to dentistry	These and other oral medications should not be administered to patients who are unconscious or unable to swallow Choking and aspiration can occur in such situations

Level 2 (noncritical drugs)

Drug	Adverse reactions	Precautions/Notes
Anticonvulsant: Diazepam	**General:** Drowsiness, fatigue, ataxia **CV:** bradycardia, cardiovascular collapse, hypertension **CNS:** Confusion, depression, slurred speech, syncope **Hema:** Venous thrombosis, phlebitis at site of injection **Resp:** depressed respiration, apnea	Although seizures can be brought under control promptly, a significant proportion of patients experience a return of seizure activity, presumably due to short-lived effect of IV diazepam; clinician should be prepared to re-administer drug When used IV, solution should be injected slowly (1 min for each mL [5 mg] given); small veins, such as those on dorsum of hand or wrist should be avoided, and extreme care should be taken to avoid intra-arterial or extravascular administration
Analgesic: Morphine sulfate	**General:** Most frequently observed adverse reactions include constipation, lightheadedness, dizziness, sedation, nausea, vomiting, sweating, dysphoria and euphoria **Resp:** Most serious side effect is respiratory depression; because of delay in maximum CNS effect with IV-administered morphine (up to 30 min), rapid administration can result in overdosing	Should be administered with extreme caution in aged or debilitated patients, in patients with increased intracranial or intraocular pressure and in patients with head injury Care must be taken with patients who have decreased respiratory reserve (emphysema, severe obesity, kyphoscoliosis) Contraindicated for patients whose medical conditions would preclude IV administration of opioids: allergy to morphine or other opiates, acute bronchial asthma or upper airway obstruction Should be limited to use by those familiar with management of respiratory depression; facilities where morphine sulfate is administered must be equipped with resuscitative equipment, oxygen, injectable naxolone and other resuscitative drugs

Continued on next page

Table 15.4 (cont.)
Injectable and Noninjectable Emergency Drugs: Adverse Reactions, Precautions and Contraindications

Type of drug	Adverse reactions	Precautions/contraindications
		Level 2 (noncritical drugs) (cont.)
Vasopressor, sympathomimetic agent: Methoxamine	**General:** Contains potassium bisulfite, a bisulfite that can cause allergic-type reactions, including anaphylactic symptoms and life-threatening or less severe asthmatic episodes, in certain susceptible people; sulfite sensitivity is seen more frequently in asthmatic than in nonasthmatic patients **CV:** Excessive blood pressure elevations, particularly with high dosage, ventricular ectopic beats **CNS:** Headache (often severe), anxiety **GI:** Nausea, vomiting (often projectile) **Integ:** Sweating, pilomotor response	Like other vasopressor agents, should be used with caution in patients with hyperthyroidism, bradycardia, partial heart block, myocardial disease or severe arteriosclerosis; caution should be exercised to avoid overdosage, which can cause undesirable high blood pressure and/or bradycardia; bradycardia can be abolished with atropine Contraindicated in patients who have severe hypertension or who are hypersensitive to methoxamine Administration of methoxamine to patients receiving monoamine oxidase inhibitors, tricyclic antidepressants or oxytocic agents (such as vasopressin or certain ergot alkaloids) can result in potentiation of pressor effect
Antihypoglycemic: Glucagon	**GI:** occasional nausea and vomiting, which can also occur with hypoglycemia	Helpful in treating hypoglycemia only if liver glycogen is available; is of little or no help for people who are in a state of starvation or for patients with adrenal insufficiency or chronic hypoglycemia; 50% dextrose should be considered for management of hypoglycemia in these situations Should be administered cautiously to patients with a history suggestive of insulinoma and/or pheochromocytoma; IV administration of glucagon will produce initial increase in blood glucose, but in patients with insulinoma, glucagon's ability to cause an insulin release can subsequently produce hypoglycemia; patient who is developing symptoms of hypoglycemia after a dose of glucagon should be given glucose orally, IV or by lavage, whichever is most appropriate Stimulates release of catecholamines, so should be used with caution in patients with pheochromocytoma because it could cause tumor to release catecholamines and thus produce sudden and marked increase in blood pressure Contraindicated in patients with known sensitivity to it or in patients with pheochromocytoma

Category and drug	Adverse reactions	Precautions/contraindications
Anti-inflammatory adrenal corticosteroid: Hydrocortisone sodium succinate	Adverse reactions are extremely rare when adrenal corticosteroids are used in acute emergency situations; most significant adverse reactions to administration of adrenal corticosteroids are observed after use in long-term treatment	For patients receiving corticosteroid therapy who are subjected to unusual stress, increased dosage of rapidly acting corticosteroids before, during and after unusual stressful situation is indicated
Antihypertensive, antianginal, β-adrenergic blocking agents: Esmolol, labetalol	**CV:** Most important adverse reaction is hypotension; symptomatic hypotension (dizziness, diaphoresis) occurs in 12% of patients receiving esmolol; asymptomatic hypotension occurs in 25% of patients; symptomatic postural hypotension occurs in 58% of patients receiving IV labetalol permitted to assume an erect posture within 3 h of administration, with increased sweating in 4%; peripheral ischemia occurs in 1% of patients, whereas less than 1% of patients experience pallor, flushing, bradycardia (heart rate < 50 beats per minute), chest pain, syncope, pulmonary edema or heart block **CNS:** Dizziness and somnolence occur in 3% of patients on esmolol and 9% with labetalol; confusion, headache and agitation in about 2% and fatigue in 1% of patients on esmolol **GI:** Nausea was reported in 7% of patients on esmolol, with vomiting in 1%; of patients on labetalol, 13% reported nausea and 4% reported vomiting; virtually all adverse reactions to esmolol and labetalol are dose-related **Resp:** Bronchospasm, wheezing, dyspnea, nasal congestion, rhonchi and rales have been reported in less than 1% of patients	**Esmolol:** Infusion concentrations of 20 mg/mL of esmolol are associated with more serious venous irritation, including thrombophlebitis, than concentrations of 10 mg/mL; extravasation of 20 mg/mL can lead to a serious local reaction and possible skin necrosis; care should be taken when administering esmolol intravenously because sloughing of the skin and necrosis have been reported in association with infiltration and extravasation of intravenous infusions **Esmolol:** 20-50% of patients treated with esmolol have experienced hypotension, generally defined as systolic pressure less than 90 mmHg and/or diastolic pressure less than 50 mmHg; about 12% of patients have been symptomatic (diaphoresis or dizziness) **Labetalol:** Symptomatic postural hypotension was observed in 58% of patients allowed to assume an upright position within 3 h of receiving IV injection **Labetalol and esmolol:** Increased risk of severe anaphylactic reaction in susceptible patients, who may prove unresponsive to doses of epinephrine usually used to treat allergic reactions **Labetalol and esmolol:** Are both contraindicated in patients with sinus bradycardia, heart block greater than first degree, cardiogenic shock or overt heart failure; labetalol also contraindicated in patients with bronchial asthma Sympathetic stimulation is necessary for supporting circulatory function in congestive heart failure, and β blockade with either esmolol or labetalol carries potential hazard of further depressing myocardial contractility and precipitating more severe failure; continued depression of myocardium with β-blocking agents over period of time can, in some cases, lead to cardiac failure Patients with bronchospastic diseases should, in general, not receive β-blockers
Anticholinergic, antiarrhythmic agent: Atropine	**General:** Adverse effects most often are a result of excessive dosage: palpitation, dilated pupils, difficulty in swallowing, hot, dry skin, thirst, dizziness, restlessness, tremor, fatigue and ataxia; toxic doses can lead to marked palpitation, restlessness and excitement, hallucinations, delirium and coma **CV:** Depression and circulatory collapse occur with severe intoxication; blood pressure declines and death due to respiratory failure can ensue as consequence of paralysis and coma	Should be administered with caution in all patients aged > 40 y; conventional systemic doses can precipitate acute glaucoma in susceptible patients, convert partial organic pyloric stenosis into complete urinary retention in patients with prostatic hypertrophy or cause inspiration of bronchial secretions and formation of dangerous viscid plugs in patients with chronic lung disease Except in doses ordinarily used for preanesthetic medication, is generally contraindicated for patients with glaucoma, pyloric stenosis or prostatic hypertrophy Is a highly potent drug, and due care is essential to avoid overdosage, especially with IV administration; children are more susceptible than adults to toxic effects of anticholinergic agents

Continued on next page

Table 15.4 (cont.)

Injectable and Noninjectable Emergency Drugs: Adverse Reactions, Precautions and Contraindications

Type of drug	Adverse reactions	Precautions/contraindications
Level 2 (noncritical drugs) (cont.)		
Respiratory stimulant: Aromatic ammonia, spirits of ammonia	**Resp:** May induce brochospasm in asthmatics and others with chronic lung disease	Contraindicated in patients with chronic obstructive pulmonary disease or asthma because it can precipitate bronchospasm resulting from its irritating effects on the mucous membranes of the upper respiratory tract
Level 3 (advanced cardiac life support drugs)		
Endogenous catecholamine: Epinephrine (1:10,000)	None that would indicate against use	Should not be mixed in same infusion bag with alkaline solutions such as sodium bicarbonate because solutions will increase rate of epinephrine's auto-oxidation; this is not of clinical significance when epinephrine is administered by IV bolus; epinephrine's positive inotropic and chronotropic effects can precipitate or exacerbate myocardial ischemia; doses in excess of 20 µg/min or 0.3 mg/kg/min frequently produce hypertension in patients who are not receiving CPR
May induce or exacerbate ventricular ectopy, especially in patients who are receiving digitalis
Anticholinergic, antiarrhythmic agent: Atropine	**General:** Adverse effects most often are a result of excessive dosage: palpitation, dilated pupils, difficulty in swallowing, hot, dry skin, thirst, dizziness, restlessness, tremor, fatigue and ataxia; toxic doses can lead to marked palpitation, restlessness and excitement, hallucinations, delirium and coma

CV: Depression and circulatory collapse occur with severe intoxication; blood pressure declines and death due to respiratory failure can ensue as consequence of paralysis and coma | Should be administered with caution in all patients aged > 40 y; conventional systemic doses can precipitate acute glaucoma in susceptible patients, convert partial organic pyloric stenosis into complete urinary retention in patients with prostatic hypertrophy or cause inspiration of bronchial secretions and formation of dangerous viscid plugs in patients with chronic lung disease
Except in doses ordinarily used for preanesthetic medication, is generally contraindicated for patients with glaucoma, pyloric stenosis or prostatic hypertrophy
Is a highly potent drug, and due care is essential to avoid overdosage, especially with IV administration; children are more susceptible than adults to toxic effects of anticholinergic agents |

Name	Adverse effects	Precautions/contraindications
Injectable antiarrhythmic agent: Lidocaine	**General:** Adverse reactions similar to those of other amide local anesthetic agents; reactions usually dose-related, resulting from high plasma levels caused by excessive dosage, rapid absorption or inadvertent intravascular injection, or can result from patient's hypersensitivity, idiosyncrasy or diminished tolerance **CV:** Usually depressant: bradycardia, hypotension and CV collapse, which can lead to cardiac arrest; allergic reactions to amide anesthetics are extremely rare **CNS:** Reactions most common when lidocaine is used for ventricular arrhythmias; reactions can be either excitatory or depressant or both: lightheadedness; nervousness; apprehension; euphoria; confusion; dizziness; drowsiness; tinnitus; blurred or double vision; vomiting; sensations of heat, cold, or numbness; twitching; tremors; convulsions; unconsciousness; respiratory depression and arrest	Caution should be employed when using lidocaine HCl in patients with severe liver or kidney disease as accumulation of the drug or its metabolites can occur Should be used with caution in the treatment of patients with hypovolemia, severe congestive heart failure, shock and all forms of heart block Is contraindicated in patients with known history of hypersensitivity to amide-type local anesthetics To manage possible adverse reactions, resuscitative equipment, oxygen and other resuscitative drugs should be immediately available when lidocaine is used
Injectable antiarrhythmic agent: Procainamide	**CV:** Hypotension and serious cardiac rhythm disturbances such as ventricular asystole or fibrillation more common after IV administration **CNS:** Dizziness or giddiness, weakness, mental depression and psychosis with hallucinations	Patients should be closely observed for possible hypersensitivity reactions immediately after start of procainamide therapy, especially if sensitivity to procaine or local anesthetic is suspected Contraindicated in patients with complete heart block or to patients with allergy to procaine or other ester-type local anesthetics Contains sodium metabisulfite, a sulfite that can cause allergic-type reactions, including anaphylactic symptoms and life-threatening or less severe asthmatic episodes, in certain susceptible people; sulfite sensitivity is seen more frequently in asthmatic patients than in those without asthma

Continued on next page

Table 15.4 (cont.)

Injectable and Noninjectable Emergency Drugs: Adverse Reactions, Precautions and Contraindications

Type of drug	Adverse reactions	Precautions/contraindications
		Level 3 (advanced cardiac life support drugs) (cont.)
Antiarrhythmic agent: Bretylium tosylate	**CV:** Hypotension and postural hypotension **GI:** Nausea and vomiting (in about 3% of patients primarily after rapid IV administration)	Should be diluted for IV use; one vial or ampule of bretylium should be diluted with minimum of 50 mL of dextrose 5% injection or sodium chloride injection before IV use; rapid IV administration can cause severe nausea and vomiting; therefore, diluted solution should be administered over period > 8 min; however, when treating existing ventricular fibrillation, bretylium tosylate should be administered as rapidly as possible and can be given without being diluted No contraindications to the use of bretylium tosylate in patients with ventricular fibrillation or life-threatening refractory ventricular arrhythmias Administration regularly results in postural hypotension, subjectively recognized by dizziness, lightheadedness, vertigo or faintness; some degree of hypotension is present in about 50% of patients when supine; due to initial release of norepinephrine from adrenergic postganglionic nerve terminals by bretylium, transient hypertension or increased frequency of ventricular premature complexes and other arrhythmias may occur in some patients
Antiarrhythmic agent: Verapamil	**CV:** Angina pectoris, atrioventricular dissociation, chest pain, claudication, myocardial infarction, palpitation, purpura and syncope **CNS:** Cerebrovascular accident, confusion, equilibrium disorders, insomnia, muscle cramps, paresthesia, psychotic symptoms, shakiness and somnolence **GI:** Diarrhea, dry mouth, GI distress, gingival hyperplasia	Because verapamil is highly metabolized by the liver, should be administered cautiously to patients with impaired hepatic function Contraindicated in patients with severe left ventricular dysfunction, hypotension (systolic pressure less than 90 mmHg or cardiogenic shock, "sick sinus syndrome," second- or third-degree atrioventricular block, patients with atrial flutter or atrial fibrillation and an accessory bypass tract (for example, Wolff-Parkinson-White and Lown-Ganong-Levine syndromes) and patients with known hypersensitivity to verapamil Use should be avoided in patients with severe left ventricular dysfunction or moderate-to-severe symptoms of cardiac failure and in patients with any degree of ventricular dysfunction if they are receiving a β-adrenergic blocker; occasionally can produce decrease in blood pressure below normal levels, which can result in dizziness or symptomatic hypotension **Overdosage:** Treat all verapamil overdoses as serious and maintain observation for at least 48 h under continuous hospital care

Drug		
Alkalinyzing agent: Sodium bicarbonate	**General:** Overly aggressive use can result in metabolic alkalosis (associated with muscular twitching, irritability and tetany) and hypernatremia	None as used in cardiac arrest
Calcium salt: Calcium chloride	**General:** Rapid injection may cause complaints of tingling sensations, calcium taste, sense of oppression or "heat wave"	If heart is beating, rapid administration of calcium can slow cardiac rate Can produce vasospasm in coronary and cerebral arteries
Level 4 (antidotal drugs)		
Narcotic antagonist: Naloxone	**General:** Abrupt reversal of narcotic depression can result in nausea, vomiting, sweating, tachycardia, increased blood pressure and tremulousness; administration of larger-than-necessary doses of naloxone can result in significant reversal of analgesia and in excitement in postsurgical patients **CV:** Hypotension, hypertension, ventricular tachycardia and fibrillation and pulmonary edema	In addition to naloxone, other resuscitative measures (such as maintenance of a patent airway, artificial ventilation, cardiac massage and vasopressor agents) should be available and employed, when needed, to counteract acute narcotic poisoning Hypotension, hypertension, ventricular tachycardia and fibrillation, and pulmonary edema have been reported in postoperative patients, most of whom had preexisting CV disorders or received drugs that may have similar adverse CV effects; therefore, naloxone should be used with caution in patients with preexisting cardiac disease or patients who have received potentially cardiotoxic drugs Contraindicated in patients with known hypersensitivity Should be administered cautiously to patients who are known to be or suspected to be physically dependent on opioids; in such cases, abrupt and complete reversal of narcotic effects can precipitate acute abstinence syndrome; after satisfactory response to naloxone, patient should be kept under continued observation and repeat doses should be administered, as needed, because duration of action of some narcotics can exceed that of naloxone; naloxone is not effective against respiratory depression caused by use of nonopioid drugs

Continued on next page

Table 15.4 (cont.)

Injectable and Noninjectable Emergency Drugs: Adverse Reactions, Precautions and Contraindications

Type of drug	Adverse reactions	Precautions/contraindications
		Level 4 (antidotal drugs) (cont.)
Benzodiazepine antagonist: Flumazenil	**CNS:** Serious adverse reactions have occurred in all clinical settings, with convulsions most commonly reported; has been associated with onset of convulsions in patients who are relying on benzodiazepine effects to control seizures, are physically dependent on benzodiazepines or who have ingested large doses of other drugs	**Use in resedation:** Improves alertness of patients recovering from procedure involving sedation or anesthesia with benzodiazepines, but should not be substituted for adequate period of postprocedure monitoring; availability of flumazenil does not reduce risks associated with use of large doses of benzodiazepines for sedation; patients should be monitored for resedation, respiratory depression or other persistent or recurrent agonist effects for adequate period after administration; resedation is least likely in cases in which flumazenil is administered to reverse low dose of short-acting benzodiazepine (< 10 mg midazolam) and is most likely in cases in which a large single or cumulative dose of a benzodiazepine has been given in the course of a long procedure along with neuromuscular-blocking agents and multiple anesthetic agents
		Use in ambulatory patients: Effects can wear off before a long-acting benzodiazepine is completely cleared from body; in general, if a patient shows no signs of sedation within 2 h after 1-mg dose of flumazenil, serious resedation at a later time is unlikely; adequate period of observation must be provided for any patient in whom either a long-acting benzodiazepine (such as diazepam) or large doses of a short-acting benzodiazepine (such as > 10 mg midazolam) have been used
		Contraindicated in patients with known hypersensitivity to flumazenil or to benzodiazepines, patients who have been given benzodiazepines for control of a potentially life-threatening condition (such as control of intracranial pressure or status epilepticus) and patients who show signs of serious cyclic antidepressant overdose
		Has been associated with seizures, most frequently in patients who have been receiving benzodiazepines for long-term sedation or in overdose cases in patients who are showing signs of a serious cyclic antidepressant overdose; practitioners should individualize dosage and be prepared to manage seizures; patients receiving flumazenil to reverse benzodiazepine effects should be monitored for resedation, respiratory depression or other residual effects for up to 120 min based on dose and duration of effect of benzodiazepine used

Pharmacology

Injectable Drugs

Level 1 (Basic, Critical Drugs)

Epinephrine (1:1,000): Epinephrine, a sympathomimetic drug, acts on both α– and β– receptors. It is the most potent α– receptor agonist available. Clinical actions of benefit during anaphylaxis include increased systemic vascular resistance, increased arterial blood pressure, increased coronary and cerebral blood flow and bronchodilation.

Histamine blockers (diphenhydramine and chlorpheniramine): Histamine blockers appear to compete with histamine for cell-receptor sites on effector cells. These drugs also have anticholinergic and sedative properties.

Level 2 (Noncritical Drugs)

Anticonvulsant (diazepam): Diazepam, an anticonvulsant that appears to act on parts of the limbic system, thalamus and hypothalamus, induces calming effects.

Analgesic (morphine sulfate): Morphine exerts its primary effects on the CNS and organs containing smooth muscle. Pharmacological effects include analgesia, drowsiness, euphoria (mood alteration), reduction in body temperature (at low doses), dose-related respiratory depression, interference with adrenocortical response to stress (at high doses) and reduction of peripheral resistance with little or no effect on the cardiac index.

Vasopressor (methoxamine): Methoxamine is an α-receptor stimulant that produces a prompt and prolonged rise in blood pressure after parenteral administration. Methoxamine differs from most other sympathomimetic amines by having a predominantly peripheral action and lacking inotropic and chronotropic effects. Methoxamine also has less arrhythmogenic potential than other sympathomimetic amines and rarely causes ventricular tachycardia, fibrillation or increased sinoatrial rate. A decrease in heart rate may occasionally be noted as the blood pressure increases. This is thought to be caused by a carotid sinus reflex. Methoxamine's pressor action appears to be due to peripheral vasoconstriction rather than to a centrally mediated effect. Methoxamine also increases venous pressure.

Antihypoglycemic (glucagon, dextrose 50%): Glucagon, which causes an increase in blood glucose concentration, is used to treat hypoglycemia. It is effective in small doses, and no evidence of toxicity has been reported with its use. Glucagon acts only on liver glycogen by converting it to glucose. Intravenous administration of 50% dextrose also can be used to manage hypoglycemia.

Anti-inflammatory adrenal corticosteroid (hydrocortisone sodium succinate): Hydrocortisone sodium succinate has the same metabolic and anti-inflammatory actions as hydrocortisone. After intravenous administration of hydrocortisone sodium succinate, demonstrable effects are evident within 1 h and persist for a variable period. The preparation is also rapidly absorbed after IM administration.

Antihypertensive, antianginal, β-adrenergic blocking agents (esmolol, labetalol): Esmolol is a β-1-selective (cardioselective) adrenergic receptor blocking agent with rapid onset, a very short duration of action and no significant membrane-stabilizing or intrinsic sympathomimetic (partial agonist) activities at therapeutic doses. Esmolol inhibits β-1-receptors located chiefly in cardiac muscle. At higher doses it can inhibit β-2 receptors located chiefly in the bronchial and vascular musculature. Clinical actions include a decrease in heart rate, increase in sinus cycle length, prolongation of sinus node recovery time, prolongation of the A-H interval during normal sinus rhythm and during atrial pacing and an increase in the antegrade Wenckebach cycle length.

Labetalol combines both selective competitive α-1-adrenergic blocking and nonselective competitive β-adrenergic blocking activity. Blood pressure is lowered more when the patient is in the standing rather than in the supine position, and symptoms of postural hypotension can occur. During intravenous dosing, the patient should not be permitted to move to an erect position unmonitored until ability to do so has been established. Labetalol is metabolized primarily through conjugation to glucuronide metabolites.

Anticholinergic, antiarrhythmic (atropine): Though commonly classified as an anticholinergic drug, atropine is more precisely an antimuscarinic agent. Atropine-induced parasympathetic inhibition can be preceded by a transient phase of stimulation. This is most notable in the heart where small doses often first slow the rate before the more characteristic tachycardia develops due to inhibition of vagal control. Compared with scopolamine, atropine's actions on the heart, intestine and bronchial smooth muscle are more potent and longer-lasting. Also unlike scopolamine, atropine, in clinical doses, does not depress the central nervous system, but may stimulate the medulla and higher cerebral centers.

Adequate doses of atropine abolish various types of reflex vagal cardiac slowing, or asystole. It also prevents or eliminates bradycardia, or asystole produced by injection of choline esters, anticholinesterase agents or other parasympathomimetic drugs, and cardiac arrest produced by vagal stimulation. Atropine can also lessen the degree of partial heart block when vagal activity is an etiologic factor.

Systemic doses can slightly raise systolic and diastolic pressures and can produce significant postural hypotension. Such doses also slightly increase cardiac output and decrease central venous pressure. Occasionally, therapeutic doses dilate cutaneous blood vessels, particularly in the blush area, producing atropine flush, and can cause atropine fever owing to suppression of sweat gland activity in infants and small children.

Atropine disappears from the blood rapidly after administration and is metabolized primarily by enzymatic hydrolysis in the liver.

Level 3 (Advanced Cardiac Life-Support Drugs)
Endogenous catecholamine (epinephrine [1:10,000]): Epinephrine is an endogenous catecholamine with both α- and β-adrenergic activity. Clinical actions of benefit during cardiac arrest include increased systemic vascular resistance, increased arterial blood pressure, increased heart rate, increased coronary and cerebral blood flow, increased myocardial contraction and increased myocardial oxygen requirements and increased automaticity.

Anticholinergic, antiarrhythmic (atropine): See description above.

Antiarrhythmic (lidocaine): Lidocaine suppresses ventricular arrhythmias primarily by decreasing automaticity, by reducing the slope of Phase 4 diastolic depolarization. Its local anesthetic properties also may help to depress ventricular ectopy after acute myocardial infarction. During acute myocardial ischemia, the threshold for the induction of ventricular fibrillation is reduced. Some studies have shown that lidocaine elevates the fibrillation threshold; therefore, elevation of the fibrillation threshold correlates closely with blood levels of lidocaine.

Lidocaine usually does not affect myocardial contractility, arterial blood pressure, atrial arrhythmogenesis or intraventricular conduction. It can, on occasion, facilitate atrioventricular conduction.

Antiarrhythmic (procainamide): Procainamide effectively suppresses ventricular ectopy and may be effective when lidocaine has not achieved suppression of life-threatening ventricular arrhythmias. Procainamide suppresses Phase 4 diastolic depolarization reducing the automaticity of ectopic pacemakers. Procainamide also slows intraventricular conduction.

Antiarrhythmic (bretylium tosylate): Bretylium is a quaternary ammonium compound with both adrenergic and direct myocardial effects. Initially, bretylium releases norepinephrine from adrenergic nerve endings in direct relation to its concentration at the adrenergic terminal. These sympath-omimetic effects, which persist for approximately 20 min, consist of transient hypertension, tachycardia and, in some patients, increases in cardiac output. Subsequently, inhibition of norepinephrine release from peripheral adrenergic terminals results in adrenergic blockade, which generally begins 15 to 20 min after injection and peaks 45 to 60 min later. During this time, clinically significant hypotension may develop, especially with changes in position. In addition, as bretylium blocks the uptake of norepinephrine into adrenergic nerve terminals, it potentiates the actions of exogenous catecholamines.

Bretylium elevates the ventricular fibrillation threshold; it also increases the action potential duration and effective refractory period without changes in the heart rate. Bretylium does not suppress Phase 4 depolarization or the spontaneous firing of Purkinje's fibers. The restoration of injured myocardial cell electrophysiology toward normal, as well as the increase of the action potential duration and effective refractory period without changing their ratio to each other, may be important factors in suppressing the reentry of aberrant impulses and decreasing induced dispersion of local excitable states.

Antiarrhythmic (verapamil): Verapamil is a calcium ion influx inhibitor (slow-channel blocker or calcium-ion inhibitor) that exerts its pharmacological effects by modulating the influx of ionic calcium across the cell membrane of the arterial smooth muscle as well as in conductile and contractile myocardial cells.

Alkalinyzing agent (sodium bicarbonate): Intravenous sodium bicarbonate therapy increases plasma bicarbonate, buffers excess hydrogen ion concentration, raises blood pH and reverses the clinical manifestations of acidosis. Administration of sodium bicarbonate does not facilitate ventricular defibrillation or survival in patients who have had a cardiac arrest.

Calcium salt (calcium chloride): Calcium ions increase the force of myocardial contraction. Calcium's positive inotropic effects are modulated by its action on systemic vascular resistance. Calcium can either increase or decrease systemic vascular resistance.

Level 4 (Antidotal Drugs)

Narcotic antagonist (naloxone): Naloxone prevents or reverses the effects of opioids, including respiratory depression, sedation and hypotension. It can also reverse the psychotomimetic and dysphoric effects of agonist-antagonists such as pentazocine.

As a "pure" narcotic antagonist, naloxone does not produce respiratory depression, psychotomimetic effects or pupillary constriction. In the absence of narcotics or agonistic effects of other narcotic antagonists, naloxone exhibits essentially no pharmacological activity.

Naloxone is a competitive antagonist for opioid receptor sites. The onset of action after IV administration is apparent within 2 min, with an only slightly slower onset after subcutaneous or IM administration. Duration depends on the route of administration; IM administration produces a more prolonged effect than IV administration. The need for repeated doses of naloxone depends on the dose, route of administration and the type of narcotic being antagonized.

Naloxone is rapidly distributed in the body and is metabolized in the liver.

Benzodiazepine antagonist (flumazenil): Flumazenil, which antagonizes the actions of benzodiazepines on the central nervous system, competitively inhibits the activity at the benzodiazepine recognition site on the GABA/benzodiazepine receptor complex. Flumazenil has little or no agonist activity in man. Flumazenil does not antagonize the central nervous system effects of drugs effecting GABA-ergic neurons by means other than the benzodiazepine receptor (that is, ethanol, barbiturates or general anesthetics) and does not reverse the effects of opioids.

Flumazenil antagonizes sedation, impairment of recall and psychomotor impairment produced by benzodiazepines in healthy human volunteers. The duration and degree of reversal of benzodiazepine effects are related to the dose and plasma concentration of flumazenil as well as that of the sedating benzodiazepine. Onset of reversal is usually evident within 1 to 2 min after the injection is completed. An 80% response is reached within 3 min, with peak effect noted at 6 to 10 min.

Noninjectable Drugs

Level 1 (Basic, Critical Drugs)

Vasodilators (nitroglycerin): The primary action of the vasodilator nitroglycerin is to relax vascular smooth muscle. Although venous effects predominate, nitroglycerin produces, in a dose-related manner, dilation of both venous and arterial beds. It decreases venous return to the heart and reduces systemic vascular resistance and arterial pressure. These effects lead to a decrease in myocardial oxygen consumption, resulting in a more favorable supply-demand ratio and the cessation of anginal discomfort.

Bronchodilator (albuterol): Compared with isoproterenol, albuterol has a preferential effect on β-2-adrenergic receptors. β-2-adrenergic receptors are the predominant receptors in bronchial smooth muscle. Recent data indicate that β-adrenergic receptors also exist in the human heart in a concentration from approximately 10 to 50%. The action of albuterol is attributable, at least in part, to stimulation through β-adrenergic receptors of ATP to cyclic-AMP. Increased cyclic-AMP levels are associated with bronchial smooth muscle relaxation and the inhibition of the release of mediators of immediate hypersensitivity from cells, especially mast cells.

Albuterol has a greater effect on the respiratory tract, in the form of bronchial smooth muscle relaxation, while producing fewer CV side effects than most bronchodilators at comparable doses. However, in some patients, albuterol, like other bronchodilators, can produce significant CV effects, such as increased pulse rate, blood pressure, symptoms such as palpitation and tremor, and/or electrocardiographic changes.

Antihypoglycemics (orange juice, regular [not diet] soft drinks): Antihypoglycemics are rapidly absorbed sources of glucose for the management of hypoglycemia.

Level 2 (Noncritical Drugs)

Respiratory stimulant (aromatic ammonia, spirits of ammonia): Ammonia, which is a noxious-smelling vapor, acts by irritating the mucous membrane of the upper respiratory tract, thereby stimulating the respiratory and vasomotor centers of the medulla. This, in turn, increases respiration and blood pressure.

Suggested Readings

Fast TB, Martin MD, Ellis TM. Emergency preparedness: a survey of dental practitioners. JADA 1986;112:499-501.

Malamed SF. Managing medical emergencies. JADA 1993;124:40-53.

Office anesthesia evaluation manual. 4th ed. Rosemont, Ill.: American Association of Oral and Maxillofacial Surgeons; 1991.

Chapter 16.

Managing Medical Emergencies in the Dental Office

Stanley F. Malamed, D.D.S.

Medical emergencies can and do occur in the dental office. Table 16.1 presents data obtained from dentists in two independent surveys, in which a total of 4,309 dentists reported 30,608 emergency situations having arisen in their practices during a 10-year period. The reported emergencies spanned a wide array, from usually benign but pressing problems such as syncope to catastrophic events such as cardiac arrest.

Given that medical emergencies do occur in the practice of dentistry, it is important for all members of the dental office staff to be able to rapidly recognize and to efficiently manage such potential problems. Taking the following measures should help dental staff members prepare for managing emergency situations:

- take American Heart Association or American Red Cross training in basic life support at the health care provider level;
- develop an in-office emergency response team that participates in regular simulated emergency drills;
- keep well informed about the availability of outside emergency assistance, such as that available by dialing 9-1-1;
- have emergency drugs and equipment available in the dental office.

Unfortunately, when emergencies occur, it is not always possible to immediately determine the precise nature of the problem. For example, a patient may report that he or she is having difficulty breathing, not suffering

from an asthmatic attack or hyperventilation, or the initial complaint may be of a "tightness in my chest," not "I am suffering an anginal attack" or a myocardial infarction.

In the following discussion, the recognition and management of medical emergencies is based on clinical signs and symptoms that are commonly presented. Six categories are noted, including

- unconsciousness;
- altered consciousness;
- convulsions;
- respiratory distress;
- drug-related emergencies (allergy and overdose);
- chest pain.

Remember P,A,B,C,D in Emergencies

To facilitate recall under times of duress, management of medical emergencies should be based on a concept of simplicity.

The following five steps are to be followed, in sequence, for all emergency situations:

- P (position),
- A (airway),
- B (breathing),
- C (circulation),
- D (definitive care).

P,A,B,C, are the steps of basic life support and are used to ensure the adequate delivery of blood containing oxygen to the brain. Once this is completed, then D—definitive care—can be implemented. This involves diagnosing

Table 16.1

A 10-Year Incidence of Emergency Situations Reported by Private Practice Dentists*

Type of emergency	Number of situations reported
Syncope	15,407
Mild allergic reaction	2,583
Angina pectoris	2,552
Postural hypotension	2,475
Seizures	1,595
Asthmatic attack (bronchospasm)	1,392
Hyperventilation	1,326
"Epinephrine reaction"	913
Insulin shock (hypoglycemia)	890
Cardiac arrest	331
Anaphylactic reaction	304
Myocardial infarction	289
Local anesthetic overdose	204
Acute pulmonary edema (heart failure)	141
Diabetic coma	109
Cerebrovascular accident	68
Adrenal insufficiency	25
Thyroid storm	4
TOTAL	30,608

* Information taken from Fast TB, Martin MD, Ellis TM. Emergency preparedness: a survey of dental practitioners. JADA 1986;112:499-501; and Malamed SF. Managing medical emergencies. JADA 1993;124:40-53.

the problem and, if possible, administering appropriate drug therapy (see Chapter 15) or seeking assistance in managing the problem.

Remembering P,A,B,C,D can save a life. The following explanations describe in more depth each step of the basic life support sequence. This information provides direction for the dentist who encounters a medical emergency in the office, whether the victim (be it a patient or staff member) is conscious or unconscious.

P: Position the Patient

Unconscious Patient

Since the most common cause of unconsciousness is a drop in blood pressure (hypotension), the supine position with feet elevated 10 to 15 degrees is recommended (at least initially) for all unconscious patients. This position ensures an increased return of blood to the heart and improved delivery of blood to the brain.

Conscious Patient

In a conscious patient suffering a medical emergency, the heart is still functioning at least adequately; thus, positioning of the conscious person during a medical emergency is based solely on patient comfort. Asthmatics and patients complaining of chest pain will usually be more comfortable if permitted to sit upright.

A: Airway

Unconscious Patient

Performing a head tilt–chin lift maneuver (one hand on the patient's forehead, the other hand on the tip of the patient's chin, lifting the chin upwards while tilting the head upwards) is necessary because in 80% of unconscious patients, the airway becomes totally obstructed by the tongue as its muscles relax and it falls into the pharynx.

Conscious Patient

In the conscious patient who can speak, airway management is unnecessary.

B: Breathing

Unconscious Patient

Assessment of ventilatory adequacy is necessary, using the "look, listen and feel" technique. If spontaneous ventilation is absent, rescue breathing must be started.

Conscious Patient

In the conscious patient who can speak, ventilatory management is unnecessary.

C: Circulation

Unconscious Patient

The carotid pulse is palpated for 5-10 s; if it is absent, chest compression is started.

Conscious Patient

In the conscious patient who can speak, chest compression is unnecessary.

D: Definitive Care

Definitive care consists of drug administration, seeking medical assistance in managing the problem, or both. If the doctor is certain of the diagnosis and has appropriate drugs available, then drug administration is warranted. If any doubt exists concerning the nature of the problem, do not administer any drug other than oxygen. **Note:** When in doubt, do not medicate.

Assistance should be obtained at any time the doctor feels it is needed, including if there is any doubt as to the nature of the emergency situation or if there is any doubt as to whether appropriate drugs or equipment are available, or are definitely not available.

Specific Emergencies

The remainder of this chapter covers specific emergency conditions:

- unconsciousness,
- altered consciousness,
- seizures,
- respiratory distress,
- allergy,
- local anesthetic overdose,
- chest pain.

Unconsciousness

A definition of unconsciousness is lack of response to sensory stimulation. Syncope—also known as vasodepressor syncope, vasovagal syncope and fainting—remains the most common emergency seen in dental practice. It develops when the patient's body, responding to a real or perceived "fight-or-flight–type" stressful situation, directs blood into the skeletal muscles of the legs and arms of a patient seated upright or standing. In the absence of movement (for example, in the "macho male who can take it like a man" who sits still and doesn't inform the doctor of his anxiety, fear or pain), blood remains in the legs; as a result, the circulating blood volume, cardiac output and cerebral blood flow all decrease. The brain is unable to function normally in the absence of an adequate blood flow (decreased glucose and oxygen supplies) and the signs and symptoms associated with syncope develop. These include pallor, nausea, sweating, feeling dizzy or faint and, finally, the loss of consciousness.

Managing the Unconscious Patient: What to Do

Position the Patient
Critical step: position the patient supine (horizontal) with his or her feet elevated slightly (10 to 15 degrees) to increase blood flow to the brain.

Airway
Critical step: maintain airway patency with head tilt–chin lift positioning.

Breathing
Assess breathing: breathing is usually present in syncope. If not, ventilate with two full breaths.

Circulation
Assess circulation: palpable pulse should be present. In syncope, bradycardia is normally present with a heart rate of 20 to 30 beats per min.

Recovery of consciousness in syncope is usually quite rapid (approximately 10-15 s) after proper positioning and airway management.

Definitive Care
- Loosen any tight clothing, such as collars and ties.
- Administer oxygen.
- Aromatic ammonia vaporole crushed and held beneath the patient's nose can help speed recovery.
- Monitor and record vital signs. For example, blood pressure typically will be lower than baseline and bradycardia will be present. In this case, return of vital signs to baseline will be quite gradual.
- Further dental care at this appointment should be postponed. Dismiss patient in the care of a responsible adult, preferably a friend or relative. Do not permit a post-syncopal patient to drive a car or leave the office unescorted. Recovery from a period of syncope, however brief its duration, requires up to 24 h.

Important Points
- Because of the extremely brief duration of unconsciousness (approximately 10-15 s) seen with proper management of syncope, activation of emergency medical services is rarely necessary.
- When unconsciousness persists for more than 15 s after positioning and maintenance of the airway, emergency medical services (EMS) should be called immediately, as syncope is unlikely to be the cause.
- Inadequate airway management during syncope or during any period of unconsciousness leads to tonic-clonic seizure activity, as the brain becomes progressively more hypoxic and finally anoxic. **Note:** positioning (to increase cerebral blood flow) and airway management (to ensure that cerebral blood contains O_2) are the critical steps in management of any unconscious patient.
- Healthy children do not faint. Healthy children do not sit in a dental chair and "take it

like a man," they behave like children. Movement of arms, legs and body maintain an adequate return of blood to the heart and brain, even when a patient may be seated upright. When a child appears to "faint," the steps P,A,B,C,D must be followed and EMS called immediately.

Altered Consciousness

Our definition of altered consciousness is a conscious patient acting strangely. There are several causes of altered consciousness, including cerebrovascular accident (stroke), hyperthyroidism, hypothyroidism and drug ingestion, with hypoglycemia being the one most commonly encountered in the dental office.

With recent changes in the management of Type I diabetes requiring the more frequent injection of insulin, it is estimated that the incidence of hypoglycemic episodes will increase threefold. When the brain is deprived of adequate glucose, it is unable to function normally, producing clinical signs and symptoms of hypoglycemia: a mentally confused appearance (which may be mistaken for inebriation, but can be differentiated in part because there is no alcohol odor on the breath), cool moist skin, a mild tremor, headache and a feeling of hunger. If severe, hypoglycemia can lead to the loss of consciousness (**Note:** For treatment, see "Managing the Unconscious Patient: What to Do" in the previous section; however, be advised that the patient will not regain consciousness in approximately 10 s as with vasodepressor syncope, and be sure to activate EMS.) Hypoglycemia can also lead to seizures. (**Note:** For treatment, see "Managing Seizures: What to Do" in next section.)

Managing Altered Consciousness: What To Do

Position the Patient
Position the patient comfortably; upright or semireclined is usually preferred.

Note: Conscious patients may be positioned in the most comfortable position during emergency situations. Unconscious patients are always (at least initially) placed supine with their feet elevated slightly.

Airway
The airway is adequately maintained by the conscious hypoglycemic patient.

Breathing
Breathing is adequately maintained by the conscious hypoglycemic patient.

Circulation
Circulation is adequately maintained by the conscious hypoglycemic patient.

Definitive Care
- If the patient is a known diabetic (look for Medic-Alert bracelet, check medical history, ask), ask if he or she has eaten or administered insulin recently.
- In absence of a history of diabetes, continue to next step.
- Administer sugar orally: suggestion— fruit juices or soft drinks, 4 oz every 5-10 min for 30 min **Note:** For most Type I diabetics who are hypoglycemic, drinking orange juice is the most rapid means of alleviating the signs and symptoms of hypoglycemia, with sucking on candy the second fastest.
- Monitor and record vital signs: blood pressure is typically at or near baseline and heart rate is rapid during hypoglycemia.
- If signs and symptoms resolve completely, dental treatment may continue if both the doctor and the patient are agreeable.
- The patient may be dismissed alone if, in the doctor's opinion, all signs and symptoms have resolved. If any doubt remains, discharge him or her into the custody of a responsible adult.
- Before dismissing the patient, determine a cause for the reaction (for example, "I didn't eat before the dental appointment") and modify future care to minimize this risk.

- If symptoms do not resolve following administration of oral sugar, activate EMS.
- If consciousness is lost, repeat P,A,B,C,D protocol and activate EMS procedures.

Important Points

- Never administer oral sugar to an unconscious patient.
- Whenever a diabetic patient exhibits the signs and symptoms listed above, assume hypoglycemia and administer sugar-rich liquids.

Seizures

The definition of seizures is generalized skeletal muscle contractions. **Note:** Seizure and convulsion are synonyms. Epilepsy implies recurrent, discrete seizures in which there is a disturbance of movement, sensation, behavior or consciousness.

The person most likely to have a seizure in the dental environment will be the patient or staff member with a history of epilepsy with poorly controlled seizures or a person with well-controlled epilepsy who is fearful of dentistry.

Local anesthetic overdose is another possible, though unlikely, cause of general tonic-clonic seizures, or GTCSs. GTCSs are present in about 90% of epileptics. Several distinct phases of the GTCS exist as follows.

1. Prodromal Phase

A prodromal phase, consisting of the aura, lasting from a few s to several h prior to the next phase. The aura serves as warning to the patient and doctor that the seizure has begun. Determine a patient's aura at a preliminary visit.

2. Tonic Phase

The patient loses consciousness and a brief (10-20 s) phase of generalized muscle rigidity (the tonic phase) is observed. The patient may arch his or her back and emit the strange crowing sound (the "epileptic cry") as air is expelled from the lungs.

3. Clonic Phase

The clonic phase, a phase of repetitive generalized skeletal muscle contraction and relaxation, usually lasts from 2 to 5 min. Muscle contraction may be violent or barely perceptible with intermediate gradations. The cardiovascular, respiratory and central nervous systems are all stimulated at this time.

4. Postictal Phase

Muscle contraction ends as the postictal phase—a stage of CNS, cardiovascular and respiratory system depression lasting from 10 to 30 min—begins. The patient is sleeping (physiological sleep) deeply and is difficult to arouse. Snoring may be heard, indicating partial airway obstruction. Gurgling, indicating fluid (vomitus, secretions, blood) in the airway may also be heard. Full recovery from GTCS requires up to 3 h.

Important Point

Status epilepticus is an acutely life-threatening situation in which a seizure is continuous for more than 5 min or when a seizure stops and returns before the patient regains consciousness.

Managing Seizures: What to Do

If a seizure occurs during dental treatment, leave the patient in the dental chair and remove all dental equipment from the mouth as expeditiously as possible. Then follow P,A,B,C,D as described below.

Position the Patient

Position the patient; all unconscious patients are to be placed in the supine position with their feet elevated slightly. **Note:** Elevation of the feet may be extremely difficult to accomplish during a seizure, but as the patient's blood pressure is quite elevated at this time, foot elevation is not critical.

Airway

The airway is usually adequately maintained by the patient during a GTCS. Little or no treatment is usually necessary by the rescuer.

Breathing

Breathing is usually adequate during a GTCS. Little or no airway management is necessary by the rescuer.

Circulation

Circulation is adequately maintained by the patient during a GTCS. Little or no treatment is usually necessary by the rescuer.

Definitive Care

- Activate EMS procedure as soon as the seizure begins.
- Protect victim from injury during clonic phase of seizure. **Note:** Gently hold arms and legs, permit limited movement, but do not restrain patient and prevent movement.

Important Point

Do not attempt to put anything into the mouth of a convulsing person. Most injury to victims of seizures occurs during the clonic phase as rescuers attempt to insert objects into the mouth (for example, tongue depressors wrapped in gauze) to "protect the victim" from injury. Fewer than 50% of persons suffering GTCS suffer any intraoral injury when left alone, with injury limited to soft-tissue bruising of the cheek, lateral border of the tongue or both.

Postseizure Phase

When seizures cease, P,A,B,C must be repeated.

Position the Patient

In the dental chair, maintain the patient in a supine position with his or her feet elevated. If lying on the floor, the patient must be turned onto his or her side after the seizure. This position aids in maintaining a patent airway.

Airway

Snoring is frequently present, thus requiring head tilt–chin lift positioning. If necessary, the patient may be repositioned supine and then given the head tilt–chin lift positioning. If a gurgling sound is heard, suctioning of the pharynx is necessary.

Breathing

Breathing is normally present.

Circulation

Adequate circulation is normally present in the postictal phase.

Definitive Care

Talk to the patient, explaining that "you are in the dental office, have had a seizure, and everything is OK." In the postictal phase, patients are disoriented and sleeping deeply. If a companion has accompanied the patient to the office, have the companion talk to the patient as the patient will respond more quickly to a familiar voice.

Recovery and Discharge

EMS is summoned at the start of the seizure for two reasons.

First, not all seizures stop within 5 min. Continuing seizures (status epilepticus) are life-threatening and mandate the administration of intravenous anticonvulsants (for example, diazepam or midazolam). Unless specifically trained in management of apneic patients, never consider the administration of anticonvulsant drugs. Emergency medical personnel are trained to administer anticonvulsants and to ventilate a nonbreathing patient.

Second, most patients (especially those with epilepsy) may be discharged in the care of a responsible adult after having seizures. However, where there is no history of seizures or where seizures last longer than 5 min, hospitalization may be required. Summoning medical assistance at the onset of seizures ensures their prompt arrival on the scene and an accurate evaluation of the postictal patient.

Respiratory Distress

Our definition of respiratory distress is a conscious patient's having difficulty breathing.

Possible causes of respiratory distress in a dental care situation include bronchospasm, hyperventilation and acute pulmonary edema. Whatever the actual cause of the respiratory problem (the actual cause may not be immediately obvious), it is important that the conscious patient who is having difficulty breathing (likely to be quite apprehensive as a result) be managed expeditiously. Initial steps in management of respiratory distress are uniform (see "Managing Bronchospasm: What to Do" below).

Bronchospasm, the acute manifestation of asthma, is the most common cause of respiratory distress in dentistry. Acute episodes of bronchospasm are usually quite easily managed; however, bronchospasm is considered to be life-threatening when it persists despite the administration of two doses of the patient's bronchodilating aerosol drug. **Note:** This is termed status asthmaticus. The incidence of asthma and the number of deaths from status asthmaticus have greatly increased in the past two decades. A bronchodilating aerosol inhaler should be included in the basic emergency drug kit. Asthmatic patients should be reminded to bring their own inhaler with them to every dental appointment. During an acute episode, the asthmatic patient will demonstrate difficulty in breathing. Wheezing is likely to be heard, along with breathing in short gasping inspirations and long noisy (wheezing) expirations. Sweating and flushing of the face and upper torso may be observed, along with use of accessory muscles of respiration.

When respiratory distress could be related to aspiration of a dental restorative material, a chest radiograph should be ordered to determine if the foreign body is in the bronchi or lungs. When foreign body aspiration is considered a possibility, immediate referral to a physician is important. If the foreign body is not in the lung, a gastrointestinal series of radiographs might be of value. However, for many patients, fecal recovery can be considered.

Managing Bronchospasm: What to Do

Position the Patient
Position the patient comfortably: patients in bronchospasm almost universally prefer the upright position.

Airway
The airway is adequately maintained during bronchospasm.

Breathing
Breathing is normally adequate during bronchospasm but is associated with the sound of wheezing (indicative of a partially obstructed airway produced by spasm of bronchial smooth muscle).

Circulation
Circulation is adequately maintained during bronchospasm. Blood pressure is usually slightly elevated while the heart rate is at baseline or slightly elevated.

Definitive Care
- Administer bronchodilator. The patient's bronchodilator aerosol inhaler should be given to the patient. Permit asthmatic patients to administer the drug themselves, as they are accustomed to doing so. The acute episode will terminate within minutes, with the wheezing resolving and the work of breathing lessening.
- Administer oxygen. Oxygen is of secondary importance to the bronchodilator and is usually not necessary; however, should the episode continue or if cyanosis appears, oxygen should be administered.

Recovery and Discharge
Once the typical acute episode of bronchospasm has passed, the patient essentially returns to a "normal state." If both the doctor and the patient agree, the planned dental treatment can proceed. Determine the cause of the episode (for example, sight of the dental syringe or a bloody gauze) and modify

future treatment to minimize the likelihood of a recurrence.

The patient may be dismissed alone after the episode only if the doctor feels that recovery is complete.

Allergy

Allergy is a potentially life-threatening reaction. Fortunately, most allergy involves only the skin, producing itching, hives, rash and possibly edema. Signs and symptoms of allergy are produced by the chemical mediators of allergy, primarily histamine, released into tissue and circulating throughout the body. Other mediators include slow-reacting substance of anaphylaxis (SRS-A); eosinophilic chemotactic factor of anaphylaxis; and others. The rate of release of these chemicals, as well as the sites of their distribution, determine the severity of the allergic reaction. It is essential that allergy be treated aggressively. In general, the faster the onset of signs and symptoms, the more rapidly they progress and the more severe the reaction will become. The usual progression of a severe anaphylactic reaction is skin → eyes, nose, GI → respiratory system → cardiovascular system. The following section describes proper management of a mild reaction.

Managing Mild Systemic Allergic Skin Reaction: What to Do

Airway, breathing and circulation must be evaluated to determine if the allergic skin reaction has progressed to involve either the respiratory system or the cardiovascular system. If the reaction involves either the cardiovascular or respiratory systems, management should proceed as described in the following section on anaphylaxis.

Position the Patient

Position the patient comfortably. The conscious patient suffering from a systemic skin reaction will usually be comfortable if seated upright or semireclined.

Airway

The patient experiencing a mild systemic allergic skin reaction can usually speak without difficulty. A high-pitched "crowing sound" is indicative of soft-tissue edema at the level of the larynx (laryngeal edema) and represents a life-threatening situation. If laryngeal edema is present, EMS must be activated immediately.

Breathing

In most patients with systemic skin reactions, breathing sounds will be normal. The presence of wheezing and of labored breathing indicates respiratory involvement—bronchospasm—necessitating activation of EMS and the administration of a bronchodilator (see "Respiratory Distress" section earlier in chapter).

Circulation

The cardiovascular system is rarely affected in an allergic skin reaction. However, if large amounts of chemical mediators are released into the cardiovascular system, vasodilation occurs, resulting in hypotension and tachycardia. The patient may feel faint or lose consciousness. Basic management of the unconscious patient is required (see "Unconsciousness" section earlier in chapter).

In a systemic skin reaction with neither respiratory nor cardiovascular involvement, there is no immediate need to contact EMS, but definitive treatment must continue.

Definitive Care

- Administer oxygen.
- Administer histamine blocker. Parenteral administration of a histamine blocker is required to manage a systemic skin reaction and to minimize the risk of its progressing to involve either the respiratory or cardiovascular systems. Diphenhydramine (50 mg) or chlorpheniramine (10 mg) are administered either IV or IM (into either

the mid-deltoid or vastus lateralis muscles).

- Permit the patient to recover. Following IM administration, histamine blockers require approximately 10-30 min to alleviate itching (the same response occurring within 2-4 min after IV administration). The skin reaction (hives) will remain.

Discharge of the Patient

The patient may be permitted to leave the dental office after being observed for at least 1 h if there is no evidence of a return or progression of the signs and symptoms.

Prescription

Prescribe oral histamine blockers for 3 days.

Note: Allergy must be treated aggressively. Whenever parenteral histamine blockers are administered, a 3-day regimen of an oral histamine blocker should be prescribed.

Managing Anaphylactoid Systemic Allergic Reaction: What to Do

Our definition of anaphylaxis is a patient experiencing a rapid-onset systemic allergic reaction involving either the respiratory system (dyspnea, wheezing), the cardiovascular system (tachycardia, hypotension) or both; this patient is in urgent need of emergency medical care.

Position the Patient

The patient, though conscious, typically exhibits signs of hypotension. Positioning is predicated on the maintenance of adequate blood flow to the brain; therefore, the supine position with feet elevated slightly is recommended, if possible. Modification might be necessary if respiratory distress is severe.

Airway

The airway need not be maintained as the patient is conscious and is communicating normally.

Breathing

Breathing is often adequate in this patient, although there is evidence of some respiratory compromise in wheezing and dyspnea.

Circulation

A palpable carotid pulse is usually present, although the rate may be rapid and the feel of the pulse "weak."

Definitive Care

- Activate EMS. When an allergic reaction involves either breathing, the cardiovascular system, or both, emergency assistance should be sought immediately.
- Administer epinephrine. Epinephrine must be administered IM as soon as possible during acute allergic reactions. Using the preloaded syringe of 1:1,000 epinephrine, a dose of 0.3 mg (0.3 mL) is administered IM in the mid-deltoid, vastus lateralis or sublingual areas. The latter is preferred to the former as the sublingual region is more vascular, resulting in a more rapid absorption of the epinephrine.
- Administer oxygen.
- Monitor and record vital signs. Blood pressure, heart rate and rhythm, and respiratory rate and quality are monitored and recorded throughout the reaction.
- Readminister epinephrine, if needed. Epinephrine in a 0.3 mg dose is administered to the patient every 5 min until the clinical signs of bronchospasm and hypotension are relieved. Breathing should sound more normal (a soft whooshing sound) and the patient should no longer exhibit labored breathing. The pulse rate will remain elevated (epinephrine produces tachycardia) but the strength of the pulse will improve (stronger). Blood pressure will increase. Itching and hives will remain.
- Administer a histamine blocker. After relief of the respiratory and cardiovascular signs and symptoms, a histamine blocker is administered parenterally. Diphenhydramine or chlorpheniramine administered IM or IV will minimize the risk of a recurrence of cardiovascular and respiratory symptoms and will alleviate the itching.
- When emergency medical technicians

(EMTs) arrive, the patient will be monitored aggressively (ECG, pulse oximetry), an IV infusion will be started and additional drugs administered. These might include additional histamine blockers and corticosteroids. The patient will usually require hospitalization for a period of time for observation and additional management.

Important Points

- The more rapid the onset of signs and symptoms, the more aggressively the allergic reaction must be treated.
- Allergic reactions involving the respiratory system, the cardiovascular system, or both, are life-threatening.
- Whenever allergic reactions involve the respiratory or the cardiovascular systems, aggressive management is essential to help ensure a positive outcome. The immediate administration of epinephrine is usually critical to success.

Local Anesthetic Overdose

Local anesthetic overdose is most likely to develop from the overadministration of the drug to a smaller, lighter-weight patient, such as a child or an elderly adult.

Peak blood levels of local anesthetic after intraoral administration develop in approximately 5-10 min. As anesthetic blood levels increase, signs and symptoms of increasing CNS stimulation can be noted (paradoxically, these are caused by a progressive depression of the CNS), including increased talkativeness, increased apprehension, slurred speech and stuttering. With further increase in anesthetic blood levels, muscular twitching and, finally, generalized convulsions are observed.

Rapid IV administration of local anesthetics can also induce seizures. The onset of the seizure will be almost immediate, within seconds of the anesthetic's IV administration.

Local anesthetic-induced seizures will continue until the local anesthetic blood level falls below the "seizure threshold" for that particular anesthetic. Of significance is the fact that acidosis lowers the seizure threshold of local anesthetics. During seizures, lactic acid is produced as a result of muscular contraction, excessive carbon dioxide is retained and hypoxia occurs. The result is acidosis and a prolongation of the seizure. Airway management and adequate ventilation are absolutely critical in management of local anesthetic-induced seizures.

Managing Local Anesthetic Overdose: What to Do

Position the Patient

The unresponsive patient having a local anesthetic-induced seizure should be placed in the supine position.

Airway

The airway is usually adequately maintained during local anesthetic-induced seizures, but head tilt–chin lift positioning should be performed to ensure airway patency.

Breathing

Breathing is usually adequately maintained during local anesthetic-induced seizures. Oxygen should be administered to the patient during a local anesthetic-induced seizure to minimize the risk of hypoxia, hypercapnia and acidosis.

Circulation

Circulation is usually adequately maintained during the seizure

Important Point

Because acidosis lowers the seizure threshold during local anesthetic-induced seizures, the provision of adequate airway maintenance and ventilation is critical to a successful outcome. A number of devices are available for emergency use to aid in airway maintenance and should be included in an office emergency kit (if the doctor is trained in their use). Oxygen is the most important drug in managing local anesthetic overdose.

Definitive Care

- Activate EMS. Emergency assistance should be summoned whenever a serious adverse reaction occurs after drug administration.
- Manage seizures (see "Seizures" section earlier in chapter). Seizures will cease when local anesthetic blood level falls below its seizure threshold. The post-seizure stage is similar to that of GTCS (CNS, CVS and respiratory depression), except that the patient will usually not be disoriented or mentally confused.
- Basic life support should be administered as indicated below.

Airway

Airway may require head tilt–chin lift positioning.

Breathing

Breathing may be depressed or absent, necessitating supplemental oxygen or controlled ventilation.

Circulation

Hypotension and tachycardia usually will be evident.

Recovery and Discharge

Patients who have had a serious local anesthetic overdose will usually be hospitalized for definitive treatment and for a period of observation.

Chest Pain

The two most likely causes of chest pain in the dental office are angina pectoris and acute myocardial infarction (heart attack). It is often difficult to distinguish between the two conditions at the onset of "the pain," so initial management is directed at the more frequently occurring and easily treated cause: angina pectoris.

Managing Angina Pectoris: What to Do

Patients who have a history of stable angina pectoris are able to tell the doctor that "I am having an anginal attack," greatly simplifying diagnosis and management. Initially, the pain is described by the patient as a pressure, a heavy weight, a constricting feeling or a burning between the shoulder blades, substernally or radiating to the left neck, left mandible or epigastric region (stomach).

Anginal pain is alleviated by rest (3-8 min) or, more promptly, by administration of nitrates (nitroglycerin). Shortness of breath may also occur during the episode. In patients who have no history of chest pain, immediate activation of EMS procedures is recommended.

Position the Patient

A conscious patient experiencing "chest pain" will almost always be more comfortable in an upright sitting position. As long as consciousness remains, this position is acceptable.

Airway

Airway is adequate.

Breathing

Breathing is adequate.

Circulation

Circulation should be monitored. Blood pressure may be near baseline, elevated slightly or somewhat lower. The heart rate will usually be increased with possible cardiac dysrhythmias noted.

Definitive Care

- Administer nitroglycerin. The patient's nitroglycerin should be used, with the patient self-administering his or her normal dose, usually 1 to 3 sublingual tablets or 1 to 3 translingual sprays. **Note:** Nitroglycerin alleviates anginal pain within 1-2 min, and the pain should not return.
- If chest pain subsides and does not return, dental treatment may continue after determining the cause of the acute episode (for example, inadequate pain control or severe dental anxiety). Modification of

future dental care may be warranted.

- If the patient's nitroglycerin tablets are administered and the chest pain is not alleviated, administer a second dose using the nitroglycerin spray from the office emergency drug kit. If the chest pain subsides and does not return, urge the patient to get a "fresh supply" of nitroglycerin immediately.

- Where there is no history of chest pain or angina and the patient experiences the aforementioned episode, treatment will be similar (steps P,A,B,C,D above), with the exception that EMS should be summoned immediately. A patient suffering an initial episode of "chest pain" will usually be extremely frightened, feeling certain that "This is it, the big one!" EMT management usually will include transportation to the hospital for further diagnosis of the patient's cardiovascular condition.

- If chest pain subsides after nitroglycerin administration and subsequently returns, EMS should be summoned immediately. Treatment proceeds as described in the next section—"Managing Acute Myocardial Infarction: What to Do."

Important Point
Chest pain alleviated by nitroglycerin that returns is not anginal. Manage it as though it was an acute myocardial infarction.

Managing Acute Myocardial Infarction: What to Do

Anginal pain is almost always precipitated by an acute episode that increases the workload of the myocardium from such things as fear, pain or exertion. Conversely, 55% of myocardial infarcts occur when the patient is at rest. Although the pain associated with acute myocardial infarction, or MI, is often indistinguishable from anginal pain at the onset, MI is of longer duration, is more severe and does not respond well or at all to nitroglycerin.

The myocardium becomes ischemic during an MI, decreasing cardiac output and leading to signs and symptoms indicative of inadequate blood flow: pallor, sweating, nausea, lightheadedness, shortness of breath, generalized weakness, cool moist skin of an ashen-gray color and cyanosis of mucous membranes. Acute dysrhythmias (bradycardias, tachycardias, PVCs, ventricular tachycardia and ventricular fibrillation) and a very intense, crushing chest pain are all associated with MI.

Position the Patient
The upright position is normally favored by the patient experiencing crushing chest pain. If blood pressure decreases or if consciousness is lost, the supine position with feet elevated slightly must be assumed immediately.

Airway
The airway is usually maintained by the patient.

Breathing
Spontaneous ventilation is usually present.

Circulation
Monitor blood pressure and heart rate and rhythm. Blood pressure is usually decreased slightly or may be close to baseline during acute MI. The heart rate may vary from baseline to extremely slow to extremely rapid. Irregularities in the rhythm may be evident. The heart functions as a pump, circulating blood to the cells of the body. As long as there is a palpable (carotid) pulse and the patient remains conscious, the pump is still functional.

Definitive Care
- Administer oxygen via nasal cannula or nasal hood at a 4-6 L/min flow rate.
- Summon EMS, and perform the following procedures while awaiting EMS arrival.
- Administer nitroglycerin. Administer a dose of two translingual sprays of nitroglycerin from the office emergency kit supply.
- Continue to administer oxygen.
- Administer one aspirin tablet (81 to 325 mg). Recent evidence indicates that chewing an aspirin, permitting it to be absorbed through the oral soft tissues, has

a potentially beneficial effect in aiding in the recanalization of the coronary artery that has become occluded by a thrombus; 81 mg (a "baby aspirin") is as effective as 325 mg (an adult aspirin). Do not swallow the aspirin, as this will delay onset of its thrombolytic actions.

- Loosen constricting clothing (such as ties, collars).
- Monitor and record vital signs.
- Alleviate pain. Traditionally, pain of myocardial infarction has been managed with intravenous morphine (2 to 5 mg every 5 to 15 min). The combination of nitrous oxide (35%) and oxygen (65%) has been shown to be equianalgesic with morphine in managing the pain of MI. Additionally, nitrous oxide at a 35% concentration is a sedative, relaxing a scared patient, while the 65% oxygen is more than three times the ambient oxygen concentration.

- Should the patient lose consciousness, reassess P,A,B,C and implement as necessary.
- On arrival, the EMTs will initiate monitoring (for example, electrocardiogram and pulse oximeter), an intravenous infusion, will administer appropriate advanced cardiac life support (ACLS) drugs and will transport the patient to the hospital emergency department for definitive management.

Suggested Readings

American Heart Association. Textbook of advanced cardiac life support. Dallas: American Heart Association; 1987.

Blakeslee S. Doctors announce new way to forestall effect of diabetes. New York Times; 1993;June 14:1,9.

Bosco DA, Haas DA, Young ER, Harrop KL. An anaphylactoid reaction following local anesthesia: a case report. Anesth Pain Control Dent 1993;2(2):87-93.

Fast TB, Martin MD, Ellis TM. Emergency preparedness: a survey of dental practitioners. JADA 1986;112:499-501.

Roberge RJ, Maciera-Rodriguez L. Seizure-related oral lacerations: incidence and distribution. JADA 1985; 111:279.

Thompson PL, Lown B. Nitrous oxide as an analgesic in acute myocardial infarction. JAMA 1976;235:924.

Section II.

Drugs Used in Medicine: Treatment and Pharmacological Considerations for Dental Patients Receiving Medical Care

Chapter 17.

Cardiovascular Drugs

Steven Ganzberg, D.M.D., M.S.

Cardiovascular disease affects one in six men and one in seven women aged 45-64 y in the United States. The incidence increases to one in three people aged > 65 y. A wide array of medications, with considerably different mechanisms of action, are prescribed to treat these disorders. Primary mechanisms involve the renin-angiotensin system mediated via renal mechanisms and nervous system control via adrenergic supply. Not surprisingly, medications to treat hypertension modify these systems or their sequelae.

This chapter will discuss the medications used for the following cardiovascular disorders: arrhythmias, congestive heart failure, angina, hypertension and atherosclerosis. This chapter is organized by drug class and provides a brief explanation of each.

Special Dental Considerations

Before performing any dental procedure with a patient who has cardiovascular disease, the dentist should evaluate the patient's blood pressure, heart rate and regularity of rhythm. Any change in medication regimen should be reviewed. It is important for patients to take their cardiovascular medications at their usual scheduled time, irrespective of a dental appointment, to minimize the possibility of rebound hypertension or tachycardia. The dentist should take special precautions to minimize the stress or pain of a dental procedure so that adverse cardiovascular responses are, in turn, minimized.

Many of these drugs can cause orthostatic hypotension. After supine positioning, the dentist should have the patient sit in the dental chair for 1-2 min and likewise monitor the patient when he or she is standing. Use of epinephrine or levonordefrin in local anesthetic solutions should be minimized and extra care should be taken with aspiration to avoid intravascular injection. If local anesthetic solutions containing epinephrine are deemed necessary, it has been recommended that no more than 40 µg of epinephrine (0.04 mg or approximately two 1.8-cubic-centimeter cartridges of local anesthetic with 1:100,000 epinephrine) should be used for successive dental anesthetic injections in patients with cardiovascular disease. Vital sign monitoring may be of value between injections for selected patients with severe disease. Additional injections of local anesthetic with epinephrine can be given after approximately 5-10 min if vital signs are satisfactory. The use of gingival retraction cord with epinephrine is absolutely contraindicated in all patients with cardiovascular disease; this cord should be used with extreme caution, if at all, in other patients.

Patients taking some cardiovascular medications may also be taking anticoagulants. Therefore, before dental procedures involving bleeding are performed, consultation with the patient's physician may be indicated to adjust the anticoagulant dose as discussed in Chapter 22, Hematologic Drugs.

Antiarrhythmic Drugs

In cardiac arrhythmia, some aspect of normal cardiac electrophysiology is disturbed. This may manifest in one or more of the following: the sinoatrial (SA) node, atrioventricular (AV) node, Bundle of His, Purkinje fibers or in cardiac muscle itself. Antiarrhythmic drugs modify aberrant electrophysiological processes to help restore or improve either an unacceptable rate, unacceptable rhythm or both.

See Table 17.1 for basic information on antiarrhythmic drugs.

Table 17.1
Antiarrhythmic Drugs: Dosage Information

Generic name	Brand name(s)	Dosage range	Interactions with other drugs
Class IA			
Disopyramide	Norpace	150-200 mg q 6 h	Excessive quantities of either local anesthetic or epinephrine/levonordefrin can precipitate arrhythmia
			These patients should avoid anticholinergics and sedating antihistamines
			Hepatic microsomal enzyme inducers, such as barbiturates, may increase metabolism of disopyramide
Procainamide	Procan, Promine, Pronestyl	500-1,000 mg q 4-6 h	Excessive quantities of either local anesthetic or epinephrine/levonordefrin can precipitate arrhythmia
			Avoid use of anticholinergics and sedating antihistamines
Quinidine gluconate, quinidine sulfate	Cardoquin, Cinquin, Duraquin, Novoquinidin [CAN], Quinalan, Quinidex, Quiniglute, Quinora	**Quinidine gluconate:** 324-660 mg q 6-12 h **Quinidine sulfate:** 200-600 mg q 6-8 h	Excessive quantities of either local anesthetic or epinephrine/levonordefrin can precipitate arrhythmia
			Avoid use of anticholinergics and sedating antihistamines if possible
			Hepatic microsomal enzyme inducers, such as barbiturates, may increase metabolism of quinidine
			Medications containing potassium, such as IV penicillin G potassium, may potentiate quinidine effects
Class IB			
Lidocaine (cardiac)	Xylocaine, Xylocard	**IV only:** 0.75-3.0 mg/kg	Not applicable; used only in emergency situations
Mexiletine	Mexitil	200-400 mg q 8 h	Hepatic enzyme inducers, such as barbiturates, may decrease plasma levels

Continued on next page

Table 17.1 (cont.)

Antiarrhythmic Drugs: Dosage Information

Generic name	Brand name(s)	Dosage range	Interactions with other drugs
Class IB (cont.)			
Phenytoin	Dilantin, Diphenylan, Phenytex	**IV only:** 50-100 mg q 10 min; maximum 50 mg/kg	**Acetaminophen (prolonged use):** Increased risk of hepatic toxicity **Aspirin:** Increased plasma concentration **CNS depressants:** Increased sedative effects **Corticosteroids, benzodiazepines, barbiturates:** Increased metabolism **Fluconazole, ketaconazole, metronidazole:** Decreased metabolism and increased plasma concentration **Lidocaine (high dose):** Increased risk of cardiac arrhythmia
Tocainide	Tonocard	400-600 mg q 8 h	Hepatic enzyme inducers, such as barbiturates, may decrease plasma levels
Class IC			
Encainide	Encaid	25-50 mg q 8 h	Hepatic enzyme inducers, such as barbiturates, may decrease plasma levels
Flecainide	Tambocor	50-200 mg q 12 h	Hepatic enzyme inducers, such as barbiturates, may decrease plasma levels
Class II			
β-blockers	See Table 17.5, Adrenergic Blocking Agents	See Table 17.5, Adrenergic Blocking Agents	See Table 17.5, Adrenergic Blocking Agents
Class III			
Amiodarone	Cordarone	200-1,600 mg q day	Lidocaine or vasoconstrictors may produce hypotension and/or bradycardia
Bretylium	Bretylate, Bretylol	**For IV use:** 5-10 mg/kg	Increased toxicity with other antiarrhythmic agents
Sotalol	Betapace	80-160 mg q 12 h	See Table 17.5, Adrenergic Blocking Agents
Class IV			
Calcium channel blockers	See Table 17.7, Calcium Channel Blockers	See Table 17.7, Calcium Channel Blockers	See Table 17.7, Calcium Channel Blockers

[CAN] indicates a drug available only in Canada.

Special Dental Considerations

If dental patients have been taking these drugs for long periods and their symptoms are under adequate control, the management of these patients in an outpatient dental setting without continuous cardiac monitoring is generally acceptable. Hypotension is commonly encountered. Quinidine is used for several arrhythmias, but commonly for atrial fibrillation. Other Class I and Class III agents are frequently administered either intravenously or orally for severe cardiac arrhythmias such as ventricular tachycardia. Class II and Class IV agents can be used for either hypertension or arrhythmia control. The dentist should consider ECG and continual vital-sign monitoring for patients with serious arrhythmias. In addition, the dentist should follow the recommendations listed under Special Dental Considerations at the beginning of this chapter for all drugs in this category.

Use of large quantities of injected local anesthetics may have additive and possibly detrimental cardiac effects. Use of epinephrine or levonordefrin in local anesthetic solutions should be minimized and extra care should be taken with aspiration to avoid intravascular injection.

Most Class I and Class III agents may rarely cause leukopenia, thrombocytopenia or agranulocytosis. Consider medication-induced adverse effects if gingival bleeding or infection occurs. Elective dental treatment should be deferred if hematologic parameters are compromised.

Quinidine and amiodarone can cause bitter or altered taste. Amiodarone can cause facial flushing.

In orofacial pain management, oral analogues of lidocaine, such as mexiletine, have been reported to be of some use in certain neuropathic pain states. The dentist using these drugs as therapeutic agents is presumed to be proficient in prescribing and managing these medications.

Drug Interactions of Dental Interest

The use of local anesthetics with or without vasoconstrictors is described earlier under Special Dental Considerations. There may be additive anticholinergic effects, such as dry mouth and constipation, with anticholinergic drugs and some sedating antihistamines. Barbiturates, especially when chronically administered, may induce hepatic enzymes and decrease the plasma levels of many antiarrhythmics. Neuromuscular blockade during general anesthesia may be prolonged. Phenytoin interactions are covered in Chapter 20, Neurological Drugs, although this agent is typically used as an antiarrhythmic only acutely for digitalis overdose.

Laboratory Value Alterations

- Most Class I and Class III agents may rarely cause leukopenia, thrombocytopenia, or agranulocytosis. Bleeding times may be affected.
- Quinidine may cause anemia.
- Disopyramide may lower blood glucose levels.

Pharmacology

The antiarrhythmic drugs, classified in four groups from Class I to Class IV, modify the aberrant electrophysiological process to help restore more normal rate and rhythm. The classification of antiarrhythmic drugs is based on the predominant electrophysiological effect of each drug on the various components of the cardiac conduction system in regard to automaticity, refractoriness and responsiveness. Examples of conditions in which these drugs are useful include atrial fibrillation and other atrial arrhythmias, emergency treatment of ventricular fibrillation, ventricular arrhythmias (including premature ventricular contractions, or PVCs), ventricular tachycardia and drug-induced arrhythmias.

Cardiac Glycosides

These drugs are used mainly to treat congestive heart failure and certain cardiac arrhythmias such as atrial fibrillation. The two commonly used drugs in this category include digoxin and digitoxin.

See Table 17.2 for basic information on cardiac glycosides.

Special Dental Considerations

Increased gag reflex is possible. Bright dental lights may not be tolerated. In addition, the dentist should follow the recommendations listed under Special Dental Considerations at the beginning of this chapter for drugs in this category.

Drug Interactions of Dental Interest

Use of epinephrine or levonordefrin in local anesthetic solutions should be minimized and extra care should be taken with aspiration to avoid intravascular injection.

Use of erythromycin may increase digitalis absorption.

Hepatic enzyme inducers (such as barbiturates), especially when used chronically, may increase digitalis metabolism.

Sudden increases in potassium, such as through rapid IV administration of penicillin G potassium or succinylcholine, may precipitate digitalis-induced arrhythmia.

Pharmacology

These drugs increase the force of cardiac contraction and decrease heart rate. By these mechanisms, an enlarged heart is allowed to function more efficiently and its size may be reduced. Because of the rate-slowing effects of these drugs, they are also used to treat specific supraventricular tachycardias. The primary mechanisms of action include inhibition of the sodium-potassium adenosinetriphosphatase, or ATPase, pump and increases in the availability of myocardial Ca^{++} ions intracellularly.

Antianginal Drugs

Angina pectoris, literally "pain in the chest," usually results from a lack of adequate oxygen for myocardial need (ischemia) secondary to coronary atherosclerosis. There are

Table 17.2

Cardiac Glycosides: Dosage Information

Generic name	Brand name(s)	Dosage range	Interactions with other drugs
Digoxin	Lanoxin, Lanoxicaps	50-350 µg (0.05-0.35 mg) q 12-24 h	Excessive epinephrine or levonordefrin in local anesthetic solutions may produce arrhythmia Erythromycin may increase digitalis absorption Hepatic enzyme inducers, such as barbiturates, may increase digitalis metabolism, especially in chronic use Sudden increases in potassium, such as by rapid IV administration of penicillin G potassium or succinylcholine, may precipitate digitalis-induced arrhythmia
Digitoxin	Crystodigin, Digitaline	50-300 µg (0.05-0.3 mg) q day	See note above

three types of angina—chronic stable exertional angina, Prinzmetal's angina and unstable angina. Chronic stable exertional angina usually occurs in patients when activity is such that myocardial oxygen requirement exceeds supply. These patients typically carry sublingual tablet or spray nitroglycerin, which usually aborts attacks. Prinzmetal's angina is angina at rest. Unstable angina is, as the name implies, new-onset angina or worsening angina in a patient who was previously stable. No elective dental procedures should be performed for patients with unstable angina until medically stabilized.

Immediate-acting nitrates, long-acting nitrates, β-blockers and calcium channel blockers are used in the management of angina.

See Table 17.3 for basic information on antianginal drugs.

Table 17.3
Antianginal Drugs: Dosage Information

Generic name	Brand name(s)	Dosage range	Interactions with other drugs
Nitroglycerin	Deponit, Klavikordal, Nitrogard, Nitrolingual, Nitrocad, Nitroglyn, Nitrolin, Nitrospan, Nitronet, Nitrong, Nitrol, Nitrostat, Nitroject, Nitro-Dur, Nitrodisc, Tridil	**Sublingual:** 0.15-0.6 mg/dose **Buccal:** 1 mg q 5 h **Extended oral:** 2.5-9 mg q 8-12 h **Transdermal, patch:** 0.1-0.6 mg/day **Topical, ointment:** 15-30 mg q 8-12 h	Opioids may have added hypotensive effects Epinephrine and levonordefrin in local anesthetic solutions may contribute to onset of angina
Isosorbide dinitrate	Dilatrate SR, Iso-Bid, Isordil, Isotrate, Sorbitrate	**Oral, tablets:** 5-40 mg q 6 h **Oral, extended-release tablets:** 40-80 mg q 8-12 h **Sublingual or buccal:** 2.5-5 mg q 2-3 h	See note above
Erythrityl tetranitrate	Cardilate	5-10 mg q 6-8 h	See note above
Pentaerythritol tetranitrate	Duotrate, Pentylan, Peritrate	**Oral, capsules and extended-release tablets:** 30-80 mg q 12 h **Oral, tablets:** 10-20 mg q 6 h	See note above
β-blockers	See Table 17.5, Adrenergic Blocking Agents	See Table 17.5, Adrenergic Blocking Agents	See Table 17.5, Adrenergic Blocking Agents
Calcium channel blockers	See Table 17.7, Calcium Channel Blockers	See Table 17.7, Calcium Channel Blockers	See Table 17.7, Calcium Channel Blockers

Special Dental Considerations

Patients with angina who are taking sublingual nitroglycerin on an as-needed basis should have this medication available at all dental appointments. In the event of chest pain during a dental visit, the prompt use of nitroglycerin is indicated. Supplemental oxygen and vital-sign monitoring is appropriate. Nitroglycerin in the dentist's emergency kit should be checked regularly, as its shelf life is generally short. This is especially true of sublingual nitroglycerin tablets after the container has been opened.

In addition, the dentist should follow the recommendations listed under Special Dental Considerations at the beginning of this chapter.

Nitroglycerin may cause flushing of the face, headache and xerostomia.

Drug Interactions of Dental Interest

Use of epinephrine or levonordefrin in local anesthetic solutions should be minimized and extra care should be taken with aspiration to avoid intravascular injection. Opioids may have added hypotensive effects.

Laboratory Value Alterations

- Use of nitrate-based antianginal agents may increase the risk of methemoglobinemia. Pulse oximetry may overestimate oxygen saturation.

Pharmacology

Four types of drugs are used to treat angina. The nitrates, typified by nitroglycerin, are direct-acting vasodilators. A dual effect of increased coronary blood flow to ischemic areas, coupled with reduction in venous tone leading to decreased myocardial workload account for nitroglycerin's antianginal activity. Long-acting nitrates, such as isosorbide dinitrate, are also somewhat effective; however, tolerance to these agents limits their long-term value. β-blockers, which block adrenergic responses, may be helpful in treating angina by decreasing myocardial rate and workload. Calcium channel blockers cause vasodilation and slow the heart rate, thus decreasing anginal attacks. Lastly, antiplatelet and anticoagulation agents, such as aspirin, may be of value in preventing myocardial infarction.

Antihypertensive Drugs

Hypertension is common in the American population, affecting 15-20% of people. The risk of hypertension increases dramatically with age. Physiological blood pressure regulation is a complex interrelationship of multiple overlapping systems. Generally, ACE inhibitors or diuretics are considered first-line agents. Other medications—such as β-blockers, calcium channel blockers, α-blockers and direct-acting vasodilators—are then used, alone or in combination, to control blood pressure. The patient taking multiple antihypertensive agents should be considered at increased risk of experiencing a hypertensive or hypotensive crisis.

Additionally, many of these drugs are used to treat orofacial pain conditions. β-blockers and calcium channel blockers are used to manage migraine and other conditions. Verapamil is used for prevention of cluster headache. β-blockers and α-blockers are used in the management of complex regional pain syndrome (sympathetically maintained pain). Intravenous phentolamine is currently being used as a diagnostic tool to help determine if pain is being influenced by the sympathetic nervous system. Clonodine is used for a variety of painful conditions. The dentist using these drugs as therapeutic agents is presumed to be proficient in prescribing and managing these medications.

Diuretics

Diuretic drugs generally exert an antihypertensive effect by increasing sodium and water excretion, thus decreasing blood volume. This decrease in blood volume decreases arterial tone and reduces myocardial workload.

These drugs are commonly first-line agents and frequently are combined with other anti-hypertensives.

See Table 17.4 for basic information on diuretics.

Special Dental Considerations

Potassium-sparing diuretics may rarely cause agranulocytosis and thrombocytopenia. Consider medication-induced adverse effects if gingival bleeding or infection occurs. In addition, some patients taking diuretics may experience xerostomia, which may require special dental care.

In addition, the dentist should follow the recommendations listed under Special Dental Considerations at the beginning of this chapter.

Drug interactions of dental interest

NSAIDs may antagonize natriuresis and the antihypertensive effects of some diuretics. Diflunisal, specifically, may increase the plasma concentration of hydrochlorothiazide. Excessive use of epinephrine or levonordefrin in local anesthetic solutions may antagonize the antihypertensive effects of these agents. All diuretics, except potassium-sparing agents, may enhance neuromuscular blockade during general anesthesia.

Laboratory value alterations

- Loop diuretics and thiazide diuretics can increase blood glucose levels.
- Potassium-sparing diuretics may rarely cause agranulocytosis and thrombocytopenia.

Pharmacology

The site of action of these drugs can be any portion of the kidney from the glomerulus to the distal tubule. Modulation of electrolyte and water reabsorption are common mechanisms of action. It should be noted that patients may be taking these drugs for conditions other than essential hypertension such as renal failure, glaucoma or congestive heart failure. A thorough health history review should provide the necessary information.

Table 17.4

Diuretics: Dosage Information

Generic name	Brand name(s)*	Dosage range	Interactions with other drugs
Diuretics, loop			
Furosemide	Lasix, Myrosemide, Novosemide, Uritol, Furoside	20-120 mg/day	**All diuretics:** NSAIDs may antagonize the diuretic effect, leading to fluid retention or loss of blood pressure control Excessive use of epinephrine or levonordefrin in local anesthetic solutions may antagonize antihypertensive effects **All diuretics except potassium-sparing:** Enhanced neuromuscular blockade possible
Ethacrynic acid	Edercin	50-400 mg/day	See note above
Bumethanide	Bumex	0.5-2 mg q 8-12 h	See note above

Continued on next page

Table 17.4 (cont.)

Diuretics: Dosage Information

Generic name	Brand name(s)*	Dosage range	Interactions with other drugs
Diuretics, potassium-sparing			
Spironolactone	Aldactone, Novospiroton	25-400 mg/day	**All diuretics:** NSAIDs may antagonize the diuretic effect, leading to fluid retention or loss of blood pressure control Excessive use of epinephrine or levonordefrin in local anesthetic solutions may antagonize antihypertensive effects **All diuretics except potassium-sparing:** Enhanced neuromuscular blockade possible
Amiloride	Midamor	5-20 mg/day	See note above
Triamterene	Dyrenium	25-300 mg/day	See note above
Diuretics, thiazide			
Hydrochlorothiazide	Apo-Hydro, Diuchlor H, Esidrix, Hydro-chlor, Hydro-D, HydroDIURIL, Neo-Codema, Novo-Hydrazide, Oretic, Urozide	25-100 mg up to bid	**All diuretics:** NSAIDs may antagonize the diuretic effect, leading to fluid retention or loss of blood pressure control Excessive use of epinephrine or levonordefrin in local anesthetic solutions may antagonize antihypertensive effects **All diuretics except potassium-sparing:** Enhanced neuromuscular blockade possible
Bendroflumethiazide	Naturetin	2.5-20 mg/day	See note above
Benzthiazide	Exna, Hydrex	25-100 mg up to bid	See note above
Chlorothiazide	Diuril	250-1,000 mg/day	See note above
Chlorthalidone	Apo-Chlorthalidone, Hygroton, Novo-Thalidone, Thalitone, Uridon	25-100 mg/day OR 100-200 mg every other day	See note above
Cyclothiazide	Anhydron	1-6 mg/day	See note above
Hydroflumethiazide	Diucardin, Saluron	25-200 mg/day	See note above
Methyclothiazide	Aquatensen, Duretic, Enduron	2.5-10 mg/day	See note above
Metolazone	Diulo, Mykrox, Zaroxolyn	**Prompt release:** 0.5-1 mg/day **Extended release:** 5-20 mg/day	See note above

Drugs with the prefixes Apo-, Neo- and Novo- are available only in Canada.

Continued on next page

Table 17.4 (cont.)
Diuretics: Dosage Information

Generic name	Brand name(s)	Dosage range	Interactions with other drugs
Diuretics, thiazide (cont.)			
Polythiazide	Renese	1-4 mg/day	**All diuretics:** NSAIDs may antagonize the diuretic effect, leading to fluid retention or loss of blood pressure control Excessive use of epinephrine or levonordefrin in local anesthetic solutions may antagonize antihypertensive effects **All diuretics except potassium-sparing:** Enhanced neuromuscular blockade possible
Quinethazone	Hydromox	50-200 mg/day	See note above
Trichloromethiazide	Metahydrin, Naqua, Trichlorex	1-4 g/day	See note above
Diuretics, combination			
Amiloride + hydrochlorothiazide (HCTZ)	Moduretic	5 mg amiloride/50 mg HCTZ 1-2 times/day	**All diuretics:** NSAIDs may antagonize the diuretic effect, leading to fluid retention or loss of blood pressure control Excessive use of epinephrine or levonordefrin in local anesthetic solutions may antagonize antihypertensive effects **All diuretics except potassium-sparing:** Enhanced neuromuscular blockade possible
Spironolactone + HCTZ	Aldactazide, Spirozide	25-200 mg/day Available as 25 mg spironolactone/25 mg HCTZ and 50 mg spironolactone/50 mg HCTZ	See note above
Triamterene + HCTZ	Dyazide	37.5-300 mg/day triamterene/25-200 mg/day hydrochlorothiazide Available as 37.5 mg triamterene/25 mg HCTZ, 50 mg triamterene/25 mg HCTZ and 75 mg triamterene/50 mg HCTZ	See note above

Table 17.5

Adrenergic Blocking Agents: Dosage Information

Generic name	Brand name(s)*	Dosage range	Interactions with other drugs
Nonselective β-blockers			
Carteolol	Cartol	2.5-10 mg/day	NSAIDs may partially antagonize antihypertensive effects of these medications Clearance of injected local anesthetics from peripheral circulation may decrease Opioids may potentiate hypotensive effect of these medications Hypertension and bradycardia can occur when epinephrine or levonordefrin in local anesthetic solutions is administered to patients taking nonselective β-blockers
Oxprenolol	Trasicor	20-160 mg q 8 h	See note above
Penbutolol	Levatol	20 mg/day	See note above
Propranolol	Apo-Propranolol, Detensol, Inderal, Novopronol	80-640 mg/day	See note above
Nadolol	Corgard, Syn-Nadolol	40-240 mg/day	See note above
Pindolol	Novo-Pindol, Syn-Pindol, Visken	5-30 mg q 12 h	See note above
Sotalol	Betapace, Sotacor	80-160 mg q 12 h	See note above
Timolol	Apo-Timol, Blocadren	10-30 mg q 12 h	See note above
Cardioselective β-blockers			
Atenolol	Apo-Atenolol, Novo-Atenol, Tenormin	25-200 mg/day	NSAIDs may partially antagonize antihypertensive effects of these medications Clearance of injected local anesthetics from peripheral circulation may decrease Opioids may potentiate hypotensive effect of these medications
Esmolol	Brevibloc	**IV infusion:** 10-50 mg bolus and/or maintenance—0.05-0.2 mg/kg/min	See note above
Metoprolol	Apo-Metoprolol, Betalol, Durules, Lopressor, Novometoprolol, Toprol XL	50-400 mg/day	See note above

* Drugs with the prefixes Apo-, Novo- and Syn- are available only in Canada.

Continued on next page

Table 17.5 (cont.)

Adrenergic Blocking Agents: Dosage Information

Generic name	Brand name(s)	Dosage range	Interactions with other drugs
Cardioselective β-blockers (cont.)			
Acebutolol	Monitan, Sectrol	100-600 mg q 12 h	NSAIDs may partially antagonize antihypertensive effects of these medications Clearance of injected local anesthetics from peripheral circulation may decrease Opioids may potentiate hypotensive effect of these medications
Betaxolol	Kerlone	10-20 mg/day	See note above
Bisoprolol	Zebeta	2.5-10 mg/day	See note above
Combined α- and β-blocker			
Labetalol	Normodyne, Trandate	100-400 mg q 12 h	NSAIDs may partially antagonize antihypertensive effects of these medications Clearance of injected local anesthetics from peripheral circulation may decrease Opioids may potentiate hypotensive effect of these medications Hypotension and tachycardia can occur when epinephrine or levonordefrin in local anesthetic solutions is administered to patients taking α-blockers
α-blockers			
Phenoxybenzamine	Dibenzyline	10-40 mg q 8-12 h	**All α-blockers:** Hypotension and tachycardia can occur when epinephrine or levonordefrin in local anesthetic solutions is administered to patients taking α-blockers NSAIDs may partially antagonize antihypertensive effects of these medications Opioids may potentiate hypotensive effect of these medications
Phentolamine	Regitine	**IV only: 5** mg 1-2 h before surgery	See note above
Prazosin	Minipress (α-1 selective)	1-15 mg/day in 2-3 divided doses	See note above
Terazosin	Hytrin (α-1 selective)	1-10 mg/day	See note above

Adrenergic Blocking Agents

Adrenergic blocking agents include β-blockers, α-blockers, and combined α- and β-blockers, These drugs are used to manage hypertension by decreasing sympathetic nervous system activity.

See Table 17.5 for basic information on adrenergic blocking agents.

Special Dental Considerations

Rarely, taste changes have been reported.

In addition, the dentist should follow the recommendations listed under Special Dental Considerations at the beginning of this chapter.

Drug interactions of dental interest
Vasoconstrictors in local anesthetics.
β-blockers. Hypertension and bradycardia can occur when epinephrine or levonordefrin in local anesthetic solutions is administered to patients taking *nonselective* β-blockers. Vital sign monitoring before and after injection of local anesthetics containing vasoconstrictors is highly recommended. There is generally minimal interaction of local anesthetic solutions containing epinephrine or levonordefrin with the cardioselective β-blockers.

α-blockers. Hypotension and tachycardia can occur when epinephrine or levonordefrin in local anesthetic solutions is administered to patients taking α-blockers. Vital sign monitoring before and after injection of local anesthetics containing vasoconstrictors is highly recommended.

Combined α- and β-blocker. There is generally minimal interaction with local anesthetic solutions containing epinephrine or levonordefrin.

All adrenergic blocking agents. NSAIDs may partially antagonize the antihypertensive effects of these medications. Opioids may potentiate the hypotensive effect of these medications.

β-blockers only. These agents may decrease the clearance of injected local anesthetics from the peripheral circulation. Phenothiazines may increase the plasma concentration of both drugs.

Pharmacology

The peripheral adrenergic autonomic system principally consists of β-1, β-2, α-1 and α-2 receptors. Catecholamines, such as epinephrine and norepinephrine, act as agonists at these receptors, which have numerous physiological effects. In regard to blood pressure control,

- β-1 activity increases force and rate of cardiac contraction, thus causing tachycardia and increase in blood pressure;
- β-2 activity causes vasodilation in skeletal muscles, thus decreasing blood pressure;
- α-1 receptors cause peripheral vasoconstriction, thus causing an increase in blood pressure;
- α-2 activity causes a decrease in the release of norepinephrine, thus decreasing adrenergic tone.

Adrenergic blocking agents work on one or more of these receptors to alter the sympathetic nervous system response.

β-blockers. β-blockers provide blood pressure control by decreasing the force and rate of cardiac contraction. They are also useful in tachyarrhythmias and angina pectoris. β-blockers are either nonselective or cardioselective. The nonselective β-blockers are antagonists at both the β-1 and β-2 receptors. The cardioselective β-blockers are antagonists at predominantly the β-1 receptor. Because of this difference in receptor activity, patients taking β-1 cardioselective agents experience little interaction with epinephrine in local anesthetic solutions.

α-blockers. α-blockers block either the α-1 receptor (making them selective) or both the α-1 and α-2 receptors (making them nonselective). These drugs control blood pressure by decreasing peripheral vascular tone. Since activation of α-2 receptors decreases adrenergic tone, agents that block both α-1 and α-2 receptors may not be desirable in some patients.

Table 17.6

Direct-Acting Vasodilators: Dosage Information

Generic name	Brand name(s)	Dosage range	Interactions with other drugs
Calcium channel blockers	See Table 17.7, Calcium Channel Blockers	See Table 17.7, Calcium Channel Blockers	See Table 17.7, Calcium Channel Blockers
Hydralazine	Apresoline, Novo-Hylazin	50-75 mg q 6 h	NSAIDs may antagonize diuretic effect, leading to fluid retention or loss of blood pressure control Excessive use of epinephrine or levonordefrin in local anesthetic solutions may antagonize antihypertensive effects of these agents Opioids may potentiate hypotensive effect of these agents
Minoxidil	Loniten	10-100 mg/day	See note above
Nitrates	See Table 17.3, Antianginal Drugs	See Table 17.3, Antianginal Drugs	See Table 17.3, Antianginal Drugs

Combined α- and β-blocker. Labetalol blocks both α-1 and β-1/β-2 receptors with more activity at β-receptors than α-receptors. Labetalol, the only combined α-blocker and β-blocker, thus possesses properties of a nonselective β-blocker and a vasodilator.

Direct-Acting Vasodilators

Direct-acting vasodilators include hydralazine, minoxidil, diazoxide, nitroglycerin and derivatives, as well as the calcium channel blockers, which are discussed in a separate section below. These drugs work directly on the peripheral vasculature to decrease arterial and/or venous tone. See Table 17.6 for basic information on direct-acting vasodilators.

Special Dental Considerations

Hydralazine may, rarely, cause agranulocytosis and thrombocytopenia. The dentist should consider medication effects if gingival bleeding or infection occurs. Facial flushing may occur. Excessive facial hair growth may be seen with minoxidil.

In addition, the dentist should follow the recommendations listed under Special Dental Considerations at the beginning of this chapter.

Drug interactions of dental interest

Excessive use of epinephrine or levonordefrin in local anesthetic solutions may antagonize the antihypertensive effects of these agents. NSAIDs may partially antagonize the antihypertensive effects of these medications. Opioids may potentiate the hypotensive effect of these medications.

Laboratory value alterations

Erythrocyte concentration, hemoglobin and hematocrit may be artificially decreased due to hemodilution.

Pharmacology

These agents provide hypertension control predominantly by various direct actions on vascular smooth muscle. The mechanism of action is believed to be mediated via nitric oxide, which alters Ca^{++} dependent muscular contractility and thus produces vascular muscle relaxation.

Table 17.7

Calcium Channel Blockers: Dosage Information

Generic name	Brand name(s)*	Dosage range	Interactions with other drugs
Bepridil	Bepadin	200-400 mg/day	Excessive use of epinephrine or levonordefrin in local anesthetic solutions may antagonize antihypertensive effects of these agents

NSAIDs may partially antagonize antihypertensive effects of these medications

Opioids may potentiate hypotensive effect of these agents

Neuromuscular blockade may be intensified or prolonged |
| Diltiazem | Cardizem, Cardizem CD, Cardizem SR, Dilacor | **Oral, tablets:** 30-120 mg q 8 h

Oral, extended-release tablets: 30-60 mg/day OR 20 mg bid | See note above |
Felodipine	Renedil	5-20 mg/day	See note above
Flunarazine	Sibelium	10 mg/day	See note above
Isradipine	DynaCirc	2.5-10 mg q 12 h	See note above
Nicardipine	Cardene	20-40 mg q 8 h	See note above
Nifedipine	Adalat, Apo-Nifed, Novo-Nifedin, Nu-Nifedin, Procardia	10-30 mg q 8 h	See note above
Nimodipine	Nimotop	60 mg q 4 h	See note above
Verapamil	Calan, Calan SR, Isoptin, Novo-Veramil, Nu-Verap, Verelan	120-480 mg/day	See note above

Drugs with the prefixes Apo-, Novo- and Nu- are available only in Canada.

Calcium Channel Blockers

Calcium channel blockers are commonly prescribed antihypertensive, antianginal and antiarrhythmic agents. See Table 17.7 for basic information on calcium channel blockers.

Special Dental Considerations

Gingival enlargement can occur with these agents. Meticulous oral hygiene can reduce these effects. If gingival enlargement occurs, the patient's physician should be consulted about changing the medication to a non-calcium channel blocker. Nimodipine may cause thrombocytopenia. Other agents rarely cause blood dyscrasias. Consider medication-induced adverse effects if gingival bleeding or infection occurs.

In addition, the dentist should follow the recommendations listed under Special Dental Considerations at the beginning of this chapter.

Drug interactions of dental interest

Excessive use of epinephrine or levonordefrin in local anesthetic solutions may antagonize the antihypertensive effects of these agents. NSAIDs may partially antagonize the antihypertensive effects of these medications. Opioids may potentiate the hypotensive effect of these medications. There is a possible increased hypotensive effect with aspirin.

Pharmacology

These drugs decrease peripheral vascular tone by decreasing calcium influx in vascular smooth muscle. The antiarrhythmic effect is due primarily to decreasing the slow inward Ca^{++} current in the cardiac conduction system. The agents also depress force and rate of cardiac contraction to various degrees. For instance, verapamil and diltiazem control heart rate more effectively than nifedipine, which acts more prominently by direct vasodilation.

Drugs Acting on the Renin-Angiotensin System

These drugs are considered first-line agents in the control of hypertension. By blocking the effects of angiotensin II, a potent vasoconstrictor, these agents decrease high blood pressure in many patients. See Table 17.8

Table 17.8
Drugs Acting on the Renin-Angiotensin System: Dosage Information

Generic name	Brand name(s)	Dosage ranges	Interactions with other drugs
ACE inhibitors			
Benazepril	Lotensin	10-40 mg/day	Excessive use of epinephrine or levonordefrin in local anesthetic solutions may antagonize antihypertensive effects of these agents
			NSAIDs may partially antagonize antihypertensive effects of these agents
			Opioids may potentiate hypotensive effect of these agents
			Medications containing potassium, such as IV penicillin G potassium, may exacerbate medication-induced hyperkalemia
Captopril	Capoten	12.5-50 mg q 8 h	See note above
Enalopril	Vasotec	5-40 mg/day	See note above
Fosinopril	Monopril	10-80 mg/day	See note above
Lisinopril	Prinivil, Zestril	10-80 mg/day	See note above
Quinapril	Accupril	10-80 mg/day	See note above
Ramipril	Altace	2.5-20 mg/day	See note above
Angiotensin II receptor antagonist			
Losartan	Cozaar	25-100 mg/day	See note above

for basic information on drugs acting on the renin-angiotensin system.

Special Dental Considerations

These agents may cause neutropenia or agranulocytosis. Consider medication-induced adverse effects if gingival bleeding or infection occurs. Angioneurotic edema may occur on the face, tongue or glottis. Coughing is a common side effect. Loss of taste has been reported, but rarely.

In addition, the dentist should follow the recommendations listed under Special Dental Considerations at the beginning of this chapter.

Drug interactions of dental interest

Excessive use of epinephrine or levonordefrin in local anesthetic solutions may antagonize the antihypertensive effects of these agents. NSAIDs may partially antagonize the antihypertensive effects of these medications. Opioids may potentiate the hypotensive effect of these medications. Potassium-containing medications, such as penicillin G potassium administered IV, may exacerbate medication-induced hyperkalemia.

Laboratory value alterations

Agranulocytosis and neutropenia may occur.

Pharmacology

Under normal conditions, the reninangiotensin system provides for an increase in blood pressure when hypotension occurs. Renin released from the renal glomerulus leads to the formation of angiotensin I, which is converted to angiotensin II, primarily in the lung. Angiotensin II is a potent vasoconstrictor and also stimulates aldosterone release. The antihypertensive effect of these agents occurs when angiotensin II is blocked, either at the angiotensin II receptor or by decreased formation of angiotensin II itself. This latter effect occurs when angiotensin-converting enzyme (ACE) in the lung is inhibited, thus blocking the metabolism of angiotensin I to angiotensin II. The term "ACE inhibitor" is therefore commonly used with these medications.

Centrally Acting Antihypertensive Agents

These drugs act in the central nervous system to decrease peripheral sympathetic tone. See Table 17.9 for basic information on centrally acting antihypertensive agents.

Special Dental Considerations

A rebound hypertensive crisis may occur if patients abruptly stop taking drugs in this category prior to a dental appointment. Dental patients should be instructed to take their medications at the usual time irrespective of the time of their dental appointment.

These drugs may inhibit salivary flow. Parotid pain may occur.

In addition, the dentist should follow the recommendations listed under Special Dental Considerations at the beginning of this chapter.

Drug interactions of dental interest

Excessive use of epinephrine or levonordefrin in local anesthetic solutions may antagonize the antihypertensive effects of these agents. NSAIDs may partially antagonize the antihypertensive effects of these medications. Opioids may potentiate the hypotensive and sedative effects of these medications. Other oral or IV sedative agents may be potentiated by these agents. There may be a decreased antihypertensive effect with tricyclic antidepressants. Methyldopa may increase the anticoagulant effect of coumarin anticoagulants.

Pharmacology

The mechanism of action of these agents is chiefly via a central nervous system α-2 agonist action. As the α-2 receptor decreases adrenergic tone, there is a decrease in sympathetic outflow. This causes a decrease in blood pressure and heart rate.

Neuronal Blocking or Depleting Agents

This diverse group of drugs is rarely prescribed today due to numerous undesirable side effects and the availability of other more efficacious agents. See Table 17.10 for basic information on neuronal blocking or depleting agents.

Table 17.9

Centrally Acting Antihypertensive Agents: Dosage Information

Generic name	Brand name(s)	Dosage range	Interactions with other drugs
Clonodine	Catapress, Catapres TTS, Dixarit	**Oral—maintenance:** 0.2-0.6 mg q 6 h **Transdermal:** 0.1-0.3 mg/day	Rebound hypertensive crisis may occur if patients abruptly stop taking these agents prior to a dental appointment Excessive use of epinephrine or levonordefrin in local anesthetic solutions may antagonize antihypertensive effects of these agents NSAIDs may partially antagonize antihypertensive effects of these agents Opioids may potentiate hypotensive and sedative effects of these agents Other oral or IV sedative agents may be potentiated by these agents
Guanabenz	Wytensin	4-16 mg q 12 h	See note above
Guanfacine	Tenex	1-3 mg/day	See note above
Methyldopa	Aldomet, Apo-Methyldopa [CAN]	250-1,000 mg q 8-12 h	See note above

Table 17.10

Neuronal Blocking or Depleting Agents: Dosage Information

Generic name	Brand name(s)	Dosage range	Interactions with other drugs
Deserpidine	Harmonyl	250-500 µg (0.25-0.5 mg)/day	Neuronal blocking or depleting agents can cause administered epinephrine to have an exaggerated cardiovascular effect Blood pressure and heart rate should be carefully monitored if local anesthetic solutions containing epinephrine are deemed essential NSAIDs may partially antagonize antihypertensive effects of these medications Opioids may potentiate hypotensive and sedative effects of these agents Effects of other oral or IV sedative agents may be potentiated by these agents Phenothiazines may produce increased extrapyramidal effects

Continued on next page

Table 17.10 (cont.)

Neuronal Blocking or Depleting Agents: Dosage Information

Generic name	Brand name(s)	Dosage range	Interactions with other drugs
Guanadrel	Hylorel	15-75 mg/day	Neuronal blocking or depleting agents can cause administered epinephrine to have an exaggerated cardiovascular effect
			Blood pressure and heart rate should be carefully monitored if local anesthetic solutions containing epinephrine are deemed essential
			NSAIDs may partially antagonize antihypertensive effects of these medications
			Opioids may potentiate hypotensive and sedative effects of these agents
			Effects of other oral or IV sedative agents may be potentiated by these agents
			Phenothiazines may produce increased extrapyramidal effects
Guanethidine	Ismelin	10-50 mg/day	See note above
Rauwolfia serpentina	Raudixin, Rauval, Rauverid, Wolfina	50-200 mg/day	See note above
Reserpine	Reserfia, Serpalan, Serpasil; Novoreserpine [CAN]	100-250 µg (0.1-0.25 mg)/day	See note above

[CAN] indicates a drug available only in Canada.

Special Dental Considerations

These drugs may inhibit salivary flow.

In addition, the dentist should follow the recommendations listed under Special Dental Considerations at the beginning of this chapter.

Drug interactions of dental interest

Neuronal blocking or depleting agents can cause administered epinephrine or levonordefrin to have an exaggerated cardiovascular effect. Blood pressure and heart rate should be carefully monitored if local anesthetic solutions containing epinephrine are deemed essential. NSAIDs may partially antagonize the antihypertensive effects of these medications. Opioids may potentiate the hypotensive and sedative effects of these medications. Other oral or IV sedative agents may be potentiated by these agents. Phenothiazines may exhibit increased extrapyramidal reactions.

Pharmacology

These drugs act principally by depleting norepinephrine and other catecholamines from the adrenergic nerve endings. There is, therefore, a decrease in heart rate, force of cardiac contraction and peripheral vascular resistance. These drugs can have complex effects when initially administered.

Adverse Effects

Table 17.11 lists adverse effects of cardiovascular medications.

Table 17.11
Cardiovascular Drugs: Adverse Effects

Body system	Cardiac glycosides	Antianginal agents	Diuretics	Antihypertensive agents						
				Adrenergic blockers: β-blockers, labetalol	Adrenergic blockers: α-blockers	Direct-acting vasodilators	Calcium channel blockers	ACE inhibitors	Centrally acting antihypertensive agents	Neuronal depleters
General	Allergic reaction	Allergic reaction	Allergic reaction	Allergic reaction	Allergic reaction	Allergic reaction lymphadenopathy, systemic lupus erythematosus	Allergic reaction	Allergic reaction cough, Stevens-Johnson syndrome		
CV	Arrhythmias, including ventricular fibrillation, bradycardia	Hypotension, tachycardia	Chest pain	Bradycardia, congestive heart failure, peripheral vascular insufficiency, arrhythmias	Hypotension, tachycardia, palpitations, angina, edema	Angina, tachycardia, hypotension, sodium and water retention, edema	Angina, congestive heart failure, arrhythmias, tachycardia, bradycardia, hypotension, edema	Angioedema, hypotension, tachycardia, chest pain	Palpitations, tachycardia, hypotension, angina, congestive heart failure, water retention, Raynaud's phenomena	Angina, bradycardia, congestive heart failure, tachycardia, edema, hypotension
CNS	Drowsiness, confusion, headache	Headache	Confusion, headache	Depression, confusion, dizziness, numbness, tingling of extremities and scalp, headache, nightmares, tiredness	Dizziness, headache, fatigue	Peripheral neuritis, headache, dizziness	Dizziness, drowsiness, anxiety, depression, insomnia, headache	Headache, nightmares	Depression, dizziness, nervousness, insomnia, headache, nightmares	Drowsiness, depression, weakness, fatigue, headache

Continued on next page

EENT	Blurred vision, photophobia	Blurred vision	Ototoxicity	Blurred vision		Nasal congestion, lacrimation			Dry eyes	Tinnitus, visual changes, diplopia, blurred vision, nasal stuffiness
Endoc			Decreased libido	Decreased sexual ability	Priapism, impotence			Impotence	Decreased libido	Difficulty in ejaculation, breast enlargement, impotence
GI	Nausea, vomiting, loss of appetite, diarrhea, stomach pain	Nausea, vomiting	Stomach pain, nausea, vomiting, diarrhea, loss of appetite, cramps	Constipation, nausea, vomiting, stomach pain	Nausea, constipation	Anorexia, diarrhea, nausea, vomiting, constipation	Nausea, vomiting, diarrhea, stomach pain, constipation	Diarrhea, fatigue, nausea, bronchospasm	Nausea, vomiting, stomach cramps, constipation	Diarrhea, nausea, vomiting, constipation
GU				Increased urination	Urinary frequency		Increased urination	Abnormal urination		Nocturia
Hema			Rare leukopenia/agranulocytosis, thrombocytopenia (especially with loop diuretics), hyperuricemia, electrolyte imbalance	Leukopenia, thrombocytopenia	Lymphadenopathy	Blood dyscrasias	Hyperkalemia	Neutropenia, agranulocytosis	Hyperglycemia	Thrombocytopenia and leukopenia with guanethidine, galactorrhea

Table 17.11 (cont.)
Cardiovascular Drugs: Adverse Effects

Body system	Cardiac glycosides	Antianginal agents	Diuretics	Antihypertensive agents						
				Adrenergic blockers: β-blockers, labetalol	Adrenergic blockers: α-blockers	Direct-acting vasodilators	Calcium channel blockers	ACE inhibitors	Centrally acting antihypertensive agents	Neuronal depleters
HB			Rare hepatic dysfunction	Hepatotoxicity			Altered liver enzymes (make sure this is on lab values if you want it)	Pancreatitis		
Integ		Skin rash, flushing of face/neck, sweating, bluish extremities (may indicate overdose)	Increased sensitivity of skin to light			Allergic reaction, skin blisters		Skin rash	Itching, redness of skin, rash, sweating, alopecia	Skin rash, alopecia
Musc		Weakness		Back or joint pain			Arthritis	Joint pain		Muscle pain/tremor

Oral	Dry mouth	Dry mouth, taste changes, parotid pain	Loss of taste	Gingival enlargement, dry mouth		Dry mouth	Dry mouth, taste change		Dry mouth, bluish lips (may indicate overdose)
Renal		Water retention	Renal failure, nephrotic syndrome		Sodium and water retention, edema			Nephrolithiasis	
Resp	Shortness of breath, bronchospasm				Shortness of breath	Shortness of breath	Bronchospasm, shortness of breath, nasal congestion		

Suggested Readings

Drugs for cardiac arrhythmias. Med Lett Drugs Ther 1991;33:55-60.

Follath F. Clinical pharmacology of antiarrhythmic drugs: variability of metabolism and dose requirements. J Cardiovasc Pharmacol 1991;17 (Supplement 6):S74-S76.

Friedman L, Schron E, Yusuf S. Risk-benefit assessment of antiarrhythmic drugs: an epidemiological perspective. Drug Safety 1991;6:323-31.

Kaplan NM, ed. Clinical hypertension. 6th ed. Baltimore: Williams & Wilkins; 1994.

Laragh JH, Brenner BM, eds. Hypertension: Pathology, diagnosis, and management. New York: Raven Press; 1990.

Veterans Administration Cooperative Study Group on Antihypertensive Agents. Effects of treatment on morbidity in hypertension. JAMA 1967;202:1028-34.

Chapter 18

Respiratory Drugs

Martha Somerman, D.D.S., Ph.D.

A significant number of people in the general population have respiratory disorders that require the use of medications. Bronchial asthma is the most common respiratory disease the dentist encounters; therefore, he or she should be particularly familiar with drugs taken by patients with such conditions.

Asthma is characterized physiologically by reversible airway obstruction that results from constriction of the bronchial and bronchiolar muscles and hypersecretion of viscous mucus. Factors that can precipitate an asthmatic attack include stimuli, allergy and stress.

There are three major approaches to the treatment of asthma:

- use of anti-inflammatory drugs to reduce symptoms and bronchial hyperactivity;
- use of agents that reverse or inhibit bronchoconstriction;
- avoidance of causative factors.

Causative factors include indoor allergens and stress; thus, the dentist must be sensitive to the possibility of these factors provoking an asthmatic attack in a susceptible person while he or she is in the dental office. If a patient is using metered-dose inhalants, these inhalants should be readily accessible at his or her dental appointment.

The information in this chapter will provide summary data on special dental considerations for, use of, interactions of, adverse effects of and contraindications for drugs taken by and potentially given to people who have respiratory conditions.

When treating a patient with a respiratory condition, the dentist must determine the nature of the condition and which, if any, drugs the patient is taking for these conditions.

Corticosteroids are covered in more detail in Chapter 6, Corticosteroids, while β-blockers are covered in Chapter 17, Cardiovascular Drugs.

Tables 18.1-18.4 provide general information on drugs used for respiratory diseases, including indications, typical dosage ranges and interactions.

Special Dental Considerations

When it comes to treating patients with respiratory conditions, practitioners should keep the following important points in mind.

First, chronic obstructive pulmonary disease (COPD) is a respiratory disease of major medical concern; bronchial obstruction in this disease is irreversible, resulting in severe infections, heart disease and respiratory failure. Respiratory conditions and the use of inhalants can result in decreased salivary flow and associated problems, including caries and candidiasis. Therefore, patients should use fluoride rinses and should be observed for the need to use antifungal agents.

Reduction of stress may require the use of sedatives, especially when complex procedures are being performed. Stress reduction methods, including medications, may be required to prevent an asthmatic attack.

Table 18.1

Inhibitors of Chemical Mediators/Anti-inflammatory Drugs: Dosage Information

Generic name	Brand name(s)	Indications/uses	Dosage range	Interactions with other drugs
Corticosteroids (inhalants)				
Beclomethasone dipropionate	Beclovent, Vanceril	Chronic asthma Severe asthma, rhinitis Chronic obstructive pulmonary disease, possibly in combination with β2 adrenergic agents Not for acute treatment	**Inhalation:** Varies depending on extent of disease; usually 2 puffs tid-qid or 4 puffs bid Tablets/liquid also available	In general, more concerns of interactions with use of systemic corticosteroids (see Chapter 6, Table 6.2 for details); for example, possible interactions with acetaminophen, amphotericin B or carbonic anhydrase inhibitors, anabolic steroids, antacids, antidiabetic agents, NSAIDs, digitalis glycosides, hepatic enzyme-inducing agents, some β2-adrenergic agonists
Budesonide	Pulmicort [CAN]	Chronic asthma Severe asthma, rhinitis Chronic obstructive pulmonary disease, possibly in combination with β2 adrenergic agents Not for acute treatment	0.5-1 mg via nebulizer bid	Same as above
Flunisolide	AeroBid; Bronalide [CAN]	Chronic asthma Severe asthma, rhinitis Chronic obstructive pulmonary disease, possibly in combination with β2 adrenergic agents Not for acute treatment	2 puffs bid	Same as above
Triamcinolone acetonide	Azmacort	Chronic asthma Severe asthma, rhinitis Chronic obstructive pulmonary disease, possibly in combination with β2 adrenergic agents Not for acute treatment	2 puffs tid-qid	Same as above

[CAN] indicates a drug available only in Canada.

Continued on next page

Table 18.1 (cont.)

Inhibitors of Chemical Mediators/Anti-inflammatory Drugs: Dosage Information

Generic name	Brand name(s)	Indications/uses	Dosage range	Interactions with other drugs
Cromolyn				
Disodium cromoglycate/ cromolyn	Intal	Chronic asthma Not for acute attacks Prophylactic for exercise, cold air, environmental pollutants	Usually 2 puffs qid by metered-dose inhaler	None listed
Nedocromil sodium	Tilade; Rynacrom [CAN]	Chronic asthma Not for acute attacks Prophylactic for exercise, cold air, environmental pollutants	Usually 2 puffs qid by metered-dose inhaler	None listed

[CAN] indicates a drug available only in Canada.

Table 18.2

Bronchodilators: Dosage Information

Generic name	Brand name(s)	Indications/uses	Dosage range	Interactions with other drugs
β-adrenergic agonists				
Albuterol	Proventil, Ventolin; Novosalomol [CAN]	Usually, for acute situations with asthma and bronchospasm and to control acute symptoms, but long-acting β2 selective agonists, such as salmeterol, are used for maintenance, often in combination with inhaled steroid Epinephrine compounds have both β1 & β2 agonist activity, thus use for bronchodilation is limited	**Inhalation, metered-dose inhaler**: 2-3 puffs q 3-4 h, not to exceed 12/day	Cardiovascular effects may be potentiated in patients receiving MAO inhibitors, tricyclic depressants, sympathomimetic agents, inhaled anesthetics
Bitolterol	Tornalate	See note above	See note above	See note above
Epinephrine/ epinephrine bitartrate/epi- nephrine HCI	Bronkaid Mist; Epi Pen; Epi Pen Jr; Sus-Phrine (parenteral), Primatene Mist Asthma Haler, Medihaler-EpiAdrenalin, Sus-Phrine; Vaponefrin [CAN]	See note above	See note above	See note above

[CAN] indicates a drug available only in Canada.

Continued on next page

Table 18.2 (cont.)

Bronchodilators: Dosage Information

Generic name	Brand name(s)	Indications/uses	Dosage range	Interactions with other drugs
β-adrenergic agonists (cont.)				
Isoetharine HCl/isoetharine mesylate	Bronkosol, Bronkometer, Arm-a-Med Isoetharine, Dry-dose, Day-lute, Dispos-a Med	Usually, for acute situations with asthma and bronchospasm and to control acute symptoms, but long-acting β2 selective agonists, such as salmeterol, are used for maintenance, often in combination with inhaled steroid Epinephrine compounds have both β1 & β2 agonist activity, thus use for bronchodilation is limited	**Inhalation, metered-dose inhaler:** 1-2 puffs q 4 h **Syrup:** 2-4 mg tid or qid PRN **Solution:** Usually not more than q 4 h	Cardiovascular effects may be potentiated in patients receiving MAO inhibitors, tricyclic depressants, sympathomimetic agents, inhaled anesthetics
Metaproterenol sulfate	Metaprel, Alupent	See note above	**Inhalation, metered-dose inhaler:** 2-3 puffs q 3-4 h, not to exceed 12/day	See note above
Pirbuterol acetate	Maxair	See note above	See note above	See note above
Salmeterol	Serevent	See note above	See note above	See note above
Terbutaline	Brethine, Bricanyl, Brethaire	See note above	See note above	See note above
Xanthines				
Aminophylline (theophylline ethylenediamine-xanthine), phyllocontin, somophyllin - DF, somophyllin, dyphylline; parolon [CAN]	Dilor, Dyflex, Lu Fyllin, Neothylline; Protophyline [CAN]	Usually chronic asthma and in combination with other asthmatic agents	See note above	Can alter metabolism of many other drugs and also other drugs may alter metabolism **Benzodiazepines:** Sedative effects may be decreased **Halothane & CNS stimulants:** Increased risk of cardiac dysrhythmia **Barbiturates, carbamazepine, phenytoin, ketoconazole:** Decrease activity **Erythromycin, clindamycin, ciprofloxacin, alcohol:** Increase concentration

[CAN] indicates a drug available only in Canada.

Continued on next page

Table 18.2 (cont.)

Bronchodilators: Dosage Information

Generic name	Brand name(s)	Indications/uses	Dosage range	Interactions with other drugs
Xanthines (cont.)				
Theophylline	Theo-24, Slo-Phyllin, Choledyl, Oxitriphylline	Usually chronic asthma and in combination with other asthmatic agents	**Extended-release capsules or tablets:** 300-600 mg/day	Can alter metabolism of many other drugs and also other drugs may alter metabolism **Benzodiazepines:** Sedative effects may be decreased **Halothane & CNS stimulants:** Increased risk of cardiac dysrhythmia **Barbiturates, carbamazepine, phenytoin, ketoconazole:** Decrease activity **Erythromycin, clindamycin, ciprofloxacin, alcohol:** Increase concentration
Theophylline, theophylline sodium glycinate	Aquaphyllin, Bronkodyl, Quibron-T, Slo-Phyllin, Theodur Sprinkle, Theolair, Theoclear, Theostat, Slo-bid, Theovent, Theospan-SR, Respbid, Uniphyl	See note above	See note above	See note above

Table 18.3

Anticholinergic Drugs: Dosage Information

Generic name	Brand name(s)	Indications/uses	Dosage range	Interactions with other drugs
Ipratopium bromide	Atrovent	Chronic obstructive pulmonary disease (not approved by FDA for asthma, but has proven useful in older, nonatopic patients who have chronic obstruction of airflow)	2-4 puffs tid/qid	Increased effects of systemic anticholinergic drugs

Table 18.4

Evolving Respiratory Therapies: Dosage Information

Generic name	Brand name(s)	Indications/uses	Dosage range	Interactions with other drugs
Allergen avoidance/ chemicals to denature allergens	generic	Prophylaxis	Not established	Not established
DNase inhibitors (Dornase Alfa)	Pulmozyme	For treatment of cystic fibrosis to reduce respiratory infection and improve pulmonary function	**Inhalation, nebulizer:** 2.5-5 mg/day Dose for children aged < 5 y not established	Has not been studied
Immunosuppressive agents such as methotrexate	Methotrexate	Prophylaxis	Not labeled	Hepatotoxic drugs alter metabolism of methotrexate
Leukotrine antagonists and inhibitors	Zileuton (Zyflo), Zafirlukast (Accolate)	Prophylaxis and maintenance treatment of asthma	20 mg tid (Accolate) 600 mg qid (Zyflo)	Zileuton metabolized by P450 system, thus will alter metabolism of other drugs including theophylline (decreased clearance, serum levels); warfarin (increased serum levels); propranolol (increased serum levels); possibly terfenadine (Seldane and other varieties of terfenadine [antihistamine]) Patients should be monitored for hepatic toxicity

NSAIDs and aspirin are contraindicated in patients with respiratory conditions, as they may prompt an asthmatic attack. Use of nitrous oxide with these patients also should be avoided.

A semisupine chair position should be used for patients with respiratory diseases, especially for patients with COPD. To prevent orthostatic hypotension, patients should sit upright for a few minutes before being dismissed.

Inhalants that patients are using should be easily accessible during the dental appointment.

With patients receiving chronic steroid therapy, there is an enhanced concern about stress situations—such as the possibility of adrenal crisis—as well as increased susceptibility to infections.

With patients using β-adrenergic agonists, there is a concern about cardiovascular side effects. Most of the drugs in this category used to treat asthma are selective β2 adrenergic agonists and thus act as bronchodilators.

However, they do have some β1 side effects, so there is a need to be aware of possible cardiovascular side effects (for example, tachycardia and hypertension).

Drug interactions of dental interest
Avoid drugs that may precipitate an asthmatic attack: aspirin, NSAIDs and narcotics.

Special patients
As a rule, inhalants are not recommended for use in children aged < 5 y. Also, these drugs may have hepatic and renal side effects that often are of more concern with children and older adults.

Adverse Effects, Precautions and Contraindications

Table 18.5 describes adverse effects associated with steroids and β2 adrenergic blockers (whether taken orally or by inhalant route); Table 18.6 describes precautions and contraindications.

Pharmacology

Inhibitors of Chemical Mediators/Anti-Inflammatory Drugs

Cromolyn sulfate
Cromolyn sulfate has no direct bronchodilating activity, so it is active only when given by inhalation. It is thought to act by stabilizing mast cells. In addition, cromolyn also may inhibit mast cell release of histamine, leukotrienes and other inflammatory mediators and inhibit calcium influx into mast cells. The result is decreased stimuli for bronchospasm. However, as it has no bronchodilating activity, cromolyn is useful only for prophylactic treatment and not for acute situations.

Corticosteroids
See Chapter 6, Corticosteroids, for details.

Bronchodilators

β-adrenergic agonists
β-adrenergic agonists are used for treatment of acute bronchospasm. Ideal drugs act predominantly on β-2 adrenergic receptors and stimulate dilation of bronchial smooth muscles. This relaxes the airway's smooth muscle. β-adrenergic agents also inhibit release of substances from mast cells and thus prevent bronchoconstriction. Most adrenergic drugs have some β-1 activity; therefore, there is a need to monitor patients for cardiovascular effects, including increased heart force and rate of cardiac contraction. This is especially true of epinephrine. Note: Epinephrine usually is used for emergency situations such as rapid/acute asthmatic attack: in which case 0.2-0.5 mL of 1:1,000 solution is administered subcutaneously.

Xanthines
Xanthines relax bronchial smooth muscle (in both acute/chronic situations, and often in combination with other drugs). Several mechanisms for this activity have been proposed, but none have been definitively proved. These mechanisms include inhibition of phosphodiesterase, mobilization of calcium pools, inhibition of prostaglandin activity and decreased uptake of catecholamines.

Anticholinergic agents
Anticholinergic agents act on receptors to prevent smooth muscle contraction. They are marketed for inhalant treatment of chronic obstructive pulmonary disease (but this use is still under investigation).

Evolving Respiratory Therapies

New therapies continue to be targeted at decreasing inflammation. DNase inhibitors are thought to act by breaking up long extracellular DNA into smaller fragments. DNA is considered to contribute to thick sputum, especially in cystic fibrosis patients. Leukotriene antagonists and inhibitors decrease leukotriene levels and thus decrease inflammatory activity of mast cells. In the area of allergen avoidance, there have been efforts to develop products that can control dust-mite allergens and that can denature allergens.

Table 18.5

Respiratory Drugs: Adverse Effects

Body system	Cromolyn	Corticosteroids	Adrenergic agents	Xanthines	Anticholinergic agents
General	Minimal adverse effects	Owing to too-quick withdrawal: flare-up of underlying disease; acute adrenal insufficiency; also (rarely) pseudotumor cerebri	Many side effects related to ß1 effect on cardiovascular system, especially with epinephrine	Flushing	In high environmental temperatures, risk of rare increase in body temperature; geriatric or debilitated patients may respond with excitement, agitation, drowsiness or confusion
CV		*Hypertension, cardiovascular collapse*	Palpitation, tachycardia, hypotension, angina, dysrhythmias (especially with epinephrine)	Palpitation, sinus tachycardia, hypotension, other dysrhythmias	Palpitation (rare)
CNS		Behavioral disturbances (rare)	Tremors, anxiety, insomnia, restlessness, hallucinations, flushing, irritability	Anxiety, restlessness, insomnia, dizziness, convulsions, headaches, lightheadedness, muscle twitching	Anxiety, dizziness, headache
EENT		Cataracts, glaucoma, blurred vision	Dry nose, irritation of nose and throat		Blurred vision (rare)
Endoc		Growth arrest, hyperglycemia, suppression of HPA			

System					
GI	Nausea, vomiting, anorexia	Increased GI upset, nausea, vomiting, peptic ulcers	Heartburn, nausea, vomiting, diarrhea	Nausea, vomiting, anorexia, diarrhea, dyspepsia, gastric distress	Nausea, vomiting, cramps
GU	Urinary frequency, dysuria		Difficulty in urination		
Hema	*Increased susceptibility to infection*				
HB				Hepatotoxicity	
Integ	Rash, urticaria, angioedema	Acne, poor or delayed wound healing, hirsutism, striae, ecchymoses		Urticaria	Rash (rare)
Metab		Catabolism, fat redistribution			
Musc	Joint pain/swelling	Fractures, osteoporosis, muscular weakness	Muscle cramps		
Oral	Irritation, dryness of throat, burning mouth, bitter taste, possible candidiasis	Dry mouth, poor or delayed wound healing, petechiae, candidiasis	Taste changes, xerostomia, discoloration of teeth	Bitter taste, xerostomia	Xerostomia, stomatitis, metallic taste
Renal		Fluid, electrolyte abnormalities			
Resp			Bronchospasm	Increased rate of respiration	Cough, worsening of symptoms

Italics indicate information of major clinical significance.

Table 18.6

Respiratory Drugs: Precautions and Contraindications

Drug	Precautions and contraindications
Adrenergic agonists	Concern about possible β1 side effects related to effects on heart in patients with tachydysrhythmias, hypertension, severe cardiac disease
	Some agents may appear in breast milk
	Should be used cautiously with patients who have hyperthyroidism, diabetes mellitus, prostatic hypertrophy, narrow-angle glaucoma, seizures
	Pregnancy risk category: C
	Epinephrine: Contraindicated in patients taking MAO inhibitors
Anticholinergic agents	Should be used cautiously with patients who have narrow-angle glaucoma, prostatic hypertrophy, bladder neck obstruction
	Pregnancy risk category: B
	Contraindicated for children aged < 12 y
Corticosteroids	Possible bacterial/fungal infections
	Consider using semisupine position while carrying out dental treatment
	May require stress reduction
	Concern about possible adrenal crisis for patients taking high doses and/or receiving chronic therapy
	Pregnancy risk category: C
	Contraindicated for children aged < 12 y
	Contraindicated in acute situations
Cromolyn	Should be used cautiously in lactating women and in patients with hepatic disease
	Pregnancy risk category: B
	Contraindicated for children aged < 5 y
	Contraindicated in acute situations
Xanthines	Should be used cautiously in pediatric and elderly patients and patients who have congestive heart failure, cor pulmonale, hepatic disease, active peptic ulcer, diabetes, hyperthyroidism, hypertension, glaucoma, prostatic hypertrophy, tachydysrhythmias
	Pregnancy risk category: C

Italics indicate information of major clinical significance.

Suggested Readings

Abramowicz M, ed. Zafirlukast for asthma. Med Lett Drugs Ther 1996;38(990):111.

Abramowicz M, ed. Drugs for asthma. Med Lett Drugs Ther 1996;37(939):1-4.

Barnes PJ, Roger IW, Thomson NC, eds. Asthma: basic mechanisms and clinical management. 2nd ed. New York: Academic Press; 1992.

Call RS, Platt-Mills TAE. Drugs used in asthma and obstructive lung disease. In: Brody TM, Larner J, Minneman KP, Neu HC, eds. Human pharmacology: molecular to clinical. 2nd ed. St. Louis: Mosby; 1994: 775-86.

Chapter 19

Gastrointestinal Drugs

B. Ellen Byrne, R.Ph., D.D.S., Ph.D.

"Heartburn" occurs daily in approximately 7% of the population. It is a symptom of reflux esophagitis, an irritation and inflammation of the esophageal mucosa caused by the reflux of acidic stomach or duodenal contents retrograde into the esophagus. Reflux esophagitis is commonly seen in gastroesophageal reflux disease (GERD) and peptic ulcer disease (PUD), which are considered together in this chapter because the same drugs are used to treat them. Other symptoms associated with GERD include regurgitation, dysphagia, bleeding and chest pain. Regurgitation is the most specific symptom of GERD and may result in morning hoarseness, laryngitis and pulmonary aspiration.

PUD is a heterogeneous group of disorders characterized by ulceration of the upper gastrointestinal tract. Peptic ulcer disease can occur at any place in the gastrointestinal (GI) tract that is exposed to the erosive action of pepsin and acid. It can be exacerbated by stress, alcohol, cigarette smoking, some foods and aspirin and aspirinlike drugs. Medical therapy for GERD and PUD consists mainly of neutralizing the stomach contents or reducing gastric acid secretions.

Diarrhea is usually caused by infection, toxins or drugs. Antidiarrheal agents can be sold over the counter or by prescription only. Virally or bacterially induced diarrhea is usually transient and requires only a clear liquid diet and increased fluid intake. Antimicrobial therapy may be indicated. Intravenous fluids may be required if dehydration occurs.

Drug- or toxin-induced diarrhea is best treated by discontinuing the causative agent when possible. Chronic diarrhea may be caused by laxative abuse, lactose intolerance, inflammatory bowel disease, malabsorption syndromes, endocrine disorders or irritable bowel syndrome. Treatment of chronic diarrhea should be aimed at correcting the cause of diarrhea rather than alleviating the symptoms.

"Gastroparesis" is the term for disorders causing gastric stasis. Nausea, vomiting, bloating, fullness and early satiety are signs of gastroparesis. Treatment is aimed at acclerating gastric emptying. This condition is often associated with diabetes.

Crohn's disease and ulcerative colitis are considered together because the same drugs are used to treat these disorders. Crohn's disease is a chronic inflammatory disease that can affect any part of the gastrointestinal system, from mouth to anus. The etiology is unknown. The most common symptoms are abdominal pain and diarrhea. Perirectal fissure with sinus formation and strictures is common.

Ulcerative colitis is an inflammatory disease of the gastrointestinal tract that is limited to the colon and rectum. Typically, patients with ulcerative colitis present with bloody diarrhea. The disease primarily affects young adults. The etiology is unknown. Management of both Crohn's disease and ulcerative colitis is aimed at decreasing the inflammation and providing symptomatic relief.

Antidiarrheal Agents

Special Dental Considerations

There are no contraindications to the dental treatment of patients with diarrhea.

Most acute diarrhea is self-limiting. The opiates and anticholinergics used to treat diarrhea produce xerostomia, therefore, meticulous oral hygiene should be stressed. These drugs also produce drowsiness and this effect is additive with other CNS depressants, thereby producing greater drowsiness.

Drug interactions of dental interest

Drugs used to treat diarrhea include opiates and absorbents. Drug interactions of concern with opiate (narcotics) would occur if the patient took another CNS depressant drug, such as alcohol, antidepressants, antianxiety agents, anticholinergics, antihistamines or barbiturates. This combination of drugs may seriously increase the side effect of either drug.

Adsorbent drugs such as bismuth salts and cholestyramine can bind with various drugs resulting in decreased adsorption of the drug and a decreased therapeutic response. If these drugs must be taken together it is best to space dosing by 6 h.

See Table 19.1 for general information on antidiarrheal agents.

Pharmacology

Antidiarrheal agents can be divided into antibiotic and nonantibiotic drugs. Antibiotics are the mainstay of treatment of acute bacterial diarrhea. Whenever possible, antibiotics should be directed toward specific microorganisms either identified by culture or clinically suspected.

There are many commercial preparations sold for symptomatic relief of diarrhea. Controlled clinical trials have not proven the safety and effectiveness of most of them.

Adsorbents have been shown to increase stool consistency but do not decrease stool water content.

Anticholinergics relieve cramps by reducing contractile activity but have no effect on diarrhea.

Bismuth subsalicylate binds toxins and prevents bacteria from attaching to intestinal epithelium.

Cholestyramine has been shown to effectively bind *Clostridium difficile* toxins and perhaps other bacterial toxins.

The opiates have a profound effect on motility. These agents are generally contraindicated in dysentery.

In general, these nonspecific antidiarrheal agents should not be used as a substitute for oral rehydration and directed antibiotics.

Table 19.1

Antidiarrheal Agents: Dosage Information

Generic name	Brand name(s)	Dosage range (daily)	Interactions with other drugs
		Adsorbents	
Bismuth subsalicylate	Pepto-Bismol, Bismatrol Extra Strength, Pepto-Bismol Maximum Strength	524-4,200 mg	**Decreased effects:** tetracyclines, uricosurics **Increased effects:** aspirin, warfarin, anticoagulants, antidiabetic agents, oral or insulin

Continued on next page

Table 19.1 (cont.)
Antidiarrheal Agents: Dosage Information

Generic name	Brand name(s)	Dosage range (daily)	Interactions with other drugs
Adsorbents (cont.)			
Cholestyramine	Questran, Questran Light	4-24 g	Concurrent use of cholestyramine may decrease absorption of fat-soluble vitamins, digoxin, diuretics, penicillin G, tetracyclines, coumadin, anticoagulants, vancomycin, thyroid hormones, phenylbutazine
Kaolin/pectin	Kaopectate, Kao-Span, K-P, Kapectolin	1.2-9 g; 60-120 mL after each loose bowel movement	Decreased absorption of orally administered clindamycin, tetracycline, penicillamine, digoxin, anticholinergics, antidyskinetics, lincomycins, loxapine, phenothiazines, thioxanthenes
Opiates			
Codeine	Generic	60-120 mg	Increased effects with CNS depressants
Diphenoxylate HCl and atropine sulfate	Lomotil, Lofene, Logen, Locomot, Lonox, VI-Atro	15-20 mg; maintenance: 5 mg	Increases effects with CNS depressants, anticholinergics May cause drowsiness Avoid alcoholic beverages May suppress respiration in elderly, very ill, or patients with respiratory problems
Loperamide	Imodium A-D, Kaopectate II, Maalox Anti-Diarrheal, Pepto Diarrhea Control	4-16 mg	Concurrent use with opioid analgesic may increase risk of severe constipation
Paregoric	Generic	5-40 mL (equivalent to 2-16 mg of anhydrous morphine)	At high doses, produces effects of opiates—dizziness, faintness, lightheadedness, antidiuretic effect, CNS effects, hypotension, ureteral spasm, xerostomia

Crohn's Disease and Ulcerative Colitis Drugs

Special Dental Considerations

There are no contraindications to the dental treatment of patients with Crohn's disease. The leukopenic and thrombocytopenic effects of sulfasalazine may increase the incidence of certain microbial infections, delay healing and increase gingival bleeding. If a patient has leukopenia or thrombocytopenia, dental treatment should be deferred until laboratory counts have returned to normal. Patients treated with corticosteroids are likely to have a decreased resistance to infection and a poor wound healing response. Actual and potential sources of infection in the mouth should be treated promptly. If surgical procedures are necessary, they should be as atraumatic, conservative and aseptic as possible. Prophylactic antibiotic coverage should be considered in most cases. Adrenal suppression owing to the administration of corticosteroids is also a consideration. Depending on the dose and length of treatment, the patient may require an increased dose of corticosteroids before undergoing stressful dental treatment.

For patients with ulcerative colitis, use of antibiotics may aggravate the problem.

Antibiotics most often associated with ulcerative colitis are broad-spectrum penicillins.

Drug interactions of dental interest

See Table 19.2 for general information on Crohn's disease and ulcerative colitis drugs.

Pharmacology

Crohn's disease is a chronic inflammatory

Table 19.2

Crohn's Disease and Ulcerative Colitis Drugs: Dosage Information

Generic name	Brand name(s)	Dosage range (daily)	Interactions with other drugs
Antibiotics			
Metronidazole	Flagyl, Metric 21, Protostat, generic	1,500-2,000 mg	**Antabuse reaction:** alcohol and alcohol-containing products
			Potentiates effects of anticoagulants
			Concurrent use of cimetadine may result in decreased serum metronidazole concentrations
			Should not be used concurrently with or 2 w after administration of disulfiram in alcoholic patients; may result in confusion and psychotic reactions
Bowel disease suppressant			
Sulfasalazine	Azulfidine	1-4 g; maintenance 2 g	Increases half-life of oral hypoglycemics (chlorpropamide, acetohexamide), anticoagulants, anticonvulsants, hemolytics, hepatotoxic medications, methotrexate, phenylbutazone, sulfin pyrazone
Corticosteroids			
Prednisone	**Syrup:** Liquid Pred **Tablets:** Meticorten, Orasone, Deltasone, Predicen-M, Sterapred, Sterapred DS	5-60 mg up to 250 mg	Decreases effect of salicylates Decreased effect with barbiturates, phenytoin, ritampin
Immunosuppressants			
Azathioprine	Imuran	1-5 mg/kg/day **Initial dose:** Up to 2.5 mg/kg/day **Maintenance dose:** Reduced from initial dose to minimum effective dose	Allopurinol increases azathioprine activity and toxicity Concurrent administration with immunosuppressants may increase risk of infection and development of neoplasms Vaccines should not be administered for 3-12 mo after use

condition of the gastrointestinal tract. Current therapy is directed at reducing inflammation and providing systematic relief. Initial treatment includes sulfasalazine antibiotics and nutritional support. Sulfasalazine (through its active component 5-aminosalicylic acid [5-ASA]) exerts an anti-inflammatory effect on the colon. Metronidazole is most commonly used and likely functions by reducing bacterial endotoxin and granuloma formation.

Second-line therapy includes the use of corticosteroids for reduction of inflammation followed by the use of immunomodulating drugs, such as azothioprine, which also reduce inflammation.

Gastric Motility Disorder (Gastroparesis) Drugs

Special Dental Considerations

There are no contraindications to the dental treatment of patients with gastroparesis.

Drug interactions of dental interest

Drugs which treat gastroparesis increase gastrointestinal mobility and decrease gastric emptying time. Oral absorption from the stomach may be decreased while absorption from the small intestine may be enhanced.

Cisapride is contraindicated with the macrolide antibiotics clarithromycin, erythromycin and troleandomycin. These antibiotics inhibit the hepatic metabolism of cisapride, resulting in cardiotoxicity.

See Table 19.3 for general information on gastric motility disorder drugs.

Pharmacology

Diabetic gastroparesis is a common GI complication of diabetes mellitus. Caused by delayed gastric emptying, the symptoms range from early satiety and bloating to severe gastric retention with nausea, vomiting and abdominal pain. Impaired gastric emptying is caused by abnormal motility of the stomach or a reduction in motor activity in the intestine. Metoclopramide affects gut motility through indirect cholinergic stimulation of the gut muscle, whereas cisapride stimulates GI motility by enhancing the physiological release of acetylcholine in GI smooth muscle.

Gastroesophageal Reflux Disease and Peptic Ulcer Disease Drugs

Special Dental Considerations

There are no contraindications to the dental treatment of patients with GERD or PUD; however, drugs that cause gastrointestinal injury should be avoided in patients with GERD or PUD. These drugs include erythromycin, aspirin, corticosteroids and nonsteroidal anti-inflammatory agents. Dental patients with GERD should be kept in a semisupine chair position for patient comfort because of the reflux effects of this disease. Xerostomia is a common side effect of the anticholinergic agents and meticulous oral hygiene must be emphasized. Many anticholinergic agents also induce orthostatic or postural hypotension. Therefore, dental patients treated with one of these agents should remain in the dental chair in an upright position for several minutes before being dismissed.

Drug interactions of dental interest

Drugs used to treat GERD and PUD include antacids, H_2 histamine receptor antagonists and anticholinergics.

Antacids potentially interfere with the absorption of many drugs by forming a complex with these drugs or by altering gastric pH. Antacids containing metal cations (Mg^{2+}, Ca^{2+}, Al^{3+}) have a strong affinity for tetracycline, and response to the antibiotic can vary according to the extent of the complex.

Antacids increase the intragastric pH, and this can decrease the absorption of drugs that require an acidic environment for dissolution and absorption. Conversely, enteric-coated drugs such as erythromycin may be released prematurely.

Table 19.3

Gastric Motility Disorder (Gastroparesis) Drugs: Dosage Information

Generic name	Brand name(s)	Dosage range (daily)	Interactions with other drugs
Cisapride	Propulsid	60 mg q day (20 mg tid)	Because of increased gastrointestinal mobility and decreased gastric emptying time, absorption of oral medicaments from the stomach may be decreased, while absorption from the small intestine may be enhanced
			Decreased effect: anticholinergics
			Contraindicated for concomitant use with clarithromycin, erythromycin, troleandomycin, fluconazole, itraconazole, ketoconazole, miconazole; potentially fatal owing to increased plasma concentrations of cisapride
Metoclopramide HCl	**Syrup:** Reglan, generic **Tablets:** Clopra, Octamide, Reclomide, Reglan, generic	40 mg q day (10 mg qid)	Because of increased gastrointestinal mobility and decreased gastric emptying time, absorption of oral medications from stomach may be decreased, while absorption from small intestine may be enhanced
			Enhanced CNS depression with opiate analgesics and alcohol

Most of these drug-antacid interactions can be minimized by administering each drug 2 h from the other.

The H_2 histamine receptor antagonist cimetadine can bind to the cytochrome P450 mixed-function oxidase system and can inhibit the biotransformation of drugs by the liver. This results in inhibition of metabolism and increased serum drug concentrations of the drug not metabolized. Serum levels of some benzodiazepines (diazepam, alprazolam, chlorodiazepoxide, midazolam, triazolam) have been shown to increase, resulting in enhanced sedation.

Anticholinergics can decrease gastric emptying time, which can increase the amount of drug absorbed or increase the degradation of a drug in the stomach, thus decreasing the amount of drug absorbed. Overall, this interaction appears to have minor significance.

See Table 19.4 for general information on GERD and PUD drugs.

Pharmacology

H_2 histamine receptor antagonists are effective for short-term treatment of GERD and PUD. These agents prevent histamine-induced acid release by competing with histamine for H_2 receptors.

Proton-pump inhibitors (such as omeprazole) act by irreversibly blocking the H^+/K^+-ATPase pump. It markedly inhibits both basal and stimulated gastric acid secretion.

Antacids act by neutralizing gastric acid and thus raising the gastric pH. This has the effect of inhibiting peptic activity, which practically ceases at pH 5. The antacids in common use are salts of magnesium and aluminum. Magnesium salts cause diarrhea and aluminum salts cause constipation, so mixtures of the two are used to maintain bowel function.

Table 19.4

Gastroesophageal Reflux Disease and Peptic Ulcer Disease Drugs: Dosage Information

Generic name	Brand name(s)	Dosage range (daily)	Interactions with other drugs
Antacids			
Aluminum salts	Alternagel, Alu-Cap, Aluminum Hydroxide Gel, Alu-Tab, Amphojel, Phosphaljel	10-60 mL; 300-10,080 mg	Decreased absorption of tetracyclines, digoxin, indomethacin, or iron salts, benzodiazepines
Calcium salts	Camalox, Robalate, Tums, Mylanta Soothing Lozenges, Mylanta, Mylanta DS, Marblen	2-16 tablets (500-10,000 mg)	Decreased absorption of tetracyclines
Magnesium salts and aluminum salts	Maalox TC, Delcid, Gelusil II, Maalox, Mylanta, Riopan, Gelusil, Mylanta DS, Aludrox, Milk of Magnesia	10-80 mL; 400-9,600 mg	Decreased absorption of tetracyline, digoxin
Anticholinergic acids			
Pirenzepine [CAN]	Gastrozepin [CAN]	100-150 mg	May cause blurred vision; with anticholinergics, possible decrease in gastric emptying time, which changes amount of drug absorbed (overall, this interaction is of minor significance)
Propantheline bromide	Pro-Banthine	22.5-120 mg	May delay absorption of concurrently ingested drugs
			Excessive cholinergic blockade may occur if given with belladonna alkaloids, synthetic or semisynthetic anticholinergics, antihistamines, phenothiazines, tricyclic antidepressants, or other psychoactive drugs
			Increases intraocular pressure if given with corticosteroids
Mepenzolate bromide	Cantil	100-200 mg	May cause blurred vision; with anticholinergics, possible decrease in gastric emptying time, which changes amount of drug absorbed (overall, this interaction is of minor significance)
Methscopolamine bromide	Pamine	10-20 mg	May cause blurred vision; with anticholinergics possible decrease in gastric emptying time, which changes amount of drug absorbed (overall this interaction is of minor significance)

[CAN] indicates a drug available only in Canada.

Continued on next page

Table 19.4 (cont.)

Gastroesophageal Reflux Disease and Peptic Ulcer Disease Drugs: Dosage Information

Generic name	Brand name(s)	Dosage range (daily)	Interactions with other drugs
H₂ histamine receptor antagonists			
Cimetidine	Tagamet	800-1,200 mg	Reduced absorption of ketoconazole, reduced hepatic clearance of lidocaine, benzodiazepines, metronidazole, warfarin-type anticoagulants, phenytoin, propanolol, nifedipine (chlordiazepoxide, diazepam), certain tricyclic antidepressants, theophylline
Famotidine	Pepcid, Pepcid AC	**Pepsid:** 40-640 mg, **Pepcid AC:** 10-20 mg	None
Nizatidine	Axid	150-300 mg	Only in very high doses of aspirin (3,900 mg/day), elevated serum salicylate levels seen with 150 mg bid nizatidine
Ranitidine	Zantac	150-600 mg	None
Miscellaneous			
Metoclopramide HCl	Reglan	40-60 mg	Opiate analgesics increase CNS depression
			GI motility affects antagonized by anticholinergics and narcotic analgesics
			Additive sedative effects with alcohol, sedatives, hypnotics, narcotics or tranquilizers
			Use cautiously, if at all, with monoamine oxidase inhibitors
			May decrease absorption of digoxin
			May increase rate and/or extent of absorption of acetaminophen, tetracycline, levodopa, ethanol and cyclosporine
Misoprostol	Cytotec	400-800 µg	Increases diarrhea when given with magnesium-containing antacids
Omeprazole	Prilosec	20-40 mg; up to 360 mg in pathological hypersecretory conditions	Decreases effect of ketoconazole; increases effect of benzodiazepines, digoxin, phenytoin and warfarin
Sucralfate	Carafate	2-4 g	If taken concurrently, decreases absorption of tetracycline, cimetidine, digoxin, fluoroquinolone antibiotics, ketoconazoles, l-thyroxine, phenytoin, quinidine, ranitidine, theophylline

Drugs that protect the mucosa can do so by either forming a protective physical barrier over the surface of the ulcer (sucralfate) or enhancing or augmenting endogenous prostaglandins (misoprostol) to promote bicarbonate and mucin release and inhibit acid secretion.

Anticholinergic agents (such as propantheline bromide) have played a limited role in the treatment of PUD by inhibiting vagally stimulated gastric acid secretion. These agents are not considered first-line agents for treatment of PUD.

Adverse Effects, Precautions and Contraindications

Adverse effects are provided in Table 19.5. Gastrointestinal drug precautions and contraindications are provided in Table 19.6.

Suggested Readings

Tatro DS, ed. Drug interactions facts: facts and comparisons. St. Louis: A Wolters Kluwer; 1995.

Young LY, Koda-Kimble MA, eds. Applied therapeutics: The clinical use of drugs. 6th ed. Vancouver, Wash.: Applied Therapeutics; 1995.

Table 19.5

Gastrointestinal Drugs: Adverse Effects

Body system	Antidiarrheal agents	Crohn's disease and ulcerative colitis drugs	Gastric motility disorder (gastroparesis) drugs	Gastroesophageal reflux disease and peptic ulcer disease drugs
General	**Bismuth subsalicylate:** Anxiety, confusion **Opiates:** Headache	**Azathioprine:** Pancreatitis **Corticosteroids:** Insomnia, depression, flushing **Metronidazole:** Headache **Sulfasalazine:** Agranulocytosis; Stevens-Johnson syndrome	**Cisapride:** Headache **Metoclopramide:** Drowsiness, restlessness, agranulocytosis, extrapyramidal effects	**Anticholinergics:** Hyperpyrexia **H$_2$ histamine receptor antagonists:** Dizziness, headache, drowsiness **Metoclopramide:** Weakness, restlessness, drowsiness, insomnia, depression **Misoprostol:** Headache **Omeprazole:** Headache
CV	**Opiates:** Angioneurotic edema	**Corticosteroids:** Hypertension	**Cisapride:** Tachycardia	**Anticholinergics:** Circulatory collapse, hypotension, tachycardia **Omeprazole:** Edema, tachycardia, bradycardia
CNS	**Opiates:** Sedation, drowsiness, depression	**Corticosteroids:** Nervousness **Metronidazole:** Dizziness, convulsions		**Anticholinergics:** Delirium, hallucinations, psychosis **Metoclopramide:** Restlessness, drowsiness, insomnia, depression **Omeprazole:** Dizziness **Sucralfate:** Drowsiness, dizziness
EENT	**Bismuth subsalicylate:** Buzzing in ears			**Anticholinergics:** Blurred vision

GI	**Bismuth subsalicylate:** fecal impactions may occur in infants and debilitated patients **Cholestyramine:** Constipation, nausea and vomiting, irritation of perianal area **Kaolin/pectin:** Constipation, fecal impaction **Opiates:** Nausea and vomiting	**Azathioprine:** Nausea and vomiting **Metronidazole:** Nausea and vomiting, pseudo-membranous colitis **Sulfasalazine:** Bleeding ulcers, nausea and vomiting	**Cisapride:** Diarrhea **Metoclopramide:** Diarrhea	**Antacids:** Constipation, stomach cramps; magnesium salts–diarrhea; calcium salts–constipation, flatulence **Anticholinergics:** Constipation **H$_2$ histamine receptor antagonists:** Diarrhea, nausea and vomiting **Metoclopramide:** Nausea, diarrhea **Misoprostol:** Diarrhea, constipation, nausea, vomiting, abdominal pain **Omeprazole:** Nausea, vomiting, diarrhea, constipation, irritable colon **Sucralfate:** Constipation, nausea, vomiting
GU	**Opiates:** Urinary retention			**Anticholinergics:** Urinary retention
Hema		**Corticosteroids:** Thrombocytopenia **Sulfasalazine:** Leukopenia, neutropenia, thrombocytopenia **Metronidazole:** Leukopenia **Azathioprine:** Leukopenia, thrombocytopenia		
HB		**Sulfasalazine:** Renal failure **Azathioprine:** Hepatotoxicity, jaundice		
Integ	**Cholestyramine:** Rash, irritation of skin	**Corticosteroids:** Poor wound healing, petechiae		
Musc				**Omeprazole:** Back pain; muscle, joint and leg pain

Continued on next page

Table 19.5 (cont.)

Gastrointestinal Drugs: Adverse Effects

Body system	Antidiarrheal agents	Crohn's disease and ulcerative colitis drugs	Gastric motility disorder (gastroparesis) drugs	Gastroesophageal reflux disease and peptic ulcer disease drugs
Oral	**Opiates:** Xerostomia **Bismuth subsalicylate:** Discoloration of tongue (darkening due to bismuth) **Cholestyramine:** Irritation of tongue	**Corticosteroids:** Xerostomia, oral candidiasis **Sulfasalazine:** Stomatitis, glossitis **Metronidazole:** Xerostomia, metallic taste, glossitis, stomatitis, change in taste **Azathioprine:** Stomatitis, oral ulcerations	**Cisapride:** Xerostomia **Metoclopramide:** Xerostomia	**Antacids:** Aluminum hydroxide–chalky taste **Anticholinergics:** Xerostomia **Metoclopramide:** Xerostomia **Omeprazole:** Xerostomia, taste alterations **Sucralfate:** Metallic taste, xerostomia
Resp	**Kaolin/pectin:** Pneumoconiosis if large amounts inhaled			**Omeprazole:** Cough

Table 19.6

Gastrointestinal Drugs: Precautions and Contraindications

Drug category	Precautions and contraindications
Antidiarrheals	**Opiates:** Use cautiously in patients who have hepatic disease, renal disease, severe liver disease, glaucoma, electrolyte imbalances or who are nursing mothers or children < 2 y; pregnancy risk category C
	Adsorbents
	Bismuth subsalicylate: Subsalicylates should be used with caution if patient is taking aspirin because of possible additive toxicity; use with caution in children < 3 y; do not use subsalicylates in patients with influenza or chicken pox because of risk of Reye's syndrome
	Kaolin/pectin: May mask dehydration, may make recognition of parasitic causes of diarrhea more difficult; check with physician if diarrhea not controlled within 48 h and/or if fever develops
	Cholestyramine: Use with caution in patients with constipation; pregnancy risk category C
Crohn's disease and ulcerative colitis drugs	**Corticosteroids:** Use cautiously in patients with diabetes mellitus, glaucoma, osteoporosis, renal disease, peptic ulcer, congestive heart failure
	Sulfasalazine: Use cautiously in patients with hypersensitivity to sulfonamides or salicylates or impaired renal or hepatic function or are nursing mothers; pregnancy risk category B
	Metronidazole: Use cautiously in patients who have *Candida* infections or are pregnant; pregnancy risk category B
	Azathioprine: Use cautiously in patients who have severe hepatic and renal disease; pregnancy risk category D
Gastric motility disorder drugs	**Metoclopramide:** Use cautiously in patients who have epilepsy, gastrointestinal hemorrhage, mechanical obstruction; pregnancy risk category B
	Cisapride: Use cautiously in patients who have gastrointestinal hemorrhage, mechanical obstruction, perforation; pregnancy risk category C; potentially fatal with mycins (for example, erythromycin, clindamycin) and antifungal azoles (fluconazole, ketoconazole, miconazole, itraconazole)
Gastroesophageal reflux disease and peptic ulcer disease drugs	**H₂ histamine receptor antagonists:** May cause agitation, reduce dosage in hepatic/renal disease; American Academy of Pediatrics has recommended that cimetidine not be taken by lactating mothers; pregnancy risk category B
	Antacids: Aluminum hydroxide—prolonged administration or large doses may cause hypophosphatemia.
	Magnesium salts—use with caution in patients with renal impairment
	Calcium salts—use with caution in patients who are taking digitalis or have congestive heart failure or renal failure
	Anticholinergic agents: May cause agitation, mental confusion; may inhibit lactation; pregnancy risk category C
	Miscellaneous
	Sucralfate: Use not established in children; pregnancy category B
	Metoclopramide: Should be used cautiously in patients with Parkinson's disease; dose should be modified for patients with renal failure; pregnancy risk category B
	Omeprazole: Pregnancy risk category C
	Misoprostol: Safety and efficacy not established in children < 18 y; use with caution in elderly patients and patients with renal impairment; pregnancy risk category X

Chapter 20

Neurological Drugs

Steven Ganzberg, D.M.D., M.S.

Patients who are receiving ongoing treatment of neurological conditions consult the dentist for oral healthcare. One of the more common neurological conditions dentists see among these patients is seizure disorders; but they also may encounter other conditions such as Parkinson's disease, multiple sclerosis, Alzheimer's disease, myasthenia gravis and other myopathies, spasticity resulting from spinal cord injury, and poststroke syndrome, among others. Long-term medication management is common. The dentist may also prescribe neurological drugs for treatment of pains of neuropathic origin as well as for primary headache syndromes, such as migraine, cluster and tension-type headaches. For general information on neurological drugs, see Tables 20.1-20.5.

Patients presenting with neurological conditions should have their condition and level of disease control (for example, quality of seizure control) reviewed. If warranted, delay in elective dental treatment may be prudent pending medical consultation. Vital signs, including respiratory status, should be evaluated preoperatively. Adverse effects are provided in Table 20.6 and precautions/contraindications in Table 20.7.

Anticonvulsant Drugs

Anticonvulsant drugs are typically used to control epilepsy, a convulsive disorder characterized by intermittent excessive discharges of neurons. This dysregulation of neural function is frequently associated with altered or lost consciousness. Seizure disorders have been characterized as generalized, including tonic-clonic (grand mal) seizures, absence, partial, atonic and unclassified. Specific anticonvulsant agents have been shown to be superior for some types of seizures.

In orofacial pain management, anticonvulsants are useful in treating trigeminal neuralgia and other posttraumatic trigeminal neuropathies. Carbamazepine, phenytoin, valproic acid and its derivatives, and clonazepam (as well as baclofen, an antispastic), have been reported to be useful. A newer anticonvulsant, gabapentin, is also being investigated in this regard. Certain anticonvulsants have been reported to provide some benefit for migraine headache as well. These medications have numerous side effects, some life-threatening. The dentist prescribing an anticonvulsant drug is presumed to have established a proper diagnosis and to be fully aware of the drug's interactions, adverse effects and contraindications.

See Table 20.1 for basic information on anticonvulsant drugs.

Special Dental Considerations

Many anticonvulsants can cause blood dyscrasias, xerostomia and/or Stevens-Johnson syndrome. These drugs should be considered in the differential diagnosis of oral lesions if signs or symptoms warrant it. Valproic acid/divalproex sodium may inhibit platelet aggregation. Acetazolamide can cause taste changes and perioral numbness or tingling.

Table 20.1

Anticonvulsant Drugs: Dosage Information

Generic name	Brand name(s)*	Dosage range (daily)	Interactions with other drugs
Acetazolamide	Acetazolam, Apo-Acetazolamide, Dazamide, Diamox, Storzolamide	375-1,000 mg	**Aspirin:** Risk of salicylate toxicity
Carbamazepine	Apo-Carbamazepine, Epitol, Novocarbamaz, Tegretol	200-1,600 mg	**Acetaminophen (prolonged use):** Increased risk of hepatic toxicity **CNS depressants:** Increased sedative effects **Corticosteroids:** Increased metabolism **Propoxyphene, erythromycin/clarithromycin:** Decreased metabolism, increased risk of toxicity
Clonazepam	Klonopin	1.5-20 mg	**CNS depressants (for example, alcohol, opioids and sedative antihistamines):** May potentiate sedative side effects
Diazepam	Apo-Diazepam, D-Val, Novodipam, Valium, Valrelease, Vivol, Zetran	0.1 mg/kg IV for emergency treatment of seizures **Oral, extended-release capsules:** 15-30 mg/day **Oral, solution or tablets:** 2-10 mg bid-qid **Injection—preoperative:** 5-10 mg	**CNS depressants (for example, alcohol, opioids and sedative antihistamines):** May potentiate sedative side effects
Ethosuximide	Zarontin	500-1,500 mg	**Acetaminophen (prolonged use):** Increased risk of hepatic toxicity **CNS depressants:** Increased sedative effects **Corticosteroids:** Increased metabolism
Ethotoin	Peganone	500-3,000 mg	**Acetaminophen (prolonged use):** Increased risk of hepatic toxicity **Aspirin:** Increased plasma concentration **CNS depressants:** Increased sedative effects **Corticosteroids, benzodiazepines, barbiturates:** Increased metabolism **Fluconazole, ketaconazole, metronidazole:** Decreased metabolism and increased plasma concentration **Lidocaine (high dose):** Increased risk of cardiac arrhythmia

* Drugs with the prefixes Apo- and Novo- are available only in Canada.

Continued on next page

Table 20.1 (cont.)
Anticonvulsant Drugs: Dosage Information

Generic name	Brand name(s)	Dosage range (daily)	Interactions with other drugs
Gabapentin	Neurontin	300-3,600 mg	**CNS depressants:** Increased sedative effects
Lamotrigine	Lamictal	50-500 mg/day **With valproic acid:** 25-200 mg/day	**Acetaminophen:** Decreased effect **CNS depressants:** Increased sedative effects
Mephenytoin	Mesantoin	50-1,200 mg	**Acetaminophen (prolonged use):** Increased risk of hepatic toxicity **Aspirin:** Increased plasma concentration **CNS depressants:** Increased sedative effects **Corticosteroids, benzodiazepines, barbiturates:** Increased metabolism **Fluconazole, ketaconazole, metronidazole:** Decreased metabolism and increased plasma concentration **Lidocaine (high dose):** Increased risk of cardiac arrhythmia
Mephobarbital	Mebaral	200-600 mg	**CNS depressants:** Increased sedative effects **Corticosteroids:** Increased metabolism
Metharbitol	Gemonil	100-800 mg	**CNS depressants:** Increased sedative effects **Corticosteroids:** Increased metabolism
Methsuximide	Celontin	300-1,200 mg	**Acetaminophen (prolonged use):** Increased risk of hepatic toxicity **CNS depressants:** Increased sedative effects **Corticosteroids:** Increased metabolism
Paramethadione	Paradione	900-2,400 mg	**CNS depressants:** Increased sedative effects
Phenacemide	Epiclase, Phenurone, Phetylureum	500-5,000 mg	**CNS depressants:** Increased sedative effects
Phenobarbital	Ancalixir, Barbita, Luminal, Solfoton	60-250 mg	**CNS depressants:** Increased sedative effects **Corticosteroids:** Increased metabolism

Continued on next page

Table 20.1 (cont.)

Anticonvulsant Drugs: Dosage Information

Generic name	Brand name(s)	Dosage range (daily)	Interactions with other drugs
Phensuximide	Milontin	500-3,000 mg	**Acetaminophen (prolonged use):** Increased risk of hepatic toxicity **CNS depressants:** Increased sedative effects **Corticosteroids:** Increased metabolism
Phenytoin	Dilantin, Diphenylan, Phenytex	200-600 mg	**Acetaminophen (prolonged use):** Increased risk of hepatic toxicity **Aspirin:** Increased plasma concentration **CNS depressants:** Increased sedative effects **Corticosteroids, benzodiazepines, barbiturates:** Increased metabolism **Fluconazole, ketaconazole, metronidazole:** Decreased metabolism and increased plasma concentration **Lidocaine (high dose):** Increased risk of cardiac arrhythmia
Primidone	Apo-Primidone [CAN], Mysoline, Myidone, Sertan	100-2,000 mg	**Acetaminophen (prolonged use):** Increased risk of hepatic toxicity **CNS depressants:** Increased sedative effects **Corticosteroids:** Increased metabolism
Trimethadione	Tridione, Tridione Dulcets	900-2,400 mg	**CNS depressants:** Increased sedative effects
Valproic acid, divalproex sodium	Depakene, Depakote	5-60 mg/kg/day	**Aspirin/NSAIDs:** Increased risk of bleeding **CNS depressants:** Increased sedative effects

Drug interactions of dental interest

Anticonvulsants are frequently sedating. Sedative agents, including opioids, may potentiate this effect.

Many anticonvulsants induce hepatic microsomal enzymes, causing decreased effectiveness or shorter duration of action of certain concomitantly prescribed drugs. Patients taking anticonvulsants may experience increased metabolism of concomitantly administered corticosteroids, benzodiazepines and barbiturates, a situation that leads to decreased effectiveness of these agents.

Prolonged use of acetaminophen may increase the risk of anticonvulsant-induced hepatic toxicity.

Propoxyphene, erythromycin and clarithromycin may result in decreased metabolism of carbamazepine and increased risk of toxicity.

Fluconazole, ketaconazole and metronidazole may result in decreased metabolism of phenytoin and related hydantoins and increased risk of toxicity. Aspirin may increase plasma concentrations of hydantoins, thereby leading to toxicity. For phenytoin, high doses of lidocaine may have additive cardiac depressant effects.

Laboratory Value Alterations

- With most anticonvulsants (except benzodiazepines, acetazolamide and gabapentin): leukopenia, thrombocytopenia, anemia or pancytopenia is possible.
- With hydantoin derivatives: increase in serum glucose possible.
- With acetazolamide: increase in serum glucose is possible.
- With valproic acid/divalproex sodium: bleeding time is increased.

Special Patients

Pediatric patients

Pediatric patients taking hydantoin derivatives are more prone than adults to gingival enlargement, coarsening of facial features (widening of nasal tip, thickening of lips) and facial hair growth.

Pharmacology

Their primary action is to prevent the spread of abnormal neuronal depolarization from an epileptic focus without completely suppressing that focus. The pharmacological mechanisms of action are varied but generally involve, alone or in combination, stabilization of neuronal sodium channels, increasing γ–aminobutyric acid (GABA) tone, alteration of excitatory amino acid neurotransmission and alteration of calcium ion influx.

Antimyasthenic Drugs

Myasthenia gravis is a progressive disease characterized by a decreased number of functional acetylcholine receptors at the neuromuscular junction, resulting in muscular weakness. Drugs to combat this disease impair acetylcholinesterase, the enzyme that degrades acetylcholine, thus increasing the relative concentration of available acetylcholine.

See Table 20.2 for basic information on antimyasthenic drugs.

Special Dental Considerations

Monitor vital signs, including respiratory status, prior to dental treatment.

Table 20.2

Antimyasthenic Drugs: Dosage Information

Generic name	Brand name(s)	Dosage range (daily)	Interactions with other drugs
Ambenonium	Mytelase Caplets	15-200 mg	**Anticholinergics:** Should not be used without medical consultation **Lidocaine:** High doses may cause decreased muscle function
Neostigmine	Prostigmin	30-150 mg	**Anticholinergics:** Should not be used without medical consultation **Lidocaine:** High doses may cause decreased muscle function
Pyridostigmine	Mestinon, Regonol	60-1,500 mg	**Anticholinergics:** Should not be used without medical consultation **Lidocaine:** High doses may cause decreased muscle function

After supine positioning, the dentist should evaluate the patient for possible postural hypotension by having him or her sit in the dental chair for a minute or two and then evaluating him or her when standing.

These drugs may cause increased salivation. Anticholinergics are generally contraindicated.

Drug interactions of dental interest
There may be a reduced rate of metabolism of ester local anesthetics.

High doses of local anesthetic may depress muscle function.

Pharmacology
Antimyasthenic drugs increase the amount of acetylcholine present at the neuromuscular junction by inhibition of acetylcholinesterase, the enzyme that degrades acetylcholine. The increase in acetylcholine concentration improves muscular function.

Antiparkinsonism Drugs
Parkinson's disease is a central nervous system disorder characterized by resting tremor, frequently accompanied by involuntary mouth and tongue movements, rigidity of the limbs and trunk, postural instability and bradykinesia including loss of facial expressions (masklike facies). Drooling is common due to swallowing incoordination. A relative imbalance between dopamine, acetylcholine and GABA neurotransmission in the basal ganglia and related areas plays a significant role in the pathophysiology of this disorder. Antiparkinsonism drugs attempt to alter this neurotransmitter imbalance.

See Table 20.3 for basic information on antiparkinsonism drugs.

Special Dental Considerations
Many of these drugs can cause xerostomia. The dentist should consider them in the

Table 20.3
Antiparkinsonism Drugs: Dosage Information

Generic name	Brand name(s)*	Dosage range (daily)	Interactions with other drugs
Drugs acting on acetylcholine			
Benztropine	Apo-Benztropine, Cognetin, PMS-Benztropine	1-6 mg	**Phenothiazines, butyrophenones, metoclopramide, and other dopamine antagonists:** Contraindicated in Parkinson's disease
Biperiden	Akineton	2-16 mg	**Anticholinergics:** Additive oral drying effect **CNS depressants:** Increased sedative effects with anticholinergics **Phenothiazines, butyrophenones, metoclopramide, and other dopamine antagonists:** Contraindicated in Parkinson's disease
Diphenhydramine	Benadryl, multiple OTC agents	100-300 mg	**CNS depressants:** CNS and respiratory depressive effects increase with administration of other CNS depressants **MAO inhibitors:** May increase anticholinergic effects
Ethopropazine	Parsidol, Parsitan	50-600 mg	**Phenothiazines, butyrophenones, metoclopramide, and other dopamine antagonists:** Contraindicated in Parkinson's disease

* Drugs with the prefixes Apo- and PMS- are available only in Canada.

Continued on next page

Table 20.3 (cont.)

Antiparkinsonism Drugs: Dosage Information

Generic name	Brand name(s)	Dosage range (daily)	Interactions with other drugs
Drugs acting on acetylcholine (cont.)			
Orphenadrine	Banflex, Disipal, Flexoject, Marflex, Myolin, Myotrol, Noradex, Norflex, Orflagen	150-250 mg	**Phenothiazines, butyrophenones, metoclopramide, and other dopamine antagonists:** Contraindicated in Parkinson's disease
Procyclinide	Kemadrin, PMS-Procyclinide [CAN], Procyclid	7.5-20 mg	See note above
Trihexyphenidyl	Aparkane, Apo-Trihex [CAN], Artane, Trihexane, Trihexy	10-15 mg	See note above
Drugs acting on dopamine			
Amantadine	Symmetrel	100-400 mg	**Phenothiazines, butyrophenones, metoclopramide, and other dopamine antagonists:** Contraindicated in Parkinson's disease
Bromocriptine	Parlodel	1.25-40 mg	See note above
Carbidopa-Levodopa	Sinemet	30 mg/200 mg-300 mg/2,000 mg	**Phenothiazines, butyrophenones, metoclopramide, and other dopamine antagonists:** Contraindicated in Parkinson's disease **Vasoconstrictors:** Less likely than levodopa to stimulate interaction
Levodopa	Dopar, Larodopa	500-8,000 mg	**Phenothiazines, butyrophenones, metoclopramide, and other dopamine antagonists:** Contraindicated in Parkinson's disease **Anticholinergics:** May have additive oral drying effects **Vasocontrictors in local anesthetic solution:** May have exaggerated effects
Pergolide	Permax	0.05-5 mg	**Phenothiazines, butyrophenones, metoclopramide, and other dopamine antagonists:** Contraindicated in Parkinson's disease
Selegiline	Eldepryl, Deprenyl, Novo-Selegiline [CAN]	10 mg	**Meperidine (and possibly other opioids):** May cause hypertensive crisis

Continued on next page

Table 20.3 (cont.)

Antiparkinsonism Drugs: Dosage Information

Generic name	Brand name(s)	Dosage range (daily)	Interactions with other drugs
Miscellaneous			
Clonazepam	Klonopin	0.5-20 mg	**CNS depressants (for example, alcohol, opioids and sedating antihistamines):** May potentiate sedative side effects
			See Chapter 21, Psychoactive Drugs, for more information
Nadolol	Corgard	40-240 mg/day	NSAIDs may partially antagonize antihypertensive effects of these medications
			Clearance of injected local anesthetics from peripheral circulation may decrease
			Opioids may potentiate hypotensive effect of these medications
			Hypertension and bradycardia can occur when epinephrine or levonordefrin in local anesthetic solutions is administered to patients taking nonselective β-blockers
			For more information, see Chapter 17, Cardiovascular Drugs
Propranolol	Apo-Propranolol [CAN], Detensol, Inderal, Novo-Pranol [CAN]	80-640 mg/day	See note above
			For more information, see Chapter 17, Cardiovascular Drugs

[CAN] indicates a drug available only in Canada.

differential diagnosis of caries, periodontal disease or oral candidiasis.

If newly diagnosed mouthing movements (involuntary mouth and tongue movements and/or drooling) are seen, which may indicate a serious medication side effect, consultation with the patient's physician may be appropriate.

Selegiline may cause circumoral burning.

The dentist should monitor the patient's vital signs during all dental visits. After supine positioning, the dentist should ask the patient to sit upright in the dental chair for a minute or two and then monitor the patient when standing.

Drug interactions of dental interest

Patients taking levodopa and high doses of selegiline may have an exaggerated hemodynamic response to vasoconstrictors in local anesthetic solutions. The dentist should employ careful aspiration technique with limited vasoconstrictor (0.04 mg epinephrine). Additional vasoconstrictor may be used after monitoring of vital signs.

Dopamine antagonist medications, such as chlorpromazine, metoclopramide, and promethazine, which may be prescribed for nausea are contraindicated in patients with Parkinson's disease.

Anticholinergics may have an additive oral drying effect and should be used with caution.

In patients taking high doses of selegiline, meperidine (and possibly other opioids) may cause a hyperthermic and possibly hypertensive crisis.

Pharmacology

Parkinson's disease is classically character-ized by an imbalance in dopaminergic and cholinergic neurotransmission with contribu-tions involving GABA neurotransmission in the nigrastriatum. Medications that act on dopamine increase its availability either by increasing the concentration of dopamine precursors (levodopa), decreasing the break-down of precursors (carbidopa), acting as agonists at the dopamine receptor (bromo-criptine, pergolide and amantadine) or decreasing the degradation of dopamine by MAO-B (selegiline). Anticholinergic drugs, or antihistamines with some degree of anti-cholinergic activity, decrease cholinergic tone by blocking cholinergic receptors and improv-ing the balance between dopaminergic and cholinergic transmission. GABA agonists such as clonazepam and other drugs, such as β-blockers, are also useful in some cases.

Antispastic Drugs

Patients taking antispastic drugs typically have spinal cord or other central nervous system lesions. Spasticity can occur in some neuro-logical disorders, such as multiple sclerosis.

Baclofen may also be effective for the treatment of trigeminal neuralgia and other trigeminal neuropathies.

See Table 20.4 for basic information on antispastic drugs.

Special Dental Considerations

Baclofen may cause dry mouth. Dantrolene can rarely cause blood dyscrasias. The dentist should consider these drugs in the differential diagnosis if oral signs and symptoms war-rant it. Tizanidine may cause hypotension.

Drug interactions of dental interest

These drugs may be sedating. Sedative agents, including opioids, may potentiate this effect.

Laboratory value alterations
- Dantrolene may rarely cause blood dycrasias.

Pharmacology

Antispastic drugs work directly on the mus-cle by decreasing calcium release from the sarcoplasmic reticulum (dantrolene), in the CNS by increasing GABA tone (baclofen) or by an α-2 agonist effect (tizanidine).

Vascular Headache Suppressants

There are numerous conditions that cause headache or facial pain. The majority of patients who list headache as a primary condition on the medical history will be diagnosed with migraine, tension-type or cluster headache. Numerous drugs are used to treat these conditions. They can be divided into symptomatic medications, abortive medications and preventive medications. Symptomatic medications include analgesics and antiemetics, both of which have been

Table 20.4

Antispastic Drugs: Dosage Information

Generic name	Brand name(s)	Dosage range (daily)	Interactions with other drugs
Baclofen	Alpha-Baclofen, Lioresal	15-80 mg	**CNS depressants:** Increased sedative effects
Dantrolene	Dantrium (also used for malig-nant hyperthermia)	25-400 mg/day	**CNS depressants:** Increased sedative effects
Tizanidine-HCl	Zanaflex	8-24 mg/day	**CNS depressants:** Increased sedative effects

covered in other chapters and will not be listed here. These drugs generally are taken intermittently for severe head pain, as continued use can aggravate headache conditions.

Abortive medications include those drugs which, when taken at onset of or during a severe headache (such as migraine or cluster headache), will arrest the headache process and in some cases the associated symptoms (such as nausea and photophobia). These medications include ergotamines, sumatriptan, isometheptene mucate combinations and in some cases phenothiazines. These medications can have adverse cardiovascular consequences, but because they generally are taken on an intermittent basis not associated with a dental visit, they should not be of concern in dental care.

Preventive medications are varied and frequently draw from other drug categories. Various cardiovascular medications—including calcium channel blockers and β-blockers—are used for management of chronic headache. Likewise, most antidepressants and some anticonvulsants have been used for headache prevention.

Neuropathic facial pains, if they respond to medical treatment, are usually treated with anticonvulsant or antidepressant medications. Specific conditions may respond to

Table 20.5

Vascular Headache Suppressants (Indicated for Headache Only): Dosage Information

Generic name	Brand name(s)	Dosage range (daily)	Interactions with other drugs
Dihydroergotamine	DHE-45	**IM or SC:** 1 mg; maximum 3 mg/day **IV:** 1 mg slow, maximum 2 mg/day	**Vasoconstrictors:** Increased hypertensive effect if used chronically
Ergotamine tartrate and caffeine	Cafergot, Ercaf, Ergocaff, Gotamine, Wigraine	1-2 mg at onset of headache; maximum 6 mg/day; not to be used more than 2 days/w	See note above
Ergotamine tartrate	Ergomar, Ergostat, Gynergen, Medihaler Ergotamine	1-2 mg at onset of headache; maximum 6 mg/day; not to be used more than 2 days/w, preferably at least 5 days apart	See note above
Isometheptene mucate, dichlorphenazone, acetaminophen	Midrin	4-8 capsules/day	See note above
Methysergide maleate	Sansert	4-6 mg	See note above
Sumatriptan succinate	Imitrex	6 mg SC at onset of headache; 25-100 mg orally at onset of headache	See note above

baclofen, α-blockers or clonidine.

See Table 20.5 for basic information on vascular headache supressants. A thorough discussion of the pharmacological management of headache and facial pain is beyond the scope of this book. Headache suppressant medications, which have not been covered elsewhere in this text, will be presented.

Special Dental Considerations

Abortive headache medications are used only when needed for moderate-to-severe headache and generally not on the day of a dental appointment. If ergot preparations or sumatriptan are used shortly before a dental appointment, vasoconstrictor precautions similar to those for hypertensive patients should be followed. For preventive medications—for example, antidepressants, anticonvulsants or antihypertensives—the dentist should follow precautions listed for that specific category of drug.

The dentist who undertakes primary treatment of head and face pain is presumed to have established a proper diagnosis and to be fully aware of the interactions, adverse effects and contraindications of headache medications.

Drug interactions of dental interest

Ergot derivatives may have hypertensive effects, in which case vasoconstrictors in local anesthetic solutions should be used cautiously.

For preventive medications, see the appropriate drug category.

Laboratory value alterations

- For preventive medications, see the appropriate drug category.
- Methysergide may cause blood dyscrasias.

Pharmacology

Numerous drugs are used for the management of headache and facial pain. The pharmacology reflects the condition that is to be treated. For example, migraine headache is thought to involve abnormal serotonergic transmission. Varied medications, such as antidepressants, ergots and specific antihistamines, alter serotonin neurotransmission and can be effective in the acute or preventive treatment of migraine. Trigeminal neuralgia responds to anticonvulsant medications by decreasing hyperactive neuronal function.

Treatment of headache and facial pain is beyond the scope of this text. For a more complete review of the pharmacological basis of headache and facial pain management, consult appropriate references.

Adverse Effects, Precautions and Contraindications

Table 20.6 presents adverse effects of neurological drugs; Table 20.7 presents precautions and contraindications.

Table 20.6

Neurological Drugs: Adverse Effects

Body system	Anticonvulsant drugs	Antimyasthenic drugs	Antiparkinsonism drugs	Antispastic drugs	Vascular headache suppressants
General	Allergic reaction		If noticeable mouthing movements occur, consultation with patient's physician regarding this medication-related side effect may be appropriate	Allergic reaction	

Continued on next page

Table 20.6 (cont.)

Neurological Drugs: Adverse Effects

Body system	Anticonvulsant drugs	Antimyasthenic drugs	Antiparkinsonism drugs	Antispastic drugs	Vascular headache suppressants
CV	Hypotension, bradycardia, arrhythmia	Hypotension, bradycardia, heart block, arrhythmia, cardiac arrest	**Dopamine agonists:** orthostatic hypotension, arrhythmias, hypertension, Raynaud's phenomena **Anticholinergics:** hypotension, tachycardia, ventricular fibrillation	Hypotension	Cardiac fibrosis, valvular thickening, hypertension, tachycardia, arrhythmias
CNS	Dizziness, drowsiness, sedation, headache, insomnia, slurred speech, trembling, paresthesia	Increased muscarinic and nicotinic effects; dizziness, confusion, weakness	**Dopamine agonists:** involuntary movements, anxiety, dizziness, confusion, headache, dyskinesia, insomnia, mood change **Anticholinergics:** ataxia, drowsiness, nervousness, hallucinations, weakness, decreased sweating	Drowsiness, vertigo, dizziness, insomnia, euphoria, excitement, slurred speech, weakness, fatigue, headache	Headache, dizziness, confusion, drowsiness, tremor
EENT	Hiccups, diplopia, photophobia	Increased nasal discharge Increased lacrimation, miosis, blurred vision	**Dopamine agonists:** stuffy nose, dry nose, blepherospasm, blurred vision **Anticholinergics:** dry nose, blurred vision, mydriasis, eye pain	Tinnitus, nasal congestion, blurred vision, mydriasis	
Endoc	Hypoventilation, respiratory depression		**Anticholinergics:** decreased breast milk production		
GI	Nausea, vomiting, dyspepsia, anorexia, weight loss, constipation	Nausea, vomiting, diarrhea	**Dopamine agonists:** nausea, vomiting, dyspepsia, anorexia, weight loss, constipation, abdominal cramps, GI bleeding **Anticholinergics:** nausea, vomiting	Nausea, vomiting, constipation	Nausea, vomiting
GU		Urinary frequency/urgency	**Dopamine agonists:** urinary retention, difficulty in urinating **Anticholinergics:** urinary retention, difficulty in urinating	Urinary frequency	

Continued on next page

Table 20.6 (cont.)

Neurological Drugs: Adverse Effects

Body system	Anticonvulsant drugs	Antimyasthenic drugs	Antiparkinsonism drugs	Antispastic drugs	Vascular headache suppressants
Hema	Aplastic anemia, agranulocytosis, thrombocytopenia, exacerbation of porphyria, decreased platelet aggregation, blood dyscrasias (with paramathadione, trimethadione, phenytoin, mephenytoin, ethotoin, ethosuximide, methsuximide, phensuximide, mephobarbitol, metharbitol, phenobarbitol, carbamazepine, primidone, phenacemide, divalproex sodium and valproic acid)		**Dopamine agonists:** anemia, leukopenia, neutropenia for amantadine only	Blood dyscrasias (dantrolene only)	Blood dycrasias
HB	Hepatitis			Elevated liver enzymes	Retroperitoneal fibrosis
Integ	Skin rash, Stevens-Johnson syndrome, urticaria	Rash, flushing	**Dopamine agonists:** skin rash, increased sweating **Anticholinergics:** skin rash	Rash	Rash, flushing, hair loss
Musc	Weakness	Weakness	**Dopamine agonists:** leg cramps, dyskinesia	Weakness	Muscle and joint pain
Oral	Dry mouth, glossitis	Increased salivation	Many of these drugs can cause xerostomia **Dopamine agonists:** dry mouth, involuntary mouth movements, drooling, altered taste **Anticholinergics:** dry mouth	Dry mouth, taste changes	
Resp	Hypoventilation, respiratory depression	Respiratory depression, bronchospasm			

Table 20.7

Neurological Drugs: Precautions and Contraindications

Drug category	Precautions and contraindications
Anticonvulsants	Monitor vital signs, including respiratory status, prior to dental appointments Blood dyscrasias may occur Should be prescribed cautiously for patients taking CNS depressants because of additive sedative effects
Antimyasthenic drugs	Monitor vital signs, including respiratory status, prior to dental appointments After supine positioning, evaluate the patient for possible postural hypotension while he or she sits in the dental chair for a minute or two and likewise when standing Anticholinergic agents should be prescribed only upon consultation with physician Should be prescribed cautiously for patients taking CNS depressants because of possible respiratory depression
Antiparkinsonism drugs	After supine positioning, the dentist should ask the patient to sit in the dental chair for a minute or two and then should evaluate the patient when standing for possible postural hypotension Dopamine antagonist medications that may be prescribed for nausea—such as chlorpromazine, metoclopramide and promethazine—are contraindicated in patients with Parkinson's disease
Antispastic drugs	Should be prescribed cautiously for patients taking CNS depressants because of possible respiratory depression
Vascular headache suppressants	Vasoconstrictors: Should be used with caution owing to hypertensive effect of vascular headache suppressants

Suggested Readings

Calne DB, Treatment of Parkinson's disease. New Eng J Med 1993;329:1021-7.

Fraser AD. New drugs for the treatment of epilepsy. Clinical Biochem 1996:29(2):97-110.

McQuay H, Carrol D, et al. Anticonvulsant drugs for the management of pain: a systematic review. Br Med J 1995;311(7012):1047-52.

Millard CB, Broomfield CA. Anticholinesterases: medical applications of neuro-chemical principles. J Neurochem 1995;64(5):1909-18.

Saper JR, Siberstein S, et al. Handbook of headache management. Baltimore: Williams & Wilkins; 1993.

The United States Pharmacopeial Convention, Inc. Drug information for the health care professional. 17th ed. Rockville, Md.: The United States Pharmacopeial Convention, Inc.; 1997.

Chapter 21

Psychoactive Drugs

Steven Ganzberg, D.M.D., M.S.

Approximately one out of every three people will suffer from a mental illness at some point in his or her life. Many of these people will be placed on psychoactive drugs, which may influence dental management. Psychiatric medications include antidepressant, antianxiety, antipsychotic and antimanic drugs as well as sedatives and "sleeping pills" and drugs for attention deficit/hyperactivity disorders and other illnesses.

When treating a patient taking psychoactive medications, common sense dictates that members of the dental team should take care in their personal interactions with the patient. Efforts to minimize anxiety, although routine in dental practice, should be given high priority.

General psychiatric drug information is provided in Tables 21.1-21.6. Adverse effects of psychiatric drugs are provided in Table 21.7; precautions and contraindications are provided in Table 21.8.

Use of Psychoactive Drugs in Dental Practice

The prescription of psychoactive agents by dentists is indicated for a number of conditions, including acute anxiety associated with dental or oral surgery, management of bruxism and management of various orofacial pain conditions. These agents also have a place in dentistry for sedation and general anesthesia; this use is covered in Chapter 3, General Anesthetics.

Anxiety associated with dental or oral surgery
The benzodiazepines are generally regarded as the drugs of choice for oral preoperative anxiolysis in dental practice. These drugs have a high margin of safety, especially when used as a single dose 1 h before a dental visit. Diazepam has historically been used in this regard, but with the advent of newer agents with different phamacokinetic properties, other agents may be preferred. Diazepam is an inexpensive drug, with a rapid onset of action and a long half-life with active metabolites. At a dose of 5-10 mg, 1 h before a dental appointment, most adult patients will have some element of anxiolysis without significant sedation.

Another drug, triazolam, has a more rapid onset of action and the shortest half-life of any oral benzodiazepine, 1.5-5 h without active metabolites. This agent may provide less postoperative sedation, which may be desirable. The typical adult oral preoperative anxiolytic dosage for triazolam would be 0.25 mg 1 h before the dental appointment.

The intravenous drug midazolam has a similar pharmacokinetic profile to that of triazolam. Although not yet FDA-approved as an oral drug, this route of administration has been used for pediatric sedation. Flurazepam, at 15-30 mg, may also be an acceptable agent based on its pharmacokinetic profile (half-life 2.3 h, peak plasma concentration 0.5-1 h), but this drug also has active metabolites.

With any of these agents, there should be minimal, if any, respiratory or cardiac depression when used alone. In elderly, medically compromised or smaller adult patients, the lower dose range should be prescribed initially. Some patients may experience significant sedation even at low doses. If oral premedication is prescribed, the patient must have a responsible adult escort present at all times until the effects of the sedative have worn off sufficiently. Patients who have taken an oral sedative before a dental appointment must not drive to or from the dental office. Patients should be cautioned about lingering sedative effects during the day and to avoid other CNS depressants such as alcohol and opioids.

Management of nocturnal bruxism

If an acute anxiety-producing circumstance leads to severe bruxism, a short course of a benzodiazepine at bedtime can be efficacious. Typically, diazepam 5-10 mg at bedtime has been used owing to its muscle relaxing properties and anxiolytic effect. Other benzodiazepines are also effective. In general, this type of benzodiazepine use should be limited to no more than 2 w to avoid issues of dependence, rebound insomnia and alteration of sleep architecture. Benzodiazepines are relatively contraindicated in a depressed patient unless approved by the patient's psychiatrist in advance. Patients should be cautioned about lingering sedative effects during the day and to avoid other CNS depressants such as alcohol and opioids.

The tricyclic antidepressants have come into increasing use for the long-term management of nocturnal bruxism unresponsive to intraoral orthotic therapy. Although not fully understood, bruxism appears to occur during transitional stages of sleep or during rapid-eye-movement (REM) sleep. The tricyclic antidepressants decrease the number of awakenings, shorten time spent in transitional stages of sleep, increase stage III and IV sleep, and markedly decrease time spent in REM sleep. These effects may be beneficial for some patients with bruxism. Common agents used include amitriptyline, nortriptyline or doxepin. These drugs are usually started at 10 mg at bedtime and gradually titrated upward every few days. It is uncommon for most patients to require more than 50 mg at bedtime, which is substantially below the effective dose for use as an antidepressant.

These drugs are not benign. They have significant anticholinergic and antihistaminic side effects. They can cause cardiac dysrhythmias and may lower seizure threshold. In patients aged > 40 y, pretreatment electrocardiogram evaluation may be appropriate. The dentist prescribing antidepressants for this use is presumed to have established a proper diagnosis and to be fully aware of the drug's interactions, adverse effects and contraindications. When used as antidepressants, these drugs should be prescribed only by clinicians who have had special training in the diagnosis and management of depression.

Management of orofacial pain

Psychotropic drugs have a long history of use for chronic pain conditions. A full listing of indications and prescribing information is not appropriate for this text. For the properly trained dentist, the use of psychoactive drugs is appropriate for the management of orofacial conditions such as primary headaches, neuropathic and musculoskeletal pains.

Antidepressants are commonly used for a variety of chronic pain conditions (including myofascial pain syndrome and migraine headache). Phenothiazines can be a useful adjunct for some types of neuropathic pains and lithium is indicated for cluster headaches. The dentist using these drugs as therapeutic agents is presumed to be proficient in prescribing and managing these medications.

Antianxiety Agents

Anxiety is a state of uneasiness of mind that resembles fear, but usually has no identifiable source. Anxiety has both physical and mental aspects. The anxious patient may be tachycardic, nauseated, diaphoretic or light-headed. Although a patient may be diagnosed with a generalized anxiety disorder, at times clearly defined categories of anxiety apply. These categories include phobia, agoraphobia, panic attacks, obsessive-compulsive disorder, posttraumatic stress disorder and performance anxiety. Benzodiazepines, gamma-aminobutyric acid-A (GABA$_A$) agonists, are typically prescribed for these disorders.

The development of dependence may limit the long-term use of these drugs in some patients. Oral overdose of benzodiazepines is rarely fatal unless combined with other central nervous system depressants such as opioids, barbiturates or alcohol. Another drug without dependence-producing characteristics, the selective serotonin agonist buspirone, may be effective for some generalized anxiety disorders.

β-blockers have more recently been prescribed as an adjunct to benzodiazepine treatment and for control of performance anxiety. Antidepressants are frequently prescribed for patients with coexisting anxiety

Table 21.1
Antianxiety Agents: Dosage Information

Generic name	Brand name(s)*	Dosage range (daily)	Interactions with other drugs
Benzodiazepines			
Alprazolam	Alprazol, Alprazolam Intensol, Apo-Alpraz, Nu-Alpraz, Xanax, Xanax TS, generic	0.75-4 mg	CNS depressants (for example, alcohol, opioids and sedating antihistamines) may potentiate sedative side effects
Bromazepam	Lectopam	6-30 mg	CNS depressants (for example, alcohol, opioids and sedating antihistamines) may potentiate sedative side effects
Chlordiazepoxide	Apo-Chlordiazepoxide, Libritabs, Librium, Novopoxide, Poxi, Solium, generic	20-100 mg	Decreased metabolism with cimetidine and erythromycin CNS depressants (for example, alcohol, opioids and sedating antihistamines) may potentiate sedative side effects
Clonazepam	Klonopin; PMS-Clonazepam, Rivotril	1.5-20 mg	CNS depressants (for example, alcohol, opioids and sedating antihistamines) may potentiate sedative side effects
Clorazepate	Apo-Chlorazepate, Gen-XENE, Novo-Clopate, Transene-SD, Tranxene, Tranxene T-Tab, generic	15-90 mg	CNS depressants (for example, alcohol, opioids and sedating antihistamines) may potentiate sedative side effects

Continued on next page

Table 21.1 (cont.)
Antianxiety Agents: Dosage Information

Generic name	Brand name(s)*	Dosage range (daily)	Interactions with other drugs
Benzodiazepines (cont.)			
Diazepam	Apo-Diazepam, Diazepam, D-Val, Novodipam, PMS-Vivol, Valium, Valrelease, Zetran; Diazemuls	2-40 mg	Decreased metabolism with cimetidine and erythromycin Decreased clearance with SSRI antidepressants
Halazepam	Paxipam	60-160 mg	CNS depressants (for example, alcohol, opioids and sedating antihistamines) may potentiate sedative side effects
Ketazolam	Loftran	15-30 mg	CNS depressants (for example, alcohol, opioids and sedating antihistamines) may potentiate sedative side effects
Lorazepam	Ativan, Lorazepam Intensol; Apo-Lorazepam, Novo-Lorazepam, Nu-Loraz	2-9 mg	CNS depressants (for example, alcohol, opioids and sedating antihistamines) may potentiate sedative side effects Increased effect with morphine, MAO inhibitors, loxapine, tricyclic antidepressants
Oxazepam	Serax, generic; Novoxapam, Apo-Oxazepam	30-120 mg	CNS depressants (for example, alcohol, opioids and sedating antihistamines) may potentiate sedative side effects Increased toxicity with anticoagulants, alcohol, tricyclic antidepressants, sedative hypnotics, MAO inhibitors
Prazepam	Centrax, generic	20-60 mg	CNS depressants (for example, alcohol, opioids and sedating antihistamines) may potentiate sedative side effects Increased toxicity with anticoagulants, alcohol, tricyclic antidepressants, sedative hypnotics, MAO inhibitors
Nonbenzodiazepines			
Buspirone	BuSpar	15-60 mg	CNS depressants (for example, alcohol, opioids and some antihistamines) may potentiate sedative side effects
Hydroxyzine	Anxanil, Apo-Hydroxyzine, Atarax, E-Vista, Hydroxacen, Hydroxyzin, Hyzine-50, Novo-Multipax, Quiess, Vistaril, Vistazine-50, Vistaject-25 or -50	**Oral:** 50-100 mg dose **IM:** 50-100 mg, repeated as needed q 4-6 h	Increased toxicity with CNS depressants and anticholinergics

* Drugs with the prefixes Apo-, Novo- and Nu- are available only in Canada.

and depression. The antihistamine hydroxyzine is sometimes used for selected cases of anxiety disorders and as an oral agent for pediatric sedation for dental treatment.

See Table 21.1 for general information on antianxiety agents. Other agents listed as sleep adjuncts, although not FDA-approved for treatment of anxiety, may be prescribed for these disorders. More information on sleep adjuncts appears later in this chapter.

Special Dental Considerations

These drugs may cause xerostomia and should be considered in the differential diagnosis of caries, periodontal disease or candidiasis.

These drugs may cause orthostatic hypotension. After supine positioning, the dentist should ask the patient to sit upright in the dental chair for a minute or two and then monitor the patient when standing.

If these drugs are used for oral preoperative anxiolysis for dental procedures, a competent adult should drive the patient to and from the dental office. Assistance to and from the dental chair may be needed, especially for elderly patients.

Drug interactions of dental interest

CNS depressants will have an additive effect with concomitantly administered CNS depressants.

Absorption of diazepam and chlordiazepoxide is delayed with antacids.

The metabolism of chlordiazepoxide, diazepam and triazolam is decreased if they are administered with cimetidine and erythromycin.

The clearance of diazepam is decreased if it is administered with selective serotonin reuptake inhibitor (SSRI) antidepressants.

Special patients

In elderly, medically compromised or smaller adult patients, the lower dose range should be prescribed initially. Some of these patients may experience significant sedation even at low doses.

Pharmacology

These agents are mainly benzodiazepines, which act at the GABA$_A$ receptor, a gated chloride-ion channel that has specific benzodiazepine and barbiturate receptor sites. Binding of benzodiazepines to the receptor complex opens the chloride channel to facilitate GABA receptor transmission. GABA is the main inhibitory neurotransmitter of the central nervous system. Activity of the GABA system provides antianxiety, sedative, anticonvulsant, amnestic and muscle-relaxing actions. Long-term use of benzodiazepines can lead to a withdrawal syndrome if abruptly discontinued. The sedative and antianxiety effects of these drugs are used to advantage in promoting short-term sleep improvement. These drugs are hepatically metabolized to active or inactive metabolites for excretion in the bile or urine.

Buspirone, a serotonin (5HT1$_A$) receptor partial agonist with weak dopamine receptor activity, has shown some utility in the management of generalized anxiety. Its onset of action is delayed, thus making this drug a poor choice for management of acute anxiety.

The antihistamines hydroxyzine and diphenhydramine are seldom-used older agents that have sedative and anticholinergic effects independent of GABA action.

Antidepressants

Depression is a common mental illness that will affect at least 5 percent of the population at some time in life. A great number of these patients will be placed on antidepressants. Antidepressants are classified as heterocyclic (tricyclic, tetracyclic), monoamine oxidase inhibitors (MAOI), selective serotonin reuptake inhibitors (SSRI), and other miscellaneous agents. These drugs work by affecting neurotransmitter balance between serotonin, norepinephrine and, in some cases, dopamine in the central nervous system.

Implications in dental and oral surgery

revolve around the use of vasoconstrictors in local anesthetics, medication side effects and issues of patient management.

See Table 21.2 for basic information on antidepressants and for epinephrine/levonordefrin interaction information.

Special Dental Considerations

Most of these drugs cause decreased salivary flow. Consider in the differential diagnosis of caries, periodontal disease or oral candidiasis.

These drugs, in rare cases, cause blood dyscrasias and should be considered in the differential diagnosis of oral signs and symptoms.

Many of these drugs can cause orthostatic hypotension. After supine positioning, the dentist should ask the patient to sit upright in the dental chair for a minute or two and then monitor the patient when standing.

Amoxapine, and less commonly other antidepressants, can cause tardive dyskinesia or extrapyramidal symptoms, which are manifested as involuntary oral or facial movements. Management of bruxism, occlusal adjustments and bite registrations may be difficult to obtain. If newly diagnosed mouthing movements (involuntary mouth and tongue movements and/or drooling) are seen, which may indicate a serious medication side effect, consultation with the patient's physician may be appropriate.

Vanlafaxine can, rarely, cause trismus.

Drug interactions of dental interest

There has been much misunderstanding about the use of local anesthetics with epinephrine for patients taking antidepressants. Local anesthetics with epinephrine are not absolutely contraindicated for any patient taking any antidepressant—including tricyclic or MAOI agents, both of which increase the concentration of norepinephrine in the synaptic cleft. The potential concern is that these drug combinations might lead to a hypertensive crisis. Because a major route of exogenously administered catecholamine metabolism involves catechol-O-methyl transferase (COMT), use of epinephrine or levonordefrin in patients taking MAOIs is not thought to be as great a risk as has been assumed in the past, although a hypertensive crisis still may occur. Antidepressants that block norepinephrine reuptake (tricyclics, tetracyclics, venlafaxine, nefazodone) also could cause unwanted cardiovascular effects when epinephrine- or levonordefrin-containing local anesthetics are administered. It is prudent, therefore, to monitor vital signs for dental patients taking antidepressants that affect norepinephrine reuptake blockade or MAO-A activity.

It is reasonable to administer no more than 40 μg of epinephrine in local anesthetic solutions (approximately one cartridge of local anesthetic with 1:50,000 epinephrine, two cartridges with 1:100,000 epinephrine, four cartridges with 1:200,000 epinephrine or two cartridges of local anesthetic with 1:20,000 levonordefrin) within a short period with careful aspiration technique. Additional anesthetic with vasoconstrictor may be administered if vital signs are acceptable. This may be particularly important in patients taking venlafaxine, which has been noted to produce a sustained increase in diastolic blood pressure and heart rate as a relatively common side effect. No vasoconstrictor contraindication exists for the SSRI antidepressants. Gingival retraction cord with epinephrine is contraindicated for all patients taking antidepressants other than SSRI and should be used with caution, if at all, in other patients.

Anticholinergics and antihistamines should be used cautiously due to additive xerostomia and CNS sedative effects.

CNS depressants (for example, alcohol, opioids and benzodiazepines) may potentiate sedative side effects.

Meperidine and dextromethorphan are specifically contraindicated in patients taking MAOIs. Hypermetabolic crisis may occur. Caution with other opioids is warranted.

Table 21.2
Antidepressants: Dosage Information

Generic name	Brand name(s)	Dosage range (daily)	Interactions with other drugs
		Miscellaneous	
Bupropion	Wellbutrin	200-450 mg	May induce hepatic microsomal enzymes; metabolism of many drugs may be increased
Mirtazapine	Remeron	7.5-45 mg	Monitor vital signs for possible hypertensive crisis Administer no more than 40 µg epinephrine in local anesthetic solutions (two cartridges of 2% lidocaine with 1:100,000 epinephrine or its equivalent) within short period with careful aspiration technique; additional anesthetic with vasoconstrictor may be administered if vital signs are acceptable
Nefazodone	Serzone	200-600 mg	CNS depressants (for example, alcohol, opioids and benzodiazepines) may potentiate sedative side effects Monitor vital signs for possible hypertensive crisis Administer no more than 40 µg epinephrine in local anesthetic solutions (two cartridges of 2% lidocaine with 1:100,000 epinephrine or its equivalent) within short period with careful aspiration technique; additional anesthetic with vasoconstrictor may be administered if vital signs are acceptable May inhibit metabolism of terfenadine/astemizole, which can lead to cardiac dysrhythmias Decreased metabolism of triazolam/alprazolam **Anticholinergics and antihistamines:** May produce additive xerostomia and CNS sedative effects
Venlafaxine	Effexor	75-375 mg	Monitor vital signs for possible hypertensive crisis Administer no more than 40 µg epinephrine in local anesthetic solutions (two cartridges of 2% lidocaine with 1:100,000 epinephrine or its equivalent) within short period with careful aspiration technique; additional anesthetic with vasoconstrictor may be administered if vital signs are acceptable

Continued on next page

Table 21.2 (cont.)

Antidepressants: Dosage Information

Generic name	Brand name(s)	Dosage range (daily)	Interactions with other drugs
Monoamine oxidase inhibitors			
Isocarboxazid	Marplan	10-60 mg	Monitor vital signs for possible hypertensive crisis
			Administer no more than 40 μg epinephrine in local anesthetic solutions (two cartridges of 2% lidocaine with 1:100,000 epinephrine or its equivalent) within short period with careful aspiration technique; additional anesthetic with vasoconstrictor may be administered if vital signs are acceptable
			CNS depressants (for example, alcohol, opioids and benzodiazepines) may potentiate sedative side effects
			Meperidine is contraindicated, as it may cause hypermetabolic crisis; caution with other opioids is warranted
			Anticholinergics and antihistamines: relatively contraindicated owing to additive xerostomia and other CNS effects
Phenelzine	Nardil	15-90 mg	See note above
Tranylcypromine	Parnate	10-60 mg	See note above
Selective serotonin reuptake inhibitors			
Fluoxetine	Prozac	20-80 mg	Anticholinergics and antihistamines may produce additive xerostomia and other CNS effects (especially paroxetine and trazadone)
			CNS depressants (for example, alcohol, opioids and benzodiazepines) may potentiate sedative side effects
			The elimination time of some benzodiazepines, especially diazepam, can be increased
			No vasoconstrictor interaction
Fluvoxamine	Luvox	50-300 mg	See note above
Paroxetine	Paxil	10-50 mg	See note above
Sertraline	Zoloft	50-200 mg	See note above
Trazodone	Desyrel, Trazon, Trialodine, generic	50-600 mg	See note above

Continued on next page

Table 21.2 (cont.)

Antidepressants: Dosage Information

Generic name	Brand name(s)*	Dosage range (daily)	Interactions with other drugs
Tetracyclic agent			
Maprotiline	Ludiomil, generic	25-225 mg	Monitor vital signs for possible hypertensive crisis
			Administer no more than 40 µg epinephrine in local anesthetic solutions (two cartridges of 2% lidocaine with 1:100,000 epinephrine or its equivalent) within short period with careful aspiration technique; additional anesthetic with vasoconstrictor may be administered if vital signs are acceptable
			CNS depressants (for example, alcohol, opioids and benzodiazepines) may potentiate sedative side effects
			Anticholinergics and antihistamines may provide additive xerostomia and CNS sedative effects
Tricyclic agents			
Amitriptyline	Apo-Amitriptyline, Elavil, Endep, Levate, Novotriptyn, generic	10-300 mg	Monitor vital signs for possible hypertensive crisis
			Administer no more than 40 µg epinephrine in local anesthetic solutions (two cartridges of 2% lidocaine with 1:100,000 epinephrine or its equivalent) within short period with careful aspiration technique; additional anesthetic with vasoconstrictor may be administered if vital signs are acceptable
			CNS depressants (for example, alcohol, opioids and benzodiazepines) may potentiate sedative side effects
			Anticholinergics and antihistamines may provide additive xerostomia and CNS sedative effects
Amoxapine	Asendin, generic	100-300 mg	See note above
Clomipramine	Anafranil	75-250 mg	See note above
Desipramine	Norpramin, Pertofrane, generic	100-300 mg	See note above
Doxepin	Novo-Doxepin, Sinequan, Triadapin, generic	75-300 mg	See note above

Continued on next page

Table 21.2 (cont.)

Antidepressants: Dosage Information

Generic name	Brand name(s)*	Dosage range (daily)	Interactions with other drugs
Tricyclic agents (cont.)			
Imipramine	Apo-Imipramine, Impril, Norfranil, Novopramine, Tipramine, Tofranil, generic	75-300 mg	Monitor vital signs for possible hypertensive crisis
			Administer no more than 40 µg epinephrine in local anesthetic solutions (two cartridges of 2% lidocaine with 1:100,000 epinephrine or its equivalent) within short period with careful aspiration technique; additional anesthetic with vasoconstrictor may be administered if vital signs are acceptable
			CNS depressants (for example, alcohol, opioids and benzodiazepines) may potentiate sedative side effects
			Anticholinergics and antihistamines may provide additive xerostomia and CNS sedative effects
Nortriptyline	Aventyl, Pamelor, generic	75-150 mg	See note above
Protriptyline	Vivactil; Triptil [CAN]	5-60 mg	See note above
Trimipramine	Rhotrimine, Surmontil, generic; Apo-Trimip, Nova-Tripramine	50-200 mg	See note above

* Drugs with the prefixes Apo-, Nova- and Novo- are available only in Canada.

Tricyclic antidepressants (which might be used for bruxism) are contraindicated with MAOIs and should be used cautiously with SSRIs unless their use is cleared by a psychiatrist.

The anticoagulant effect of coumarin agents is increased when most antidepressants, including tricyclic agents, are administered concomitantly.

Antidepressants may lower the seizure threshold.

The therapeutic effect of tricyclic antidepressants may be decreased by concurrent administration of barbiturates, anticonvulsants or other hepatic-enzyme–inducing drugs.

With cimetidine, fluoxetine, methylphenidate and some estrogens (oral contraceptives), there is increased plasma concentration of trycyclic antidepressants.

Laboratory value alterations
- Blood glucose levels may increase or decrease.
- ECG changes are possible with tricyclic antidepressants, especially with pre-existing conduction abnormalities.

Special patients
Side effects, such as dry mouth and orthostatic hypotension, are more pronounced in elderly patients.

Pharmacology
Antidepressants affect mood by altering the

balance between serotonin, norepinephrine and dopamine in critical brain centers. Antidepressants, in general, increase the availability of neurotransmitters in the synaptic cleft, causing changes in the post-synaptic receptor. These changes take some time to develop, thus accounting for the delay in action of 2-4 w or longer for these drugs' mood-altering effects to become apparent. Due to the side-effect profile of many of the tricyclic and MAOI agents, the SSRIs are frequently chosen as first-line therapy for depression. In pain management, both norepinephrine and serotonin reuptake blockade appears to be important for an analgesic effect, so the tricyclics remain the preferred initial agents. Analgesia occurs well before the antidepressant effect and at low doses that are not effective for management of depression in many chronic pain patients.

The heterocyclic (tricyclic and tetracyclic) and selective serotonin reuptake inhibitor (SSRI) antidepressants block the reuptake of the neurotransmitters into the presynaptic neuron, a partial mechanism by which neurotransmitter activity is modulated. The SSRIs, as their name implies, affect only serotonin reuptake. Because of the receptor selectivity of these agents, they generally possess the fewest side effects of any antidepressant type. The heterocyclic (tricyclic, tetracyclic) antidepressants affect norepinephrine and serotonin, as well as a number of other important neurotransmittors but to varying degrees. Amoxapine possesses strong dopamine reuptake blocking effects. The MAOIs block the action of MAO-A, an enzyme found in the presynaptic neuron, which degrades serotonin and norepinephrine after reuptake. Buproprion is a weak reuptake blocker of dopamine and, to a lesser extent, norepinephrine and serotonin. Vanlafaxine and nefazadone both block reuptake of norepinephrine and serotonin but have slightly different side-effect profiles than the tricyclic agents. Mirtazapine is an α-2 antagonist affecting norepinephrine and, indirectly, serotonin.

Antimanic/Bipolar Disorder Drugs

Mania is a state of excessive excitement or enthusiasm and is frequently associated with hyperactivity or aggressive behavior. Approximately 90% of people who experience mania alternate these experiences with episodes of depression; this condition is termed "bipolar disorder" (manic-depression). Lithium carbonate is usually the drug of choice, although the anticonvulsants carbamazepine and divalproex sodium are also used.

See Table 21.3 for general information on antimanic/bipolar disorder drugs.

Special Dental Considerations: Lithium

Lithium can cause decreased salivary flow. Consider in the differential diagnosis of caries, periodontal disease or oral candidiasis.

Lithium can cause blood dycrasias and should be considered in the differential diagnosis of oral signs and symptoms.

Lithium can cause orthostatic hypotension. The dentist should monitor vital signs and, after supine positioning, ask the patient to sit upright in the dental chair for a minute or two and then monitor the patient when standing.

Drug interactions of dental interest: Lithium
Vasoconstrictors in local anesthetics should be used with caution owing to lithium's hypotensive effects.

Opioids, alcohol and other hypotension-producing agents have additive hypotensive effects.

NSAIDs, including aspirin, increase lithium's plasma concentration because of decreased renal clearance and should be prescribed, if at all, in consultations with the patient's psychiatrist.

Metronidazole increases plasma lithium concentration because of decreased renal clearance.

Table 21.3

Antimanic/Bipolar Disorder Drugs: Dosage Information

Generic name	Brand name(s)	Dosage range (daily)	Interactions with other drugs
Carbamazepine	Atretol, Epitol, Tegretol; Apo-Carbamazepine [CAN], Novo-Carbamaz [CAN], Nu-Carbamazepine [CAN], Tegretol Chewtabs [CAN]	200-1,200 mg or 60 mg/kg/day	**Acetaminophen (prolonged use):** Increased risk of hepatic toxicity **CNS depressants:** Increased sedative effects **Corticosteroids:** Increased metabolism **Propoxyphene, erythromycin/ clarithromycin:** Decreased metabolism, increased risk of toxicity
Divalproex	Depakote, Depakote Sprinkle; Epival [CAN]	500-4,000 mg	**Aspirin/NSAIDs:** Increased risk of bleeding **CNS depressants:** Increased sedative effects
Lithium	Carbolith, Cibalith-S, Duralith, Eskalith, Eskalith CR, Lithane, Lithizine, Lithobid, Lithonate, Lithotabs, generic	600-2,400 mg	**With NSAIDs, metronidazole, chlorpromazine:** Increased serum lithium concentration **With succinylcholine:** Prolonged paralysis may occur

[CAN] indicates a drug available only in Canada.

Tricyclic antidepressants (which may be used for bruxism) may lead to manic episodes.

Laboratory value alterations: Lithium
• Blood glucose may be increased.

Pharmacology

Lithium remains the primary treatment for prevention of mania and treatment of bipolar disorder. Although the mechanism of action is incompletely understood, the mood-stabilizing effects may be due to enhancement of the Na^+/K^+ ATPase pump, catecholamine neurotransmission, interference with inositol turnover in the brain or decreased activity of cyclic AMP. Lithium, a monovalent cation, is almost completely dependent on renal excretion for elimination. Coadministered drugs that affect renal function, such as NSAIDs, can increase the plasma concentration of this agent, which has a narrow therapeutic range of plasma concentration.

Other agents useful for the treatment of mania, such as valproic acid and carbamazepine, also have poorly understood mechanisms of action. The anticonvulsant mechanism of these agents is discussed in Chapter 20, Neurological Drugs.

Antipsychotic Agents

The term "psychotic" refers to behavior in which a person cannot distinguish between the real and the unreal. Although a psychotic state denotes mental illness, it does not identify the etiology, such as schizophrenia, major depression, brain tumor or adverse drug reaction. Hallucinations, delusions and thought disorders are characteristic of a psychotic state. Antipsychotic drugs are prescribed to help patients organize chaotic and disorganized thinking. In the past, the terms "major tranquilizers" (denoting prominent sedative side effects) and "neuroleptics"

Table 21.4

Antipsychotic Agents: Dosage Information

Generic name	Brand name(s)	Dosage range (daily)	Interactions with other drugs
Benzoxazole			
Risperidone	Risperdal	1-16 mg	**With epinephrine/levonordefrin:** Many antipsychotics can cause α-adrenergic receptor blockade; use of epinephrine-containing local anesthetic solutions may cause hypotension and tachycardia
			Monitor vital signs for possible hypertensive crisis
			Administer no more than 40 µg epinephrine in local anesthetic solutions (two cartridges of 2% lidocaine with 1:100,000 epinephrine or its equivalent) within short period with careful aspiration technique; additional anesthetic with vasoconstrictor may be administered if vital signs are acceptable
			With CNS depressants (alcohol, opioids, barbiturates): Additive sedative effects
			With anticholinergic drugs: Additive anticholinergic effects
Butyrophenone			
Haloperidol	Haldol, generic; Apo-Haloperidol [CAN], Novo-peridol [CAN], Peridol [CAN]	1-100 mg	**With epinephrine/levonordefrin:** Many antipsychotics can cause α-adrenergic receptor blockade; use of epinephrine-containing local anesthetic solutions may cause hypotension and tachycardia
			Monitor vital signs for possible hypertensive crisis
			Administer no more than 40 µg epinephrine in local anesthetic solutions (two cartridges of 2% lidocaine with 1:100,000 epinephrine or its equivalent) within short period with careful aspiration technique; additional anesthetic with vasoconstrictor may be administered if vital signs are acceptable
			With CNS depressants (alcohol, opioids, barbiturates): Additive sedative effects
			With anticholinergic drugs: Additive anticholinergic effects

[CAN] indicates a drug available only in Canada.

Continued on next page

Table 21.4 (cont.)

Antipsychotic Agents: Dosage Information

Generic name	Brand name(s)	Dosage range (daily)	Interactions with other drugs
		Dibenzoxapines	
Loxapine	Loxitane, Loxitane C, Loxitane IM; Loxapac [CAN]	30-250 mg	**With epinephrine/levonordefrin:** Many antipsychotics can cause α-adrenergic receptor blockade; use of epinephrine-containing local anesthetic solutions may cause hypotension and tachycardia Monitor vital signs for possible hypertensive crisis Administer no more than 40 μg epinephrine in local anesthetic solutions (two cartridges of 2% lidocaine with 1:100,000 epinephrine or its equivalent) within short period with careful aspiration technique; additional anesthetic with vasoconstrictor may be administered if vital signs are acceptable **With CNS depressants (alcohol, opioids, barbiturates):** Additive sedative effects **With anticholinergic drugs:** Additive anticholinergic effects
Clozapine	Clozaril	25-900 mg	See note above
Olanzapine	Zyprexa	10-100 mg	See note above
		Diphenylbutyl	
Pimozide	Orap	1-20 mg	**With epinephrine/levonordefrin:** Many antipsychotics can cause α-adrenergic receptor blockade; use of epinephrine-containing local anesthetic solutions may cause hypotension and tachycardia Monitor vital signs for possible hypertensive crisis Administer no more than 40 μg epinephrine in local anesthetic solutions (two cartridges of 2% lidocaine with 1:100,000 epinephrine or its equivalent) within short period with careful aspiration technique; additional anesthetic with vasoconstrictor may be administered if vital signs are acceptable **With CNS depressants (alcohol, opioids, barbiturates):** Additive sedative effects **With anticholinergic drugs:** Additive anticholinergic effects

[CAN] indicates a drug available only in Canada.

Continued on next page

Table 21.4 (cont.)

Antipsychotic Agents: Dosage Information

Generic name	Brand name(s)	Dosage range (daily)	Interactions with other drugs
Indole derivatives			
Molindone	Moban Concentrate; Fluanoxol Depot [CAN]	20-225 mg	**With epinephrine/levonordefrin:** Many antipsychotics can cause α-adrenergic receptor blockade; use of epinephrine-containing local anesthetic solutions may cause hypotension and tachycardia Monitor vital signs for possible hypertensive crisis Administer no more than 40 µg epinephrine in local anesthetic solutions (two cartridges of 2% lidocaine with 1:100,000 epinephrine or its equivalent) within short period with careful aspiration technique; additional anesthetic with vasoconstrictor may be administered if vital signs are acceptable **With CNS depressants (alcohol, opioids, barbiturates):** Additive sedative effects **With anticholinergic drugs:** Additive anticholinergic effects
Phenothiazines			
Chlorpromazine	Largactil, Ormazine, Thorazine, Thorazine Concentrate, Thorazine Spansule, Thor-prom, generic; Chlorpromanyl-40 [CAN], Chlorpromanyl-5 [CAN], Largactil Liquid [CAN], Novo-Chlorproamzine [CAN]	30-1,000 mg	**With epinephrine/levonordefrin:** Many antipsychotics can cause α-adrenergic receptor blockade; use of epinephrine-containing local anesthetic solutions may cause hypotension and tachycardia Monitor vital signs for possible hypertensive crisis Administer no more than 40 µg epinephrine in local anesthetic solutions (two cartridges of 2% lidocaine with 1:100,000 epinephrine or its equivalent) within short period with careful aspiration technique; additional anesthetic with vasoconstrictor may be administered if vital signs are acceptable **With CNS depressants (alcohol, opioids, barbiturates):** Additive sedative effects **With anticholinergic drugs:** Additive anticholinergic effects
Thioridazine	Apo-Thioridazine [CAN], Mellaril, Mellaril Concentrate, Mellaril-S, PMS Thioridazine [CAN], generic	20-800 mg	See note above

Continued on next page

Table 21.4 (cont.)
Antipsychotic Agents: Dosage Information

Generic name	Brand name(s)	Dosage range (daily)	Interactions with other drugs
Phenothiazines (cont.)			
Mesoridazine	Serentil, Serentil Concentrate	25-150 mg	**With epinephrine/levonordefrin:** Many antipsychotics can cause α-adrenergic receptor blockade; use of epinephrine-containing local anesthetic solutions may cause hypotension and tachycardia Monitor vital signs for possible hypertensive crisis Administer no more than 40 µg epinephrine in local anesthetic solutions (two cartridges of 2% lidocaine with 1:100,000 epinephrine or its equivalent) within short period with careful aspiration technique; additional anesthetic with vasoconstrictor may be administered if vital signs are acceptable **With CNS depressants (alcohol, opioids, barbiturates):** Additive sedative effects **With anticholinergic drugs:** Additive anticholinergic effects
Trifluoperazine	Solazine, Stelazine, Terfluzine	1-40 mg	See note above
Fluphenazine	Modecate, Moditen, Permitil, Prolixin	2.5-20 mg	See note above
Perphenazine	Trilafon	4-64 mg	See note above
Acetophenazine	Tindal	40-120 mg	See note above
Pericyazine	Neuleptil	5-60 mg	See note above
Pipotiazine	Piportal L4	50-150 mg/q 4 w (parenteral only)	See note above
Thiopropazate	Dartal [CAN]	20-100 mg	See note above
Thioproperazine	Majeptil [CAN]	5-90 mg	See note above
Triflupromazine	Vesprin	80-150 mg (parenteral only)	See note above
Prochlorperazine	Stemetil, Vesprin	10-150 mg	See note above
Promazine	Promazine, Sparine	40-1,000 mg	See note above
Methotrimeprazine	Norinan, Levoprome	5-100 mg	See note above

[CAN] indicates a drug available only in Canada.

Continued on next page

Table 21.4 (cont.)

Antipsychotic Agents: Dosage Information

Generic name	Brand name(s)	Dosage range (daily)	Interactions with other drugs
Thioxanthene			
Chlorprothixene	Taractan	75-600 mg	**With epinephrine/levonordefrin:** Many antipsychotics can cause α-adrenergic receptor blockade; use of epinephrine-containing local anesthetic solutions may cause hypotension and tachycardia Monitor vital signs for possible hypertensive crisis Administer no more than 40 μg epinephrine in local anesthetic solutions (two cartridges of 2% lidocaine with 1:100,000 epinephrine or its equivalent) within short period with careful aspiration technique; additional anesthetic with vasoconstrictor may be administered if vital signs are acceptable **With CNS depressants (alcohol, opioids, barbiturates):** Additive sedative effects **With anticholinergic drugs:** Additive anticholinergic effects
Thiothixene	Intensol, Navane, Thiothixine HCl, generic	6-60 mg	See note above
Flupenthixol	Fluanxol [CAN]	3-12 mg	See note above
Tricyclic agents			
Carbamazepine	Atretol, Epitol, Tegretol; Apo-Carbamazepine [CAN], Novo-Carbamaz [CAN], Nu-Carbamazapine [CAN], Tegretol Chewtabs [CAN]	200-1,200 mg	**Acetaminophen (prolonged use):** Increased risk of hepatic toxicity **CNS depressants:** Increased sedative effects **Corticosteroids:** Increased metabolism **Propoxyphene, erythromycin/clarithromycin:** Decreased metabolism, increased risk of toxicity

[CAN] indicates a drug available only in Canada.

(denoting parkinsonian-like side effects) were used, but the term "antipsychotic" is now preferred.

See Table 21.4 for general information on antipsychotic agents.

Special Dental Considerations

Many of these drugs can cause decreased salivary flow, and should be considered in the differential diagnosis of caries, periodontal disease or oral candidiasis.

These drugs can cause blood dycrasias (although this is less likely with risperidone and molindone). The dentist should consider this in the differential diagnosis of oral signs and symptoms.

Many of these drugs can cause orthostatic hypotension. After supine positioning, the dentist should ask the patient to sit upright in the dental chair for a minute or two and then monitor the patient when standing.

Extrapyramidal effects can cause involuntary oral or facial movements (although this is less likely with risperidone and clozapine). Management of bruxism, occlusal adjustments and bite registrations may be difficult. If newly diagnosed oral movements (involuntary mouth and tongue movements and/or drooling) are seen, this may indicate a serious medication side effect and the need for consultation with the patient's physician.

Drug interactions of dental interest

With epinephrine/levonordefrin: Many antipsychotics can cause α-adrenergic receptor blockade. Use of epinephrine-containing local anesthetic solutions may cause hypotension and tachycardia. It is prudent, therefore, to monitor vital signs for dental patients taking these medications. It is reasonable to administer no more than 40 μg of epinephrine in local anesthetic solutions (approximately one cartridge of local anesthetic with 1:50,000 epinephrine, two cartridges with 1:100,000 epinephrine, four cartridges with 1:200,000 epinephrine or two cartridges of local anesthetic with 1:20,000 levonordefrin) within a short period with careful aspiration

technique. Additional anesthetic with vasoconstrictor may be administered if vital signs are acceptable.

CNS depressants such as alcohol, opioids and barbiturates have additive sedative effects.

Anticholinergic drugs have additive anticholinergic effects.

Tricyclic antidepressants (which may be used for bruxism) have additive anticholinergic effects; combined use of these drugs can lead to alteration of plasma concentration of either drug. Also, there is a possible increased risk of neuroleptic malignant syndrome.

Laboratory value alterations

- ECG changes (Q, T wave changes, QT interval, ST depression, AV conduction changes) are possible.

Special patients

If antipsychotic drugs are being used in elderly patients for an antiemetic effect, lower doses should be used.

Pharmacology

All antipsychotic drugs appear to produce reduction of dopamine synaptic activity in limbic forebrain centers as a common pathway of antipsychotic activity. It appears that action at the dopamine-2 receptor is particularly important. Some of the newer agents, such as clozapine, also have significant influences at serotonergic receptors as well, which suggests that other neurotransmitters also play a role in affected midbrain dopamine neurotransmisson. Many of the side effects of these drugs relate to interaction at other receptor sites. α-adrenergic receptor blockade (causing orthostatic hypotension, reflex tachycardia and epinephrine interactions), antihistaminic effects (causing sedation and weight gain) and anticholinergic effects (causing dry mouth, constipation, tachycardia and difficulty in focusing the eyes) are common with many of these drugs.

Because these drugs produce effects on nigrostriatal pathways, an important area in Parkinson's disease, side effects such as tardive dyskinesia and neuroleptic malignant syndrome can occur with these agents. Other extrapyramidal reactions, such as akathisia (restlessness usually associated with some component of motor hyperactivity) or acute dystonic reactions such as oculogyric crisis (uncontrolled eye, face, or neck movements), can occur. Bruxism or other excessive oral movement disorders can be a drug-induced side effect.

These drugs typically undergo extensive hepatic metabolism by oxidation and glucuronidation to inactive metabolites, which are then excreted in the urine.

Drugs Used for Attention Deficit/Hyperactivity Disorder

Hyperactive children have difficulty keeping still for even a few minutes or may display impulsive behaviors. Children with attention deficit disorder (ADD) have difficulty concentrating on tasks and are easily distracted. These diagnoses should not be cavalierly applied to any child who is difficult to manage or is distracted easily; rather, a thorough medical and psychiatric evaluation, including an evaluation of the child's psychosocial functioning, is needed to render the diagnosis of ADD and/or hyperactivity. Interestingly, stimulant medications, with or without psychotherapy, are frequently used for treatment. There is increasing recognition of this disorder in adults.

See Table 21.5 for general information on drugs used for attention deficit/hyperactivity disorder.

Special Dental Considerations

Determine if the patient is taking any drug for attention deficit disorder or narcolepsy. Monitor vital signs due to sympathomimetic effects.

Many of these drugs can cause decreased salivary flow and should be considered in the differential diagnosis of caries, periodontal disease or oral candidiasis.

These drugs can rarely cause blood dyscrasias and should be considered in the differential diagnosis of oral signs and symptoms.

Drug interactions of dental interest

Vasoconstrictors in local anesthetics have possible additive sympathomimetic effects. Depending on vital signs, it is reasonable to administer no more than 40 µg of epinephrine in local anesthetic solutions (approximately one cartridge of local anesthetic with 1:50,000 epinephrine, two cartridges with 1:100,000 epinephrine, four cartridges with 1:200,000 epinephrine or two cartridges of local anesthetic with 1:20,000 levonordefrin) within a short period with careful aspiration technique. If vital signs warrant it, less vasoconstrictor should be used. Additional anesthetic with vasoconstrictor may be administered if vital signs are acceptable after a short period.

Tricyclic antidepressants (which may be used for bruxism) should be used with caution, because their metabolism is decreased by methylphenidate. Increased sympathomimetic effects are possible when tricyclic antidepressants are prescribed to patients taking dextroamphetamine because of norepinephrine reuptake blockade by tricyclics.

Anticholinergics have additive oral drying effects.

Meperidine is contraindicated due to the MAO-inhibitory effect of dextroamphetamine.

Pharmacology

Methylphenidate and pemoline appear to act by blocking dopamine reuptake. These drugs increase children's ability to pay attention and decrease their motor restlessness. Dextroamphetamine is a sympathomimetic amine that blocks the reuptake of dopamine and norepinephrine, inhibits MAO and releases catecholamines. Because of the stimulant effects, use of these drugs may result in weight loss, insomnia and tachycardia. These effects are particularly prominent with dextroamphetamine. These drugs are also used to treat narcolepsy.

Sleep Adjuncts

Sleep disorders include disorders in initiating or maintaining sleep, disorders of excessive

Table 21.5
Drugs Used for Attention Deficit/Hyperactivity Disorder: Dosage Information

Generic name	Brand name(s)	Dosage range (daily)	Interactions with other drugs
Dextroamphetamine	Dexedrine, Dexedrine Spansule, Dextrostat, generic	5-60 mg	Can interact with vasoconstrictors in local anesthetic solutions; therefore, reasonable approach is to monitor vital signs for possible hypertensive crisis and administer no more than 40 µg epinephrine in local anesthetic solutions (two cartridges of 2% lidocaine with 1:100,000 epinephrine or its equivalent) within short period with careful aspiration technique; additional anesthetic with vasoconstrictor may be administered if vital signs are acceptable; if preoperative vital signs warrant, smaller quantities of vasoconstrictor or no vasoconstrictor may be indicated; additional anesthetic with vasoconstrictor may be administered if vital signs are acceptable **Meperidine:** Contraindicated in patients taking dextroamphetamine
Methylphenidate	Ritalin, Ritalin-SR, generic; PMS-Methylphenidate [CAN]	10-90 mg	Monitor vital signs for possible hypertensive crisis Administer no more than 40 µg epinephrine in local anesthetic solutions (two cartridges of 2% lidocaine with 1:100,000 epinephrine or its equivalent) within short period with careful aspiration technique; additional anesthetic with vasoconstrictor may be administered if vital signs are acceptable
Pemoline	Cylert	37.5-112.5 mg	Can interact with vasoconstrictors in local anesthetic solutions (to a lesser extent than methylphenidate and dextroamphetamine); therefore, reasonable approach is to administer no more than 40 µg epinephrine in local anesthetic solutions (two cartridges of 2% lidocaine with 1:100,000 epinephrine or its equivalent) within a short period with careful aspiration technique; if preoperative vital signs warrant, smaller quantities of vasoconstrictor or no vasoconstrictor may be indicated; additional anesthetic with vasoconstrictor may be administered if vital signs are acceptable

[CAN] indicates a drug available only in Canada.

Table 21.6

Sleep Adjuncts: Dosage Information

Generic name	Brand name(s)	Dosage range (daily)*	Interactions with other drugs
Benzodiazepines			
Alprazolam	Alprazolam Intensol, Apo-Alpraz [CAN], Novo-Alprazol [CAN], Nu-Alpraz [CAN], Xanax, Xanax TS, generic	0.75-4 mg	CNS depressants (for example, alcohol, opioids and sedating antihistamines) may potentiate sedative side effects Delayed absorption with antacids for chlordiazepoxide and diazepam **Chlordiazepoxide, diazepam:** Decreased metabolism with cimetidine and erythromycin
Bromazepam	Lectopam	6-30 mg	CNS depressants (for example, alcohol, opioids and sedating antihistamines) may potentiate sedative side effects
Diazepam	Apo-Diazepam [CAN], D-Val, PMS-Diazepam [CAN], Novodipam [CAN], Vivol [CAN], Valrelease, Valium, Zetran; Diazemuls [CAN]	4-40 mg	Decreased metabolism with cimetidine and erythromycin Decreased clearance with SSRI antidepressants
Estazolam	ProSom	1-2 mg	CNS depressants (for example, alcohol, opioids and sedating antihistamines) may potentiate sedative side effects
Flurazepam	Dalmane, generic; Apo-Flurazepam [CAN], Novoflupam [CAN], Somnol [CAN]	15-30 mg	CNS depressants (for example, alcohol, opioids and sedating antihistamines) may potentiate sedative side effects
Lorazepam	Apo-Lorazepam [CAN], Ativan, Novo-Lorazam [CAN], Nu-Loraz [CAN]	2-4 mg	CNS depressants (for example, alcohol, opioids and sedating antihistamines) may potentiate sedative side effects
Nitrazepam	Mogadon [CAN]	5-10 mg	CNS depressants (for example, alcohol, opioids and sedating antihistamines) may potentiate sedative side effects
Quazepam	Doral	7.5-15 mg	CNS depressants (for example, alcohol, opioids and sedating antihistamines) may potentiate sedative side effects
Temazepam	Restoril	7.5-15 mg	CNS depressants (for example, alcohol, opioids and sedating antihistamines) may potentiate sedative side effects

Continued on next page

Table 21.6 (cont.)

Sleep Adjuncts: Dosage Information

Generic name	Brand name(s)	Dosage range (daily)*	Interactions with other drugs
Benzodiazepines (cont.)			
Triazolam	Halcion; Apo-Triazo [CAN], Gen-Triazolam [CAN], Novo-Triolam [CAN], Nu-Triazo [CAN]	0.125-0.5 mg	Decreased effect with phenytoin, phenobarbitol; increased effect with CNS depressants, cimetidine, erythromycin
Nonbenzodiazepines			
Diphenhydramine	Benadryl, Compoz, Diphen, Nidryl, Nordryl, Nytol	25-100 mg	CNS depressants (for example, alcohol, opioids and some antihistamines) may potentiate sedative side effects
Zolpidem	Ambien	10-20 mg	CNS depressants (for example, alcohol, opioids and some antihistamines) may potentiate sedative side effects
Zopicione [CAN]	Imovane [CAN]	3.75-7.5 mg	CNS depressants (for example, alcohol, opioids and some antihistamines) may potentiate sedative side effects

[CAN] indicates a drug available only in Canada.
* Dosage listed is single adult dose at bedtime.

somnolence, disorders of sleep-wake schedule and parasomnias (including nocturnal bruxism). Disorders of initiating and maintaining sleep are by far the most common complaints and will be addressed in this section.

The benzodiazepines, $GABA_A$ agonists, are the drugs most commonly prescribed for insomnia. Unfortunately, prolonged use can interfere with normal sleep architecture and be detrimental in the long term. The FDA indication for these drugs is for short-term use only, although they are frequently prescribed for many months or years. Dependence and rebound insomnia are frequently observed. Nevertheless, for short-term use, these agents are generally effective.

A recently introduced nonbenzodiazepine $GABA_A$ agonist, zolpidem, produces less disruption of sleep architecture and may have some effect in treating bruxism. The more sedating tricyclic antidepressants and trazadone

also have been used for some patients who require long-term treatment, as have sedating antihistamines. The older barbiturate drugs, such as secobarbital and pentobarbital, are rarely used today for insomnia.

See Table 21.6 for general information on sleep adjuncts.

Special Dental Considerations

These drugs can cause xerostomia. The dentist should consider this in the differential diagnosis of caries, periodontal disease or candidiasis.

These drugs may cause orthostatic hypotension. The dentist should monitor vital signs and, after supine positioning, ask the patient to sit upright in the dental chair for 1-2 min and then monitor the patient when standing.

If these drugs are used for preoperative anxiolysis for dental procedures, ensure that a competent adult drives the patient to and from the dental office. Assistance to and from the dental chair may be needed, especially for elderly patients.

Drug interactions of dental interest

CNS depressants will have an additive effect with concomitantly administered CNS depressants.

Diazepam and chlordiazepoxide have delayed absorption with antacids.

The metabolism of chlordiazepoxide, diazepam and triazolam is decreased if they are administered with cimetidine and erythromycin.

The clearance of diazepam is decreased if it is administered with SSRI antidepressants.

Special patients

In elderly, medically compromised or smaller adult patients, the lower dose range should be prescribed initially. Some of these patients may experience significant sedation even at low doses.

Pharmacology

See the description for antianxiety agents above.

Adverse Effects, Precautions and Contraindications

Table 21.7 provides adverse effects and Table 21.8 provides precautions and contraindications of psychoactive drugs.

Suggested Readings

American Psychiatric Association. Diagnostic and statistical manual of mental disorders (DSM-IV). 4th ed. Washington, D.C.: American Psychiatric Association; 1994.

Brown RS, Bottomley WK. The utilization and mechanism of action of tricyclic antidepressants in the treatment of chronic facial pain: a review of the literature. Anes Prog 1990:37:223-9.

Eschalier A, Mestre C, Dubray C, Ardid D. Why are antidepressants effective as pain relief? CNS Drugs 1994:2:261-7.

Mortimer AM. Newer and older antipsychotics: a comparative review of appropriate use. CNS Drugs 1994; 2:381-6.

Okeson JP, ed. Orofacial pain: guidelines for assessment, diagnosis and management. Lombard, Ill.: Quintessence; 1996.

Tucker GJ. Psychiatric disorders in medical practice. In: Wyngaarden JB, Smith LH Jr., Bennett JC, eds. Cecil textbook of medicine. 19th ed. Philadelphia: Saunders; 1992.

The United States Pharmacopeial Convention. Drug information for the health care professional. 17th ed. Rockville, Md.: The United States Pharmacopeial Convention, Inc.; 1997.

Table 21.7

Psychoactive Drugs: Adverse Effects

Body system	Antianxiety agents and sleep adjuncts	Antidepressants —tricyclic, tetracyclic	Antimanic/bipolar disorder drugs	Antipsychotics	Drugs used for attention deficit/hyperactivity disorder	MAO inhibitors	Miscellaneous antidepressants (nefazadone, vanlafaxine, buproprion, mirtazapine)	SSRI antidepressants
General	Pain on injection of diazepam or lorazepam, physical and psychological dependence		Lithium: Bluish discoloration of fingers and toes			Peripheral edema, chest pain, headache, increased sweating, increased appetite, weight gain, fatigue	Headache, chest pain, peripheral edema, increased sweating	Chills, fever, joint/muscle pain, allergic reaction, swollen glands, headache, increased sweating, decreased appetite/weight, chest pain, weakness
CV	Hypotension, bradycardia, syncope	Arrhythmias, tachycardia, bradycardia, hypotension	Tachycardia, bradycardia, irregular pulse	Hypotension, tachycardia	Tachycardia, hypertension, hypotension, arrhythmias	Hypotension, tachycardia, hypertension, bradycardia, hypertension, dysrhythmias	Palpitations, hypertension, tachycardia, increased diastolic pressure and heart rate (vanlafaxine), hypotension	Tachycardia

Continued on next page

Table 21.7 (cont.)
Psychoactive Drugs: Adverse Effects

Body system	Antianxiety agents and sleep adjuncts	Antidepressants —tricyclic, tetracyclic	Antimanic/bipolar disorder drugs	Antipsychotics	Drugs used for attention deficit/hyperactivity disorder	MAO inhibitors	Miscellaneous antidepressants (nefazodone, vanlafaxine, buproprion, mirtazapine)	SSRI antidepressants
CNS	Drowsiness, amnesia, confusion, ataxia, dizziness, paradoxical excitement, depression, sweating, ataxia, headache, parasthesias	Anticholinergic effects; confusion, fatigue, seizures, delirium, hallucinations, nervousness, anxiety, restlessness, fine tremor, extrapyramidal symptoms, neuroleptic malignant syndrome	Lethargy, dizziness, trembling of hands, pseudotumor cerebri, fatigue, trembling, weakness	Akathisia, loss of balance, dizziness, fine tremor of hands/fingers, decreased seizure threshold, decreased sweating, psychotic behavior, memory loss, tardive dyskinesia, neuroleptic malignant syndrome	Agitation, nervousness, insomnia, drowsiness, headache, Tourette's syndrome, increased sweating	Orthostatic hypotension, sympathetic stimulation, parkinsonian syndrome, shakiness, trembling	Abnormal thinking, agitation, confusion, worsening depression, insomnia, orthostatic hypotension, mania, anxiety, trismus	Mania, hypomania, seizures, insomnia, sedation
Endoc	Irregular menses, decreased libido	Syndrome of inappropriate antidiuretic hormone	Diabetes insipidus, polydipsia, symptoms of hypothyroidism	Galactorrhea, impaired temperature regulation, priapism, menstrual changes, decreased libido, breast pain/swelling	Retarded growth, increase or decrease in libido	Decreased libido, decreased sexual ability, syndrome of inappropriate antidiuretic hormone	Sexual dysfunction, menstrual changes	Decreased libido, priapism (trazadone), hypoglycemia

System								
EENT	Blurred vision, diplopia, ear ringing, hyperacusis, nasal congestion	Blurred vision, eye pain, ear ringing	Visual problems	Blurred vision, cornea/lens changes, dry eyes, pigmentary retinopathy, nasal congestion	Blurred vision	Photophobia, blurred vision	Ear pain, ringing of ears, rhinitis, eye pain, blurred vision, pharyngitis	Vision changes
GI	Diarrhea, nausea, vomiting, appetite changes	Constipation, weight gain	Diarrhea, nausea, weight gain	Nausea, vomiting, stomach pain, constipation, weight gain	Nausea, vomiting, weight loss, anorexia, GI pain, diarrhea	Diarrhea, nausea, vomiting, constipation	Constipation, dyspepsia	Nausea, vomiting, constipation
GU		Difficulty in urinating, sexual dysfunction, gynecomastia, galactorrhea	Urinary urgency, renal disease	Difficulty in urinating			Urinary retention or frequency, vaginitis	Frequent urination, hyponatremia
Hema	Rare blood dyscrasias	Blood dyscrasias including aganulocytosis, leukopenia, thrombocytopenia	Leukocytosis	Blood dyscrasias	Blood dyscrasias including thrombocytopenia, leukopenia and anemia	Anemia, leukopenia	Thrombocytopenia, leukopenia	

Continued on next page

Table 21.7 (cont.)
Psychoactive Drugs: Adverse Effects

Body system	Antianxiety agents and sleep adjuncts	Antidepressants—tricyclic, tetracyclic	Antimanic/bipolar disorder drugs	Antipsychotics	Drugs used for attention deficit/hyperactivity disorder	MAO inhibitors	Miscellaneous antidepressants (nefazadone, vanlafaxine, buproprion, mirtazapine)	SSRI antidepressants
HB	Hepatic dysfunction	Cholestatic jaundice		Cholestatic jaundice, hepatotoxicity	Elevated liver enzymes	Hepatitis		
Integ	Rash, dermatitis	Alopecia, photosensitivity	Rash, eruptions	Photosensitivity, rash, itching	Rash		Itch/rash	Rash, hives, itching, flushing/redness of skin (including face/neck)
Musc	Rigidity, tremor	Fine tremor	Weakness, rigidity, tremor, twitching	Dystonic reactions			Neck rigidity	
Oral	Dry mouth	Dry mouth, tardive dyskinesia (especially amozapine) glossitis	Impaired taste, xerostomia	Dystonic oral/facial movements, dry mouth, tardive dyskinesia	Dry mouth		Taste changes, xerostomia, stomatitis, glossitis	Taste changes, xerostomia
Resp	Decrease in respiratory rate or apnea (with high dose or with other CNS depressants)	Asthma					Dyspnea, cough, bronchitis	Difficulty in breathing

Table 21.8

Psychoactive Drugs: Precautions and Contraindications

Drug category	Precautions/contraindications
Antidepressants	
General	Except for SSRIs, antidepressants can interact with vasoconstrictors in local anesthetic solutions, so it is prudent to monitor vital signs for dental patients taking these drugs; reasonable approach is to administer no more than 40 μg of epinephrine in local anesthetic solutions (approximately one cartridge of local anesthetic with 1:50,000 epinephrine, two cartridges with 1:100,000 epinephrine, four cartridges with 1:200,000 epinephrine or two cartridges of local anesthetic with 1:20,000 levonordefrin) within short period with careful aspiration technique; additional anesthetic with vasoconstrictor may be administered if vital signs are acceptable
	Can cause orthostatic hypotension; therefore, after supine positioning, dentist should ask patient to sit upright in the dental chair for 1-2 min and then monitor patient when standing
Tricyclic agents and tetracyclic agent*	Should not be prescribed to patients who have preexisting cardiovascular disease without work-up
	Should be used cautiously, if at all, with fluoxetine
	If used in combination with other antidepressants, or possibly meperidine or dextromethorphan, may cause "serotonin syndrome," a condition of serotonin overload characterized by agitation, hyperthermia, sweating, shivering tremors, and muscle rigidity
	May cause tardive dyskinesia or neuroleptic malignant syndrome
Selective serotonin reuptake inhibitors	If used in combination with other antidepressants or possibly meperidine or dextromethorphan, may cause "serotonin syndrome," a condition of serotonin overload characterized by agitation, hyperthermia, sweating, shivering tremors, and muscle rigidity
Monoamine oxidase inhibitors	Use of MAOIs in combination with other antidepressants, or possibly meperidine or dextromethorphan, may cause "serotonin syndrome," may cause condition of serotonin overload characterized by agitation, hyperthermia, sweating, shivering tremors, and muscle rigidity
	Meperidine: Contraindicated for patients taking MAOIs
Miscellaneous (nefazadone, vanlafaxine, buproprion, mirtazapine)	Use of these antidepressants (buproprion less than others) in combination with other antidepressants, or possibly meperidine or dextromethorphan, may cause "serotonin syndrome," a condition of serotonin overload characterized by agitation, hyperthermia, sweating, shivering tremors, and muscle rigidity
	Vanlafaxine may produce sustained increased diastolic blood pressure and heart rate
	Nefazadone may increase plasma levels of terfenadine and astemizole, resulting in cardiac arrhythmias

*All heterocyclic agents are tricyclic except maprotiline, which is tetracyclic.

Continued on next page

Table 21.8 (cont.)

Psychoactive Drugs: Precautions and Contraindications

Drug category	Precautions/contraindications
Antianxiety agents	
General	Antianxiety agents, except buspirone and hydroyzine, can produce dependence and should not be prescribed for longer than 2 w unless for specific chronic pain complaints unresponsive to other treatments
	If used for an extended time, psychiatric consult may be advisable
	Should be used cautiously with other CNS depressant medications because of additive sedative effects
	Contraindicated in depressed patients without physician consultation
	Contraindicated in patients with acute narrow-angle glaucoma
Antimanic/bipolar disorder drugs	
Lithium	Lithium toxicity can occur at or near therapeutic serum concentrations
	As lithium is eliminated almost exclusively via renal mechanisms, drugs that alter renal function—such as NSAIDs—should be used cautiously, if at all
	After supine positioning, dentist should ask patient to sit upright in dental chair 1-2 min and then monitor patient when standing
Antipsychotic drugs	
General	Many antipsychotics can cause α-adrenergic receptor blockade
	Use of epinephrine-containing local anesthetic solutions may cause hypotension and tachycardia, so it is prudent to monitor vital signs for dental patients taking these drugs; reasonable approach is to administer no more than 40 μg of epinephrine in local anesthetic solutions (approximately one cartridge of local anesthetic with 1:50,000 epinephrine, two cartridges with 1:100,000 epinephrine, four cartridges with 1:200,000 epinephrine or two cartridges of local anesthetic with 1:20,000 levonordefrin) within short period with careful aspiration technique; additional anesthetic with vasoconstrictor may be administered if vital signs are acceptable
	Can cause orthostatic hypotension; therefore, after supine positioning, dentist should ask patient to sit upright in dental chair for 1-2 min and then monitor patient when standing
	Many of these drugs can cause tardive dyskinesia (involuntary movements of facial, jaw and tongue muscles); consultation with patient's psychiatrist is appropriate, especially if mouthing movements are initially emergent or particularly severe
Drugs used for attention deficit/hyperactivity disorder	
General	Monitor vital signs before and after administration of epinephrine used in local anesthetic solutions as it may have an exaggerated effect
	Meperidine: Contraindicated in patients taking amphetamines

Continued on next page

Table 21.8 (cont.)

Psychoactive Drugs: Precautions and Contraindications

Drug category	Precautions/contraindications
	Sleep adjuncts
General	Sleep adjuncts, except buspirone and hydroyzine, can produce dependence and should not be prescribed for longer than 2 w unless for specific chronic pain complaints unresponsive to other treatments
	If used for an extended time, psychiatric consultation may be advisable
	Should be used cautiously with other CNS depressant medications because of additive sedative effects
	Contraindicated in depressed patients without physician consultation
	Contraindicated in patients with acute narrow-angle glaucoma

Chapter 22

Hematologic Drugs

Angelo J. Mariotti, D.D.S., Ph.D.

Hematologic disturbances involve a wide variety of diseases that affect erythrocyte production (anemia or erythrocytosis), leukocytes (leukopenia or leukocytosis), platelets (thrombocytopenia or thrombocytosis), homeostasis (hemorrhage) and normal growth of the lymphoreticular system. Because various drugs, including hormones, growth factors, vitamins and minerals, can directly or indirectly influence the blood as well as blood-forming organs, the treatment of hematologic disorders should always be directed to the specific cause of the disorder; accordingly, proper testing is an important factor in diagnosing the hematologic disturbance.

Antianemic Agents

Special Dental Considerations

Clinical signs of iron toxicity sometimes include bluish-colored lips, fingernails or palms of hands.

Drug interactions of dental interest
Use of iron supplements reduces the absorption of tetracyclines.

Laboratory value alterations
The normal daily recommended intake of elemental iron for adolescent and adult males is 10 mg; for nonpregnant adolescent and adult females, the amount ranges from 10 to 15 mg. Common methods to ascertain iron levels in the human body usually measure iron indirectly via hemoglobin levels or hematocrits. For adult males, the normal range of hemoglobin is 14 mg/dL-18 mg/dL and the normal hematocrit is 42-52%. For adult females, the normal range of hemoglobin is 12 mg/dL-16 mg/dL and the normal hematocrit range is 37-47%. Laboratory values falling below these ranges may indicate anemia.

See Table 22.1 for general information on antianemic agents.

Pharmacology

Iron supplements provide adequate amounts of iron necessary for erythropoeisis and increased oxygen transport capacity in the blood. Epoetin alfa induces erythropoeisis by stimulating erythroid progenitor cells to divide and differentiate into mature red blood cells.

Anticoagulant Agents

Special Dental Considerations

Early signs of overdose include bleeding from noninflamed gingivae on brushing or unexplained bruising on skin or in mouth. As the risk of localized bleeding after dental procedures (such as scaling, root planing and surgical procedures) can increase in patients taking anticoagulants, the dentist should consult with the patient's physician to determine whether temporary reduction or withdrawal of the drug is advisable.

Drug interactions of dental interest
All drug interactions affecting anticoagulants have not been identified; therefore, monitoring prothrombin time (PT) is recommended when any drug is added to or withdrawn from a patient's regimen.

Special patients
Women of childbearing age should take

Table 22.1

Antianemic Agents: Dosage Information

Generic name	Brand name(s)	Indications/uses	Dosage range*	Interactions with other drugs
Epoetin alfa	Epogen, Eprex, Procrit	A recombinant protein (identical to erythropoietin) that is used to treat anemias associated with renal failure and AIDS	**Adult, initial parenteral dose:** 50-100 units/kg 3 times/w **Adult, maintenance:** Should be lowest possible dose to maintain hematocrit at appropriate level **Child aged < 12 y:** Not established	With an increase in red blood cells, iron supplements may need to be increased as well as antihypertensive agents, owing to a decrease in endogenous iron stores and increases in blood pressure, respectively
Ferrous fumarate	Femiron, Feostat, Fumerin, Hemocyte, Ircon, Neo-Fer [CAN], Novofumar, Palafer, Palmiron, Span-FF	Replacement therapy with iron supplements is used for the prevention and treatment of anemia induced by iron deficiency	**Adult, therapeutic—oral, tablets:** 200 mg tid-qid **Adult, prophylactic—oral, tablets:** 200 mg/day **Child, therapeutic—oral, tablets:** 3 mg/kg tid **Child, prophylactic—oral, tablets:** 3 mg/kg/day	Precautions should be taken not to use iron supplements concomitantly with acetohydroxamic acid, dimercaprol, etidronate, tetracyclines, alcohol, foods or medications containing bicarbonates, carbonates, oxalates or phosphates, milk or milk products, tea, whole-grain breads, coffee, calcium supplements, cimetidine, ciprofloxacin, deferoxamine, pancreatin, penicillamine, tetracycline, trientine
Ferrous gluconate	Apo-Ferrous Gluconate [CAN], Fergon, Ferralet, Fertinic, Novoferrogluc [CAN], Simron	Replacement therapy with iron supplements is used for the prevention and treatment of anemia induced by iron deficiency	**Adult, therapeutic—oral, capsules:** 325-650 mg qid **Adult, prophylactic—oral, capsules:** 325 mg/day **Child aged < 2 y:** Dosage must be individualized by physician **Child aged > 2 y, therapeutic—oral, capsules:** 16 mg/kg tid **Child aged > 2 y, prophylactic—oral, capsules:** 8 mg/kg/day	Precautions should be taken not to use iron supplements concomitantly with acetohydroxamic acid, dimercaprol, etidronate, tetracyclines, alcohol, foods or medications containing bicarbonates, carbonates, oxalates or phosphates, milk or milk products, tea, whole-grain breads, coffee, calcium supplements, cimetidine, ciprofloxacin, deferoxamine, pancreatin, penicillamine, tetracycline, trientine

[CAN] indicates a drug available only in Canada.
* Oral dosage forms for children and adults will differ depending on how drug is formulated.

Continued on next page

Table 22.1 (cont.)

Antianemic Agents: Dosage Information

Generic name	Brand name(s)	Indications/uses	Dosage range*	Interactions with other drugs
Ferrous sulfate	Apo-Ferrous Sulfate [CAN], Feosol, Fer-In-Sol, Fero-Grad, Fero-Fradumet, Ferospae, Ferralyn Lanacaps, Ferra-TD, Mol-Iron, Novoferrosulfa [CAN], PMS-Ferrous Sulfate [CAN], Slow Fe	Replacement therapy with iron supplements is used for the prevention and treatment of anemia induced by iron deficiency	**Adult, therapeutic—oral, capsules:** 300 mg bid-qid **Adult, prophylactic—oral, capsules:** 300 mg/day **Child, therapeutic—oral, capsules:** 10 mg/kg tid **Child, prophylactic—oral, capsules:** 5 mg/kg/day	Precautions should be taken not to use iron supplements concomitantly with acetohydroxamic acid, dimercaprol, etidronate, tetracyclines, alcohol, foods or medications containing bicarbonates, carbonates, oxalates or phosphates, milk or milk products, tea, whole-grain breads, coffee, calcium supplements, cimetidine, ciprofloxacin, deferoxamine, pancreatin, penicillamine, tetracycline, trientine

* Oral dosage forms for children and adults will differ depending on how drug is formulated.
[CAN] indicates a drug available only in Canada.

additional nonhormonal precautions to prevent pregnancy when using anticoagulant agents. Anticoagulant use is not recommended during pregnancy or labor and delivery.

See Table 22.2 for general information on anticoagulant agents.

Pharmacology

These agents inhibit vitamin K γ-carboxylation of procoagulation factors II, VII, IX and X in the liver. Heparin potentiates the effects of antithrombin III and neutralizes thrombin.

Antidotes

Special Dental Considerations

In most cases, patients who receive folinic acid are suffering from toxicity (symptoms such as gastrointestinal bleeding and thrombocytopenia) owing to methotrexate, pyrimethamine or trimethoprim therapy for a neoplasm.

See Table 22.3 for general information on the antidote leucovorin.

Pharmacology

The principal use of leucovorin is to circumvent the actions of dihydrofolate reductase inhibitors.

Antifibrinolytic Agent

Special Dental Considerations

Aminocaproic acid has been used for postsurgical hemorrhage after oral surgical procedures.

Drug interactions of dental interest

Aminocaproic acid and drugs containing estrogen may increase thrombus formation.

Special patients

In women using oral contraceptives, concurrent use of aminocaproic acid increases the chance of thrombus formation.

See Table 22.4 for general information on the antifibrinolytic agent aminocaproic acid.

Pharmacology

This agent inhibits the activation of plasminogen.

Table 22.2

Anticoagulant Agents: Dosage Information

Generic name	Brand name(s)	Indications/uses	Dosage range	Interactions with other drugs
Acenocoumarol [CAN]	Sintrom [CAN]	Ensures flow of blood in vessels by preventing blood clotting and lysing of thrombi	Each dose of acenocoumarol must be individualized and adjusted according to appropriate coagulation test **Adult—oral, tablets:** 8-12 mg on first day, 4-8 mg on second day **Adult, maintenance—oral, tablets:** 1-10 mg, depending on prothrombin time tests **Child:** Not established	**Following drugs can increase anticoagulant activity:** Acetaminophen, allopurinol, aminosalicylates, amiodarone, anabolic steroids, antibiotics, oral antidiabetic agents, aspirin, bromelains, cefamandole, cefoperazone, chloral hydrate, chloramphenicol, chymotrypsin, cimetidine, cinchophen, clofibrate, danzol, dextrothyroxine, diazoxide, diflunisal, disulfiram, erythromycin, ethacrynic acid, fenoprofen, gemfibrozil, glucagon, heparin, indomethacin, influenza vaccine, isoniazid, ketoconazole, meclofenamate, mefenamic acid, meperidine, methamazole, methotrexate, methyldopa, methylphenidate, metronidazole, miconazole, MAO inhibitors, nalidixic acid, nifedipine, phenylbutazone, plicamycin, propoxyphene, propylthiouracil, quinidine, quinine, salicylates, sulfinpyrazone, sulfonamides, sulindac, testolactone, thyroid hormones, tricyclic antidepressants, valproic acid, verapamil, vitamin A, vitamin E **Following drugs can decrease anticoagulant activity:** Antacids, ascorbic acid, barbiturates, carbamazepine, chlorobutanol, diuretics, estramustine, estrogens, ethchlorvynol, glutethimide, griseofulvin, laxatives, primidone, rifampin, vitamin K **Following drugs can increase or decrease anticoagulant activity:** Alcohol, cholestyramine, colestipol, contraceptives, corticotropin, cyclophosphamide, disopyramide, glucocorticoids, halperidol, mercaptopurine, phenytoin **Comments:** Oral surgical procedures can increase danger of hemorrhage from localized areas; before scaling and root planing or any surgical procedure, consultation with patient's physician is required
Anisindione	Miradon	Ensures flow of blood in vessels by preventing blood clotting and lysing of thrombi	Each dose of anisindione must be individualized and adjusted according to appropriate coagulation test **Adult and adolescent—oral, tablets:** 25-200 mg/day as indicated by prothrombin time levels **Child:** Not established	See note above

[CAN] indicates a drug available only in Canada.

Continued on next page

Table 22.2 (cont.)

Anticoagulant Agents: Dosage Information

Generic name	Brand name(s)	Indications/uses	Dosage range	Interactions with other drugs
Dicumeral	Dicumeral	Ensures flow of blood in vessels by preventing blood clotting and lysing of thrombi	Each dose of dicumeral must be individualized and adjusted according to appropriate coagulation test **Adult and adolescent—oral:** 25-200 mg/day **Child:** Not established	**Following drugs can increase anticoagulant activity:** Acetaminophen, allopurinol, aminosalicylates, amiodarone, anabolic steroids, antibiotics, oral antidiabetic agents, aspirin, bromelains, cefamandole, cefoperazone, chloral hydrate, chloramphenicol, chymotrypsin, cimetidine, cinchophen, clofibrate, danzol, dextrothyroxine, diazoxide, diflunisal, disulfiram, erythromycin, ethacrynic acid, fenoprofen, gemfibrozil, glucagon, heparin, indomethacin, influenza vaccine, isoniazid, ketoconazole, meclofenamate, mefenamic acid, meperidine, methamazole, methotrexate, methyldopa, methylphenidate, metronidazole, miconazole, MAO inhibitors, nalidixic acid, nifedipine, phenylbutazone, plicamycin, propoxyphene, propylthiouracil, quinidine, quinine, salicylates, sulfinpyrazone, sulfonamides, sulindac, testolactone, thyroid hormones, tricyclic antidepressants, valproic acid, verapamil, vitamin A, vitamin E **Following drugs can decrease anticoagulant activity:** Antacids, ascorbic acid, barbiturates, carbamazepine, chlorobutanol, diuretics, estramustine, estrogens, etchlorvynol, glutethimide, griseofulvin, laxatives, primidone, rifampin, vitamin K **Following drugs can increase or decrease anticoagulant activity:** Alcohol, cholestyramine, colestipol, contraceptives, corticotropin, cyclophosphamide, disopyramide, glucocorticoids, halperidol, mercaptopurine, phenytoin **Comments:** Oral surgical procedures can increase the danger of hemorrhage from localized areas; before scaling and root planing or any surgical procedure, a consultation with the patient's physician is required
Heparin	Calcilean, Calciparine, Hepalean, Heparin Leo, Liquaemin	Ensures flow of blood in vessels by preventing blood clotting and lysing of thrombi	Each dose of heparin must be individualized and adjusted according to appropriate coagulation test **Adult—IV:** 5,000 units, followed by 20,000-40,000 units over 24 h **Child—IV:** 50 units/kg followed by 20,000 units/m²/24 h	Glucocorticoids, ethacrynic acid, salicylates, anticoagulants (for example, coumarin, antihistamines, digitalis glycosides, nicotine, tetracyclines, streptokinase, urokinase, and so forth) may interact with heparin, aspirin, sulfinpyrazone, cefamandole, cefoperazone, plicamycin, valproic acid, chloroquine, hydroxychloroquine, methimazole, propylthiouracil, nitroglycerine, probenecid and thrombolytic agents **Comments:** Oral surgical procedures can increase the danger of hemorrhage from localized areas; before scaling and root planing or any surgical procedure, consultation with patient's physician is required

| Warfarin | Coumadin, Panwarfin, Sofarin, Warfilone | Ensures flow of blood in vessels by preventing blood clotting and lysing of thrombi | Each dose of warfarin must be individualized and adjusted according to appropriate coagulation test

Adult and adolescent—oral: 10-15 mg/day for 2-4 days, followed by 2-10 mg/day as indicated by prothrombin time levels

Child: Not established | **Following drugs can increase anticoagulant activity:** Acetaminophen, allopurinol, aminosalicylates, amiodarone, anabolic steroids, antibiotics, aspirin, bromelains, cefamandole, cefoperazone, chloral hydrate, chloramphenicol, chymotrypsin, cimetidine, cinchophen, clofibrate, danzol, dextrothyroxine, diazoxide, diflunisal, disulfiram, erythromycin, ethacrynic acid, fenoprofen, gemfibrozil, glucagon, heparin, indomethacin, influenza vaccine, isoniazid, ketoconazole, meclofenamate, mefenamic acid, meperidine, methamazole, methotrexate, methyldopa, methylphenidate, metronidazole, miconazole, MAO inhibitors, nalidixic acid, nifedipine, phenylbutazone, plicamycin, propoxyphene, propylthiouracil, quinidine, quinine, salicylates, sulfinpyrazone, sulfonamides, sulindac, testolactone, thyroid hormones, tricyclic antidepressants, valproic acid, verapamil, vitamin A, vitamin E

Following drugs can decrease anticoagulant activity: Antacids, ascorbic acid, barbiturates, carbamazepine, chlorobutanol, diuretics, estramustine, estrogens, ethchlorvynol, glutethimide, griseofulvin, laxatives, primidone, rifampin, vitamin K

Following drugs can increase or decrease anticoagulant activity: Alcohol, cholestyramine, colestipol, contraceptives, corticotropin, cyclophosphamide, disopyramide, glucocorticoids, halperidol, mercaptopurine, phenytoin

Comments: Oral surgical procedures can increase the danger of hemorrhage from localized areas; before scaling and root planing or any surgical procedure, a consultation with the patient's physician is required |

Table 22.3

Antidote: Dosage Information

Generic name	Brand name(s)	Indications/uses	Dosage range	Interactions with other drugs
Leucovorin	Wellcovorin, generic	Used in cancer chemotherapy when high doses of folic acid antagonists (that is, methotrexate, pyrimethamine or trimethoprim) are used	Various dosage regimens have been used; doctor who prescribes this medication should consult the literature, as most regimens are experimental **Adult—parenteral:** 10 mg/m² q 6 h until methotrexate blood levels fall below 5x10⁻⁸ m **Child:** Not established	Anticonvulsants (barbiturate or hydantoin), primidone and fluorouracil may interact with folinic acid

Table 22.4

Antifibrinolytic Agent: Dosage Information

Generic name	Brand name(s)	Indications/uses	Dosage range	Interactions with other drugs
Aminocaproic acid	Amicar	Used to control hemorrhage induced following surgery or by hyperfibrinolysis-induced treatment	**Adult—oral:** 5 g in first h, followed by 1 g/h for 8 h or until appropriate response is achieved **Child—oral:** 0.1 g/kg for first h, followed by 0.0333 g/kg for 24 h or until appropriate response is achieved; total dose should not exceed 18 g	Estrogens, oral contraceptives containing estrogens and factor IX complex, in combination with aminocaproic acid, may increase the potential for thrombus formation

Antithrombotic Agents

Special Dental Considerations

As increased risk of localized bleeding can occur after dental procedures (such as scaling, root planing and surgical procedures), the dentist should consider consulting the patient's physician to determine whether temporary reduction or withdrawal of the drug is advisable. It is recommended that these drugs be discontinued 10-14 days before any dental surgery. Ticlopidine also may induce neutropenia, leading to microbial infections, delayed healing and gingival bleeding. Dental work should be delayed if severe neutropenia occurs.

Drug interactions of dental interest

There are additive effects of dipyridamole with aspirin on platelet aggregation. Therefore, there is a risk of increased bleeding when these agents are used with aspirin or (nonsteroidal anti-inflammatory drugs (NSAIDs).

Laboratory value alterations

Blood pressure and bleeding times should be monitored. Normal bleeding times range between 3 and 10 min, depending on the method used to determine bleeding times. Normal neutrophil levels are 3000-7000/cm³.

See Table 22.5 for general information on antithrombotic agents.

Table 22.5

Antithrombotic Agents: Dosage Information

Generic name	Brand name(s)	Indications/uses	Dosage range	Interactions with other drugs
Dipyridamole	Apo-Dipyridamole [CAN], Dipridacot, IV Persantine, Novodipiradol [CAN], Persantine	Used in conjunction with other anticoagulants to reduce chance of clotting problems associated with prosthetic heart valves	**Adult—oral:** 75-100 mg for 4 days with concomitant administration of an anticoagulant **Child:** Not established	Nonsteroidal anti-inflammatory drugs, platelet aggregation inhibitors, aspirin, cefamandole, cefoperazone, cefotetan, pliamycin, valproic acid and thrombolytic agents may affect actions of this drug
Ticlopidine	Ticlid	Inhibits platelet aggregation and reduces chance of recurrent stroke in individuals who have had a thrombotic stroke	**Adult—oral:** 250 mg bid **Child:** Not established	Anticoagulants (for example, coumarin-derivatives), heparin, thrombolytic agents (for example, alteplase) and aspirin may increase the risk of bleeding when used with ticlopidine Antacids may decrease plasma concentrations of ticlopidine **Comments:** Prior to any dental surgery, patients should discontinue use of ticlopidine for 10-14 days In an emergency, the transfusion of fresh platelets may rectify hemostatic problems; in addition, ticlopidine may induce neutropenia and patient may elicit gingival bleeding, delayed healing and susceptiblity to infections; blood tests should be considered to determine neutrophil content and work delayed until blood counts return to normal

[CAN] indicates a drug available only in Canada.

Pharmacology

These agents either decrease or increase platelet aggregation.

Nutritional Supplements

Special Dental Considerations

Anemic patients may exhibit pallor in the mouth. Cyanocobalamin and folic acid are dietary supplements used to treat anemia.

Drug interactions of dental interest

Antibiotics can interfere with the assay of serum vitamin B$_{12}$ concentrations or serum folic acid concentrations. Sulfonamides will inhibit the absorption of folate.

See Table 22.6 for general information on nutritional supplements.

Pharmacology

These supplements provide adequate amounts of vitamin K or folic acid to prevent anemia.

Thrombolytic Agents

Special Dental Considerations

These agents are used intensively for short periods in a hospital setting; therefore, drug interactions are not normally observed in a dental office.

Drug interactions of dental interest

Antibiotics (cefamandole, cefoperazone, cefotetan), aspirin and NSAIDs may increase the risk of bleeding when used in conjunction with thrombolytic agents.

See Table 22.7 for general information on thrombolytic agents.

Table 22.6

Nutritional Supplements: Dosage Information

Generic name	Brand name(s)	Indications/uses	Dosage range	Interactions with other drugs
Cyanocobalamin	Anacobin, Bedoz, Cobex, Crystamine, Crysti-12, Cyanoject, Cyomin, Rubion, Rubramin, Rubramin PC, generic	For prevention or treatment of pernicious anemia	**Adult—oral:** 0.001 mg/day, not to exceed 0.025 mg/day **Child aged ≤ 1 y—oral:** 0.0007 mg/day **Child aged > 1 y—oral:** 0.001 mg/day	Alcohol, aminosalicylates, colchicine, ascorbic acid and folic acid may reduce plasma concentration of cyanocobalamin Antibiotics can interfere with assay of serum vitamin B$_{12}$ concentrations
Folic acid	Apo-Folic [CAN], Folvite, Novo-Folacid [CAN]	Replacement therapy with folic acid is used for prevention and treatment of anemia induced by folic acid deficiency	**Adult, as dietary supplement—oral:** 0.1 mg/day **Adult, for initial treatment of folic acid deficiency—oral:** 0.25-1 mg/day **Adult, for maintenance treatment of folic acid deficiency—oral:** 0.4 mg/day **Child, as dietary supplement—oral:** 0.1 mg/day **Child, for initial treatment of folic acid deficiency—oral:** 0.25-1 mg/day **Child, for maintenance treatment of folic acid deficiency—oral:** 0.1-0.4 mg/day, depending on child's age	Analgesics, anticonvulsants (hydantoin), carbamazepine, estrogens, aluminum- or magnesium-containing antacids, antibiotics, chlestyramine, methotrexate, pyrimethamine, triamterene, trimethoprim, sulfonamides and zinc supplements have been indicated to interact with folic acid

[CAN] indicates a drug available only in Canada.

Pharmacology

These agents activate the endogenous fibrinolytic system by converting plasminogen to plasmin.

Adverse Effects, Precautions and Contraindications

Dental care professionals should be aware of the possible adverse effects of hematologic drugs (Table 22.8), as well as precautions and contraindications for their use (Table 22.9).

Suggested Readings

Becker RC, Gore JM. Cardiovascular therapies in the 1990s. An overview. Drugs 1991;41:345-57.

Corbett NE, Peterson GM. Review of the initiation of anticoagulant therapy. J Clin Pharm Ther 1995;20(4):221-4.

Freedman MD. Pharmacodynamics, clinical indications, and adverse effects of heparin. J Clin Pharmacol 1992;32:584-96.

Haines ST, Bussey HI. Thrombosis and the pharmacology of antithrombotic agents. Ann Pharm 1995;29:892-905.

Stringer KA. Beyond thrombolysis: other effects of thrombolytic drugs. Ann Pharm 1994;28:752-6.

Workman ML. Anticoagulants and thrombolytics: what's the difference? AACN Clin Issues 1994;5:26-35.

Table 22.7

Thrombolytic Agents: Dosage Information

Generic name	Brand name(s)	Indications/uses	Dosage range*	Interactions with other drugs
Alteplase, recombinant	Activase, Activase rt-PA, Lysatec rt-PA	Lysis of occluding thrombi in arterial or venous vessels	**Adult > 65 kg, for coronary arterial thrombosis—IV:** 100 mg over 3 h **Child:** Not established	Anticoagulants (for example, coumarin-derivative drugs), enoxaparin, heparin, antifibrinolytic agents (for example, amino-caproic acid), antihypertensive agents, cefamandole, cefoperazone, cefotetan, plicamycin, valproic acid, corticosteroids, ethacrynic acid, salicylates, nonsteroidal anti-inflammatory drugs, aspirin, indomethacin, phenylbutazone, platelet aggregation inhibitors, sulfinpyrazone, ticlopidine and thiotepa may interfere with this drug's actions
Anistreplase	Eminase	Lysis of occluding thrombi in arterial or venous vessels	**Adult, for coronary arterial thrombosis—IV:** 30 units over 2-5 min **Child:** Not established	See note above
Streptokinase	Kabikinase, Streptase	Lysis of occluding thrombi in arterial or venous vessels	**Adult, for coronary arterial thrombosis—IV:** 1,500,000 international units **Child:** Not established	See note above
Urokinase	Abbokinase, Abbokinase Open-Cath	Lysis of occluding thrombi in arterial or venous vessels	**Adult, for coronary arterial thrombosis—IV:** 6,000 units/min **Child:** Not established	See note above

* Thrombolytic therapy should be accomplished in a hospital setting with appropriate personnel and equipment to monitor the patient. Each dose of drug must be individualized and adjusted according to the appropriate coagulation test.

Table 22.8

Hematologic Drugs: Adverse Effects

Body system	Antianemic agents	Anticoagulant agents	Antidote: Leucovorin	Antifibrinolytic agent: Aminocaproic acid	Antithrombotic agents	Nutritional supplements	Thrombolytic agents
General	**Epoetin alfa:** Chest pain **Ferrous drugs:** Soreness, contact irritation	**Heparin:** Pain, allergic reactions (anaphylaxis and anaphylactic shock), bleeding, chest pain **All other drugs in this category:** Bleeding	**Leucovorin:** Allergic reaction	Allergic reaction, unusual tiredness or weakness	**Dipyridamole:** Allergic reaction **Ticlopidine:** Bleeding complications	**Folic acid:** Allergic reaction	**All listed:** Allergic reaction, bleeding from wounds, fever, bleeding into subcutaneous spaces
CV	**Epoetin alfa:** Hypertension, tachycardia			Hypotension, thromboembolism	**Dipyridamole:** Angina pectoris		Hypotension, stroke, cholesterol or fat embolism
CNS	**Epoetin alfa:** Seizures **Ferrous drugs:** Drowsiness			Dizziness, lightheadedness	**Dipyridamole:** Dizziness, lightheadedness		
EENT				Tinnitus	**Ticlopidine:** Tinnitus		
GI	**Ferrous drugs:** Stomach pain, cramping, diarrhea, vomiting, constipation, nausea	**All but heparin:** Diarrhea, nausea		Gastrointestinal irritation (nausea, diarrhea)	**Dipyridamole:** Gastrointestinal irritation (diarrhea, nausea) **Ticlopidine:** Diarrhea, indigestion, nausea, abdominal pain		

System					
GU	**All but heparin:** Renal damage		Bladder obstruction		
Hema	**All but heparin:** Agranulocytosis			**Ticlopidine:** Agranulocytosis, thrombocytopenia	
HB	**All but heparin:** Hepatotoxicity			**Ticlopidine:** Hepatitis	
Integ	**Epoetin alfa:** Allergic reactions (rash, hives) **Ferrous drugs:** Bluish-colored lips and palms of hand; rash, hives	**Heparin:** Coldness or bluish tinge of extremities, necrosis of skin		**Ticlopidine:** Rash	**Cyanocobalamin:** Allergic reactions (rash, hives) **Folic acid:** Rash
Musc	**Ferrous drugs:** Muscle pain	**Heparin:** Peripheral neuropathy	Myopathy		
Oral	**Ferrous drugs:** Metallic taste				
Renal			Renal failure		
Resp	**Epoetin alfa:** Shortness of breath			**Dipyridamole:** Dyspnea	**Folic acid:** Bronchospasm

Table 22.9

Hematologic Drugs: Precautions and Contraindications

Antianemic agents	Anticoagulant agents	Antidote: Leucovorin	Antifibrinolytic agent: Aminocaproic acid	Antithrombotic agents	Nutritional supplements	Thrombolytic agents
Epoetin alfa: May cause increase in blood pressure; therefore, blood pressure should be monitored at frequent intervals; hypertensive patients must comply with their antihypertensive regimen Rapid rise of the hematocrit has been associated with medical problems and must be monitored twice/w Low iron levels will decrease efficacy of epoetin Renal function should be monitored in patients with impaired renal function Pregnancy risk category: C	**Acenocoumarol, anisindione, dicumeral, warfarin:** Congenital defects have been reported in pregnant women taking coumarin-like anticoagulants Owing to the deficiency of vitamin K, infants are more susceptible to anticoagulants Contraindicated in patients with history of miscarriage, aneurysm, any type of hemorrhage (for example, cerebrovascular), hypertension, hemophilia, thrombocytopenia, severe diabetes, recent childbirth, endocarditis, recent surgery (for example, ophthalmic, neurosurgery), pericarditis, impaired renal function, trauma, impaired hepatic function Pregnancy risk category: X	**Leucovorin:** May increase seizures in children Contraindicated in patients with pernicious anemia, vitamin B$_{12}$ deficiency, impaired renal function, sensitivity to folinic acid Pregnancy risk category: C	May cause hypotension and bradycardia and should be carefully considered when prescribed to patients with cardiovascular problems In a few cases, this medication has caused acute renal failure Contraindicated in patients with hypersensitivity to this medication Pregnancy risk category: C	**Dipyridamole:** Contraindicated in patients with unstable angina pectoris, collateral blood vessels and hypotension Pregnancy risk category: B	**Cyanocobalamin:** Contraindicated in patients with Leber's disease and sensitivity to this drug Pregnancy risk category: C	**All thrombolytic agents:** Contraindicated in patients with aneurysm, arteriovenous malformations, active bleeding, brain tumors, cerebrovascular accident, recent surgery, recent trauma, hypertension, anaphylaxis to streptokinase or anistreplase, recent childbirth, coagulation defects, endocarditis, mitral stenosis **Alteplase, recombinant; anistreplase; streptokinase:** Pregnancy risk category C **Urokinase:** Pregnancy risk category B

Ferrous fumarate, ferrous gluconate, ferrous sulfate: Tumors have been reported at injection site for iron dextran

Use of iron supplements is contraindicated in patients with hemochromatosis, hemosiderosis, hemolytic anemia, thalassemia, alcoholism, asthma, hepatitis, kidney disease, enteritis, colitis, peptic ulcer, rheumatoid arthritis, allergy to iron

Pregnancy risk category: C

Heparin: Geriatric women (aged > 60 y) may be more susceptible to bleeding during therapy

May cause osteoporosis in lactating women

Contraindicated in patients with history of miscarriage, aneurysm, any type of hemorrhage (for example, cerebrovascular), hypertension, hemophilia, thrombocytopenia, severe diabetes, recent childbirth, endocarditis, recent surgery (for example, ophthalmic, neurosurgery), pericarditis, impaired renal function, trauma, impaired hepatic function

Pregnancy risk category: C

Ticlopidine: Use should be discontinued 10-14 days before any surgical procedure

Contradindicated in patients with active bleeding, hemophilia, hemapoietic disorders (for example, neutropenia), impaired hepatic function, gastrointestinal ulceration, recent surgery, recent trauma, impaired renal function and sensitivity to this drug

Pregnancy risk category: B

Folic acid: Contraindicated in treatment of pernicious anemia, as irreversible neurologic problems may occur; also contraindicatedin patients with hypersensitivity to this drug

Pregnancy risk category: A

Chapter 23

Endocrine/Hormonal Drugs

Angelo J. Mariotti, D.D.S., Ph.D.

Hormones are chemical substances that are secreted from various organs into the blood stream and have specific regulatory effects on target tissues. The general functions of hormones can be divided into reproduction; growth and development; homeostasis of the internal environment; and energy production, utilization and storage.

Although the effects of hormones are diverse and complex, hormones can be divided into two broad categories according to their chemical structure: polypeptides and steroids. The polypeptides or amino acid derivates represent a majority of hormones. This category comprises hormones that are secreted from a variety of organs (such as brain, pancreas, thyroid and adrenal glands) and include large polypeptides (such as leuteinizing hormone), medium-sized peptides (such as insulin), small peptides (such as throtropin-releasing hormone), dipeptides (such as throxine) and single amino acid byproducts (such as histamine).

The remaining hormones are derivatives of cholesterol and are called steroid hormones. Similarly to the polypeptide hormones, steroid hormones are secreted from a variety of organs (such as adrenal glands, testis and ovary). But unlike the polypeptide hormones, they are more uniform in their chemical structure, because each steroid hormone must contain a cyclopentano-perhydrophenanthrene ring system (for example, estradiol).

Hormones, regardless of their chemical structure, have common characteristics. First, hormones are found in low concentrations in the blood circulation. Most polypeptide hormone concentrations in the blood range from 1 to 100 femtomolar, while thyroid and steroid hormone concentrations range between picomolar and micromolar concentrations. Second, hormones must be directed to their sites of action, and this is most commonly accomplished by special protein molecules (receptors) that recognize specific hormones. Polypeptide hormone receptors are proteins that are fixed on the cell membrane; thyroid and steroid hormone receptors are proteins located inside the cell.

Although most drugs are considered to be foreign substances to the body, naturally occurring substances such as hormones can be used as drugs and can exert important effects on the human body. Furthermore, analogs of hormones also have been synthesized to produce important therapeutic effects. In addition, various drugs affect the synthesis, secretion or degradation of hormones as well as antagonize their cellular effects (hormone antagonists).

Androgens

Special Dental Considerations
Androgens can exacerbate patients' inflammatory status, causing erythema and an increased tendency toward gingival bleeding. A controlled oral hygiene program that combines professional cleanings and plaque control will minimize androgen-induced sequelae.

Drug interactions of dental interest

Androgens are responsible for the growth and development of male sex organs and for the maintenance of secondary sexual characteristics in males. Androgens can be used for replacement therapy in androgen-deficient men or for treatment of certain neoplasms. Androgens may enhance the actions of oral anticoagulants, oral hypoglycemic agents and glucocorticoids.

See Table 23.1 for general information on androgens.

Pharmacology

Androgens bind to intracellular androgen receptors that regulate RNA and DNA in target tissues.

Estrogens

Special Dental Considerations

Estrogens can exacerbate patients' inflammatory status, causing erythema and an increased tendency toward gingival bleeding. In some instances, estrogens have been reported to induce gingival overgrowths. A controlled oral hygiene program that combines professional cleanings and plaque control will minimize estrogen-induced sequelae.

Drug interactions of dental interest

Estrogens are responsible for the growth and development of female sex organs and for the maintenance of secondary sexual characteristics in women. Estrogens can be used to treat a variety of estrogen-deficiency states, as well as for certain neoplasms. Estrogen may change the requirements for oral anticoagulants, oral hypoglycemics, insulin or barbiturates.

See Table 23.2 for general information on estrogens.

Pharmacology

Estrogens bind to intracellular estrogen receptors that regulate RNA and DNA in target tissues.

Insulin

Special Dental Considerations

Patients with diabetes mellitus are at risk of developing periodontal disease. A thorough evaluation of the mouth followed by a controlled oral hygiene program—including regular oral examinations, professional cleanings and plaque control—are recommended. Because diabetics have an increased risk of leukopenia and thrombocytopenia, an increased frequency of infection, altered wound healing and gingival bleeding is possible. Dental treatment should be delayed if leukopenia or cytopenia occurs.

People who have either insulin-dependent or noninsulin-dependent diabetes mellitus can experience untoward effects in the dental office. These can occur when a patient's insulin dose is not correctly titrated and blood glucose levels are either too low or too high. In patients whose diabetes is well-controlled by insulin (or other hypoglycemic agents), these concerns are minimized by proper medication in conjunction with proper diet.

Drug interactions of dental interest

Insulin can be used for the treatment of patients with either insulin-dependent or noninsulin-dependent diabetes mellitus. Corticosteroids may enhance blood glucose levels, and large doses of salicylates and nonsteroidal anti-inflammatory drugs may increase the hypoglycemic effect of insulin.

Laboratory value alterations

- Values for leukocytes in leukopenia: less than 4,000 cells per cubic millimeter as opposed to the normal values, 5,000-10,000 cells/mm³.
- Values for platelets in thrombocytopenia: less than 20,000 platelets/mm³ as opposed to the normal values, 150,000-350,000 platelets.

Table 23.1

Androgens: Dosage Information

Generic name	Brand name(s)	Indications/uses	Dosage range	Interactions with other drugs
Fluoxymesterone	Android-F, Halotestin	Androgens are anabolic steroid hormones used for treatment of androgen deficiency, delayed male puberty, catabolic processes, anemia as well as for treatment of some types of breast neoplasms	Drug therapy with androgens should be at lowest effective dose, with amount of drug individualized and adjusted to obtain desired effect Regular monitoring by a physician is necessary	Anticoagulants (coumarin- or indandione-derivative), oral hypoglycemics, insulin and cylcosporine may affect actions of androgens
Methyltestosterone	Android-10, Metandren, Oreton, Testred	See note above	See note above	See note above
Nandrolone	Deca-Durabolin, Durabolin, Hybolin Decanoate, Hybolin-Improved, Kabolin, Neo-Durabolic	See note above	See note above	See note above
Oxandrolone	Oxandrin	See note above	See note above	See note above
Oxymetholone	Anadrol-50, Anapolon 50	See note above	See note above	See note above
Stanozolol	Winstrol	See note above	See note above	See note above
Testosterone	Andro 100, Andro-Cyp 100, Andro-Cyp 200, Andro L.A. 100, Andro L.A. 200, Andryl 200, Delatest, Delatestryl, depAndro 100, depAndro 200, Depotest, Depo-Testosterone, Depo-Testosterone Cypionate, Duratest-100, Duratest-200, Durathate-200, Everone, Histerone-50, Histerone-100, Malogen, Malogex, T-Cypionate, Testa-C, Testamone 100, Testaqua, Testex, Testoderm, Testoject-50, Testoject-LA, Testone L.A. 200, Testred Cypionate 200, Testrin-P.A., Virilon IM	See note above	See note above	See note above

Table 23.2

Estrogens: Dosage Information

Generic name	Brand name(s)	Indications/uses	Dosage range	Interactions with other drugs
Cholortrianisene	TACE	Estrogens are steroid hormones used for treatment of estrogen deficiency, atropic vaginitis, vulvar squamous hyperplasia, menopause, uterine bleeding, osteoporosis, and some types of breast and prostatic neoplasms	Drug therapy with estrogens should be at the lowest effective dose, with amount of drug individualized and adjusted to obtain desired effect Estrogens may be administered in a cyclic or continuous regimen depending on the indication for use Regular monitoring by a physician is necessary	Bromocriptine, corticosteroids, cyclosporine, and some antibiotics may affect actions of estrogens
Conjugated estrogen	Congest, Premarin, Premarin Intravenous	See note above	See note above	See note above
Diethylstilbestrol	Honvol, Stilphostrol	See note above	See note above	See note above
Esterified estrogens	Estratab, Menest, Neo-Estrone [CAN]	See note above	See note above	See note above
Estradiol	Clinagen LA 40, Deladiol-40, Delestrogen, depGynogen, Depo-Estradiol, Depogen, Dioval 40, Dioval XX, Dura-Estrin, Duragen-20, Duragen-40, E-Cypionate, Estrace, Estraderm, Estragyn LA 5, Estra-L 40, Estro-Cyp, Estrofem, Estroject-LA, Estro-L.A., Estro-Span, Femogex, Gynogen L.A. 20, Gynogen L.A. 40, Menaval-20, Valeregen-10, Valeregen-20, Valeregen-40	See note above	See note above	See note above
Estrone	Aquest, Estragyn 5, Estro-A, Kestrone-5, Wehgen	See note above	See note above	See note above
Estropipate	Ogen, Ogen .625, Ogen 1.25, Ogen 2.5, Ortho-Est	See note above	See note above	See note above
Ethinyl estradiol	Estinyl	See note above	See note above	See note above
Quinestrol	Estrovis	See note above	See note above	See note above

[CAN] indicates a drug available only in Canada.

Signs of hypoglycemia	Signs of hyperglycemia
Anxiety	Dry mouth
Blood pressure normal or increased	Blood pressure normal or decreased
Breath normal in odor	Smell of acetone on breath
Breathing may be stertorous but at normal depth and rate	Breathing is deep and fast
Confusion, inability to concentrate	Warm and dry skin
Cool and moist skin	Loss of appetite
Hunger	Normal or depressed reflexes
Hyperactive reflexes	Lethargy
Lethargy	Gradual onset of symptoms
Rapid onset of symptoms	Rapid, normal or thready pulse
Rapid pulse	
Tired, weak	
Unsteadiness	
Vision problems	

See Table 23.3 for general information on insulin.

Pharmacology

Insulin binds to fixed receptors on the cell membrane to control the storage and metabolism of carbohydrates, proteins and lipids.

Oral Contraceptives

Special Dental Considerations

Oral contraceptives can exacerbate patients' inflammatory status, causing erythema and an increased tendency toward gingival bleeding. In some instances, oral contraceptives have been reported to induce gingival overgrowths. A controlled oral hygiene program that includes regular oral examinations, professional cleanings and plaque control will minimize the effects of oral contraceptives. These drugs can also increase the incidence of local alveolar osteitis after extraction of teeth.

Drug interactions of dental interest

Oral contraceptives are used primarily to prevent ovulation. The effectiveness of oral contraceptives may be decreased by penicillin, chloramphenicol, oral neomycin, sulfonamides, barbiturates, glucocorticoids, griseofulvin and tetracyclines.

See Table 23.4 for general information on oral contraceptives.

Pharmacology

Oral contraceptives prevent conception by suppressing ovulation, preventing nidation or slowing migration of sperm to the ovum.

Oral Hypoglycemic Agents

Special Dental Considerations

Patients with diabetes mellitus are at risk of developing periodontal disease. In patients whose diabetes is well-controlled by hypoglycemic agents, concerns are minimized with proper medication, proper diet and proper oral hygiene. It is recommended that these patients receive a thorough evaluation of the mouth followed by a controlled oral hygiene program that includes regular oral examinations, professional cleanings and plaque control. Owing to an increased risk of leukopenia and thrombocytopenia in diabetic patients, an increased frequency of infection, altered wound healing and gingival bleeding is possible. Dental treatment should be delayed if leukopenia or cytopenia occurs.

Drug interactions of dental interest

Oral hypoglycemic agents can be used only for the treatment of noninsulin-dependent diabetes mellitus. Glucocorticoids may decrease the effectiveness of oral hypoglycemic agents. Nonsteroidal anti-inflammatory drugs and salicylates may increase the risk of hypoglycemia.

Table 23.3

Insulin: Dosage Information

Generic name	Brand name(s)	Indications/uses	Dosage range	Interactions with other drugs
Extended insulin zinc	Humulin-U, Humulin U Ultralente, Lente Iletin, Lente Iletin I, Lente Iletin II, Lente Insulin, Lente L, Novolin ge Ultralente [CAN], Ultralente Insulin, Ultralente U	Insulin is used in treatment of insulin-dependent and noninsulin dependent diabetes mellitus	Amount of insulin and timing of insulin administration can vary dramatically among different patients; consequently, dosage and administration of insulin must be individualized and adjusted by physician to obtain desired blood glucose level in the patient **Adult—maintenance, SC:** 0.5-1.0 unit/kg/day	Amphetamines, baclofen, oral contraceptives, corticosteroids, danazol, dextrothyroxine, thiazide diuretics, epinephrine, estrogens, ethacrynic acid, furosemide, molindone, phenytoin, thyroid hormones and triamterene may enhance blood glucose concentrations, and dosage of either insulin or these drugs must be adjusted Alcohol, anabolic steroids, disopyramid, guanethidine, MAO inhibitors, large doses of salicylates and nonsteroidal anti-inflammatory analgesics may increase hypoglycemic effect of insulin β-adrenergic blocking agents may increase risk of either hypoglycemia or hyperglycemia
Insulin	Humulin R, Humulin-R, Insulin-Toronto, Novolin ge Toronto [CAN], Novolin R, Regular Iletin II, Regular Iletin, Regular Iletin I, Regular Iletin II, Regular Insulin, Velosulin Human	See note above	Amount of insulin and timing of insulin administration can vary dramatically among different patients; consequently, dosage and administration of insulin must be individualized and adjusted by physician to obtain desired blood glucose level in the patient	See note above

[CAN] indicates a drug available only in Canada.

Continued on next page

Table 23.3 (cont.)

Insulin: Dosage Information

Generic name	Brand name(s)	Indications/uses	Dosage range	Interactions with other drugs
Insulin zinc	Humulin L, Humulin-L, Novolin ge Lente [CAN], Novolin L	Insulin is used in treatment of insulin-dependent and noninsulin dependent diabetes mellitus	Amount of insulin and timing of insulin administration can vary dramatically among different patients; consequently, dosage and administration of insulin must be individualized and adjusted by physician to obtain desired blood glucose level in the patient	Amphetamines, baclofen, oral contraceptives, corticosteroids, danazol, dextrothyroxine, thiazide diuretics, epinephrine, estrogens, ethacrynic acid, furosemide, molindone, phenytoin, thyroid hormones and triamterene may enhance blood glucose concentrations, and dosage of either insulin or these drugs must be adjusted

Alcohol, anabolic steroids, disopyramid, guanethidine, MAO inhibitors, large doses of salicylates and nonsteroidal anti-inflammatory analgesics may increase hypoglycemic effect of insulin

ß-adrenergic blocking agents may increase risk of either hypoglycemia or hyperglycemia |
| Isophane insulin | Humulin 10/90, Humulin 20/80, Humulin 30/70, Humulin 40/60, Humulin 50/50, Humulin 70/30, Humulin N, Humulin-N, Novolin 70/30, Novolin ge 10/90, Novolin ge 20/80, Novolin ge 30/70, Novolin ge 40/60, Novolin ge 50/50, Novolin ge NPH, Novolin N, NPH Iletin, NPH Iletin I, NPH Iletin II, NPH Insulin | See note above | See note above | See note above |
| Prompt insulin zinc | Semilente Insulin | See note above | See note above | See note above |

[CAN] indicates a drug available only in Canada.

Table 23.4

Oral Contraceptives: Dosage Information

Generic name	Brand name(s)	Indications/uses	Dosage range	Interactions with other drugs
Desogestrel (progestin), ethinyl estradiol (estrogen)	Desogen, Marvelon, Ortho-Cept	Oral contraceptives are a combination of estrogens and/or progestins used for prevention of pregancy	Use of oral contraceptives depends on the preparation; monophasic, biphasic and triphasic combination oral contraceptives are taken for 21 days followed by a 7-day period during which no pills are taken; progesterone-only contraceptives (see Table 23.6, Progestins) are taken daily without interruption or can be injected IMI (for example, medroxyprogesterone)	Bromocriptine, anticoagulants (coumarin- or indandione-derivative) corticosteroids, cyclosporine, tricyclic antidepressants and some antibiotics (for example, ampicillin, chloramphenicol, neomycin, penicillin V, sulfonamides, tetracyclines) may affect actions of estrogens
Ethynodiol diacetate (progestin), ethinyl estradiol (estrogen)	Demulen 1/35, Demulen 1/50, Demulen 30, Demulen 50, Nelulen 1/35E, Nelulen 1/50E	See note above	See note above	See note above
Levonorgestrel (progestin), ethinyl estradiol (estrogen)	Levlen, Mini-Ovral, Nordette, Tri-Levlen, Triphasil, Triquilar	See note above	See note above	See note above
Norethindrone (progestin), ethinyl estradiol (estrogen)	Brevicon, Brevicon 0.5/35, Brevicon 1/35, GenCept 0.5/35, GenCept 1/35, GenCept 10/11, Genora 0.5/35, Genora 1/35, Jenest, ModiCon, N.E.E. 1/35, N.E.E. 1/50, Nelova 0.5/35E, Nelova 1/35E, Nelova 10/11, Norethin 1/35E, Norinyl 1+35, Ortho 0.5/35, Ortho 1/35, Ortho 7/7/7, Ortho 10/11, Ortho-Novum 1/35, Ortho-Novum 7/7/7, Ortho-Novum 10/11, Ovcon-35, Ovcon-50, Synphasic, Tri-Norinyl	See note above	See note above	See note above
Norethindrone (progestin), mestranol (estrogen)	Genora 1/50, Nelova 1/50M, Norethin 1/50M, Norinyl 1/50, Norinyl 1+50, Ortho-Novum 0.5, Ortho-Novum 1/50, Ortho-Novum 1/80, Ortho-Novum 2	See note above	See note above	See note above

Continued on next page

Table 23.4 (cont.)

Oral Contraceptives: Dosage Information

Generic name	Brand name(s)	Indications/uses	Dosage range	Interactions with other drugs
Norethindrone acetate (progestin), ethinyl estradiol (estrogen)	Loestrin 1/20, Loestrin 1.5/30, Minestrin 1/20	Oral contraceptives are a combination of estrogens and/or progestins used for prevention of pregancy	Use of oral contraceptives depends on the preparation; monophasic, biphasic and triphasic combination oral contraceptives are taken for 21 days followed by a 7-day period during which no pills are taken; progesterone-only contraceptives (see Table 23.6, Progestins) are taken daily without interruption or can be injected IMI (for example, medroxyprogesterone)	Bromocriptine, anticoagulants (coumarin- or indandione-derivative) corticosteroids, cyclosporine, tricyclic antidepressants and some antibiotics (for example, ampicillin, chloramphenicol, neomycin, penicillin V, sulfonamides, tetracyclines) may affect actions of estrogens
Norgestimate (progestin), ethinyl estradiol (estrogen)	Cyclen, Ortho-Cyclen, Ortho Tri-Cyclen, Tri-Cyclen	See note above	See note above	See note above
Norgestrel (progestin), ethinyl estradiol (estrogen)	Lo/Ovral, Ovral	See note above	See note above	See note above

Table 23.5

Oral Hypoglycemic Agents: Dosage Information

Generic name	Brand name(s)*	Indications/uses	Dosage range	Interactions with other drugs
Acetohexamide	Dimelor, Dymelor	Oral hypoglycemics are used in treatment of noninsulin-dependent diabetes mellitus	Amount of oral hypoglycemic agents and timing of administration of oral hypoglycemic agents can vary dramatically among different patients; consequently, dosage, administration and type of oral hypoglycemic agents must be individualized and adjusted by physician to obtain desired blood glucose level in patient	Blood glucose concentrations may be increased with concomitant use of oral hypoglycemic agents and adrenocorticoids, amphetamines, anticonvulsants (for example, hydantoin), baclofen, bumetanide, calcium channel blocking agents, chlorthalidone, oral contraceptives, danazol, dextrothyroxine, epinephrine, ethacrynic acid, furosemide, glucagon, molindine, large doses of salicylates, thiazide diuretics, thyroid hormones and triamterene

Blood glucose concentrations may be decreased with concomitant use of oral hypoglycemic agents and androgens, allopurinol, nonsteroidal anti-inflammatory drugs, insulin, chloramphenicol, clofibrate, MAO inhibitors, salicylates and sulfonamides

β-adrenergic blocking agents may increase risk of either hypoglycemia or hyperglycemia |
Chlorpropamide	Chlorpropamide	See note above	See note above	See note above
Glipizide	Glucotrol	See note above	See note above	See note above
Glyburide	Albert Glyburide, Apo-Glyburide, DiaBeta, Euglucon, Gen-Glybe, Glynase PresTab, Micronase, Novo-Glyburide	See note above	See note above	See note above
Tolazamide	Tolamide, Tolinase, Tol-Tab	See note above	See note above	See note above
Tolbutamide	Apo-Tolbutamide, Mebenol, Novo-Butamide, Orinase	See note above	See note above	See note above

Drugs with the prefixes Apo- and Novo- are available only in Canada.

Laboratory value alterations

- Values for leukocytes in leukopenia: less than 4,000 cells per cubic millimeter as opposed to the normal values, 5,000-10,000 cells/mm³.
- Values for platelets in thrombocytopenia: less than 20,000 platelets/mm³ as opposed to the normal values, 150,000-350,000 platelets

See Table 23.5 for general information on oral hypoglycemic agents.

Pharmacology

Oral hypoglycemics lower blood glucose levels by stimulating the functioning of β cells of the pancreatic islets to secrete insulin.

Progestins

Special Dental Considerations

Progestins can exacerbate patients' inflammatory status, causing erythema and an increased tendency toward gingival bleeding. In some instances, progestins have been reported to induce gingival overgrowths. A controlled oral hygiene program that includes regular oral examinations, professional cleanings and plaque control will minimize the effects of progestins.

Drug interactions of dental interest

Progestins are responsible for maintenance of the female reproductive system in pregnant and nonpregnant women. Progestins are used for the treatment of certain female

Table 23.6

Progestins: Dosage Information

Generic name	Brand name(s)	Indications/uses	Dosage range	Interactions with other drugs
Hydroxyprogesterone	Hy/Gestrone, Hylutin, Pro-Depo, Prodrox, Pro-Span	Progestins are steroid hormones used for treatment of female hormonal imbalances, endometriosis, contraception, maintenance of pregancy as well as for treatment of uterine corpus, metastatic endometrial and metastatic renal carcinomas	Drug therapy with progestins should be at lowest effective dose, with amount of drug individualized and adjusted to obtain desired effect; regular monitoring by a physician is necessary	Bromocriptine in combination with progestins may cause amenorrhea or galactorrhea
Medroxyprogesterone	Amen, Curretab, Cycrin, Depo-Provera, Provera	See note above	See note above	See note above
Megestrol	Megace	See note above	See note above	See note above
Norethindrone	Aygestin, Micronor, Morlutate, Norlutin, Nor-QD	See note above	See note above	See note above
Norgestrel	Ovrette	See note above	See note above	See note above
Progesterone	Gesterol 50	See note above	See note above	See note above

hormone imbalances as well as for the treatment of some neoplasms. Drug interactions with progestins are limited and involve drugs not normally prescribed by dentists.

See Table 23.6 for general information on progestins.

Pharmacology

Progestins bind to intracellular progesterone receptors that regulate RNA and DNA in target tissues.

Thyroid Hormones

Special Dental Considerations

Well-controlled hypothyroid or hyperthyroid patients can receive any dental treatment. Dental treatment should be delayed in thyroid patients whose symptoms are not appropriately controlled pharmacologically.

Drug interactions of dental interest

Thyroid hormones, a mixture of liothyroxin and levothyroxine, are necessary for the homeostasis of the human body. Liothyroxin and/or levothyroxine are used for replacement therapy in patients with diminished thyroid function. Glucocorticoids and sympathomimetic agents may interfere with the actions of the drugs.

See Table 23.7 for general information on thyroid hormones.

Table 23.7

Thyroid Hormones: Dosage Information

Generic name	Brand name(s)	Indications/uses	Dosage range	Interactions with other drugs
Levothyroxine	Eltroxin, Leo-T, Levoxine, Synthroid	Thyroid hormones include natural and synthetic products used for treatment of hypothyroidism (replacement therapy), suppression of goiter growth and some thyroid neoplasms	Thyroid hormone therapy is generally begun with low doses and gradually increased, with amount of drug individualized and adjusted to obtain euthyroid state **Adult, maintenance:** 60-120 mg/day	Glucocorticoids, anticoagulants, cholestyramine, colestipol, estrogens, ketamine, maprotiline and sympathomimetics may interfere with actions of these drugs
Liothyronine	Cytomel	See note above	Thyroid hormone therapy is generally begun with low doses and gradually increased, with the amount of drug individualized and adjusted to obtain euthyroid state	See note above
Liotrix	Thyrolar	See note above	See note above	See note above
Thyroglobulin	Proloid	See note above	See note above	See note above
Thyroid	Armour Thyroid, Thyrar, Thyroid Strong, Westhroid	See note above	See note above	See note above

Table 23.8
Endocrine/Hormonal Drugs: Adverse Effects

Body system	Androgens	Estrogens	Insulin	Oral contraceptives	Oral hypoglycemics	Progestins	Thyroid hormones
General	Edema	Edema, anorexia, headache	Untoward effects of insulin occur when patient's insulin dose is not correctly titrated and blood glucose levels are either too low or too high, allergy	Edema, anorexia, headache, fever	Untoward effects of oral hypoglycemics occur when the individual's dose is not correctly titrated and blood glucose levels are either too low or too high, allergy	Edema, fever	Allergy
CV					Increased risk of cardiovascular mortality, congestive heart failure (chlorpropamide only)		
CNS				Mental depression		Mental depression	Pseudotumor cerebri
Endoc	**Only in males:** Breast soreness, gynecomastia, priapism, nonspecific acute epididymitis, prostatic carcinoma, benign prostatic hypertrophy **Only in females:** ammenorrhea, oligomenorrhea	Breast pain or tenderness, gynecomastia, amenorrhea, breakthrough bleeding, menorrhagia	Insulin resistance	Breast pain or tenderness, gynecomastia, amenorrhea, breakthrough bleeding, menorrhagia, changes in vaginal bleeding pattern, galactorrhea		Changes in vaginal bleeding pattern, galactorrhea	Hyperthyroidism

GI	Gastrointestinal irritation, diarrhea	Diarrhea, abdominal cramping, nausea	Diarrhea, abdominal cramping, nausea	Constipation, diarrhea, nausea	
GU	Bladder irritability (only in males)			Antidiuretic effect (chlorpropamide only), impaired renal function	
Hema	Erythrocytosis	Thromboembolism	Thromboembolism	Eosinophilia, agranulocytosis, aplastic anemia, bone marrow depression	Thromboembolic disorders
HB	Hepatic dysfunction; hepatic necrosis		Hepatitis, gallbladder obstruction		Hepatitis, gallbladder obstruction
Integ	Acne, increased hair growth in pubic region	Fat atrophy at injection site and fat hypertrophy	Acne, increased body and facial hair		Acne, increased body and facial hair
Oral	Gingival inflammation and bleeding	Gingival inflammation and bleeding	Gingival inflammation and bleeding		Gingival inflammation and bleeding

Table 23.9

Endocrine/Hormonal Drugs: Precautions and Contraindications

Drug category	Precautions/contraindications
Androgens	Increased risk of hepatic neoplasms with long-term, high-dose therapy
	In children, androgens can cause precocious puberty in boys, virilization in girls and premature closure of epiphyseal plates
	Precautions should be taken when administering androgens to patients with cardiac failure, cardi-renal disease, nephritis, nephrosis, myocardial infarction, diabetes mellitus, impaired hepatic function, hyperglycemia and benign prostatic hypertrophy
	Pregnancy risk category: X
	Contraindicated in patients taking other potentially hepatotoxic drugs
	Contraindicated in male patients with breast cancer or prostatic cancer
Estrogens	Increased risk of endometrial cancer in postmenopausal women
	In children, estrogens can cause precocious puberty in girls and prematurely close the epiphyseal plates
	Precautions should be taken when administering estrogens to patients with endometriosis, gallstones, hepatic dysfunction, hypercalcemia, thromboembolic disorders and uterine fibroids
	Pregnancy risk category: X
	Contraindicated in patients with breast cancer, neoplasms of reproductive organs or undiagnosed vaginal bleeding
Insulin	Should be used cautiously with patients who have high fever, hyperthyroidism, severe infections, diabetic ketoacidosis, trauma or surgery, hypothyroidism, diarrhea, nausea and impaired renal function
	Pregnancy risk category: A
Oral contraceptives	Increased risk of hepatic cancer in women using these drugs for > 8 y
	In children, oral contraceptives can cause precocious puberty in girls and prematurely close epiphyseal plates
	Should be used cautiously with patients who have endometriosis, gallstones, hepatic dysfunction, hypercalcemia, mental depression, hypertension, hepatic dysfunction, renal dysfunction and uterine fibroids
	Pregnancy risk category: X
	Contraindicated in patients with breast cancer, neoplasms of the reproductive organs, hepatic tumors, cerebrovascular disease, cholestatic jaundice, thromboembolic disorders or undiagnosed vaginal bleeding
Oral hypoglycemics	Should be used cautiously with patients who have adrenal insufficiency, pituitary insufficiency, high fever, impaired thyroid function, impaired hepatic function, impaired renal function and malnourishment
	Pregnancy risk category: C
	Contraindicated in patients with acidosis, severe burns, diabetic coma, severe infections, and major surgery or trauma

Continued on next page

Table 23.9 (cont.)

Endocrine/Hormonal Drugs: Precautions and Contraindications

Drug category	Precautions/contraindications
Progestins	Should be used cautiously with patients who have asthma, cardiac insufficiency, epilepsy, diabetes mellitus, hyperlipemia, mental depression and thromboembolic disorders
	Pregnancy risk category: X
	Contraindicated in patients with breast cancer or cancer of reproductive organs, hepatic disease, incomplete abortion, suspected pregnancy and undiagnosed vaginal bleeding
Thyroid hormones	Should be used cautiously with patients who have adrenocortical insufficiency, cardiovascular disease, hyperthyroidism, pituitary insufficiency or thyrotoxicosis
	Pregnancy risk category: A

Pharmacology

Thyroid hormones bind to intracellular thyroid hormone receptors that regulate catabolic and anabolic effects necessary for homeostasis.

Adverse Effects, Precautions and Contraindications

Table 23.8 presents adverse effects of endocrine/hormonal drugs; Table 23.9 presents precautions and contraindications.

Suggested Readings

Galloway JA, Hooper SA, Spradlin CT, et al. Biosynthetic human proinsulin. Review of chemistry, in vitro and in vivo receptor binding, animal and human pharmacology studies, and clinical trial experience. Diabetes Care 1992;15:666-92.

Gray H, O'Rahilly S. Toward improved glycemic control in diabetes. What's on the horizon? Arch Intern Med 1995;155:1137-42.

Ilarde A, Tuck M. Treatment of non-insulin-dependent diabetes mellitus and its complications. A state of the art review. Drugs Aging 1994;4:470-91.

Johnson JL, Felicetta JV. Hypothyroidism: a comprehensive review. J Am Acad Nurse Pract 1992;4:131-8.

Mariotti A. Sex steroid hormones and cell dynamics in the periodontium. Crit Rev Oral Biol Med 1994;5:27-53.

Shepard AR, Eberhardt NL. Molecular mechanisms of thyroid hormone action. Clin Lab Med 1993;13:531-41.

Chapter 24

Connective-Tissue Disorder and Musculoskeletal Relaxant Drugs

Martha Somerman, D.D.S., Ph.D.

Patients with connective-tissue/musculoskeletal diseases also often have associated oral symptoms. Some of the general characteristics related to connective-tissue diseases affect the skin, making it tight, drawn or affected by a rash disorder. The posture may be altered, with the loss of specific movements in the arms, hands, fingers and jaw. In addition, the joints may be swollen or inflamed with associated redness and pain. Because of this and because dentists may use muscle relaxants as an adjunct in the treatment of certain patients, dentists must be able to recognize clinical symptoms—especially oral symptoms—of connective-tissue/musculoskeletal diseases. Dentists should also be able to order biopsies where appropriate, as well as be familiar with other medical/diagnostic tests and select appropriate medications for treatment of specific disorders/diseases. This chapter focuses on drugs used for treatment of connective-tissue/musculoskeletal disorders.

General Treatment

For skin or mucosal lesions of nonviral nature, creams, lotions or ointments containing corticosteroids are often used (see Chapter 6, Corticosteroids, for details). In general, creams and lotions are preferred for moist areas because of their drying properties. Ointments retard drying, so they are used for their occlusive properties; they can be used on areas of dry skin. The more potent topical agents should be considered for recalcitrant and/or severe lesions and short-term treatment. Examples of situations in which these topical agents are used are lichen planus, psoriasis, pemphigus, pemphigoid and lupus erythematosus (LE). It is recommended that a biopsy be performed before dental treatment to determine the nature of the lesions. Steroids should not be used for virus-associated lesions.

In addition to steroids, topical antibiotics can be used for minor wounds, as can antiseptic cleansers such as povidone-iodine and chlorhexidine. Also, antihistamines (diphenhydramine HCl) can be used as a rinse for relief of certain allergic reactions. Furthermore, antimalarial drugs (such as hydroxychloroquine sulfate) have been reported to have benefits in the treatment of certain diseases and associated lesions, such as lupus erythematosus, rheumatoid arthritis, osteoarthritis and inflammation associated with joint prostheses. These act by a variety of mechanisms, including decreasing neutrophils' locomotion and decreasing complement-dependent antigen-antibody reactions. The exact reason why these compounds work in treating lupus erythematosus and rheumatoid arthritis is not understood; nevertheless, they are used for these purposes, sometimes in combination with steroids and/or NSAIDs. Yet another agent that has been used (but not approved) for pemphigus, pemphigoid, LE and malaria is dapsone, which is used to treat leprosy.

Nonviral ulcers, such as aphthous ulcers, can be treated with topical and (in very severe situations) systemic corticosteroids and immunosuppressants or both, when indicated. Importantly, if lesions are severe enough to warrant systemic therapy, a consultation with a physician or an oral medicine specialist may be in order. The FDA recently approved amlexanox for use in treatment of aphthous ulcers (see Chapter 8, Antifungal and Antiviral Agents, for further details).

Connective-Tissue Disorder Drugs

Connective-tissue disorder drugs included here are those associated with the more common connective-tissue disorders: LE, psoriasis and rheumatoid disorders, including gout and gouty arthritis. Also included are drugs used to treat oral lesions associated with lichen planus, pemphigus and pemphigoid. Unfortunately, the etiologies of these diseases remain unknown, and patients with these diseases appear to develop autoimmune reactions. Hence, drug therapy is often palliative and directed at controlling the immune response.

Common Connective-Tissue Disorders

Lupus Erythematosus

Lupus erythematosus is a relatively common autoimmune disorder whose exact cause remains unknown. There are two very dissimilar forms of this disease: chronic discoid lupus erythematosus (CDLE), a chronic form of the disease, and systemic lupus erythematosus (SLE), a systemic and more severe form. Certain drugs—hydralazine, procainamide, isoniazid, anticonvulsants, chlorpromiazine, penicillamine—can induce lupus-like syndromes; however, they do not seem to exacerbate existing LE, and symptoms disappear when the drug is discontinued.

Clinically, CDLE patients usually have an erythematous cutaneous rash, often involving the cheeks and the bridge of the nose in a "butterfly pattern" (in the areas most exposed to the sun). Oral lesions may include hyperkeratosis, ulceration and erythema. Biopsy may be required to rule out other diseases.

SLE, often seen in young women, is associated with malaise, joint pains, fever, rash, weight loss, kidney and CNS involvement and heart and pulmonary activity. Differential diagnosis is aided by noting that 90% of SLE patients exhibit antinuclear antibodies. Oral manifestations include erosive and vesiculobullous lesions and erythema.

Dentists should avoid any situation that may provoke acute outbreak, such as elective surgery, stress and use of certain drugs. The dentist should consult a physician before prescribing medications for these patients.

Psoriasis and Associated Syndromes/Diseases

The exact cause of psoriasis remains to be defined, but it appears to be multifactorial in nature, with approximately one-third of patients having a genetic predisposition to the condition. The condition can begin at any age, with a prevalence of 2% in the general population. The lesions are erythematous papules and plaques with associated silvery scales that resemble mica. The areas in which lesions most commonly appear are elbows and knees. The goal of treatment is to decrease epidermal proliferation and resulting inflammation. When possible, topical treatment with steroids is used, often in combination with topical tars or anthralin preparations. With severe disease, antimetabolites and antimitotic agents such as methotrexate (10-25 mg/w) are used.

Reiter's syndrome

Reiter's syndrome, whose cause is unknown, is often confused with psoriasis, but a possible oral clue of Reiter's syndrome includes presence of asymptomatic erosions on the tongue and buccal mucosa. Both psoriasis and Reiter's syndrome are associated with arthritis. When treatment is warranted, it usually is limited to topical steroids and antihistamines.

Lichen planus

Lichen planus, whose cause is unknown, is postulated to be an autoimmune-genetic predisposition. Lichen planus lesions range from white lacelike patterning to more erosive lesions surrounded by radiating white striae. Lesions are most often noted on buccal mucosa, gingiva and tongue and less frequently on the lips and palate. Biopsy is required to rule out other etiologies, including maligancy, LE and candidiasis. Treatment usually is limited to topical steroids, but severe lesions may require more aggressive systemic treatment.

Erythema multiforme

Erythema multiforme appears to be an acute self-limited skin/mucous membrane disease. Lesion severity varies from a few lesions to widespread vesiculobullous form (Stevens Johnson syndrome). Various treatments, including sulfonamides (Dapsone) and NSAIDs, have been recommended.

Pemphigus and Pemphigoid

Pemphigus

Pemphigus is used to define a group of chronic blistering skin diseases in which autoantibodies are directed against keratinocytes, resulting in loss of epidermal cell-to-cell adhesion and thus causing acantholysis. IgG autoantibodies take on a unique pattern in affected cell membranes and are found in patients' serum. Oral lesions are frequent in pemphigus vulgaris. General management includes systemic corticosteroids; for severe cases, 80 mg/day or higher may be required. Biopsy is required.

Pemphigoid

Pemphigoid, or bullous pemphigoid, is seen in older adults and is characterized clinically by erythematous macules, papules and urticarial plaques with serpiginous configuration. Most patients have circulating autoantibodies directed against the epithelial basement membrane zone, with linear deposition of IgG and C3 in this zone. Immunofluorescence assay is used to provide a differential diagnosis. Treatment includes systemic steroids limited to the lowest dose possible.

Rheumatologic Disorders

Numerous diseases are associated with the presence of rheumatoid factor. These include the rheumatic diseases: rheumatoid arthritis, Sjögren's syndrome, systemic LE, gouty arthritis, polymycositis/dermatomyositis, mixed connective-tissue disease and scleroderma. Other conditions associated with rheumatoid factor include infectious diseases (such as hepatitis and tuberculosis), malignancies (such as multiple myeloma) and sarcoidosis; in addition, this factor occurs in some normal adults and older people. When treating patients with such disorders, dentists should be aware of possible drug-associated concerns, patients' functional inabilities and oral-associated lesions.

Patients need to be monitored carefully, with frequent recall visits required for monitoring caries and periodontal disease in patients who are less capable of performing oral home care. Fluoride rinses should be used in these situations.

For patients with a history of ankylosing spondylitis, concerns for the dentist—in addition to medications the patient is taking—include inflammation of joints (usually spine and limbs) with ankylosis and possibly TMJ inflammation.

Osteoarthritis is yet another degenerative joint disease that may affect the mouth. In addition, patients with gouty arthritis may have joint-associated pain. Gout results from increased serum levels of monosodium urate, which result in deposits of urate crystals in joints and soft tissues. The joints most commonly affected include the metatarsephaloangeal, midfoot, ankles, knees, fingers, wrists and elbows; however, other joints—including the TMJ—may be affected.

In addition, an excessive urinary excretion of uric acid is found in gout. Thus, patients with gout experience recurrent attacks of acute arthritis, as well as chronic arthritis and nephropathy owing to urate/uric acid crystallization. Gouty arthritis is noted most frequently in men in the fourth through sixth decades of life and is also noted, with less frequency, in postmenopausal women. Persistent gout results in clinical palpable tophi and also erosions in bone, as noted in radiographic analysis.

Management of gout includes diet modification and prophylactic therapy, including drugs targeted at decreasing inflammation (NSAIDs, corticosteroids), treating acute gouty arthritis (colchicine) and lowering urate/uric acid levels (probenecid, allopurinol).

Tables 24.1-24.2 provide a list of the drugs more commonly used to treat connective-tissue/musculoskeletal disorders and includes specific disorders, drug indications and dosage ranges.

Table 24.1

Connective-Tissue Disorder Drugs: Dosage Information

Generic name	Brand name(s)	Indications/uses	Dosage range	Interactions with other drugs
Aspirin/NSAIDs	Many available—see Chapter 4, Analgesics	Alleviate pain and inflammation	Lowest dose possible	Aspirin and NSAIDs affect liver metabolism
Capsaicin	Zostrix-OTC	Used topically for pain associated with postherpetic neuralgia, rheumatoid arthritis (RA), osteoarthritis, diabetic neuropathy, postsurgical pain (unlabeled use for psoriasis)	Apply to affected area 3-4 times/day	Not reported
Colchicine	Colchicine	Acute gouty arthritis, anti-inflammatory agent	1-2 mg/day in 2-3 divided doses	May reduce absorption of vitamin B_{12}
Corticosteroids	See Table 24.2, Topical Corticosteroids, and Chapter 6, Corticosteroids			
Gold salts	Auralate, Myochrysine, Solganal	Progressive RA	10-50 mg q 3-4 w (maintenance)	Not reported
Hydroxy-chloroquine	Plaquenil	RA, osteoarthritis, joint prostheses, malaria (suppress & treat acute attacks), lupus erythematosus (LE)	Maintenance dose of 1-2 tablets/day for RA and LE, up to 6.5 mg/kg/day	Not reported
Methotrexate	Folex, Rheumatrex	RA, psoriatic arthritis, psoriasis, dermatomyositis	10-25 mg once/w OR 2.5-5 mg q 12 h for 3 doses/w	Drugs altering liver metabolism will alter metabolism of methotrexate

Continued on next page

Table 24.1 (cont.)

Connective-Tissue Disorder Drugs: Dosage Information

Generic name	Brand name(s)	Indications/uses	Dosage range	Interactions with other drugs
Penicillamine D	Cuprimine, Depen	Wilson's disease, cystinuria, RA; used as a chelating agent	0.5-1.5 g/day	Interacts with several drugs, including iron and bone-marrow depressants

Contraindicated in combination with gold compounds or phyenylbutazone owing to potentiation of serious hemotologic and/or renal adverse reactions |
| Probenecid | Benemid, Probalan; Benuryl [CAN] | Hyperuricemia (lowers uric acid) | 250 mg bid/w

250-500 mg/day to max of 2-3 g/day | May prolong penicillin levels

Effect may be decreased when coadministered with salicylates

Increased toxicity of acyclovir, thiopental, benzodiazepines, dapsone, sulfonyl ureas, zidovudine |

[CAN] indicates a drug available only in Canada.

Table 24.2

Topical Corticosteroids (Examples): Information*

Potency	Generic name	Brand name(s)	Content/form
High	Clobetasol	Temovate	15 or 45 g
Medium-high	Betamethasone 0.05%	Alphatrex, Diprosone	15 or 45 g
	Desoximetasone 0.25%	Topicort	**Cream:** 15-, 60-, 1,800-g tube

Ointment: 15-, 60-g tube

Gel: 15-, 60-g tube |
| | Fluocinonide 0.05% | Lidex Gel | **Cream/ointment:** 15-, 20-, 60-g tube

Solution: 15-120 mL |
| | Halcinonide 0.1% | Halog Cream | **Ointment:** 15-, 240-g tube

Solution: 20, 60 mL |

* See Chapter 6, Corticosteroids, for complete details.

Continued on next page

Table 24.2 (cont.)

Topical Corticosteroids (Examples): Information*

Potency	Generic name	Brand name(s)	Content/form
Medium a	Triamcinolone acetonide 0.5%	Aristocort cream, ointment Aristocort A cream Kenalog cream, ointment	15, 60 g
Medium b	Desoximetasone 0.05%	Topicort LP	**Cream:** 15-, 60-g tube
	Fluocinonide 0.025%	Synalar	**Ointment:** 15-, 425-g tube
	Triamcinolone acetonide 0.1%	Kenalog	**Ointment:** 15-, 60-g tube, 240-g jar
Medium c	Fluocinolone acetonide 0.025%	Synalar cream	**Cream:** 15-, 425-g tube
	Triamcinolone acetonide 0.1%	Aristocort	**Cream:** 15-, 1,520-g tube
		Kenalog	**Lotion:** 0.1% in 15-, 60-g tube **Cream:** 0.1% in 15-, 240-g tube **Ointment:** 0.025% in 15-, 240-g tube
		Trymex	**Cream:** 0.1% in 15-, 480-g tube **Ointment:** 0.025% in 15-, 80-g tube
Low a	Fluocinolone acetonide 0.01%	Synalar	**Cream:** 15-, 425-g tube **Solution:** 20-, 60-mL vial
		Fluonid cream	**Cream:** 15-, 60-g tube
	Triamcinolone acetonide 0.025%	Aristocort cream	**Cream:** 15-, 240-g tube
		Kenalog cream	**Cream:** 15-, 240-g tube
		Trymex	**Cream:** 15-, 480-g tube

See Chapter 6, Corticosteroids, for complete details.

Continued on next page

Table 24.2 (cont.)

Topical Corticosteroids (Examples): Information*

Potency	Generic name	Brand name(s)	Content/form
Low b	Betamethasone 0.2%	Celestone cream	**Cream:** 15-g tube
	Dexamethasone 0.1%	Decadermgel	**Cream:** 15-, 30-g tube
	Hydrocortisone 1%, 2.5%	Hytone, Texacort	**Solution:** 1% in 15-, 60-g vial (Texacort)
			Cream, ointment, lotion: 2.5% in 1-, 4-oz tube (Hytone)
		Synacort cream	15-, 60-g tube
		Lacticare HC lotion	2-, 4-oz tube
		Nutracort	**Cream:** 30-, 60-g tube
			Lotion: 4-oz tube
	Methylprednisolone 0.25%	Medrol cream	**Cream:** 7.5-, 45-g tube

* See Chapter 6, Corticosteroids, for complete details.

Special Dental Considerations

Management

For most patients with arthritic autoimmune diseases, treatment ranges from protective to preservation of joints: weight loss, physical therapy to specific drugs to decrease pain and inflammation. Pain medications include analgesics and NSAIDs. In addition, acetic acid anti-inflammatory drugs such as indomethacin, sulindac and tolmetin have been used to treat osteoarthritis, ankylosing spondylitis and gouty arthritis. Topical capsaicin also has been used for osteoarthritis (see Table 24.1). (Capsaicin depletes and prevents accumulation of substance P at sensory nerve terminals, thereby decreasing pain.) Intra-articular steroid injections have been used, with caution, for joint pain and are not recommended for treatment of TMDs (see Chapter 6). Other medications include those targeted at altering the course of rheumatoid synovitis and thus decreasing risk of joint damage. For aggressive disease, such medications include methotrexate and injectable gold salts (whose mechanism is unknown—they may act by decreasing prostaglandin synthesis or may alter cell function by inhibiting sulfhydryl). For mild situations, medications may include hydroxychloroquine, auranofin and sulfasalazine. Other agents sometimes used include Penicillamine D, azathioprine and cyclophosphamide, but caution is needed with these because of their toxicity. The last option is surgery—joint debridement, fusion or replacement—for those with major disabilities.

Dental Considerations

The dentist must take a careful history, including details on medications, drug interactions and side effects (for instance, stomatitis occurs with many of these drugs). Furthermore, an intense maintenance program to monitor the patient's oral health may be necessary. Any oral lesions should be monitored and biopsies performed as needed.

The patient may need fluoride rinses and should be monitored for symptoms of xerostomia (such as in Sjögren's syndrome) and possible need for salivary supplements (including use of pilocarpine).

Finally, the dentist should be aware of the general concerns associated with steroid therapy (see Chapter 6, Corticosteroids, for complete details).

Drug interactions of dental interest

Some patients with connective-tissue disorders may be taking numerous medications that can interact with drugs the dentist may wish to prescribe. Therefore, it is imperative that the dentist take a detailed history that includes medications (dosage, duration).

Special patients

Differential diagnosis of oral lesions is required. Certain lesions may be more common in certain groups than in others; nevertheless, differential diagnosis still is required.

Adverse Effects, Precautions and Contraindications

Table 24.3 describes adverse effects of connective-tissue disorder drugs; Table 24.4 describes precautions and contraindications.

Pharmacology

Aspirin/NSAIDs

These drugs act by blocking various activities along the arachidonic acid pathway and also blocking inflammatory cell function, with the result being a reduction in inflammation. For further details, see Chapter 4, Analgesics.

Capsaicin

This agent depletes and prevents accumulation of substance P at sensory terminals, thereby decreasing pain.

Colchicine

This agent acts by binding to tubulin (a cellular microtubular protein), disrupting microtubules and causing loss of function of leukocytes.

Gold Salts and Methotrexate

The mechanism that makes these drugs effective immunosuppressants, and thus of value in treating arthritis, is not known. They may act by decreasing prostaglandin synthesis and/or altering cell function by inhibiting synthesis of sulfhydryl.

Hydroxychloroquine

This is an antimalarial drug that acts by inhibiting locomotion of neutrophils and chemotaxis of eosinophils.

Penicillamine D

This agent may unmask T-cell suppressor activity and thereby inhibit production of rheumatoid factor.

Probenecid

As a uricosuric agent, probenecid promotes excretion of urate by competing for the renal tubular acid transporter; the result is decreased reabsorption of urate.

Table 24.3

Common Connective-Tissue Disorder Drugs: Adverse Effects

Body system	Aspirin/ NSAIDs	Capsaicin	Colchicine	Corticosteroids	Gold salts	Hydroxy- chloroquine	Methotrexate	Penicillamine D	Probenecid
General	**Aspirin toxici- ty/intolerance:** Ringing in ears, burning in stomach or esophagus, black stools **NSAIDs:** Significant side effects (especially in older patients), are gastric ulcers; this may require additional drugs to protect against ulcers (for example, prostaglandins like misoprostol, which exerts gastric antisecre- tory effects and decreases hista- mine-stimulated acid secretion) See Chapter 4, Analgesics, for complete details	No known systemic adverse effects		Owing to too- quick withdraw- al: flare-up of underlying dis- ease; acute adrenal insuffi- ciency; also (rarely), pseudo- tumor cerebri See Chapter 6, Corticosteroids, for complete details	Skin rash, sores in mouth, kid- ney disease, blood dyscrasias		As with all immunosup- pressants, side effects can be significant and may include ulcers, skin rashes, hair loss, fetal deformity, increased sus- ceptibility to infections		

CNS	Salicylism	Myopathy, peripheral neuritis	Neuropathy	Neuromyopathy, *headache, irritability*	*Headache*		*Headache, dizziness*
CV				Cardiomyopathy			*Flushing of face*
EENT	*Ototoxicity*			Blurred vision, retinopathy, *corneal deposits,* tinnitus			
Endoc		*Azospermia*				Gynecomastia	
GI	Upset, *ulcers*	Nausea, *vomiting, anorexia,* diarrhea, abdominal pain	Enterocolitis	*Discomfort*	*Intolerance, ulcers*	*Nausea, anorexia*	*Anorexia, nausea, vomiting*
GU			Proteinuria, hematuria			*Proteinuria*	*Painful urination*
Hema	*Decrease in platelet aggregation and function, neutropenia, hemolytic anemia, thrombocytopenia*	Bone marrow suppression, agranulocytosis, aplastic anemia	Thrombocytopenia, granulocytopenia, aplastic anemia, eosinophilia	*Leukopenia, hemolytic anemia*	*Hematologic effects*	Thrombocytopenia, leukopenia, aplastic anemia	Leukopenia, hemolytic anemia, aplastic anemia

Continued on next page

Italics indicate information of major clinical significance.

Table 24.3 (cont.)
Common Connective-Tissue Disorder Drugs: Adverse Effects

Body system	Aspirin/ NSAIDs	Capsaicin	Colchicine	Corticosteroids	Gold salts	Hydroxy-chloroquine	Methotrexate	Penicillamine D	Probenecid
HB	Hepatotoxicity		Hepatotoxicity		Hepatotoxicity		*Cirrhosis, liver abnormalities,* hepatitis	Liver abnormalities	Hepatic necrosis
Integ	*Rash*	*Localized and transient burning, itching, stinging, erythema*	*Alopecia,* rash		*Rash, alopecia*	*Rash, skin hyperpigmentation*	Atypical infection, rash, alopecia	*Rash*	Rash, itching
Oral	Stomatitis				*Stomatitis*		*Stomatitis*	*Hypogeusia, stomatitis*	Sore gums
Renal	Toxicity							*Nephritis*	*Renal calculi, urate nephrotoxicity, nephrotic syndrome*
Resp	Infiltrates	Cough			Infiltrates		Pneumonitis	Toxicity	Anaphylaxis

Italics indicate information of major clinical significance.

Table 24.4

Connective-Tissue Disorder Drugs: Precautions and Contraindications

Drug category	Precautions/contraindications
Antimalarial compounds	Because of potential damage to eyes with use, frequent ophthalmological examinations are needed
Aspirin/NSAIDs	Significant side effects, ulcers, hepatotoxicity warrant caution in patients with history of ulcers and liver disease—often a problem with older patients
Capsaicin	None reported
Colchicine	Pregnancy risk category: C oral, D parenteral
Corticosteroids	Not a preferred systemic treatment due to significant side effects (see Chapter 6, Corticosteroids)
Penicillamine D	Should be used cautiously in patients with history of GI distress D-penicillamine is highly reactive with other drugs Contraindicated in pregnancy because of risk of fetal abnormalities Contraindicated in presence of renal insufficiency Contraindicated in conjunction with gold therapy, cytotoxic drugs, phenylbutazone Contraindicated for patients with lupus erythematosus
Gold salts	May take weeks for inflammation to cease
Hydroxychloroquine	Should be used cautiously in patients with history of GI distress
Methotrexate	Dose of methotrexate (the most widely used immunosuppressant) must be monitored, as this agent is extremely hepatotoxic
Probenecid	Interaction with other drugs (see Table 24.1) Pregnancy risk category: B Contraindicated with salicylates

Skeletal Muscle Relaxants

Patients with various arthritic conditions, as well as those with isolated oral-associated problems of an inflammatory nature, may require muscle relaxants. TMD can be present without underlying systemic problems. Often, TMD is associated with significant pain; thus, drugs used range from analgesics/anti-inflammatories to tranquilizer medications to muscle relaxants to moist heat for localized inflammation. In addition, the dentist may opt to use muscle relaxants for their sedative effects.

Described here are muscle relaxants that the dentist may consider when contemplating muscle relaxant therapy. For the most part, muscle relaxants should be used over a short term, as adjunctive therapy, to manage acute pain. They are often given in conjunction with analgesics and/or NSAIDs to relieve associated pain. Also, muscle relaxants can be used with certain more complex surgical procedures to reduce the amount of anesthetic agent required and thus improve the margin of safety and the patient's recovery from anesthesia. Examples of the more commonly used relaxants are provided in Table 24.5. Many of these act by interrupting transmission of signals at the interphase between skeletal muscle fibers and their associated innervating somatic nerves. There are two main classes of neuromuscular blocking agents:

- those that act as competitive antagonists, such as d-tubocuraine;
- those that have depolarizing effects, such as succinylcholine.

An additional group acts by blocking intraneuronal activity; these agents are often used for CNS disorders.

Table 24.5 provides a list of the drugs more commonly used to treat musculoskeletal disorders and includes specific disorders, drug indications and dosage ranges.

Special Dental Considerations

Patients with significant TMD pain or other associated problems may warrant examination by a specialist in this area before the dentist undertakes any intervention, including drug therapy.

Drug Interactions of Dental Interest

Centrally acting muscle relaxants interact with vascoconstrictors (such as epinephrine); thus, caution is required when using vasoconstrictors.

Centrally acting muscle relaxants cause CNS depression, so the dentist must be aware of the possibility of potentiating these effects with other medications or substances (including alcohol).

Adverse Effects, Precautions and Contraindications

Table 24.6 describes adverse effects of skeletal muscle relaxants; Table 24.7 describes precautions and contraindications.

Pharmacology

Skeletal muscle relaxants are neuromuscular blocking agents that interrupt transmission at junctions between skeletal muscle fibers and the somatic nerves innervating those fibers. They can act as competitive agonists (d-tubocurarine) or as depolarizing agents (succinylcholine) or are centrally acting agents (which act by blocking intraneuronal activity). Provided here are mechanisms of action to consider for the skeletal muscle relaxants described in this chapter.

Carisoprodol

The exact mechanism by which this agent acts as a muscle relaxant is not known, but its effects are attributed to its central depressant actions.

Cyclobenzaprine

This agent reduces tonic somatic motor activity through its action on both α and γ motor neurons. Its actions are similar to those of tricyclic antidepressants.

Methocarbamol, Chlorzoxazone, Orphenadrine

These agents reduce transmission of impulses from the spinal cord to skeletal muscles.

Table 24.5

Skeletal Muscle Relaxant Drugs: Dosage Information

Generic name*	Brand name(s)	Indications/uses	Dosage range	Interactions with other drugs
Carisoprodol	Sodal, Soma, Soprodol	Relief of muscle spasm; nonspecific sedation; some indication that it works better in combination with aspirin/NSAIDs	**Adults:** 350-mg tablet tid	Increased CNS depression and thus caution with all agents that have CNS effects, including alcohol Use vasoconstrictors with caution; avoid retraction cord containing epinephrine
Chlorzoxazone	Blanex, Chlorofon-F, Flexaphen, Lobac, Miflex, Mus-Lac, Paraflex, Parafon Forte, Pargen Fortified, Polyflex, Skelex	Relief of muscle spasm; may be used in combination with aspirin or NSAIDs	**Adult:** 250-270 mg tid-qid	See note above
Cyclobenzaprine HCl	Flexeril, Cycoflex; Novo-Cycloprine [CAN]	Relief of muscle spasm; may be used in combination with aspirin or NSAIDs	**Adult:** 20-40 mg/day, not to exceed 2-3 g/w	See note above
Methocarbamol	Delaxin, Marbaxin, Robamol, Robaxin	Relief of muscle spasm	1-4.5 g/day in 3-6 divided doses	See note above
Orphenadrine citrate	Banflex, Flexon, Norflex, Marflex, Noradex, Orflagen, O-Flex, K-Flex; Myolin [CAN]	Treatment of muscle spasm; may be used in combination with aspirin or NSAIDs	100 mg bid	See note above

* Also available in combinations with analgesics.
[CAN] indicates a drug available only in Canada.

Table 24.6

Skeletal Muscle Relaxant Drugs: Adverse Effects

Body system	Carisoprodol	Chlorzoxazone	Cyclobenzaprine HCL	Methocarbamol	Orphenadrine citrate
CV	Postural hypotension, tachycardia		Tachycardia, dysrhythmia, postural hypotension	Postural hypotension, bradycardia	
CNS	*Dizziness, weakness, drowsiness, headache, tremors, depression, insomnia, ataxia, irritability*		*Headache, dizziness, weakness, drowsiness*	*Dizziness, weakness, drowsiness, seizures*	
EENT	Diplopia, temporary loss of vision	Burning of eyes	Diplopia, *temporary loss of vision*	Diplopia, temporary loss of vision, blurred vision, nystagmus	*Blurred vision,* increased intraocular pressure
GI	Nausea, vomiting, hiccups, epigastric distress	Nausea, vomiting	Nausea, vomiting, hiccups	Nausea, vomiting, hiccups	Nausea, vomiting
GU			Urinary retention	Black, brown, green urine	Urinary hesistancy
Hema				Hemolysis	Aplastic anemia
Integ	Rash, pruritis, fever, facial flushing	Angioedema	Rash, facial flushing	Rash	Rash, pruritis
Musc		Trembling	Muscle weakness		
Oral			Altered taste, dry mouth	Metallic taste	Dry mouth
Resp		Shortness of breath			Nasal decongestion

Italics indicate information of major clinical significance.

NOTE: As the muscle relaxants listed here are all centrally acting, side effects noted for one drug can be anticipated for all drugs listed, where reactions for one drug vs. another may be more or less remarkable.

Table 24.7

Skeletal Muscle Relaxant Drugs: Precautions and Contraindications

Drug category	Precautions/contraindications
Carisoprodol	Should be used cautiously in elderly patients or patients who have renal disease, hepatic disease or addictive personalities
	Pregnancy risk category: C
	Contraindicated in patients with hypersensitivity to carisoprodol, meprobamate
	Contraindicated in patients with intermittent porphyria
Chlorzoxazone	Should be used cautiously with lactating women, elderly patients and patients who have hepatic disease
	Pregnancy risk category: C
	Contraindicated for patients who have hypersensitivity to chlorzoxazone
	Contraindicated for patients who have impaired hepatic function
Cyclobenzaprine HCl	Should be used cautiously with elderly patients and patients who have renal disease, hepatic disease, glaucoma, urinary hesitancy, or addictive personalities; also with patients who are taking MAO inhibitors
	Vasoconstrictors should be used with caution
	Pregnancy risk category: B
	Contraindicated for concomitant use with epinephrine retraction cord
	Contraindicated in patients with hypersensitivity, cardiovascular disease and intermittent porphyria thyroid disease and in children aged < 12 y
Methocarbamol	Should be used cautiously in patients who have renal disease, hepatic disease, addictive personality, myasthemia gravis or epilepsy
	Pregnancy risk category: C
	Contraindicated in patients with hypersensitivity to methocarbamol or intermittent porphyria
Orphenadrine citrate	Should be used cautiously with children, lactating women and patients who have cardiac disease
	Pregnancy risk category: Not listed
	Containdicated in hypersensitivity, narrow-angle glaucoma, GI obstruction, myasthenia gravis, stenosing peptic ulcer

Suggested Readings

Kaufman RL, Baldassare AR, Fiechtner JJ. Guidelines for reviewers of rheumatic disease care. Council on Rheumatic Care, American College of Rheumatology. 3rd ed. Atlanta: American College of Rheumatology; 1992.

McCarthy GM, McCarty DJ. Effect of topical capsaicin in the therapy of painful osteoarthritis of the hands. J Rheumatol 1992;19:604-7.

Rosenberg SW, Arm RN. Clinician's guide to treatment of common oral conditions. 4th ed. New York: American Academy of Oral Medicine; 1997:1-28.

Sonis ST, Faxio RC, Fang L. Principles and practice of oral medicine. 2nd ed. Philadelphia: WB Saunders Co.; 1995.

Chapter 25

Therapeutics in Renal and Hepatic Disease

B. Ellen Byrne, R.Ph., D.D.S., Ph.D.

The dosage of many drugs that are normally cleared by the kidney must be adjusted in patients with renal disease, as well as those with hepatic disease. If such adjustments are not made, drug accumulation and toxicity are likely to occur during renal dysfunction. The goal of therapy in a patient with renal impairment is to achieve unbound drug serum concentrations similiar to those that have been associated with optimal response in patients with normal renal function. Drug dosage in those with renal failure can be accomplished by one of two methods:

- keeping the dose the same and lengthening the dosing interval (interval prolongation method); or
- reducing the dose and keeping the dose interval constant (dose reduction method).

The interval prolongation method is convenient because the same doses used in patients with normal renal function are given less frequently. This method is most practical for drugs with long half-lives; however, this approach may result in marked fluctuations in high and low serum concentration and should be avoided where the drug has a narrow therapeutic index. The dose reduction method allows the drug to be given at the usual intervals but in less convenient doses. More constant serum concentrations are achieved with this method. This may be more beneficial in instances in which it is desirable to maintain concentrations above a given threshold.

No controlled studies have been performed to establish the relative efficacy of these two methods for drug-dose alterations in patients with renal insufficiency. And as neither of these two dosage adjustment methods is optimal for all agents, clinicians often will combine these two approaches by giving lower doses at a less prolonged dosing interval.

Drug dosage adjustments for hepatically eliminated drugs in patients with liver disease or dysfunction are difficult to predict. This is due to the complexity of hepatic metabolism, which involves numerous metabolic pathways that are variably affected in hepatic dysfunction. In renal disease, creatinine serves as an endogenous marker to predict the clearance of renally eliminated drugs. Unfortunately, in hepatic dysfunction, there are no reliable endogenous markers to accurately predict a drug's hepatic clearance. Because of this difficulty in predicting hepatic drug clearance, unnecessary and potentially hepatotoxic medications are best avoided. When drug therapy is indicated with agents that undergo hepatic elimination, it is prudent to use the lowest doses possible to achieve the desired therapeutic effect. The use of serum drug concentrations is necessary when treating patients with liver failure.

Special Dental Considerations
Drug interactions of dental interest
Patients with renal disease usually receive a large variety of drugs. This creates great potential for numerous drug interactions. For example, one drug may displace another drug from protein binding sites. This increases the free unbound fraction of the

drug and also increases its pharmacological activity. This also will change the amount of drug to be dialyzed. Before adding any drug to a patient's drug regimen, the dentist should review the drug combinations and screen for adverse interactions.

Laboratory value alterations

Aberrant renal function test results can be caused by medications. The consequences of this can be costly, time-consuming and misleading to the dentist, resulting in deleterious clinical results.

- Serum creatinine: aspirin competes with receptors for creatinine secretion, causing increased creatinine.
- Urate: increases with administration of salicylates and acetaminophen (nonenzymatic analytical method).
- Urine color: changes with administration of metronidazole (darkens on standing).
- Urine protein: false positive reaction occurs with administration of salicylates, cephalosporin or penicillin.

Drug dosing in renal impairment

The drugs listed in Table 25.1 include drugs that could be given by the dentist. The drugs have been listed in alphabetical order independent of their classification of use. The brand names given are only representative, not all-inclusive. A brief summary of the route of elimination—that is, renal excretion, hepatic metabolism, presence of active metabolites— for each drug is also provided. The half-life (t ½) of drug elimination from the body is given for people with normal renal function and for anephric patients, those with end-stage renal disease (creatinine clearance [CrCl] < 10 mL/min). Dosing guidelines for three categories of renal disease are included. Dosing recommendations for the category "CrCl > 50 mL/min" usually represent normal dosage regimens. The effect of dialysis on drug removal is also described.

Suggested Readings

Aweeka FT. Appendix: drug reference table. In: Schrier RW, Gambertoglio JG, eds. Handbook of drug therapy in liver and kidney disease. Boston: Little, Brown; 1991: 285-371.

Aweeka FT. Drug dosing in renal failure. In: Young L, Koda-Kimble MA, eds. Applied therapeutics: the clinical use of drugs. 6th ed. Vancouver, Wash.: Applied Therapeutics Inc.; 1995:32.1-32.21.

Benet LZ, Williams RL. Appendix II: design and optimization of dosage regimens. In: Bennett WM. Guide to drug dosage in renal failure. Clin Pharmacokinet 1988; 15:326-51.

Goodman Gilman A, et al., eds. Goodman and Gilman's the pharmacological basis of therapeutics. New York: Pergamon Press; 1990:1650-1737.

Table 25.1

Drug Dosing in Renal Impairment: General Information

Generic name	Brand name(s)	Metabolism and elimination	Normal (t ½[h])*	Anephric (t ½[h])	Dose change with renal failure (CrCl† >50 mL/min)††	Dose change with renal failure (CrCl 10-50 mL/min)	Dose change with renal failure (CrCl <10 mL/min)	Effect of dialysis	Dose change in liver failure
Acetaminophen	Tylenol	Hepatic conjugation, oxidated metabolites are hepatotoxic; 3% excreted unchanged	1.9-2.5	1.9-2.5	q 4-6 h	q 4-6 h	q 4-6 h	Slightly/moderately dialyzed	Avoid
Acyclovir	Zovirax	76-82% excreted unchanged renally; 14% hepatic metabolism	1.5-3.3	20	No change	q 12-24 h	50% every 24 h	Dialyzed	No change
Amoxicillin	Amoxil, Apo-Amoxi [CAN], Novamoxin, Nu-Amoxi [CAN], Trimox, Wymox	Hepatic metabolism 12-28%; 50-88% excreted unchanged	0.5-2.3	7-20	No change	q 6-12 h	q 12-14 h	Moderately dialyzed	No change
Ampicillin	OmniPen, PrinciPen, Totcillin, Apo-Ampi [CAN], Novo-Ampicillin [CAN]	76-88% excreted unchanged; 12-24% metabolism	0.5-1.5	20	No change	q 6-12 h	q 12-18 h	Moderately dialyzed	No change
Carbamazepine	Tegretol	Extensive metabolism; renal excretion; 1-2% unchanged and active metabolites	10-20	Half-life unknown in patient without kidney function	No change	No change	No change	Slightly dialyzed	Decrease

Cefaclor		70% excreted unchanged; <10% hepatic metabolism	0.6-1.0	1.5-4.7	No change	50-100% every 8 h	25-50% every 8-12 h	Moderately dialyzed	No change
Cephalexin	Keflex, C-Lexin, generic	85-95% excreted unchanged	1.0-1.9	20-40	No change	q 12 h	q 24 h	Moderately dialyzed	No change
Chloral hydrate	Noctec, generic	Rapidly metabolized to active trichloroethanol	7-14	Half-life unknown in patient without kidney function	q 24 h	Avoid	Avoid	Dialyzed	Decrease
Chlordiazepoxide	Librium, Libritabs, generic	Hepatic metabolism to active metabolites < 1% excreted unchanged	5-30	No change	q 6-8 h	q 6-8 h	q 12 h	Not/slightly dialyzed	Decrease
Clavulanic acid with amoxicillin	Augmentin	34-52% excreted unchanged; 26% unchanged in feces	0.8-1.2	2.6-4.0	No change	q 8 h	q 12-24 h	Dialyzed	No change
Clindamycin	Cleocin, generic	85% hepatic metabolism to active and inactive metabolites; 10% excreted unchanged in urine and 5% in feces	2-4	1.6-3.4	No change	No change	No change	Not dialyzed	Decrease

Continued on next page

[CAN] indicates a drug available only in Canada.
* Half-life in hours.
† CrCl: creatinine clearance.
†† mL/min: milliliters per minute.

Table 25.1 (cont.)

Drug Dosing in Renal Impairment: General Information

Generic name	Brand name(s)	Metabolism and elimination	Normal (t ½[h])*	Anephric (t ½[h])	Dose change with renal failure (CrCl† >50 mL/min)††	Dose change with renal failure (CrCl 10-50 mL/min)	Dose change with renal failure (CrCl <10 mL/min)	Effect of dialysis	Dose change in liver failure
Codeine phosphate, codeine sulfate	generic	Hepatic metabolism; 5-17% excreted unchanged	2.5-3.5	No change	No change	Decrease dose 25%	Decrease dose 50%	Unknown	Decrease
Diazepam	D-Val, Diazepam Intensol, Valium, Valrelease, generic	Hepatic metabolism to active metabolites via N-demethylation and hydroxylation; renal excretion	20-70	37	q 8 h	q 8 h	q 8 h	Not dialyzed	Decrease
Doxycycline	Doxy Film, Monodox, Doxy-Caps, Doryx, Vibramycin, Vibratabs, generic	10-20% hepatic metabolism; 30% intraluminal gut wall; 20-26% excreted unchanged renally; 20-40% in feces	14-24	14-36	No change	No change	No change	Not dialyzed	Decrease
Erythromycin	E-Mycin, Ery-Tab, Erythro, Erythrocin, generic	Hepatic metabolism 85-95% to inactive metabolites; 5-15% excreted unchanged	1.5-30	4-6	No change	No change	No change	Slightly dialyzed	Decrease
Ibuprofen	Advil*, Excedrin IB, Ibuprin, Motrin, Rufen	Hepatic metabolism 40-60% excreted in urine as unchanged drug and metabolites	2	2	No change	No change	No change	Not dialyzed	Unknown

Ketoconazole	Nizoral	51% hepatic metabolism; 45% excreted unchanged in feces and 3% unchanged renally	3-8	3-8	No change	No change	No change	Not dialyzed	Decrease
Lorazepam	Ativan, generic	Extensive glucuronide conjugation in the liver; excreted renally	8-24	28	q 8 h	q 8 h	q 8 h	Not/slightly dialyzed	Decrease
Meperidine	Demerol	Hepatic hydrolysis and conjugation, active normeperidine metabolite, 10% excreted unchanged	3.2	Half-life unknown in patient without kidney function	q 3-4 h	q 6 h (decrease dose 25%)	q 8 h (decrease dose 50%)	Unknown	Decrease
Metronidazole	Flagyl, Metric 21, Protostat, generic	Hepatic oxidation and glucuronide conjugation; 60-80% renal excretion, 20% excreted unchanged	8	q 8 h	q 8 h	q 8-12 h	q 12-24 h	Rapidly dialyzed	Decrease
Minocycline	Minocin, generic	60-75% hepatic metabolism; < 10% excreted unchanged renally; 20-34% excreted in feces	11-26	14-30	No change	No change	No change	Not dialyzed	Decrease

Continued on next page

★ indicates a drug bearing the ADA Seal of Acceptance.
* Half-life in hours.
† CrCl: creatinine clearance.
†† mL/min: milliliters per minute.

Table 25.1 (cont.)
Drug Dosing in Renal Impairment: General Information

Generic name	Brand name(s)	Metabolism and elimination	Normal (t ½[h])*	Anephric (t ½[h])	Dose change with renal failure (CrCl† > 50 mL/min)††	Dose change with renal failure (CrCl 10-50 mL/min)	Dose change with renal failure (CrCl < 10 mL/min)	Effect of dialysis	Dose change in liver failure
Morphine	Astramorph PF Injection, Duramorph Injection, Infumorph Injection, MS Contin, Oramorph, Rescudose, Roxanol	Hepatic metabolism; 85% renal excretion, 10% excreted unchanged	2-3	2-3	No change	Decrease dose 25%	Decrease dose 50%	Unknown	Decrease
Naloxone	Narcan Injection ★	Rapidly metabolized via N-dealkylation and glucuronidation, 70% renal excretion within 72 h	1.0-1.5	Half-life unknown in patient without kidney function	No change	No change	No change	Unknown	No change
Naproxen	Aleve, Anaprox, Anaprox DS EC-Naprosyn, Naprosyn	Hepatic metabolism in inactive metabolites; < 1% excreted unchanged in urine	10-18	10-18	No change	No change	No change	Not dialyzed	Decrease
Oxazepam	Serax, generic	Extensive glucuronide conjugation in the liver; renal and fecal excretion	4-25	24-91	q 8 h	q 8 h	q 8 h	Not dialyzed	No change

Drug	Trade names	Metabolism	Half-life		Dose			Dialysis	
Penicillin G	Pentids, Bicillin L-A, Permapen, Wycillin, generic	Hepatic metabolism 19%; 50% excreted unchanged	0.4-0.9	6-19	No change	50-100% every 8-12 h	25-50% every 12 h	Moderately dialyzed, 30-50 mL/min	No change
Penicillin V potassium	Beepen-VK, Betapen-VK, Ledercillin VK, Pen.Vee K	Hepatic metabolism <30%; mostly renal	0.5-1	Unknown	q 6 h	q 6 h	q 6-8 h	Unknown	No change
Pentazocine	Talwin, Talwin-Nx	Hepatic metabolism; hydroxylation 2-15% excreted changed	2	2-3	No change	Decrease dose by 25%	Decrease dose by 50%	Unknown	Decrease
Pentobarbital	Nembutal, generic	Hepatic hydroxylation; <1% excreted unchanged	18-48	27	q 8-24 h	q 8-24 h	q 8-24 h	Slightly dialyzed	Decrease
Phenobarbital	Solfoton, Barbita, generic	Hepatic metabolism; renal excretion; 10-40% unchanged and active metabolites	100	Half-life unknown in patient without kidney function	No change	No change	Slight decrease	Moderately dialyzed	Decrease
Propoxyphene	Darvon	30-70% first-pass metabolism; 7% excreted unchanged	9-15	12-20	q 4 h	q 4 h	Avoid	Not dialyzed	Decrease
Salicylates (aspirin)	Aspiritab, Bayer, Empirin, Norwich, St. Joseph, Anacin	Converted to salicylic acid by peripheral enzymes; hepatic metabolism of salicylic acid	2-20 (dose-dependent)	2-20 (dose-dependent)	q 4 h	q 4-6 h	Avoid	Dialyzed	Avoid

Continued on next page

★ indicates a drug bearing the ADA Seal of Acceptance.
* Half-life in hours.
† CrCl: creatinine clearance.
†† mL/min: milliliters per minute.

Table 25.1 (cont.)
Drug Dosing in Renal Impairment: General Information

Generic name	Brand name(s)	Metabolism and elimination	Normal (t ½[h])*	Anephric (t ½[h])	Dose change with renal failure (CrCl† >50 mL/min)††	Dose change with renal failure (CrCl 10-50 mL/min)	Dose change with renal failure (CrCl <10 mL/min)	Effect of dialysis	Dose change in liver failure
Temazepam	Restoril	Extensive conjugation to inactive metabolites	10-15	10-15	q 12 h	q 12 h	q 12 h	Unknown	No change
Tetracycline	Achromycin V, Sumycin, Tetracyn	48-70% excreted unchanged renally; < 30% excreted through hepatic/biliary/fecal route	6-15	33-80	q 6 h	Avoid	Avoid	Slightly dialyzed	Use with caution
Thiopental (IV)	Pentothal, Thiopentone, generic	Hepatic metabolism; renal elimination is minimal	10	6-18	No change	No change	Decrease dose by 25%	Unknown	Decrease
Triazolam	Halcion	Extensive glucuronide conjugation to slightly active metabolites; little renal excretion, fecal excretion	2.3-2.8	Half-life unknown in patient without kidney function	q 12 h	q 12 h	q 12 h	Unknown	No change

* Half-life in hours.
† CrCl: creatinine clearance.
†† mL/min: milliliters per minute.

Chapter 26.

Drugs for Neoplastic Disorders

Martha Somerman, D.D.S., Ph.D.

Stomatotoxicity is a common finding in patients who are undergoing radiotherapy or cancer chemotherapy. Most antitumor agents have a low therapeutic index. They often act by interfering with the cell replicatory cycle and are targeted at rapidly dividing cells, including tumor cells, as well as some normal rapidly proliferating cells. Normal cells and tissues often affected by chemotherapy include bone marrow, hematopoietic cells, gonads, gastrointestinal tract lining and hair follicles. The major methods of treating malignant neoplasms are surgery, radiotherapy and/or chemotherapy. In addition, immunotherapy is being explored, but it is still primarily at the investigational stage.

Dentists should take a thorough health history and review drug considerations before planning and delivering dental treatment to patients being treated for neoplastic disorders.

Oral side effects are a frequent occurrence for patients receiving treatment for cancer. Side effects are related both to the patient's status (for example, age, disease and oral health before and during therapy) and to therapy modalities, including specific type of drugs, dose and frequency of treatment. In younger patients (aged < 12 y), 90% develop oral side effects, whereas in the general population of patients, about 40% to 50% do so. This probably is related to the higher mitotic index of "normal" cells in younger patients. Oral complications may be a direct effect of the neoplasm, a direct effect of the drug or an indirect effect of the drug or the cancer

related to changes in other organs, most specifically myelosuppression.

In general, oral complications are most frequently observed in myelosuppressive diseases (for example, leukemia and lymphoma). Patients with gastrointestinal tract neoplasms also have a high frequency of oral complications. And, without white blood cells, the body has no protection against bacteria in the mouth. Thus, patients with poor oral hygiene and untreated odontogenic and periodontal infections will have an increased incidence of oral complications during therapy-induced myelosuppression.

Some chemotherapeutic agents are more likely to have direct effects on oral tissue than others. For example, antimetabolites such as methotrexate, which block DNA synthesis, have a tendency to induce mucositis. Combined treatment—radiation therapy and chemotherapy—tends to enhance the incidence and severity of oral complications induced by therapy. In addition, these therapies reduce the volume and alter the composition of saliva, as well as disrupt oral microflora. Disruption of normal flora allows for overgrowth of opportunistic organisms, including candidiasis.

Oral Complications Associated With Cancer Therapy

Oral toxicities include gingival bleeding, ulcers, mucositis (with risk of candidiasis), xerostomia, osteoradionecrosis, loss of taste and caries. The incidence of oral problems increases with pre-existing disease. Thus, it is imperative that the physician and the dentist work as a team to provide the best care for the patient, including visits prior to chemotherapy/radiation therapy.

Bone marrow transplantation

Patients receiving allogeneic bone marrow transplant have an added risk of side effects that can result from graft-vs.-host disease. Where immunocompetent donor cells react against anergic cells of the recipient, the tissues most affected include mouth, skin, liver and lungs. Oral changes most commonly include a clinical resemblance to lichen planus. Other changes include salivary-gland–induced xerostomia. Oral lesions respond to steroid therapy, where use of topical vs. systemic therapy is based on the severity of lesions.

Infection

Bacterial, fungal and viral infections of the mouth may be encountered. The most frequent site of infection reported for the granulocytopenic cancer patient is the mouth. Proper diagnosis and treatment is needed to prevent systemic involvement, which is often fatal.

Signs and symptoms of infection include pain, fever and lesions of the teeth, mucosa, gingiva, and salivary glands (most commonly the parotid).

Fungal infections, such as *Candida albicans*, are a common danger in compromised patients. Fungal overgrowth can spread to other tissues. Antifungal agents have been prescribed, as a prophylactic measure, to myelosuppressed patients to reduce the frequency and severity of oral candidiasis even before fungal infections appear. (A sample dosage would be nystatin 200,000-400,000 units qid.) However, this use is controversial. Other therapies used, especially on appearance of infection, include clotrimazone (10-mg tablets 5 times/day for 2 w), nystatin suspension in ice cubes, ketoconazole tablets, gentian violet (the taste and color of which are objectionable to some patients) and

fluconazole tablets. With spread of a fungal infection, hospitalization and more aggressive therapy (for example, IV amphotericin B) are required.

Viral infections also occur in patients undergoing cancer therapy. Most common are the herpes simplex virus (HSV); herpes zoster; and recurrent herpes infection. Viral infections can manifest as crops of vesicular lesions: intraorally, most frequently on the palate; extraorally, most frequently on the lips and under the nose. Patients may also have fever and lymphadenopathy. Treatment is palliative. The prophylactic use of acyclovir is suggested for the markedly myelosuppressed cancer patient. Due to increased susceptibility to infections, including bacterial, certain mouthrinses may be of benefit, such as chlorhexidine and povidone-iodine.

Mucositis

Mucositis is the most common form of direct stomatoxicity. It is characterized by painful diffuse ulcerations of nonkeratinized oral mucosa, typically 5-7 days after therapy. Palliative treatment may include topical anesthetics such as 2% viscous lidocaine (xylocaine viscous); dyclonine hydrochloride (Dyclone); rinsing with diphenhydramine HCl (Benadryl elixir); coating agents such as aluminum hydroxide, magnesium hydroxide and simethicone (Mylanta, Gelusil, Maalox) and attapulgite (Kaopectate, Rheaban); benzocaine (Orabase with benzocaine), benzonatate (Tessalon Perles) or diphenhydramine-lidocaine mixes; soothing the mucosa with ice chips and popsicles (possibly containing nystatin); systemic analgesics; and mouthrinses such as chlorhexidine, povidone-iodine and dyclonine HCl (Dyclone-local anesthetic).

Neurotoxicity

Plant alkaloids may produce neurotoxicity, which may result in odontogenic pain if oral nerves are involved. Neurotoxicity—which accounts for about 6% of all oral-associated problems—is not as common as other oral problems and consists of pulpitislike constant pain (especially in the mandibular molars). Palliative treatment, including analgesics and anti-inflammatory agents, is recommended. Symptoms typically disappear after therapy is discontinued.

Thrombocytopenia-associated oral bleeding
Usually when there is a platelet count less than 20,000 cells/mm³, it is possible to see spontaneous gingival bleeding and submucosal bleeding, as well as postoperative hemorrhage. Patients with profound thrombocytopenia require daily oral evaluation for hemorrhage. Platelet transfusions may be required. Also, adequate oral hygiene must be maintained in order to control spontaneous hemorrhage related to gingivitis/ periodontitis.

Xerostomia
Xerostomia can be eased by artificial saliva substitutes (Xero-lube, Salivart, Moi-Stir, Mouth-Kote, Optimoist, Saliva substitute); lemon-glycerin swabs; sucrose-free lemon drops; fluoride mouthrinses; sugarless chewing gum; and pilocarpine. Also, the dentist should advise the patient to decrease his or her intake of caries-inducing foods and should place him or her on a schedule of frequent recall visits to monitor oral hard and soft tissue disease.

Management of the Dental Patient Receiving Cancer Chemotherapy

Provided below is an outline of procedures that should be considered in the management of patients with cancer.

Table 26.1 presents general information on antineoplastic and related drugs.

Special Dental Considerations

All patients undergoing cancer therapy must be monitored carefully by the dentist for increased incidence of oral infections and then treated accordingly, as discussed above.

Patients receiving chronic drug therapy may exhibit symptoms of blood dyscrasias, which can include infection, bleeding and poor healing. Because of dyscrasias, the dentist should avoid prescribing products that contain aspirin or NSAIDs. Such patients should be placed on a frequent recall schedule because of their increased risk of infection and for evaluation of their healing response. The dentist should determine why the patient is taking a specific drug, as this—in addition to the physician's report— may help the dentist understand the nature of the disease and anticipate potential oral side effects. Palliative treatment may be needed if stomatitis occurs. Antibiotic agents may be required for more complex dental procedures.

Dental Management and Prevention Protocol in Patients Receiving Cancer Chemotherapy

Pretreatment evaluation
- Medical history
- Oral examination
- Radiographs
- Consultations as needed
- Current drugs

Pretreatment therapy
- Oral hygiene instruction
- Treatment and/or removal of infected teeth (i.e., hopeless teeth should be extracted)
- Elimination of faulty or sharp restorations or prostheses
- Scaling and root planing as needed

Prevention during therapy
- Meticulous oral hygiene protocol: Brushing, flossing, use of rubber tip when white blood cell count is > 1,000 cells/mm³ and platelet count is > 50,000 cells/mm³; with profound myeolosuppression, use of gauze sponge for débridement; daily use of fluoride rinses; use of chlorhexidine or povidone- iodine when needed
- Avoidance of mouthwashes containing alcohol or undiluted hydrogen peroxide
- Prophylactic use of antifungal rinses or lozenges
- Removal of prostheses
- Limitation of food intake to soft foods during periods of myelosuppression or stomatotoxicity
- Limitation of sucrose intake
- Frequent oral evaluation

Table 26.1

Antineoplastic Agents and Related Drugs: Dosage Information

Generic name	Brand name(s)	Dosage range	Interactions with other drugs
Alkylating agents			
Carmustine (nitrosourea)	BiCNU	150-200 mg/m² body surface q 6-8 w	Nephrotoxic and hepatotoxic drugs will alter metabolism of carmustine
Cisplatin	Platinol	10-120 mg/m² body surface q 3-4 w	Nephrotoxic and hepatotoxic drugs will alter metabolism of cisplatin
Melphalan (nitrogen mustard)	Alkeran	16 mg/m² body surface q 2 w for 4 doses	Myelosuppressive drugs
Antimetabolites			
Methotrexate	Folex, Rheumatrex	30-40 mg/m² body surface/w and higher	Drugs altering liver metabolism
Hormonal agents			
Tamoxifen	Nolvadex; Alpha-Tamoxifen, Apo-Tamox [CAN], Novo-Tamoxifen [CAN], Tamofen, Tamone [CAN]	**As adjunctive treatment for breast cancer:** 10-20 mg bid	**Warfarin:** Tamoxifen increases anticoagulant effects Hepatotoxic and nephrotoxic drugs will alter metabolism of tamoxifen **Cyclosporine:** Levels may be increased by tamoxifen
Plant alkaloids			
Paclitaxel	Taxol	**For metastatic carcinoma of the ovary or metastatic breast cancer:** 135-170 mg/m² body surface over 1-24 h q 3 w; to avoid anaphylaxis, administer with corticosteroid, H₁ antagonist or H₂ antagonist	Increased toxicity in combination with bone-marrow depressants, live virus vaccines

[CAN] indicates a drug available only in Canada.

Drug Interactions of Dental Interest

While no direct interactions with antineoplastic agents have been reported, consultation with a physician is recommended. Specific drug interactions are shown in Table 26.1.

Laboratory value alterations

Before treating a patient who is undergoing cancer therapy, the dentist must establish his or her health status, including CBC.

Special patients

Young patients undergoing chemotherapy are more susceptible to oral lesions than older adults. Thus, this may require careful explanation of the need for excellent oral care, as well as increased recall visits, judicious home care and use of fluoride rinses.

Patient Monitoring: Aspects to Watch

- Disease control: Medical consultation may be required to assess this

- Blood dyscrasias: In a patient with symptoms of these, the dentist should request a medical consultation for blood studies and postpone dental treatment until normal values are re-established

Adverse Effects and Precautions

The major concern for dentists in treatment of patients undergoing cancer therapy is to limit oral complications, which may include use of antibiotics, analgesics, anti-inflammatory agents and antifungal agents. Table 26.2 presents adverse effects of one or two selected antineoplastic agents in each category; Table 26.3 lists precautions and contraindications. Listed below are other antineoplastic drugs that patients may be taking.

Pharmacology

In general, alkylating agents, intercalators and antibiotics damage or disrupt DNA, block

---

Antineoplastic Drugs

Alkylating agents

Nitrogen mustards
- Mechlorethamine HCl (nitrogen mustard, HN$_2$, HCl)
- Melphalan: L-phenylalanine, L-PAM, chlorambucil
- Cyclophosphamide
- I fosfamide

Nitrosoureas
- Carmustine (BCNU)
- Lomustine (CCNU)

Others
- Cisplatin (cis-diamminedichloro-platinum)
- Carboplatin (cis-dichloro-trans-hydroxybisiso-propylamine)
- Platinum IV
- Busulfan
- Dacarbazine (DTIC)
- Procarbazine
- Triethylenethiophosphoramide (thio-TEPA)

Antimetabolites
- Methotrexate (MTX)
- Mercaptopurine (6-MP)
- Thioguanine (6-TG)
- Fluorouracil (5-FU)
- Cytarabine (cytosine arabinoside, ara-C)
- Trimetrexate
- Pentostatin (2-deoxycoformycin)

Antibiotics
- Daunorubicin (daunomycin)
- Doxorubicin
- Idarubicin
- Bleomycin
- Dactinomycin (actinomycin D)
- Mitomycin C
- Plicamycin

Hormonal agents
- Prednisone
- Tamoxifen
- Flutamide
- Leuprolide
- Goserelin

Plant alkaloids
- Vincristine
- Vinblastine
- Etoposide (VP-16)
- Teniposide (VN-26)
- Paclitaxel

Others
- Asparaginase
- Hydroxyurea

Adapted from Sluzo J, Larner JM. Clinical effects and antineoplastic drugs. In: Brody TM, Larner J, Minneman KP, Neu HC, eds. Human pharmacology: molecular to clinical. 2nd ed. St. Louis: Mosby; 1994:591-5.

Table 26.2
Antineoplastic Agents and Related Drugs: Adverse Effects

Body system	Alkylating agents			Antimetabolites	Hormonal agents	Plant alkaloids
	Carmustine (nitrosourea)	Cisplatin	Melphalan (nitrogen mustard)	Methotrexate	Tamoxifen	Paclitaxel
CV		Bradycardia, arrhythmias			Chest pain	Bradycardia, severe CV events
CNS		Peripheral neuropathy		Dizziness, convulsions, headache, confusion, hemiparesis, malaise, fatigue, chills, fever	Weakness, light-headedness, depression, dizziness, headache, mental confusion, hot flashes	*Cumulative neurotoxicity:* sensory neuropathy, motor neuropathy, autonomic neuropathy, myopathy
EENT		*Ototoxicity,* optic neuritis, blurred vision			**At high doses:** Ocular lesions, retinopathy, corneal opacity, blurred vision	
Endoc			Amenorrhea	Menstrual irregularities, defective spermatogenesis	Hypercalcemia	
GI	*Nausea, vomiting, diarrhea*	*Very emetogenic*	Nausea, vomiting, diarrhea	Nausea, vomiting, anorexia, diarrhea, hepatotoxicity, cramps, ulcer, gastritis, GI hemorrhage, abdominal pain, hematemesis	*Nausea, vomiting, weight gain*	*Nausea, vomiting*
GU		Hypocalcemia, hypokalemia Hypophosphatemia Hypomagnesemia	Bladder irritation	Urinary retention, renal failure, hematuria, azotemia, uric acid nephropathy	Vaginal bleeding and/or discharge, endometriosis, priapism, possible endopmetrial cancer, pruritus vulvae	

Hema	*Myelosuppression*	*Myelosuppression*	*Myelosuppression*	*Myelosuppression*	*Myelosuppression*	*Myelosuppression*

	Drug 1	Drug 2	Drug 3	Drug 4	Drug 5	Drug 6
Hema	*Myelosuppression*	*Myelosuppression*	*Myelosuppression*	*Myelosuppression*	*Myelosuppression*	*Myelosuppression*
HB	Hepatoxicity	Increased liver enzymes				*Abnormal liver function*
Integ	*Facial flushing, alopecia*	Papilledema	Alopecia, vasculitis, rash, urticaria	Rash, alopecia, dry skin, urticaria, photosensitivity, vasculitis, petechiae, ecchymosis, acne, alopecia	*Rash, alopecia*	*Dermatitis, alopecia, erythema, swelling*
Oral	*Stomatitis*	Stomatitis	Stomatitis, oral ulceration	Ulcerative stomatitis, gingivitis, bleeding		
Renal	*Nephrotoxicity*	*Nephrotoxicity*	*Nephrotoxicity*	*Nephrotoxicity*	*Nephrotoxicity*	*Nephrotoxicity*
Resp			Fibrosis, dysplasia		Pulmonary embolism	

Italics indicate information of major clinical significance.

Table 26.3

Antineoplastic Agents and Related Drugs: Precautions and Contraindications

	Alkylating agents			Antimetabolites (also see Chapter 24, Connective-Tissue Disorder and Musculoskeletal Relaxant Drugs)	Hormonal agents	Plant alkaloids
	Carmustine (nitrosourea)	Cisplatin	Melphalan (nitrogen mustard)	Methotrexate	Tamoxifen	Paclitaxel
Precautions and contraindications	No effects of concern to dentists except usual concerns of myelosuppression Nephrotoxicity Hepatotoxicity Myelosuppression Ototoxicity GI upset Pregnancy risk category: D	No effects of concern to dentists except usual concerns of myelosuppression Nephrotoxicity Hepatotoxicity Myelosuppression Ototoxicity GI upset Pregnancy risk category: D	Should be used cautiously with patients who have bone marrow depression, renal impairment Pregnancy risk category: D Contraindicated in patients with cancer who have a history of resistance to the drug; lactating women; patients with hypersensitivity to nitrogen mustards	No effects of concern to dentists except usual concerns of myelosuppression Nephrotoxicity Hepatotoxicity Myelosuppression Ototoxicity GI upset Pregnancy risk category: D	No effects of concern to dentists except usual concerns of myelosuppression Nephrotoxicity Hepatotoxicity Myelosuppression Ototoxicity GI upset Pregnancy risk category: D	No effects of concern to dentists except usual concerns of myelosuppression Nephrotoxicity Hepatotoxicity Myelosuppression Ototoxicity GI upset Pregnancy risk category: D

activity of topoisomerases or alter RNA structure. Antimetabolities block or decrease DNA synthesis. Steroids interfere with transcription, while plant alkaloids disrupt mitosis.

Patient Advice

- Patients should avoid using mouthrinses with high alcohol content because they have drying effects, which can aggravate medication-induced xerostomia.
- Daily home fluoride preparations are needed if chronic xerostomia occurs.
- Patients should use sugarless gum, sugarless lemon- or pineapple-flavored lozenges, frequent sips of water or artificial saliva substitutes if chronic xerostomia occurs.
- If a secondary oral infection occurs, which is not unusual, the patient should see the dentist immediately.
- Good oral hygiene is important in preventing soft-tissue inflammation.
- Caution must be taken to prevent injury when using oral hygiene aids.
- Palliative therapies such as topical anesthetics may be used for a sore mouth.

Suggested Readings

Consensus Development Conference on Oral Complications of Cancer Therapies: Diagnosis, prevention, and treatment. NCI Monogr 9:1-104, 1990.

Peterson DE, Schubert MM. Oral toxicity. In: Perry MC, ed. The chemotherapy source book. Baltimore: Williams and Wilkins; 1991:508-30.

Sluzo J, Larner JM. Individual antineoplastic drugs. In: Brody TM, Larner J, Minneman KP, Neu HC, eds. Human pharmacology: molecular to clinical. 2nd ed. St. Louis: Mosby; 1994:575-90.

Sluzo J, Larner JM. Clinical effects and antineoplastic drugs. In: Brody TM, Larner J, Minneman KP, Neu HC, eds. Human pharmacology: molecular to clinical. 2nd ed. St. Louis: Mosby; 1994:591-5.

Terezhalmy GT, Whitmyer CC, Markman M. Cancer chemotherapeutic agents. In: Dental Clinics of North America. Pharmacologic Management of the Medically Compromised Patient 1996;40(July); 1996:709-26.

Section III.

Drug Issues in Dental Practice

Chapter 27

Oral Manifestations of Systemic Agents

B. Ellen Byrne, R.Ph., D.D.S., Ph.D.

Many commonly prescribed medications are capable of causing adverse oral drug reactions. The oral manifestations of drug therapy are often nonspecific and vary in significance. These undesirable effects can mimic many disease processes, such as erythema multiforme. They may also be very characteristic of a particular drug reaction (as in the case of phenytoin and gingival enlargement).

Oral Manifestations

Oral manifestations can be divided into 15 broad categories: abnormal hemostasis, altered host resistance, angioedema, coated tongue (black hairy tongue), dry socket, dysgeusia (altered taste), erythema multiforme, gingival enlargement, leukopenia and neutropenia, lichenoid lesions, movement disorders, salivary gland enlargement, sialorrhea (increased salivation), soft-tissue reactions and xerostomia.

In Tables 27.1-27.15, each of the 15 oral manifestations of systemic drugs is related to specific types of drugs that may cause it. In Table 27.16, systemic drugs that may have oral manifestations are listed by their generic names and are linked to the associated manifestation(s).

Abnormal Hemostasis

Abnormal hemostasis is seen with drugs that interfere with platelet function or that decrease coagulation by depressing prothrombin synthesis in the liver. Patients using such medications require a bleeding profile before extensive dental procedures.

Altered Host Resistance

Altered host resistance occurs when the microflora of the mouth is altered, resulting in an overgrowth of organisms that are part of the normal oral flora. Bacterial, fungal and viral superinfections all occur as a result of drug therapy. Broad-spectrum antibiotics and corticosteroids, as well as xerostomia, radiation and side effects of cancer chemotherapy (and AIDS), can elicit episodes of oral candidiasis. Treatment includes elimination of the causative factor, if possible, combined with use of an antifungal agent, such as nystatin suspension, clotrimazole (Myclex) troche or ketoconazole (Nizoral) tablets. Various conditions such as diabetes, leukemia, lymphomas and AIDS can also render a patient more susceptible to oral candidal infections.

Angioedema

Angioedema is the result of drug-induced hypersensitivity reactions and can be life-threatening when it involves the mucosal and submucosal layers of the upper aerodigestive tract. Mild angioedema is treated with antihistamines. In more severe cases where the airway is threatened, the emergency treatment is managed the same way as in the case of an anaphylactic reaction.

Coated Tongue (Black Hairy Tongue)

The most common discoloration of the tongue is a condition known as black hairy tongue. This results from hypertrophy of the filiform papillae. This condition is asymptomatic. The color is usually black, but may be various shades of brown. The exact mechanism by which this condition is produced is unknown and there is no effective treatment for this condition.

Dry Socket

Dry socket, or alveolar osteitis, is the result of lysis of a fully formed blood clot before the clot is replaced with granulation tissue. The incidence of dry socket seems to be higher in patients who smoke and in female patients who take oral contraceptives. Dry socket can be minimized in patients taking oral contraceptives if extractions are performed during days 23-28 of the tablet cycle.

Dysgeusia

Dysgeusia is manifested in taste alterations; medication taste; unusual taste; bitter, peculiar and metallic taste; taste perversion; and changes in taste and distaste for food. Xerostomia, malnutrition, neurological deficiencies and olfactory deficiencies also can be responsible for taste changes. Although the operative mechanism is unclear, there is some evidence that medications alter taste by affecting trace metal ions, which interact with the cell membrane proteins of the taste pores. There is no treatment other than withdrawal of the drug.

Erythema Multiforme

Erythema multiforme is a syndrome consisting of symmetrical mucocutaneous lesions that have a predilection for the oral mucosa, hands and feet. It presents initially as erythema, and vesicles and erosions develop within hours. Erythema multiforme usually has its onset from 1-3 w after the person begins taking the offending drug. Skin lesions can have concentric rings of erythema, producing the "target" or "bull's-eye" appearance that is associated with this condition. The lesions are normally self-limiting but will persist if the patient continues to take the offending drug. Oral lesions heal without scarring.

Gingival Enlargement

Gingival enlargement has been associated with numerous types of systemic drug therapy, and usually becomes apparent in the first 3 mo after drug therapy begins. Clinically, the overgrowth starts as a diffuse swelling of the interdental papillae, which then coalesces for a nodular appearance. Many theories have been suggested to explain the overgrowth. The most attractive theory is that it is a direct effect of the drug or its metabolites on certain subpopulations of fibroblasts, which are capable of greater synthesis of protein and collagen. Many studies have shown a clear relationship between a patient's oral hygiene status and the extent of overgrowth. Also, mouth breathing and other local factors such as crowding of teeth, significantly relate to the occurrence of gingival enlargement.

Leukopenia and Neutropenia

Many drugs can alter a patient's hematopoietic status. These effects can take the form of leukopenia, agranulocytosis and neutropenia. These conditions can have a variety of effects in the mouth: increased infections, ulcerations, nonspecific inflammation, bleeding gingiva and significant bleeding after a dental procedure. Treatment includes discontinuing use of the suspected offending drug and replacing it with a structurally dissimilar agent if continued therapy is indicated.

Lichenoid Lesions

Lichenoid lesions seen with systemic use of drugs differ from actual lichen planus in that the condition resolves when the patient discontinues taking the offending drug. Patients have pain after ulcerations have developed. Buccal mucosa and lateral borders of the tongue are most often involved, and characteristic white striations (Wickham's striae) usually occur.

Movement Disorders

Movement disorders in the muscles of facial expression and mastication can be brought on by systemic drug therapy. These side effects include pseudoparkinsonism (rigidity, bradykinesia, tremor), akathisia (restlessness) and involuntary dystonic movements such as tardive dyskinesia. Tardive dyskinesia is characterized by repetitive, involuntary movements, usually of the mouth and tongue, secondary to long-term neuroleptic drug treatment. This type of movement, once developed, cannot be controlled and is usually irreversible. Tardive dyskinesia occurs in approximately 20% of all patients who take neuroleptic medications regularly. These patients may find it difficult to communicate, eat and use removable oral prostheses.

Salivary Gland Involvement

Salivary gland problems can appear as salivary gland swelling or pain and can resemble mumps. Differential diagnosis must include salivary gland infections, obstructions and neoplasms. The mechanism of salivary gland enlargement is unknown, and the treatment is discontinuing the use of the offending drug.

Sialorrhea

Any drug that works by increasing cholinergic stimulation by directly stimulating parasympathetic receptors (such as pilocarpine) or by inhibiting the action of cholinesterase (such as neostigmine) may cause sialorrhea or increased salivation.

Soft-Tissue Reactions

Soft-tissue problems include discoloration, ulcerations, stomatitis and glossitis. Gingivitis is inflammation of the gingiva, while gingival enlargement is an overgrowth of fibrous gingival tissue. Gingival overgrowth usually becomes apparent in the first 3 mo after the patient starts taking the drug and is most rapid in the first year. There are many theories on the cause of the gingival overgrowth. The most likely theory is that the drug or one of its metabolites directly stimulates a population of fibroblasts to synthesize more protein and collagen. This condition is aggravated by poor oral hygiene, mouth breathing and crowded teeth.

Xerostomia

Xerostomia, defined as dry mouth or a decrease in salivation, is a frequently reported side effect. This effect may be exaggerated during prolonged drug use by elderly people and may be even more pronounced when several drugs causing dry mouth are taken simultaneously. Possible nondrug causes of xerostomia include dehydration, salivary gland infection, neoplasm, obstruction, radiation to the mouth, diabetes mellitus, nutritional deficiencies, Sjögren's syndrome and drugs that either stimulate sympathetic activity or depress parasympathetic activity.

Table 27.1

Abnormal Hemostasis: Associated Drugs

Generic name	Brand name
Anticoagulant agents	
Heparin	Hepalean
Warfarin	Coumadin
Antithrombotic agents	
Dipyridamole	Persantine
Ticlopidine	Ticlid

Continued on next page

Table 27.1 (cont.)

Abnormal Hemostasis: Associated Drugs

Generic name	Brand name
Nonsteroidal anti-inflammatory drugs (NSAIDs)	
Aspirin	Various brand names
Diclofenac	Cataflam, Voltaren
Diflunisal	Dolobid
Etodolac	Lodine
Ibuprofen	Advil, Motrin, Nuprin, Rufen
Indomethacin	Indocin
Ketoprofen	Orudis
Ketorolac	Toradol
Meclofenamate	Meclomen
Mefenamic acid	Ponstel
Naproxen	Aleve, Anaprox, Naprosyn
Oxaprozin	Daypro
Piroxicam	Feldene
Tolmetin	Tolectin

Table 27.2

Altered Host Resistance (Microflora Imbalance): Associated Drugs

Generic name	Brand name
Antibiotics	
Aminoglycoside: Gentamicin	Garamycin
Cephalosporin: Cefaclor	Ceclor
Macrolide: Erythromycin	E.E.S., E. Mycin, Eryc
Penicillin: Amoxicillin	Amoxil

Continued on next page

Table 27.2 (cont.)
Altered Host Resistance (Microflora Imbalance): Associated Drugs

Generic name	Brand name
Antibiotics (cont.)	
Fluoroquinolone: Ciprofloxacin	Cipro
Sulfonamide: Sulfisoxazole	Gantrisin
Tetracycline	Vibramycin
Antidiabetic agent	
Insulin	Humulin
Antidiabetic (oral hypoglycemic) agents	
Acetohexamide	Dymelor
Chlorpropamide	Diabinese
Diazoxide	Proglycem
Glipizide	Glucotrol
Glyburide	DiaBeta
Metaformin	Glucophage
Tolazamide	Tolinase
Tolbutamide	Orinase
Antineoplastic agent	
Tamoxifen	Nolvadex
Corticosteroids (inhaled)	
Beclomethasone dipropionate	Beconase
Dexamethasone	Decadron Turbinaire
Flunisolide	Nasalide
Triamcinolone	Azmacort

Continued on next page

Table 27.2 (cont.)

Altered Host Resistance (Microflora Imbalance): Associated Drugs

Generic name	Brand name
Corticosteroids (oral)	
Betamethasone	Celestone
Cortisone acetate	Cortone
Dexamethasone	Decadron
Methylprednisolone	Medrol
Immunosuppressant agent	
Cyclosporin A	Sandimmune

Table 27.3

Angioedema: Associated Drugs

Generic name	Brand name
Angiotensin-converting enzyme (ACE) inhibitors (antihypertensive agents)	
Benazepril	Lotensin
Captopril	Capoten
Fosinopril	Monopril
Quinapril	Accupril
Ramipril	Altace
Antianxiety agent	
Midazolam	Versed
Antifungal agent	
Ketoconazole	Nizoral
Antirheumatic agent (disease-modifying gold compound)	
Auranofin	Ridaura

Table 27.4

Coated Tongue (Black Hairy Tongue): Associated Drugs

Generic name	Brand name
Antianxiety agents	
Diazepam	Valium
Lorazepam	Ativan
Antibiotics	
Amoxicillin	Amoxil
Amoxicillin/clavulanic acid	Augmentin
Penicillin VK	PenVeeK
Tetracycline	Robitet
Anticonvulsant agent	
Clonazepam	Klonopin
Antidepressant agents	
Amitriptyline	Elavil
Nortriptyline	Pamelor
Muscle relaxant	
Cyclobenzaprine	Flexeril
Nonsteroidal anti-inflammatory drugs (NSAIDs)	
Ketoprofen	Orudis
Urinary tract anti-infective agent	
Nitrofurantoin	Macrodantin

Table 27.5
Dry Socket (Increased Incidence): Associated Drugs

Generic name	Brand name
Oral contraceptives	
Ethinyl estradiol	Estinyl
Ethinyl estradiol and ethynodiol	Demulen
Ethinyl estradiol and levonorgestrel	Levlen, Levora, Nordette, Tri-Levlen, Triphasil
Ethinyl estradiol and norethindrone	Brevicon, Genora, Loestrin, Ortho-Novum
Ethinyl estradiol and norgestrel	Lo/Ovral, Ovral

Table 27.6
Dysgeusia (Taste Disturbances): Associated Drugs

Generic name	Brand name
Antianemic agent	
Iron	Numerous iron-containing vitamins and iron supplements
Antiarthritic (disease-modifying) agent	
Allopurinol	Zyloprim
Auranofin	Ridaura
Aurothioglucose	Solganal
Penicillamine	Cuprimine
Antibiotics	
Cefamandol	Mandol
Clarithromycin	Biaxin
Lincomycin	Lincocin
Metronidazole	Flagyl
Procaine penicillin	Wycillin
Tetracycline	Achromycin

Continued on next page

Table 27.6 (cont.)

Dysgeusia (Taste Disturbances): Associated Drugs

Generic name	Brand name
Anticonvulsant agent	
Carbamazepine	Tegretol
Antifungal agent	
Amphotericin B	Fungizone
Griseofulvin	Fulvicin
Antilipidemic agents	
Cholestyramine	Questran
Clofibrate	Atromid-S
Antineoplastic agents	
Azathioprine	Imuran
Bleomycin	Blenoxane
5-fluorouracil	Adrucil
Methotrexate	Folex
Vincristine	Oncovin
Antiparkinsonism agent	
Levodopa	Dopar
Antipsychotic agent	
Lithium	Eskalith
Antithyroid agent	
Methimazole	Tapazole
Cardiovascular agents	
Amrinone	Inocor
Bretylium	Bretylol
Captopril	Capoten

Continued on next page

Table 27.6 (cont.)

Dysgeusia (Taste Disturbances): Associated Drugs

Generic name	Brand name
Cardiovascular agents (cont.)	
Diltiazem	Cardizem
Dipyridamole	Persantine
Enalapril	Vasotec
Nifedipine	Procardia
Spironolactone	Aldactone
CNS stimulant agent	
Dextroamphetamine	Dexedrine
Dental agent	
Chlorhexidine	Peridex
Muscle relaxant agent	
Lioresal	Baclofen
Nonsteroidal anti-inflammatory drug (NSAID)	
Phenylbutazone	Butazolidin
Smoking cessation agents	
Nicotine polacrilex (chewing gum)	Nicorette
Nicotine topical patches	Habitrol, NicoDerm

Table 27.7

Erythema Multiforme: Associated Drugs

Generic name	Brand name
Antibiotics	
Clindamycin	Cleocin
Penicillin VK	V-Cillin K, Pen Vee K, Veetids
Tetracycline	Achromycin

Continued on next page

Table 27.7 (cont.)

Erythema Multiforme: Associated Drugs

Generic name	Brand name
Anticonvulsant agents	
Carbamazepine	Tegretol
Phenytoin	Dilantin
Antidiabetic (oral hypoglycemic) agent	
Chlorpropamide	Diabinese
Barbiturates	
Pentobarbital	Nembutal
Phenobarbital	Luminal
Secobarbital	Seconal
Nonsteroidal anti-inflammatory drugs (NSAIDs)	
Phenylbutazone	Butazolidin
Sulfonamides	
Sulfacytine	Renoquid
Sulfamethizole	Thiosulfil Forte
Sulfamethoxazole	Gantanol
Sulfisoxazole	Gantrisin

Table 27.8

Gingival Enlargement: Associated Drugs

Generic name	Brand name
Anticonvulsant agent	
Phenytoin	Dilantin
Cardiovascular (calcium channel blockers)	
Diltiazem	Cardizem
Nifedipine	Procardia
Immunosuppressant agent	
Cyclosporin A	Sandimmune

Table 27.9

Leukopenia and Neutropenia: Associated Drugs

Generic name	Brand name
Antibiotic	
Chloramphenicol	Chlormycetin
Antidiabetic (oral hypoglycemic) agent	
Tolbutamide	Orinase
Antiprotozoal agent	
Quinine	Quinamm
Antipsychotic agents (phenothiazines)	
Chlorpromazine	Thorazine
Chlorprothixene	Taractan
Fluphenazine	Prolixin
Haloperidol	Haldol
Mesoridazine	Serentil
Perphenazine	Trilafon

Continued on next page

Table 27.9 (cont.)

Leukopenia and Neutropenia: Associated Drugs

Generic name	Brand name
Antipsychotic agents (phenothiazines) (cont.)	
Prochlorperazine	Compazine
Promazine	Sparine
Thioridazine	Mellaril
Trifluoperazine	Stelazine
Barbiturates	
Amobarbital	Amytal
Mephobarbital	Mebaral
Pentobarbital	Nembutal
Phenobarbital	Luminal
Primidone	Mysoline
Secobarbital	Seconal
Nonsteroidal anti-inflammatory drugs (NSAIDs)	
Phenylbutazone	Butazolidin
Sulfonamides	
Sulfacytine	Renoquid
Sulfamethizole	Thiosulfil Forte
Sulfamethoxazole	Gantanol
Sulfisoxazole	Gantrisin

Table 27.10
Lichenoid Reactions: Associated Drugs

Generic name	Brand name
Angiotensin-converting enzyme (ACE) inhibitor (antihypertensive agent)	
Captopril	Capoten
Antidiabetic (oral hypoglycemic) agent	
Chlorpropamide	Diabinese
Antihypertensive agent	
Methyldopa	Aldomet
Diuretic agent	
Furosemide	Lasix
Nonsteroidal anti-inflammatory drugs (NSAIDs)	
Diflunisal	Dolobid
Flurbiprofem	Ansaid
Ibuprofen	Motrin, Advil, Nuprin, Rufen

Table 27.11
Movement Disorders: Associated Drugs

Generic name	Brand name
Antidepressant agent	
Amoxapine	Asendin
Antiparkinsonian agent	
Levodopa	Dopar, Larodopa
Antipsychotic agents (phenothiazines)	
Acetophenazine	Tindal
Chlorpromazine	Thorazine
Chlorprothixene	Taractan
Clozapine	Clozaril

Continued on next page

Table 27.11 (cont.)
Movement Disorders: Associated Drugs

Generic name	Brand name
Antipsychotic agents (phenothiazines) (cont.)	
Fluphenazine	Prolixin
Haloperidol	Haldol
Loxapine	Loxitane
Mesoridazine	Serentil
Perphenazine	Trilafon
Prochlorperazine	Compazine
Promazine	Sparine
Risperidone	Risperdal
Thioridazine	Mellaril
Thiothixene	Navane
Trifluoperazine	Stelazine

Table 27.12
Salivary Gland Involvement: Associated Drugs

Generic name	Brand name
Antihypertensive agents	
Methyldopa	Aldomet
Quanethidine	Ismelin
Antipsychotic agent	
Lithium	Eskalith
Nonsteroidal anti-inflammatory drug (NSAID)	
Phenylbutazone	Butazolidin

Table 27.13

Sialorrhea: Associated Drugs

Generic name	Brand name
Cholinergic agents	
Bethanechol	Urecholine
Tacrine	Cognex

Table 27.14

Soft-Tissue Reactions*: Associated Drugs

Generic name (reaction)	Brand name
Antiacne agent	
Isotretinoin (G)	Accutane
Antianxiety agent	
Meprobamate (S)	Equanil
Antiarthritic (disease-modifying) agent	
Auranofin (G, S)	Ridaura
Aurothioglucose (G, S)	Solganal
Gold sodium thiomalate (S)	Myochrysine
Antibiotic	
Minocycline (D)	Minocin
Ampicillin (U)	Omnipen
Anticoagulant agent	
Warfarin (U)	Coumadin
Antilipidemic agent	
Clofibrate (S)	Atromid-S

*(D): discoloration; (G): glossitis; (P): pigmentation; (S): stomatitis; (U): ulceration.

Continued on next page

Table 27.14 (cont.)

Soft-Tissue Reactions*: Associated Drugs

Generic name (reaction)	Brand name
Antihypertensive agents	
Captopril (G, S)	Capoten
Methyldopa (D)	Aldomet
Chelating agent	
Penicillamine (D)	Cuprimine
Cytotoxic agents	
Busulphan (D)	Myleran
Carboplatin (S)	Paraplastin
Carmustin (D)	BiCNU
Hydroxyurea (G, S)	Hydrea
Lomustine (S)	CeeNU
Mercaptopurine (G)	Purinethol
Methotrexate (G, S)	Folex
P-cyclophosphamide (P)	Cytoxan
Vincristine (S)	Oncovin
Heavy metals	
Lead (P)	No brand names
Mercury (P)	No brand names
Immunosuppressant agent	
Azathioprine (G, S)	Imuran

*(D): discoloration; (G): glossitis; (P): pigmentation; (S): stomatitis; (U): ulceration.

Continued on next page

Table 27.14 (cont.)

Soft-Tissue Reactions*: Associated Drugs

Generic name (reaction)	Brand name
Nonsteroidal anti-inflammatory drugs (NSAIDs)	
Aspirin (U)	Various brand names
Ibuprofen (U)	Motrin, Advil
Indomethacin (U)	Indocin
Ketoprofen (U)	Orudis
Ketorolac (U)	Toradol
Oral contraceptives	
Ethinyl estradiol (D)	Estinyl
Ethinyl estradiol/ethynodiol (D)	Demulen
Ethinyl estradiol/levonorgestrel (D)	Levlen, Levora, Nordette, Tri-Levlen, Triphasil
Ethinyl estradiol/norethindrone (D)	Brevicon, Ortho-Novum
Ethinyl estradiol/norgestrel (D)	Lo/Ovral, Ovral

*(D): discoloration; (G): glossitis; (P): pigmentation; (S): stomatitis; (U): ulceration.

Table 27.15

Xerostomia: Associated Drugs

Generic name	Brand name
Anorexiant agent	
Diethylpropion	Tenuate, Tepanil
Fenfluramine	Pondimin
Phendimetrazine	Anorex
Phentermine	Adipex-P, Fastin, Ionamin
Antiacne agent	
Isotretinoin	Accutane

Continued on next page

Table 27.15 (cont.)

Xerostomia: Associated Drugs

Generic name	Brand name
Antianxiety agents	
Alprazolam	Xanax
Chlordiazepoxide	Librium
Diazepam	Valium
Lorazepam	Ativan
Meprobamate	Equanil, Miltown
Oxazepam	Serax
Prazepam	Centrax
Anticholinergic/antispasmodic agents	
Atropine	Atropisol
Belladonna alkaloids	Bellergal
Chlordiazepoxide/clidinium	Librax
Dicyclomine	Bentyl
Hyoscyamine	Anaspaz
Hyoscyamine/atropine/phenobarbital/scopolamine	Donnatal, Kinesed
Isopropamide	Darbid
Methantheline	Banthine
Methscopolamine	Pamine
Oxybutynin	Ditropan
Oxyphencyclimine	Daricon
Propantheline	Pro-Banthine
Scopolamine	Transderm-Scop
Anticonvulsant agent	
Carbamazepine	Tegretol

Continued on next page

Table 27.15 (cont.)

Xerostomia: Associated Drugs

Generic name	Brand name
Antidepressant agents	
Amitriptyline	Elavil, Endep
Amitriptyline/perphenazine	Etrafon
Amoxapine	Asendin
Desipramine	Pertofrane, Norpramin
Doxepin	Sinequan, Adapin
Fluoxetine	Prozac
Imipramine	Tofranil
Isocarboxazid	Marplan
Maprotiline	Ludiomil
Nortriptyline	Aventyl, Pamelor
Paroxetine	Paxil
Phenelzine	Nardil
Sertraline	Zoloft
Tranylcypromine	Parnate
Trazodone	Desyrel
Antidiarrheal agents	
Diphenoxylate/atropine	Lomotil
Loperamide	Imodium AD
Antihistamines	
Astemizole	Hismanal
Brompheniramine	Dimetane
Brompheniramine/phenylpropanolamine	Dimetapp

Continued on next page

Table 27.15 (cont.)
Xerostomia: Associated Drugs

Generic name	Brand name
Antihistamines (cont.)	
Chlorpheniramine	Chlor-Trimeton
Clemastine	Tavist
Cyproheptadine	Peractin
Diphenhydramine	Benadryl
Hydroxyzine	Vistaril
Loratadine	Claritin
Promethazine	Phenergan
Terfenadine	Seldane
Tripelennamine	Pyribenzamine (PBZ)
Triprolidine/pseudoephedrine	Actifed
Antihypertensive agents	
Captopril	Capoten
Clonidine	Catapres
Enalapril	Vasotec
Guanethidine	Ismelin
Lisinopril	Zestril
Methyldopa	Aldomet
Metoprolol	Lopressor
Nadolol	Corgard
Nifedipine	Procardia
Prazosin	Minipress
Reserpine	Serpasil

Continued on next page

Table 27.15 (cont.)
Xerostomia: Associated Drugs

Generic name	Brand name
Antinausea agents	
Dimenhydrinate	Dramamine
Hydroxyzine	Atarax, Vistaril
Meclizine	Antivert
Antiparkinsonism agents	
Benztropine mesylate	Cogentin
Biperiden	Akineton
Carbidopa/levodopa	Sinemet
Ethopropazine	Parsidol
Levodopa	Larodopa, Dopar
Orphenadrine HCl	Marflex
Trihexyphenidyl	Artane
Antipsychotic agents	
Amitriptyline/perphenazine	Triavil
Chlorpromazine	Thorazine
Clozapine	Clozaril
Haloperidol	Haldol
Lithium	Eskalith
Loxapine	Loxitane
Molindone	Moban
Pimozide	Orap
Prochlorperazine	Compazine
Promazine	Sparine

Continued on next page

Table 27.15 (cont.)

Xerostomia: Associated Drugs

Generic name	Brand name
Antipsychotic agents (cont.)	
Risperidone	Risperdal
Thioridazine	Mellaril
Thiothixene	Navane
Trifluoperazine	Stelazine
Bronchodilators	
Albuterol	Proventil, Ventolin
Isoproterenol	Arm-a-Med, Isopro, Isuprel, Vapo-Iso
Decongestant agent	
Phenylpropanolamine/chlorpheniramine	Ornade
Diuretics	
Chlorothiazide	Diuril
Triamterene/hydrochlorothiazide	Dyazide, Maxzide
Furosemide	Lasix
Hydrochlorothiazide	HydroDiuril, Esidrix
Triamterene	Dyrenium
Muscle relaxant agents	
Cyclobenzaprine	Flexeril
Orphenadrine	Norflex
Narcotic analgesics	
Meperidine	Demerol
Morphine	MS Contin

Continued on next page

Table 27.15 (cont.)

Xerostomia: Associated Drugs

Generic name	Brand name
Nonsteroidal anti-inflammatory drugs (NSAIDs)	
Diflunisal	Dolobid
Fenoprofen	Nalfon
Ibuprofen	Motrin, Advil, Rufen
Naproxen	Naprosyn, Anaprox, Aleve
Phenylbutazone	Butazolidin
Piroxicam	Feldene
Sedatives	
Flurazepam	Dalmane
Temazepam	Restoril
Triazolam	Halcion
Smoking cessation agents	
Nicotine polacrilex (chewing gum)	Nicorette
Nicotine topical patches	Habitrol, NicoDerm

Table 27.16

Generic Drugs and Associated Oral Manifestations

Generic name	Brand name	Drug category	Associated manifestation(s)
Acetohexamide	Dymelor	Antidiabetic (oral hypoglycemic)	Altered host resistance
Acetophenazine	Tindal	Antipsychotic	Movement disorders
Albuterol	Proventil, Ventolin	Bronchodilator	Xerostomia
Allopurinol	Zyloprim	Antiarthritic (disease modifying)	Dysgeusia
Alprazolam	Xanax	Antianxiety	Xerostomia
Amitriptyline	Elavil, Endep	Antidepressant	Xerostomia, coated tongue
Amitriptyline/perphenazine	Etrafon, Triavil	Antidepressant, antipsychotic	Xerostomia
Amobarbital	Amytal	Barbiturate	Leukopenia and neutropenia
Amoxapine	Asendin	Antidepressant	Xerostomia, movement disorders
Amoxicillin	Amoxil	Antibiotic (penicillin)	Coated tongue, altered host resistance
Amoxicillin/clavulanic acid	Augmentin	Antibiotic	Coated tongue
Amphotericin B	Fungizone	Antifungal	Dysgeusia
Ampicillin	Omnipen	Antibiotic	Soft-tissue reaction (U)*
Amrinone	Inocor	Cardiovascular	Dysgeusia
Aspirin	Anacin, A.S.A., Ascriptin, Aspergum, Bayer Aspirin, Bufferin, Ecotrin, Empirin, Zorprin	NSAID	Soft-tissue reaction (U), abnormal hemostasis
Astemizole	Hismanal	Antihistamine	Xerostomia
Atropine	Atropisol	Anticholinergic/ antispasmodic	Xerostomia
Auranofin	Ridaura	Antiarthritic (disease modifying)	Soft-tissue reaction (G, S), dysgeusia, angioedema

indicates a soft-tissue reaction. (D): discoloration; (G): glossitis; (P): pigmentation; (S): stomatitis; (U): ulceration.

Continued on next page

Table 27.16 (cont.)

Generic Drugs and Associated Oral Manifestations

Generic name	Brand name	Drug category	Associated manifestation(s)
Aurothioglucose	Solganal	Antiarthritic (disease modifying)	Soft-tissue reaction (G, S), dysgeusia
Azathioprine	Imuran	Immunosuppressant, antineoplastic	Soft-tissue reaction (G, S), dysgeusia
Beclomethasone dipropionate	Beconase	Corticosteroid (inhaled)	Altered host resistance
Belladonna alkaloids	Bellergal	Anticholinergic/ antispasmodic	Xerostomia
Benazepril	Lotensin	ACE inhibitor	Angioedema
Benztropine mesylate	Cogentin	Antiparkinsonism	Xerostomia
Betamethasone	Celestone	Corticosteroid (oral)	Altered host resistance
Bethanechol	Urecholine	Cholinergic	Sialorrhea
Biperiden	Akineton	Antiparkinsonism	Xerostomia
Bleomycin	Blenoxane	Antineoplastic	Dysgeusia
Bretylium	Bretylol	Cardiovascular	Dysgeusia
Brompheniramine	Dimetane	Antihistamine	Xerostomia
Brompheniramine/ phylpropanolamine	Dimetapp	Antihistamine	Xerostomia
Busulphan	Myleran	Cytotoxic agent	Soft-tissue reaction (D)
Captopril	Capoten	Cardiovascular, ACE inhibitor	Xerostomia, soft-tissue reaction (G, S), dysgeusia, angioedema, lichenoid reaction
Carbamazepine	Tegretol	Anticonvulsant	Xerostomia, dysgeusia, erythema multiforme
Carbidopa/levodopa	Sinemet	Antiparkinsonism	Xerostomia
Carboplatin	Paraplastin	Cytotoxic agent	Soft-tissue reaction (S)

indicates a soft-tissue reaction. (D): discoloration; (G): glossitis; (P): pigmentation; (S): stomatitis; (U): ulceration.

Continued on next page

Table 27.16 (cont.)

Generic Drugs and Associated Oral Manifestations

Generic name	Brand name	Drug category	Associated manifestation(s)
Carmustine	BiCNU	Cytotoxic agent	Soft-tissue reaction (D)*
Cefaclor	Ceclor	Antibiotic (cephalosporin)	Altered host resistance
Cefamandol	Mandol	Antibiotic	Dysgeusia
Chloramphenicol	Chlormycetin	Antibiotic	Leukopenia and neutropenia
Chlordiazepoxide	Librium	Antianxiety	Xerostomia
Chlordiazepoxide/ clidinium	Librax	Anticholinergic/ antispasmodic	Xerostomia
Chlorhexidine	Peridex	Dental agent	Dysgeusia
Chlorothiazide	Diuril	Diuretic	Xerostomia
Chlorpheniramine	Chlor-Trimeton	Antihistamine	Xerostomia
Chlorpromazine	Thorazine	Antipsychotic	Xerostomia, leukopenia and neutropenia, movement disorders
Chlorpropamide	Diabinese	Antidiabetic (oral hypoglycemic)	Erythema multiforme, altered host resistance, lichenoid reaction
Chlorprothixene	Taractan	Antipsychotic	Leukopenia and neutropenia, movement disorders
Cholestyramine	Questran	Antilipidemic	Dysgeusia
Ciprofloxacin	Cipro	Antibiotic (fluoroquinolone)	Altered host resistance
Clarithromycin	Biaxin	Antibiotic	Dysgeusia
Clemastine	Tavist	Antihistamine	Xerostomia
Clindamycin	Cleocin	Antibiotic	Erythema multiforme
Clofibrate	Atromid-S	Antilipidemic	Soft-tissue reaction (S), dysgeusia
Clonazepam	Klonopin	Anticonvulsant	Coated tongue

*indicates a soft-tissue reaction. (D): discoloration; (G): glossitis; (P): pigmentation; (S): stomatitis; (U): ulceration.

Continued on next page

Table 27.16 (cont.)

Generic Drugs and Associated Oral Manifestations

Generic name	Brand name	Drug category	Associated manifestation(s)
Clonidine	Catapres	Antihypertensive	Xerostomia
Clozapine	Clozaril	Antipsychotic	Xerostomia, movement disorders
Cortisone acetate	Cortone	Corticosteroid (oral)	Altered host resistance
Cyclobenzaprine	Flexeril	Muscle relaxant	Xerostomia, coated tongue
Cyclosporin A	Sandimmune	Immunosuppressant	Gingival enlargement, altered host resistance
Cyproheptadine	Peractin	Antihistamine	Xerostomia
Desipramine	Pertofrane	Antidepressant	Xerostomia
Dexamethasone	Decadron, Decadron Turbinaire	Corticosteroid (oral), corticosteroid (inhaled)	Altered host resistance
Dextroamphetamine	Dexedrine	CNS stimulant	Dysgeusia
Diazepam	Valium	Antianxiety	Xerostomia, coated tongue
Diazoxide	Proglycem	Antidiabetic (oral hypoglycemic)	Altered host resistance
Diclofenac	Cataflam, Voltaren	NSAID	Abnormal hemostasis
Dicyclomine	Bentyl	Anticholinergic/ antispasmodic	Xerostomia
Diethylpropion	Tenuate, Tepanil	Anorexiant	Xerostomia
Diflunisal	Dolobid	NSAID	Xerostomia, abnormal hemostasis, lichenoid reaction
Diltiazem	Cardizem	Cardiovascular (calcium channel blocker)	Dysgeusia, gingival enlargement
Dimenhydramine	Dramamine	Antinauseant	Xerostomia
Diphenhydramine	Benadryl	Antihistamine	Xerostomia

Continued on next page

Table 27.16 (cont.)

Generic Drugs and Associated Oral Manifestations

Generic name	Brand name	Drug category	Associated manifestation(s)
Diphenoxylate/atropine	Lomotil	Antidiarrheal	Xerostomia
Dipyridamole	Persantine	Cardiovascular	Dysgeusia, abnormal hemostasis
Doxepin	Adapin, Sinequan	Antidepressant	Xerostomia
Enalapril	Vasotec	Cardiovascular	Xerostomia, dysgeusia
Erythromycin	E.E.S., E. Mycin, ERYC	Antibiotic (macrolide)	Altered host resistance
Ethinyl estradiol	Estinyl	Estrogen	Soft-tissue reaction (D)*, dry socket
Ethinyl estradiol/ethynodiol	Demulen	Oral contraceptive	Soft-tissue reaction (D), dry socket
Ethinyl estradiol/levonorgestrel	Levlen, Levora, Nordette, Tri-Levlen, Triphasil	Oral contraceptive	Soft-tissue reaction (D)*, dry socket
Ethinyl estradiol/norethindrone	Brevicon, Genora, Loestrin, Ortho-Novum	Oral contraceptive	Soft-tissue reaction (D), dry socket
Ethinyl estradiol/norgestrel	Lo/Ovral, Ovral	Oral contraceptive	Soft-tissue reaction (D), dry socket
Ethopropazine	Parsidol	Antiparkinsonism	Xerostomia
Etodolac	Lodine	NSAID	Abnormal hemostasis
5-fluorouracil	Adrucil	Antineoplastic	Dysgeusia
Fenfluramine	Pondimin	Anorexiant	Xerostomia
Fenoprofen	Nalfon	NSAID	Xerostomia
Flunisolide	Nasalide	Corticosteroid (inhaled)	Altered host resistance
Fluoxetine	Prozac	Antidepressant	Xerostomia
Fluphenazine	Prolixin	Antipsychotic	Leukopenia and neutropenia, movement disorders

indicates a soft-tissue reaction. (D): discoloration; (G): glossitis; (P): pigmentation; (S): stomatitis; (U): ulceration.

Continued on next page

Table 27.16 (cont.)

Generic Drugs and Associated Oral Manifestations

Generic name	Brand name	Drug category	Associated manifestation(s)
Flurazepam	Dalmane	Sedative	Xerostomia
Flurbiprofen	Ansaid	NSAID	Lichenoid reaction
Fosinopril	Monopril	ACE inhibitor	Angioedema
Furosemide	Lasix	Diuretic	Xerostomia, lichenoid reaction
Gentamicin sulfate	Garamycin	Antibiotic (aminoglycoside)	Altered host resistance
Glipizide	Glucotrol	Antidiabetic (oral hypoglycemic)	Altered host resistance
Glyburide	DiaBeta	Antidiabetic (oral hypoglycemic)	Altered host resistance
Gold sodium thiomalate	Myochrysine	Antirheumatic (disease modifying)	Soft-tissue reaction (S)*
Griseofulvin	Fulvicin	Antifungal	Dysgeusia
Guanethidine	Ismelin	Antihypertensive	Xerostomia
Haloperidol	Haldol	Antipsychotic	Xerostomia, leukopenia and neutropenia, movement disorders
Heparin	Hepalean	Anticoagulant	Abnormal hemostasis
Hydrochlorothiazide	HydroDIURIL, Esidrix	Diuretic	Xerostomia
Hydroxyurea	Hydrea	Cytotoxic agent	Soft-tissue reaction (G, S)
Hydroxyzine	Atarax, Vistaril	Antihistamine, antinauseant	Xerostomia
Hyoscyamine	Anaspaz	Anticholinergic/ antispasmodic	Xerostomia
Hyoscyamine/ atropine/phenobarbital/ scopolamine	Donnatal, Kinesed	Anticholinergic/ antispasmodic	Xerostomia

*indicates a soft-tissue reaction. (D): discoloration; (G): glossitis; (P): pigmentation; (S): stomatitis; (U): ulceration.

Continued on next page

Table 27.16 (cont.)

Generic Drugs and Associated Oral Manifestations

Generic name	Brand name	Drug category	Associated manifestation(s)
Ibuprofen	Advil, Motrin, Nuprin, Rufen	NSAID	Xerostomia, soft-tissue reaction (U)*, abnormal hemostasis, lichenoid reaction
Imipramine	Tofranil	Antidepressant	Xerostomia
Indomethacin	Indocin	NSAID	Soft-tissue reaction (U), abnormal hemostasis
Insulin	Humulin	Antidiabetic	Altered host resistance
Iron	Feosol	Antianemic	Dysgeusia
Isocarboxazid	Marplan	Antidepressant	Xerostomia
Isopropamide	Darbid	Anticholinergic/ antispasmodic	Xerostomia
Isoproterenol	Isoprel	Bronchodilator	Xerostomia
Isotretinoin	Accutane	Antiacne	Xerostomia, soft-tissue reaction (G)
Ketoconazole	Nizoral	Antifungal	Angioedema
Ketoprofen	Orudis	NSAID	Soft-tissue reaction (U), abnormal hemostasis, coated tongue
Ketorolac	Toradol	NSAID	Soft-tissue reaction (U), abnormal hemostasis
Lead	none	Heavy metal	Soft-tissue reaction (P)
Levodopa	Dopar, Larodopa	Antiparkinsonism	Xerostomia, dysgeusia, movement disorders
Levonorgestrel	Demulen	Oral contraceptive	Soft-tissue reaction (D), dry socket
Lincomycin	Lincocin	Antibiotic	Dysgeusia
Lioresal	Baclofen	Muscle relaxant	Dysgeusia

indicates a soft-tissue reaction. (D): discoloration; (G): glossitis; (P): pigmentation; (S): stomatitis; (U): ulceration.

Continued on next page

Table 27.16 (cont.)

Generic Drugs and Associated Oral Manifestations

Generic name	Brand name	Drug category	Associated manifestation(s)
Lisinopril	Zestril	Antihypertensive	Xerostomia
Lithium	Eskalith	Antipsychotic	Xerostomia, dysgeusia, salivary gland involvement
Lomustine	CeeNU	Cytotoxic agent	Soft-tissue reaction (S)*
Loperamide	Imodium AD	Antidiarrheal	Xerostomia
Loratadine	Claritin	Antihistamine	Xerostomia
Lorazepam	Ativan	Antianxiety	Xerostomia, coated tongue
Loxapine	Loxitane	Antipsychotic	Xerostomia, movement disorders
Maprotiline	Ludiomil	Antidepressant	Xerostomia
Meclizine	Antivert	Antinauseant	Xerostomia
Meclofenamate	Meclomen	NSAID	Abnormal hemostasis
Mefenamic acid	Ponstel	NSAID	Abnormal hemostasis
Meperidine	Demerol	Narcotic analgesic	Xerostomia
Mephobarbital	Mebaral	Barbiturate	Leukopenia and neutropenia
Meprobamate	Equanil, Miltown	Antianxiety	Xerostomia, soft-tissue reaction (S)
Mercaptopurine	Purinethol	Cytotoxic agent	Soft-tissue reaction (G)
Mercury	none	Heavy metal	Soft-tissue reaction (P)
Mesoridazine	Serentil	Antipsychotic	Leukopenia and neutropenia, movement disorders
Metaformin	Glucophage	Antidiabetic (oral hypoglycemic)	Altered host resistance
Methantheline	Banthine	Anticholinergic/ antispasmodic	Xerostomia

*indicates a soft-tissue reaction. (D): discoloration; (G): glossitis; (P): pigmentation; (S): stomatitis; (U): ulceration.

Continued on next page

Table 27.16 (cont.)

Generic Drugs and Associated Oral Manifestations

Generic name	Brand name	Drug category	Associated manifestation(s)
Methimazole	Tapazole	Antithyroid	Dysgeusia
Methotrexate	Folex	Antineoplastic	Soft-tissue reaction (G, S)*, dysgeusia
Methscopolamine	Pamine	Anticholinergic/ antispasmodic	Xerostomia
Methyldopa	Aldomet	Antihypertensive	Xerostomia, soft-tissue reaction (D), salivary gland involvement, lichenoid reaction
Methylprednisolone	Medrol	Corticosteroid (oral)	Altered host resistance
Metoprolol	Lopressor	Antihypertensive	Xerostomia
Metronidazole	Flagyl	Antibiotic	Dysgeusia
Midazolam	Versed	Antianxiety	Angioedema
Minocycline	Minocin	Antibiotic	Soft-tissue reaction (D)
Molindone	Moban	Antipsychotic	Xerostomia
Morphine	MS Contin	Narcotic analgesic	Xerostomia
Nadolol	Corgard	Antihypertensive	Xerostomia
Naproxen	Aleve, Anaprox, Naprosyn	NSAID	Xerostomia, abnormal hemostasis
Nicotine polacrilex (chewing gum)	Nicorette	Smoking cessation agent	Xerostomia, dysgeusia
Nicotine topical patches	Habitrol, NicoDerm	Smoking cessation agent	Xerostomia, dysgeusia
Nifedipine	Procardia	Cardiovascular (calcium channel blocker)	Xerostomia, dysgeusia, gingival enlargement
Nitrofurantoin	Macrodantin	Urinary tract anti-infective	Coated tongue
Nortriptyline	Aventyl, Pamelor	Antidepressant	Xerostomia, coated tongue

*indicates a soft-tissue reaction. (D): discoloration; (G): glossitis; (P): pigmentation; (S): stomatitis; (U): ulceration.

Continued on next page

Table 27.16 (cont.)

Generic Drugs and Associated Oral Manifestations

Generic name	Brand name	Drug category	Associated manifestation(s)
Orphenadrine	Norflex	Muscle relaxant	Xerostomia
Orphenadrine HCl	Marflex	Antiparkinsonism	Xerostomia
Oxaprozin	Daypro	NSAID	Abnormal hemostasis
Oxazepam	Serax	Antianxiety	Xerostomia
Oxybutynin	Ditropan	Anticholinergic/ antispasmodic	Xerostomia
Oxyphencyclimine	Daricon	Anticholinergic/ antispasmodic	Xerostomia
P-cyclophosphamide	Cytoxan	Cytotoxic agent	Soft-tissue reaction (P)*
Paroxetine	Paxil	Antidepressant	Xerostomia
Penicillamine	Cuprimine	Chelating agent, antiarthritic (disease modifying)	Soft-tissue reaction (D), dysgeusia
Penicillin G	Pfizerpen	Antibiotic	Erythema multiforme, altered host resistance
Penicillin VK	PenVeeK, V-Cillin K	Antibiotic	Coated tongue
Pentobarbital	Nembutal	Barbiturate	Leukopenia and neutropenia, erythema multiforme
Perphenazine	Trilafon	Antipsychotic	Leukopenia and neutropenia, movement disorders
Phendimetrazine	Anorex	Anorexiant	Xerostomia
Phenelzine	Nardil	Antidepressant	Xerostomia
Phenobarbital	Luminal	Barbiturate	Leukopenia and neutropenia, erythema multiforme
Phentermine	Adipex-P, Fastin, Ionamin	Anorexiant	Xerostomia
Phenylbutazone	Butazolidin	NSAID	Xerostomia, dysgeusia, leukopenia and neutropenia, salivary gland involvement, erythema multiforme

* indicates a soft-tissue reaction. (D): discoloration; (G): glossitis; (P): pigmentation; (S): stomatitis; (U): ulceration.

Continued on next page

Table 27.16 (cont.)

Generic Drugs and Associated Oral Manifestations

Generic name	Brand name	Drug category	Associated manifestation(s)
Phenylpropanolamine/ chlorpheniramine	Ornade	Decongestant	Xerostomia
Phenytoin	Dilantin	Anticonvulsant	Gingival enlargement, erythema multiforme
Pimozide	Orap	Antipsychotic	Xerostomia
Piroxicam	Feldene	NSAID	Xerostomia, abnormal hemostasis
Prazepam	Centrax	Antianxiety	Xerostomia
Prazosin	Minipress	Antihypertensive	Xerostomia
Primidone	Mysoline	Barbiturate	Leukopenia and neutropenia
Procaine penicillin	Wycillin	Antibiotic	Dysgeusia
Prochlorperazine	Compazine	Antipsychotic	Xerostomia, leukopenia and neutropenia, movement disorders
Promazine	Sparine	Antipsychotic	Xerostomia, leukopenia and neutropenia, movement disorders
Promethazine	Phenergan	Antihistamine	Xerostomia
Propantheline	Pro-Banthine	Anticholinergic/ antispasmodic	Xerostomia
Quanethidine	Ismelin	Antihypertensive	Salivary gland involvement
Quinapril	Accupril	ACE inhibitor	Angioedema
Quinine	Quinamm	Antiprotozoal	Leukopenia and neutropenia
Quinolone	Cipro	Antibiotic	Altered host resistance
Ramipril	Altace	ACE inhibitor	Angioedema
Reserpine	Serpasil	Antihypertensive	Xerostomia

Continued on next page

Table 27.16 (cont.)

Generic Drugs and Associated Oral Manifestations

Generic name	Brand name	Drug category	Associated manifestation(s)
Risperidone	Risperdal	Antipsychotic	Xerostomia, movement disorders
Scopolamine	Transderm-Scop	Anticholinergic/ antispasmodic	Xerostomia
Secobarbital	Seconal	Barbiturate	Leukopenia and neutropenia, erythema multiforme
Sertraline	Zoloft	Antidepressant	Xerostomia
Spironolactone	Aldactone	Cardiovascular	Dysgeusia
Sulfacytine	Renoquid	Sulfonamide	Leukopenia and neutropenia, erythema multiforme
Sulfamethizole	Thiosulfil Forte	Sulfonamide	Leukopenia and neutropenia, erythema multiforme
Sulfamethoxazole	Gantanol	Sulfonamide	Leukopenia and neutropenia, erythema multiforme
Sulfisoxazole	Gantrisin	Sulfonamide	Leukopenia and neutropenia, erythema multiforme, altered host resistance
Tacrine	Cognex	Cholinergic	Sialorrhea
Tamoxifen	Novadex	Antineoplastic	Altered host resistance
Temazepam	Restoril	Sedative	Xerostomia
Terfenadine	Seldane	Antihistamine	Xerostomia
Tetracycline	Achromycin, Robitet, Vibramycin	Antibiotic	Dysgeusia, coated tongue, altered host resistance
Thioridazine	Mellaril	Antipsychotic	Xerostomia, leukopenia and neutropenia, movement disorders
Thiothixene	Navane	Antipsychotic	Xerostomia, movement disorders
Ticlopidine	Ticlid	Antithrombotic	Abnormal hemostasis

Continued on next page

Table 27.16 (cont.)
Generic Drugs and Associated Oral Manifestations

Generic name	Brand name	Drug category	Associated manifestation(s)
Tolazamide	Tolinase	Antidiabetic (oral hypoglycemic)	Altered host resistance
Tolbutamide	Orinase	Antidiabetic (oral hypoglycemic)	Leukopenia and neutropenia, altered host resistance
Tolmetin	Tolectin	NSAID	Abnormal hemostasis
Tranylcypromine	Parnate	Antidepressant	Xerostomia
Trazodone	Desyrel	Antidepressant	Xerostomia
Triamcinolone	Azmacort	Corticosteroid (inhaled)	Altered host resistance
Triamterene	Dyrenium	Diuretic	Xerostomia
Triamterene/ hydrochlorothiazide	Dyazide, Maxzide	Diuretic	Xerostomia
Triazolam	Halcion	Sedative	Xerostomia
Trifluoperazine	Stelazine	Antipsychotic	Xerostomia, leukopenia and neutropenia, movement disorders
Trihexyphenidyl	Artane	Antiparkinsonism	Xerostomia
Tripelennamine	Pyribenzamine (PBZ)	Antihistamine	Xerostomia
Triprolidine/pseudoephedrine	Actifed	Antihistamine	Xerostomia
Vincristine	Oncovin	Antineoplastic (cytotoxic)	Soft-tissue reaction (S)*, dysgeusia
Warfarin	Coumadin	Anticoagulant	Soft-tissue reaction (U), abnormal hemostasis

* indicates a soft-tissue reaction. (D): discoloration; (G): glossitis; (P): pigmentation; (S): stomatitis; (U): ulceration.

Suggested Readings

Felder RS, Millar SB, Henry RH. Oral manifestations of drug therapy. Spec Care Dentist 1988;8(3):119-24.

Lewis IK, Hanlon JT, Hobbins MJ, Beck JD. Use of medications with potential oral adverse drug reactions in community-dwelling elderly. Spec Care Dentist 1993; 13(4):171-6.

Mott AE, Grushka M, Sessle BJ. Diagnosis and management of taste disorders and burning mouth syndrome. Dent Clin North Am 1993;37(1):33-71.

Walton JG. Dental disorders. In: Davies DM, ed. Textbook of adverse drug reactions. 4th ed. Oxford, England: Oxford University Press; 1991:205-29.

Zelickson BD, Rogers RS. Oral drug reactions. Dermatol Clin North Am 1987;5(4):695-708.

Chapter 28.

Infection Control Strategies for the Dental Office

Chris H. Miller, Ph.D.

Infection control primarily consists of a series of standard procedures designed to reduce the number of microbes shared among people. In the office, this involves protection of patients, protection of the dental team and protection of the people in the community from microbes in the office. Infection control is accomplished by using universal precautions and by using products, equipment and procedures that will prevent or reduce exposure of people to microbes by

- preventing contamination of objects or surfaces and
- killing microbes and/or removing them from objects or surfaces.

Infection control guidelines for dentistry have been presented by the American Dental Association and the Centers for Disease Control and Prevention. The U.S. Department of Labor has established the Bloodborne Pathogens Standard for protection of employees from exposure to pathogens present in human body fluids. This standard covers employees who could come into contact with blood and other potentially infectious body fluids (for example, saliva in dentistry) as a result of performing their jobs. It indicates that it is the employer's responsibility to protect employees from this type of occupational exposure. Compliance with this standard in dentistry involves activity in seven areas:

- preparing a written exposure control plan for the workplace;
- training employees at their initial appointment with annual updates about this standard, the spread and prevention of bloodborne diseases, hepatitis B vaccination, engineering and work practice controls, personal protective equipment, and all other exposure control policies and procedures;
- practicing universal precautions with emphasis on engineering and work practice controls; providing, using, maintaining and disposing of personal protective equipment; washing hands; minimizing spattering and spraying of blood and other body fluids; minimizing injuries caused by sharps; ensuring proper packaging of specimens, contaminated equipment and regulated waste; decontaminating surfaces soiled with blood or other body fluids; handling waste and contaminated laundry properly;
- making the hepatitis B vaccination series available to covered employees at no cost to the employees;
- making a confidential medical evaluation and follow-up available to employees who are exposed to blood or other body fluid at work;
- using warning labels, signs and/or color-coding to identify biohazards such as regulated waste and contaminated laundry;
- maintaining records of employee training and confidential employee medical records

(documentation of hepatitis B vaccination or vaccination refusal, and of postexposure medical evaluations).

Detailed descriptions of infection control procedures in dentistry can be obtained from a number of publications. Table 28.1 summarizes infection control procedures used in dentistry.

Although a considerable amount of published information about infection control in dentistry exists, this chapter provides a listing of representative infection control products and equipment. This listing is organized into five major categories based on groups of infection control procedures. These categories are presented in Table 28.2.

Table 28.1

Summary of Infection Control Procedures Used in Dentistry

Path of microbe spread	Infection control procedure to prevent spread
Patient to dental team	Wash hands
	Use gloves, mask, protective eyewear
	Use protective clothing
	Handle sharps carefully • recap needles safely • discard sharps in proper containers • use instrument cassettes to reduce instrument handling • use mechanical cleaning to reduce instrument handling • return sharps to resting position carefully • use tongs to pick up needles, scalpel blades, glass • use heavy gloves for instrument handling
	Use a rubber dam
	Have patients use an antimicrobial mouthrinse before receiving care
	Use high-volume evacuation
	Obtain immunizations
Dental team to patient	Use gloves, mask, protective clothing
	Wash hands
	Handle sharps carefully inside and outside of the mouth
	Sterilize instruments and handpieces
	Clean and disinfect contaminated surfaces
	Obtain immunizations
Patient to patient	Sterilize instruments and handpiece before reuse
	Package instruments before sterilization to maintain sterility
	Use surface covers
	Clean and disinfect contaminated surfaces
	Wash and properly glove hands
	Use disposable items (such as syringe tips, prophy angles)
	Use clean/sterile supplies
	Change mask and protective clothing
	Control retraction of water into dental unit
	Maintain quality of treatment water

Continued on next page

Table 28.1 (cont.)
Summary of Infection Control Procedures Used in Dentistry

Path of microbe spread	Infection control procedure to prevent spread
Office to community	Dispose of waste properly
	Disinfect impressions and appliances before shipping
	Decontaminate items sent out for repair
	Place specimens in proper containers before shipping
	Remove protective clothing before leaving office
	Place contaminated laundry in proper container before shipping
	Wash hands
Community to patient	Maintain quality of treatment water

Table 28.2
Major Categories of Infection Control Products

Infection control category	Infection control procedures	Table of related products
Aseptic techniques	Controlling spattering of oral fluids Controlling contamination Using disposables	Tables 28.3 and 28.4
Barrier protection	Using gloves, masks and eyewear Using protective clothing	Tables 28.5 and 28.6
Instrument processing	Cleaning, packaging, sterilizing instruments Monitoring the sterilization process	Table 28.7
Surface asepsis	Cleaning and disinfecting Covering surfaces	Table 28.8
Waste management	Identifying biohazards and containing regulated waste	Table 28.9

Understanding the philosophy of the categories listed in Table 28.2 may help clarify the reasons for the specific procedures listed.

Aseptic techniques. Aseptic techniques, in general, are aimed at reducing the spread of microbes from a potential source of contamination. The main source of microbes in the dental office is the patient's mouth. Thus, various aseptic techniques are used to limit the escape of microbes from a patient's mouth. These include the rubber dam that physically prevents most of the salivary microbes from escaping the mouth, high-volume evacuation that takes away microbes as they escape the mouth, preprocedure mouthrinsing that reduces the number of live microbes that can escape the mouth during the appointment, and disposable instruments that allow microbes on an item to be discarded so they cannot be spread to someone else. Other aseptic techniques reduce the number of microbes in treatment water, which can serve as a source of microbes. Another aseptic technique is handwashing, which is described in Chapter 9. Some procedures—such as the use of "hands-free" sink faucets—are included under aseptic techniques because they do not fit well in other categories but do interfere with the spread of microbes.

Barrier protection. Barrier protection techniques are used to prevent microbes from directly contacting our bodies. The barriers of gloves, eyewear, masks and protective clothing interfere with the transfer of the microbes from patients' mouths to one's eyes, skin, mouth, nose and clothing.

These barriers also help prevent the dental team's contact with microbes on operatory surfaces, contaminated instruments, in the air and in cleaning solutions. Gloves prevent transfer of microbes on the hands of dental team members to patients, and wearing masks keeps respiratory microbes of the dental team from reaching open tissue in patients' mouths.

Instrument processing. Instrument processing converts contaminated instruments and handpieces into sterile instruments and handpieces ready to use on another patient. It not only allows for the cleaning and sterilizing of instruments but also for the maintenance of sterility (through packaging) until the instruments are presented at chairside for the next patient. Cleaning instruments facilitates subsequent sterilization, and using an ultrasonic cleaner or a washer/disinfector (rather than hand-scrubbing) reduces the direct handling of these contaminated sharps. Packaging the rinsed and dried instruments before placing them in a sterilizer protects the instruments after they are removed from the sterilizer and during transport to chairside or

storage. The packaging maintains instrument sterility until they are used on a patient.

The cleaned and packaged instruments are heat-processed in a steam sterilizer (autoclave), a dry heat sterilizer or the unsaturated chemical vapor sterilizer. The sterilization process is monitored routinely by using spore-tests called biological indicators (BI). The BI consist of highly resistant bacterial spores of *Bacillus stearothermophilus* (used to monitor steam and unsaturated chemical vapor sterilizers) or *Bacillus subtilis* (used for monitoring the dry heat sterilizer). Chemical indicators in the form of tape, strips, tabs and special markings on packaging material indicate exposure to heat or to sterilizing conditions. These indicators identify packages that indeed have been processed through a sterilizer and are ready to use. Plastic items that are destroyed in a heat sterilizer are cleaned, rinsed, dried and sterilized by 10 h of submersion in a properly prepared glutaraldehyde solution.

Surface asepsis. There are two approaches to surface asepsis: using surface covers to prevent a surface from becoming contaminated, and cleaning and disinfecting the surface after it becomes contaminated. Surfaces with deep grooves or protected sites that cannot be effectively cleaned should be covered with a protective barrier rather than disinfected (for example, chair, view-box, some handpiece control units, and electrical/light switches or buttons; grooved knobs; three-way syringe buttons; light handles; some sink faucets; cameras; and lenses). Surfaces that are flat and smooth or easily cleanable can be cleaned and disinfected (for example, countertops, chair arms, bracket tables, trays). Usually, a combination of these two approaches is used in an office.

Waste management. The key aspect of proper waste management in the dental office is to first identify what is regulated waste (defined below); then avoid direct contact with that waste; and finally to contain the waste so that when it is treated, transported or finally discarded it will not contaminate people or surfaces.

Regulated waste in dentistry is defined by OSHA as

- liquid or semiliquid blood or saliva in dentistry;
- items contaminated with blood or saliva that would release these substances in a liquid or semiliquid state if compressed;
- items caked with dried blood or saliva that are capable of releasing these materials during handling;
- contaminated sharps; and
- pathological wastes (for example, tissue and teeth) containing blood or saliva.

The listings in Tables 28.3-28.9 provide a categorized guide to some representative infection control products and equipment. These lists do not include all infection control products or equipment. Also, the actual listing of an item does not denote its superiority to any other product listed or not listed, nor does it guarantee the availability, quality or proper functioning of the items. In some instances, identical products may be listed under different brand names.

The American Dental Association has an acceptance program for five categories of infection control products: antimicrobial mouthrinses, disposable prophy angles, handwashing agents, sterilization packaging materials and gloves. Latex gloves should not be used on patients who are allergic to latex. Handwashing agents are described in Chapter 9. Gloves and sterilization packaging materials bearing the ADA Seal of Acceptance (as of the date of this writing) are identified in these tables with a blue star ★.

Table 28.3

Asepsis: Techniques and Associated Products

Generic name	Brand name(s)	Techniques and uses
Controlling spatter		
Rubber dam	Dental Dam, Dental Dam: Non-latex, Rubber Dam	Reduces escape of microbes from patient's mouth during care
Preprocedure antimicrobial mouthrinses	Listerine ★, Peridex ★, PerioGard	Temporarily reduce the number of microbes in the patient's mouth so that fewer will escape during care
Aerosol reduction system	Safety suction	Evacuates microbes escaping from the patient's mouth in aerosols
Aerosol reduction during air-polishing	JetShield	Evacuates microbes escaping from the patient's mouth in aerosols generated by ultrasonic scaler
Controlling contamination		
Evacuation system cleaners	ProE-Vac, Purevac, Sani-Treet Plus, Surge, Turbo-Vac, Vacusol	Help clean debris from evacuation lines
Waterline filters	Clearline	Filter out microbes from dental unit water

★ indicates a product bearing the ADA Seal of Acceptance.

Continued on next page

Table 28.3 (cont.)

Asepsis: Techniques and Associated Products

Generic name	Brand name(s)	Techniques and uses
Controlling contamination (cont.)		
Dental unit clean-water delivery systems	Self-Contained Clean Water System, Self-Contained Water System	Provide for the use of water other than municipal water to improve the quality of treatment water for patient care Also provide a means of disinfecting unit waterlines
Dental unit water treatment system	Spirit S1/S2 dental unit	Adds antimicrobial chemical to the municipal water to improve microbial quality of treatment water Also provides a means of disinfecting unit waterlines
Antiretraction valve	Check valve	Needed in some dental units to reduce the retraction of water (and oral fluids) up through handpiece and three-way syringe into waterlines
Sterile water delivery systems	Sterile water system, SteriWater system, Aseptiwater system	Provide sterile water during patient care
Hands-free faucets	Aquaflow, Automatic Faucet (infrared), WaterSense controller	Reduce the chances of cross-contamination during handwashing by preventing contact with potentially contaminated faucets
Transport containers	Safe-T-Bag ICD	Allow specimens to be shipped in a safe manner

Table 28.4

Asepsis: Techniques and Associated Disposable Products

Generic name	Brand name(s)	Techniques and uses
Air/water syringe tips	Sani-Tip, Safe-Tips EZ	Eliminate the need to clean and sterilize reusable tips, which may be difficult to clean
Curing light probe	SaniCure	Eliminates the need to cover curing light tips
High-volume evacuation tips and saliva ejector tips	Evacuator/Ejector Tips, Oratip Evacuation Tips	Eliminate the need to clean and sterilize reusable tips
Eyewear	Eye Clasps	Eliminates need to decontaminate reusable eyewear; also can be used to protect patient's eyes during care

Continued on next page

Table 28.4 (cont.)

Asepsis: Techniques and Associated Disposable Products

Generic name	Brand name(s)	Techniques and uses
Napkin chains	Disposa Chain	Allow chains to be discarded along with napkin and eliminates need to clean and sterilize reusable napkin chains
Prophy angles	Densco ★, Denticator ★, Butler, Pivot, Rite-Angle, Schein, Teledyne, Young	Eliminate need to clean and sterilize reusable angles
Saliva ejector tips	Saliva ejector baskets, Saliva ejector screens	Eliminate the need to clean and decontaminate reusable tips
Vacuum traps	Dispos-a-Trap, Evacuation Screens, Solids Collector Screen	Eliminate the need to clean and decontaminate reusable traps, thus reducing chances of exposure to microbes

★ indicates a product bearing the ADA Seal of Acceptance.

Table 28.5

Barrier Protection: Gloves

Generic name	Brand name(s)	Techniques and uses
Nonsterile latex examination gloves	Aid Premium Latex Examination ★, Aladan Classic Latex Examination ★, Allerjoy Latex Examination ★, Amerglo Deluxe Latex ★, Astra Pro Disposable Latex Exam ★, Audra Latex Examination ★, Baldur Lightly Powdered Latex Examination ★, Bio-Flex Dental Examination ★, Conform Latex Medical, Cranberry Latex Examination ★, Curity Latex Examination ★, Dental Latex Examination ★, DuraFit Powder-Free Latex Procedural Exam ★, Insurex Latex Exam ★, KLH Silky Touch Latex Exam ★, Lightly Powdered Latex Exam ★, Malaytex Latex Examination ★, Marsin Latex Examination ★, Medical Dental Latex ★, Micro-Touch Latex, Neutraderm Latex Exam ★, Perfect Touch Latex Examination ★, Powder-Free Latex Examination ★, Powder Free Plus Latex ★, ProTouch Latex Examination, QualiTouch L/R Fitted Latex ★, QualiTouch Ambidextrous Latex ★, Quantum Latex Examination ★, Redwood Latex Examination★, Satin Plus Satin Finish Latex Exam ★, Savacare Latex ★, Sensi Grip Latex Examination ★, Spectrum ★, Supergloves Latex Examination ★, Tan Chong Latex Examination ★, Tri-Clean 110 Latex Exam ★, Tronex Latex Examination—Lightly Powdered ★, Uniseal Latex Examination ★, Vital Defense Latex Examination, Vital Shield Gold Non-Sterile Medical Examination ★, Waterforde Hypoallergenic Latex Examination ★, Wet-Grip Latex Exam ★	For intraoral use during nonsurgical procedures to prevent direct contact with patient's oral fluids and to protect patient from contact with microbes on hands Also may be worn to prevent contact with contamination when handling inanimate objects

★ indicates a product bearing the ADA Seal of Acceptance.

Continued on next page

Table 28.5 (cont.)

Barrier Protection: Gloves

Generic name	Brand name(s)	Techniques and uses
Sterile latex gloves	Surgeons', Classic Sterile Latex, Micro-Touch Latex Surgical, Natraflex Surgeons'	For intraoral use during surgical procedures to prevent direct contact with patient's oral fluids and to protect patient from contact with microbes on hands
Non-latex patient-care gloves	Accu-Gard Vinyl Examination, N-Dex Nitrile, ProTouch Vinyl Examination, TactyLite Non-latex, Triflex, Tru-Touch Stretch Vinyl, Vinylite	Used by those who may have a hypersensitivity to latex allergens
Overgloves	Operatory Overgloves, Overgloves, ProBarrier Glove Sox	May be used to cover up contaminated patient-care gloves when it is necessary to leave chairside and possibly touch other surfaces Are removed to expose the original patient-care gloves when returning to care for the patient, protecting surfaces and patients from unnecessary contamination
Heavy utility gloves	Asep-Gluv, Heavy Duty Nitrile, Latex Utility, Nitrile Decontamination	Used to prevent direct contact with contaminated items and surfaces during operatory clean-up and instrument processing **Note:** Heavy gloves may give the hands more protection from sharp objects, but such gloves are not puncture-proof
Glove liners	Stretch Knit All-day	Cotton gloves worn under patient care or utility gloves by those who may have skin reactions to the outer gloves

Table 28.6

Barrier Protection: Masks, Eyewear, Clothing

Generic name	Brand name(s)	Techniques and uses
Masks		
Mask, earloop	Com-Fit , Cone Classic, Ear Loop Face, Ear Loop Procedure, InstaGard, Shield High Efficiency Face, Sofloop Earloop, Vital Defense Pleated Surgical	Used to prevent sprays and spatter of blood, saliva, or other contaminated fluids from contacting mucous membranes of nose and lips Will reduce inhalation of some airborne particles Can reduce contamination of patient with respiratory particles from dental team member Are retained by two elastic bands that are placed over ears

Continued on next page

Table 28.6 (cont.)

Barrier Protection: Masks, Eyewear, Clothing

Generic name	Brand name(s)	Techniques and uses
Masks		
Mask, single retention band	Defend Conpleat, Com-Fit, Aseptex Fluid Resistant, Molded face, Shield High Efficiency Face	Retained by a single elastic band that is placed around back of head
Mask, tie-on	Barrier Extra Protection Face, Fog-Free Surgical, Tie-On Surgical	Retained by two pairs of nonelastic straps that tie in back of head
Protective eyewear		
Eyeglasses	Barrier Protective Glasses, Eyesaver glasses, Fog Free Enfog Safety Eyeglasses, ProSpec, Safety Glasses, SmartPractice Mono Lens	Used to protect eyes from sprays and spatter of blood, saliva, other contaminated fluids and from solid projectiles
Clip-on side shields	Side Shields, Disposable Side Shields	Attach to eyeglasses to prevent contamination or injury to eyes by particles entering from side
Goggles	Barrier Protective Goggles, Cover Goggles	Are more heavy-duty; fit close to skin around eyes and are frequently used over corrective glasses
Faceshields	Disposable Face Shield, ProSpec Shield, Sofloop Faceshield Plus Mask	Used to provide more protection to eyes and face usually worn instead of eyeglasses; some are attached to a mask
Protective clothing		
Disposable clothing	Barrier Scrub Apparel, Cover Gown, Criterion Shield Gown, Dental Cover Gown, Disposable Gowns, Sof-Therm Jackets	Used to prevent contaminated material from reaching work clothes, street clothes, undergarments, or skin Is changed when visibly soiled and before leaving work area and is not worn out of office
Reusable protective clothing	Various brands	Examples include uniforms, clinic coats, lab coats and gowns used to prevent contaminated material from reaching work clothes, street clothes, undergarments, skin Is changed when visibly soiled and before leaving the work area and is not worn out of the office Is handled in same manner as contaminated laundry, using personal protective equipment and leak-proof biohazard bags or containers May be laundered in office or by outside laundry service

Table 28.7

Instrument Processing: Techniques and Associated Products

Generic name	Brand name(s)	Techniques and uses
Precleaning and cleaning solutions		
Non-enzymatic solution	Dri-Clave, General Purpose Cleaner, GP Plus Ultrasonic Solution, IMS Instrument Daily Clean, Nonionic Multipurpose Ultrasonic, ProClense, Pro-Sonic, Security Cleaning Solution, UltraClean	Used to facilitate removal of blood, saliva, dental materials, other debris, and some associated microbes from instruments prior to packaging and sterilization
Enzymatic solution	Biozyme, Clean & Simple, Coezyme, Denta-zyme, Enzol, IMS Enzymax, Maxizyme, MetriZyme, ProEZ, Security Holding Solution	May facilitate removal of blood or other proteinaceous material from instruments before packaging and sterilization
Mechanical cleaners	Dental Thermal Disinfector, Biosonic Ultrasonic Cleaner, Health Sonics Ultrasonic Cleaner, Henry Schein Ultrasonic Cleaner, Pro-Sonic Cleaning System, Quantrex Ultrasonic Cleaner, Tuttnauer Ultrasonic Cleaner, Ultrasonic Cleaning System	Washer/disinfectors or ultrasonic cleaners that remove blood, saliva, dental materials, other debris and some associated microbes from instruments Used in place of the dangerous method of hand-scrubbing instruments
Rust inhibitors		
Rust inhibitors	Vapor Phase, Surgical Milk, Credo Clave	Retard corrosion of carbon steel items and surfaces to be processed through a steam sterilizer
Sterilization packaging material		
Cassettes	Instrument Cassettes, IMS Cassettes, Instrument Delivery Cassettes	Perforated metal or plastic/resin containers used to house instruments at chairside and during all of instrument processing (mechanical cleaning, rinsing, drying, packaging, sterilization, storage and distribution) Reduce dangerous direct handling of contaminated sharp instruments during processing
Paper/"plastic" pouches	Assure Plus Self-sealing ★, Assure Self-sealing ★, ATI Self-sealing, Carerite Nylon ★, Crosstex ★, Defend Self-sealing ★, Harken Assure Self-seal ★, Kenpak Self-sealing ★, Medi-Plus Self-sealing ★, Medi-Plus Sterilization ★, Patterson Self-sealing ★, Peel Vue Autoclave/Chemiclave ★, ProView Sterilization ★, Tower Dual Peel Self-sealing ★	Used with steam or unsaturated chemical vapor sterilizers Keep instruments separated and protects them from recontamination after removal from sterilizer and during storage and distribution for use on next patient "Plastic" portion allows easy identification of package contents May be self-sealing or are sealed with sterilization tape Chemical indicators are present on paper portions

★ *indicates a product bearing the ADA Seal of Acceptance.*

Continued on next page

Table 28.7 (cont.)

Instrument Processing: Techniques and Associated Products

Generic name	Brand name(s)	Techniques and uses
Sterilization packaging material (cont.)		
Nylon tubing	Nyclave (steam), DH/Nyclave (dry heat), ProPak Nylon Sterilization	Used with steam or dry heat sterilizers Keeps instruments separated and protects them from recontamination after removal from sterilizer and during storage and distribution for use on next patient Is see-through, supplied on a roll in different widths, and sealed with a heat-sealer or sterilization tape
Wraps	Sterilization Wrap	Designed specifically for wrapping instrument cassettes or other items before they are processed through a sterilizer; some wraps are for steam and others may be used in dry heat sterilizers
Other	Re-Bag	Has necessary approval to be reused if handled properly
Sterilization packaging equipment		
Heat sealers	Heat Sealer and Cutter, Nyclave Impulse Heat Sealer	Used to seal nylon tubing packaging material
Sterilizers		
Steam autoclaves	Eagle Sterilizer, Midmark, Porter Sterilizer, Statim Cassette Sterilizer, Tuttnauer, Validator Plus	Use steam under pressure to kill microbes remaining on previously cleaned and packaged instruments or other items Operate at 121°C to 134°C at exposure times ranging from 30 to 2.5 min Yield good penetration of heat into packages Cause corrosion of carbon steel items, and produce wet packs that should be dried before handling
Oven-type dry heat sterilizers	Schein dry heat sterilizer, Steri-Dent dry heat sterilizer	Use dry heat to kill microbes remaining on cleaned and packaged instruments or other items Operate at 320°F for 1-2 h; no corrosion occurs

Continued on next page

Table 28.7 (cont.)

Instrument Processing: Techniques and Associated Products

Generic name	Brand name(s)	Techniques and uses
Sterilizers (cont.)		
Rapid heat-transfer type dry heat sterilizers	Cox Rapid Heat Transfer Sterilizer, Guardian	Use circulated dry heat to kill microbes remaining on previously cleaned and packaged instruments or other items Operate at 375°F for 6-20 min; no corrosion occurs
Unsaturated chemical vapor sterilizer	Harvey Chemiclave	Uses unsaturated chemical vapors from formaldehyde and alcohol to kill microbes remaining on cleaned and packaged instruments or other items Operates at 134°C for 20 minutes; no corrosion occurs
Liquid sterilants for heat-labile plastic and rubber items		
Glutaraldehyde	Banicide (2.5% acidic), Banicide Plus (3.4 % alkaline), Cida-Steryl Plus (3.4% alkaline), Coecide XL (2.0% alkaline), Coecide XL Plus (3.4% alkaline), Cidex (2.4% alkaline), Cidex Plus (3.4% alkaline), MaxiCide (2.4% alkaline), MaxiCide Plus (3.4% alkaline), MetriCide 28 (2.5% alkaline), ProCide (2.4% alkaline), ProCide Plus(3.4% alkaline), Security (2.5% alkaline), Security (3.4 % alkaline), SmartPractice (2.5% alkaline), SmartPractice (3.4% alkaline)	Used to sterilize previously cleaned items (usually made of plastic or rubber) that will be destroyed if processed through a heat sterilizer Not recommended for use on instruments that can be heat-sterilized or as a surface disinfectant Alkaline-based brands must be prepared properly and used container dated to monitor the 14- to 30-day use life Items being processed must be previously cleaned, rinsed and dried, then completely submerged for 10 h of contact time and thoroughly rinsed Avoid contact with skin, eyes and other mucous membranes
Chemical indicators		
Integrators for steam	ProChek S, SteriGauge, Vapor Line	Chemical indicators that change color or form after certain steam sterilizer conditions (temperature, time, presence of steam) have been achieved
Process indicators	ATI (steam-tape), IMS Autoclave tape, ProChek ID (steam-tape), ATI (steam-strip), ProChek ID (steam-strip), ATI (dry heat-labels/strips), ProChek ID (dry heat-strip)	Chemicals that change color very soon after exposure to a certain temperature achieved in a sterilizer

Continued on next page

Table 28.7 (cont.)

Instrument Processing: Techniques and Associated Products

Generic name	Brand name(s)	Techniques and uses
Biological monitoring		
Mail-in spore testing service (for steam, dry heat, chemical vapor sterilizers)	ConFirm mail-in, PassPort mail-in, Monitoring Services	Use and functioning of heat sterilizers are routinely monitored by using biological indicators (highly resistant bacterial spores); some states require this spore testing weekly and others require it monthly; with a mail-in spore testing service, tests are sent to dental office, where they are routinely processed through sterilizer and mailed back to the service for analysis; service telephones office if a sterilization failure is detected and sends a written report to office on all test results
In-office spore testing systems (for steam, dry heat, chemical vapor sterilizers)	ConFirm Culture Kit/Incubator, SporView Culture Set/Incubator	Dental office purchases proper spore strips, culture tubes and proper incubator system for in-office analysis of tests
In-office spore testing (for steam)	Assert Spore vials/Incubator, Attest Spore vials/Incubator, Biosign Spore vials/Incubator, ConFirm Ampules/Incubator, Proof Plus Spore vials/Incubator, SporAmpule Ampules/Incubator, Spor-Test Spore strips/Incubator	Dental office purchases proper spore test vials and incubator for in-office analysis of tests; vials contain both the spores and the culture medium
Spore strips (*Bacillus stearothermophilus* and/or *Bacillus subtilis*)	Spore strips	Are strips of filter paper impregnated with appropriate bacterial spores and are used in spore testing sterilizers; their use requires culture tubes containing proper growth medium and an incubator
Liquid sterilants		
Glutaraldehyde concentration monitor	ProChek G, Cold Sterilog, Cidex Plus test strips	Chemically estimates concentration of alkaline glutaraldehyde sterilant being used for sterilization; with time, glutaraldehyde becomes inactivated, and this test estimates when concentration is below that which achieves sterilization

Table 28.8

Surface Asepsis: Techniques and Associated Products

Generic name	Brand name(s)	Techniques and uses
Surface disinfectants		
Chlorine-based	Dispatch	Used to disinfect surfaces that may be contaminated with microbial pathogens and/or patient materials such as blood or saliva; such surfaces may include countertops, handles, trays, supply containers and small nonsterilizable items
		Surfaces to be disinfected are to be cleaned first; disinfectants used in dentistry should at least be registered with the Environmental Protection Agency (as indicated on the product label under "Reg. No.") and be tuberculocidal
		As kill time for different microbes may vary, contact time for disinfection step should be longest microbial kill time indicated on product label for disinfection
Iodophor	Asepti-IDC, Biocide, IodoFive, Iodophor	See note above
Water-based tri-phenolics	Asepti-phene 128, Dencide, Tri-Cide	See note above
Water-based dual phenolics	BiArrest-2, Birex$_{se}$, Dual-X, Lysol I.C., Omni II, ProPhene, ProSpray, SmartPractice, Vital Defense-D	See note above
Alcohol-based phenolics	Asepti-Steryl, Citrace, Coe-Spray, DisCide, Lysol I.C.	See note above
Alcohol-based quaternary ammonium compound	Asepticare TB, Cavicide, DisCide-TB, GC Spray-Cide, MetriGuard, Precise QTB, SaniTex Plus	See note above
Surface covers		
Surface covers	Clear ProTection, Disposable Protectors, Disposa-Shield, Disposable Sleeves, ProBarrier, Sani-Shield, Surface Barriers	Used as barriers to prevent contamination of surfaces with microbes and/or patient materials such as blood or saliva; barriers are to be impervious to moisture (for example, made of plastic) and are usually used on surfaces or items that cannot easily be cleaned and disinfected (for example, knurled knobs; three-way syringe handle; electrical switches on the unit, light, chair, or radiographic unit and view-box; sink faucets; hoses; cameras); covers are carefully replaced with fresh covers between patients, surfaces that are covered need not be cleaned and disinfected between patients unless underlying surface accidentally becomes contaminated

Table 28.9

Waste Management: Techniques and Associated Products

Generic name	Brand name(s)	Techniques and uses
Sharps management		
Safety syringes	Safety Plus, UltraSafe Aspirating Syringe	Help prevent needlesticks by providing protective shield around needle
Recapping devices	Aim Safe, Monotray, ProTector Needle Sheath Prop, Protector Recapper	Help prevent needlesticks by holding (stabilizing) needle cap to allow insertion of used needle back into cap for later reuse on same patient or for removal and disposal
Waste disposal		
Sharps containers	DisposiNeedle System Sharps-a-Gator, Sharps Collector, Sharps Infectious Waste	Used to contain contaminated sharps during storage, treatment and/or transport for disposal; contaminated sharps are regulated waste and are anything that can puncture skin or that can become a sharp if broken (such as needles, scalpel blades, wire, anesthetic carpule, broken instruments, wedges)
		Sharps containers are to be puncture-resistant, leak-proof on sides and bottom, closable and color-coded red or marked with a biohazard symbol
		Should be located near where sharps are used or found; maintained in an upright position; not allowed to overflow; opened during heat-sterilization treatment; closed during transport; properly labeled with office name and address for transport in some states where indicated
Biohazard bags	Labcraft Biohazard Autoclave Bag, ProTector Infectious Waste Bags	Used to contain non-sharp solid regulated waste during storage, treatment and/or transport for disposal; examples of such waste are cotton rolls or gauze pads that are saturated or caked with blood or saliva so that liquid or semiliquid material is released when compressed; items that are merely spotted or damp with blood or saliva are not considered as regulated waste
		Should be leak-proof, closable and color-coded red or marked with a biohazard symbol; should be opened during heat-sterilization treatment, closed during transport, placed in a second appropriate biohazard bag if outside is contaminated and properly labeled with office name and address for transport in some states where indicated

Continued on next page

Table 28.9 (cont.)

Waste Management: Techniques and Associated Products

Generic name	Brand name(s)	Techniques and uses
Biohazard communication		
Signs and labels	ProTector Labels and Signage, Signs and Labels	Are used as warnings (for example, "biohazard") or for safety information (for example, "eyewash station")

Suggested Readings

ADA Council on Scientific Affairs and ADA Council on Dental Practice. Infection control recommendations for the dental office and the dental laboratory. JADA 1996;127(5):672-80.

Centers for Disease Control and Prevention. Recommended infection control practices for dentistry, 1993. MMWR 1993;41(RR-8):1-12.

Cottone JA, Terezhalmy GT, Molinari JA. Practical infection control in dentistry. Baltimore: Williams & Wilkins; 1996.

Miller CH. Infection Control. Dent Clin North Am 1996;40(2):437-56.

Miller CH, Palenik CJ. Infection control and management of hazardous materials for the dental team. St. Louis: Mosby; 1994.

U.S. Department of Labor, Occupational Safety and Health Administration. Controlling occupational exposure to bloodborne pathogens in dentistry. Washington, D.C.: U.S. Department of Labor, Occupational Safety and Health Administration; 1992: OSHA publication no. 3129.

Chapter 29.

Cessation of Tobacco Use

Martha Somerman, D.D.S., Ph.D.;
Robert E. Mecklenburg, D.D.S., M.P.H.

It is well-established that smoking is a leading cause of death in the world; it leads to nearly one of every five deaths in the United States. Tobacco use causes or contributes to various oral diseases and adverse conditions, with periodontal diseases being the most common among them. The risk is directly proportional to intensity and duration of exposure. Tobacco use adversely affects certain dental care and treatment prognoses—for example, wound healing, periodontal therapy, dental implants, cosmetic dentistry and cancer therapy. Smoking during pregnancy increases risks for fetal oral clefts and subsequent tooth anomalies. Long-term smokers often have serious health conditions that must be managed during dental treatment and may disrupt or compromise care.

Dentists may be the first health care professionals exposed to the signs and symptoms of oral cancer and other diseases that result from smoking or chewing tobacco. Signs and symptoms related to cancer may include oral sores that do not heal; lumps in the head and neck region; white, thickened patches on the oral mucosa (oral leukoplakia); gingival recession, which also results in increased tooth sensitivity and root decay; or difficulty in chewing, swallowing or moving the tongue or jaw. Additional symptoms and signs may be related to enhanced periodontal breakdown. Thus, the importance of a thorough dental examination for patients who use tobacco products cannot be overemphasized. Careful dental evaluations may decrease the chance for metastases to occur.

Some forms of oral malignancies are aggressive, so prompt diagnosis is critical. Beyond this, the correlation of smoking with certain dental diseases warrants careful evaluation of patients who use tobacco products.

All forms of tobacco contain toxins and carcinogens and produce addiction to nicotine, which is the most commonly abused drug. Once dependence is established, use continues, even when the user understands the risks involved and makes attempts to quit. Nicotine dependence is defined as a chronic, progressive, relapsing disease. Patients with this disease must be treated with these characteristics in mind.

Nicotine dependence also has been defined as a brain disease embedded in a social context. People, generally young people, begin using tobacco for sociocultural reasons. These social stimuli are soon superseded in influence by internal drug-desiring cues and drug-seeking and drug-using behavior. Thus, it is insufficient to treat nicotine-dependent patients solely with FDA-approved pharmacological agents; treatment needs to include behavioral interventions as well. Indeed, reinforcing patients' motivation to quit and helping them develop coping skills are primary services; these services sometimes are provided without pharmacological assistance, as is the case with most youths and pregnant women. However, FDA-approved pharmacological agents, when used as a supplement to recommended behavioral interventions, significantly increase long-term quit rates (6 mo or longer).

Helping patients quit is practical in every clinical condition and can be done by any clinician. A few moments of assistance from a health care practitioner can be significantly more effective than self-help methods in helping patients quit. Minimum assistance includes identifying whether patients use tobacco, advising users to stop, strengthening their commitment to quit, equipping them with coping skills needed during the quitting process and providing follow-up support. Nicotine patches, polacrilex gum, sprays, inhalers and antidepressants are to be used as adjuncts to, not substitutes for, support and follow-up programs. Some of the products available to dentists as guides to helping patients stop using tobacco include the following:

- *How to Help Your Patients Stop Using Tobacco: A National Cancer Institute Manual for the Oral Health Team*, National Cancer Institute, National Institutes of Health, Bethesda, Md.;
- *Tobacco Cessation Resource Packet and Smokeless Tobacco Resource Packet*, American Dental Association, Council on Access, Prevention and Interprofessional Relations, Chicago;
- *Helping Smokers Quit: A Guide for Primary Care Clinicians*, Agency for Health Care Policy and Research (AHCPR), Rockville, Md.;
- *Tobacco Effects in the Mouth: An NCI and NIDR Guide for Health Professionals*, National Cancer Institute, National Institutes of Health, Bethesda, Md.

The publications referenced at the end of this chapter provide further information.

This chapter provides an overview of the rationale for clinical participation in tobacco-use cessation programs and an outline for using intervention procedures.

Clinical Practice Guidelines for Tobacco-Use Cessation

It has been established that dentists are as effective as physicians and other clinicians in helping patients stop using tobacco. It is important to do so for several reasons:

- It is ethical. Many oral diseases and adverse health conditions are caused or exacerbated by tobacco use. It is a major risk factor in the development of periodontal diseases. Risk prevention and reduction meet professional criteria for beneficence and nonmalfeasance.
- It is moral. Half of the people who smoke will die of a smoking-related illness. One of every four smokers will die prematurely, losing on average two decades of life. Tobacco-use intervention services are more effective in terms of life-years saved than is any other dental service, including providing CPR and infection control. Common human decency does not permit standing passively aside when patients are at such high risk of experiencing preventable disease, disability and death.
- It is evidence-based. A large and growing body of scientific evidence shows that even minimum clinical interventions are effective; that intensive, long-duration treatments are more effective than brief treatments; and that specific pharmaceutical agents are effective components of treatment.
- It is practical. Recommended methods are brief and simple and have been shown to significantly increase patient quit rates in virtually any type of practice setting.
- It is cost-effective. Long-term tobacco users develop chronic conditions; these become patient management problems that consume time and may lead to interrupted services and eventually loss of patients owing to tobacco-related disability and death. Among tobacco-using patients, many dental treatments are not an option, have a poor prognosis and/or are at special risk of failure.

Minimum Clinical Intervention

Minimum clinical intervention consists of the following steps, as described by AHCPR:

1. Ask patients about their tobacco use. Implement an officewide system that ensures that tobacco-use status is obtained and recorded for each patient at each office visit.

2. In a clear, strong and personalized manner, urge every tobacco-using patient to quit.

3. Assist the patient with a quit plan. Advise the user to

- set a quit date, ideally within 2 w;
- inform friends, family and coworkers of plans to quit and ask for support;
- remove tobacco from home, car and workplace and avoid using it in these places;
- review previous quit attempts—what helped and what led to relapse;
- anticipate challenges—including nicotine withdrawal—particularly during the critical first few weeks.

  Give advice on successful quitting:
- total abstinence is essential—not even a single puff, dip or chew;
- drinking alcohol is strongly associated with relapse, so avoid any use of alcohol;
- having other users in the household hinders successful quitting, so seek their cooperation in not smoking in the patient's presence.

  Encourage use of an FDA-approved pharmaceutical cessation agent.
- Nicotine replacement agents are effective in reducing withdrawal symptoms during the first 2-3 mo of the quitting process. Nicotine patches approximately double long-term quit rates. Nicotine gum, nasal spray and inhalers are also effective for many patients.
- A non-nicotine tablet is effective in countering nicotine reward and withdrawal effects.
- Every patient should be offered an FDA-approved pharmaceutical cessation agent, except when such agents are medically contraindicated.

  Provide culturally and educationally appropriate materials on cessation techniques.

4. Arrange follow-up care and counseling. Schedule follow-up contacts, either in person or by telephone. A first follow-up contact should be within 2 w of the quit date, preferably during the first week, a second contact within the first month, and further follow-up contacts as needed.

- Recognize and congratulate the patient on success.
- If a lapse occurs, ask for recommitment to total abstinence. This is a common experience, as nicotine dependence is a chronic, relapsing disease.
- Remind the patient that a lapse can be used as a learning experience and review the circumstances that cause it. Assist the patient in identifying alternative behaviors.
- Identify problems encountered and anticipate challenges in the immediate future.

  Providing social support, skills training and problem-solving techniques and prescribing an FDA-approved pharmacological agent are the three most effective treatment strategies.

A more intensive tobacco-use cessation program may be offered if it is determined that such a program is appropriate. Intensive programs should offer four to seven sessions, each at least 20-30 min in length, lasting at least 2 w. Individual and group counseling are both effective. Always follow up with patients who have been referred. Follow-up should extend more than 8 w; in fact, former users need a lifetime of periodic reinforcement.

Special Considerations

1. If a tobacco user does not want to quit, the clinician should ask questions at each visit that help the patient identify reasons to quit and barriers to quitting. The clinician should pledge to assist the patient when he or she is ready to quit.

2. All treatment strategies apply as well to adolescents who use tobacco. Clinicians should be emphatic and nonjudgmental, and should personalize the encounter to the adolescent's individual situation. FDA-approved pharmacological agents may be considered for adolescents who are motivated to quit and who exhibit symptoms of nicotine dependence.

3. Fear of weight gain is an impediment to tobacco cessation for many. The clinician should inform users that some weight gain may be expected, but that it is a minor risk compared to continued tobacco use. Patients should tackle one problem at a time—first striving to feel confident that they have quit using tobacco for good, then working to reduce weight gain, if any. Use of nicotine gum may delay weight gain.

4. Pregnant women should be strongly encouraged to quit for the duration of pregnancy. Because of the serious risks of smoking to the pregnant smoker and the fetus alike, pregnant smokers should be offered intensive counseling. Minimum interventions should be offered if more intensive interventions are not feasible. The clinician should deliver a motivational message regarding the impact of tobacco use on both the pregnant smoker and the fetus. Nicotine replacement should be used during pregnancy only if the increased likelihood of tobacco-use cessation, with its potential benefits, outweighs the risk of nicotine replacement and potential concomitant smoking.

Risks associated with the use of the non-nicotine agent bupropion HCl have not been studied in humans; the teratology risk is negligible in animals.

Guides to help dentists strengthen their clinical tobacco-use cessation skills and related tobacco-use intervention materials are available from the National Cancer Institute's Cancer Information Service (1-800-4-CANCER), the National Institute of Dental Research's Oral Health Information Clearing House (301-496-4261), or the American Dental Association's Council on Access, Prevention and Professional Relations (1-312-440-2860). In addition, practitioners may obtain copies of the clinical practice guideline on smoking cessation from the Agency for Health Care Policy and Research (AHCPR) Publication Clearinghouse (1-800-358-9295).

General information on tobacco-use cessation drugs is provided in Table 29.1; more specific dosage information for transdermal nicotine systems appears in Table 29.2. Many of these products are now available over the counter.

Table 29.1

General Information: Tobacco-Use Cessation Drugs

Generic name	Brand name(s)	Indications/uses	Dosage range	Interactions with other agents
Centrally acting non-nicotine agent				
Bupropion HCl	Zyban	As part of a comprehensive behavioral tobacco-use cessation program to relieve nicotine withdrawal symptoms	150 mg/day for 3 days, then 150 mg bid for 7-12 w **Note:** Patient should choose a "stop tobacco use" date 1-2 w after use of bupropion begins, because drug takes 1 w to reach required levels for effectiveness See manufacturer's instructions	Contraindicated for simultaneous use with monoamine oxidase (MAO) inhibitors, other medications containing bupropion, alcohol, antipsychotic agents, hepatic enzyme inducers and inhibitors, levodopa; such agents may inhibit bupropion metabolism so that plasma levels increase, thereby increasing risk of seizures

Continued on next page

Table 29.1 (cont.)

General Information: Tobacco-Use Cessation Drugs

Generic name	Brand name(s)	Indications/uses	Dosage range	Interactions with other agents
Nicotine inhalation system				
Nicotine inhalation system	Nicotrol Inhaler	As part of a comprehensive behavioral tobacco-use cessation program to relieve nicotine withdrawal symptoms	10 puffs through mouthpiece Begin with 6-16 cartridges/day; after 12 (or fewer) w, reduce dose gradually Pump should be primed before use See manufacturer's instructions	Should not be used with other tobacco products owing to risk of nicotine toxicity Tobacco-use cessation, with or without nicotine replacement, may require adjustment of doses of other medications
Nicotine nasal spray				
Nicotine nasal spray	Nicotrol NS	As part of a comprehensive behavioral tobacco-use cessation program to relieve nicotine withdrawal symptoms	One spray in each nostril; patient should not sniff or inhale and should wait 2-3 min before blowing nose Pump should be primed before use See manufacturer's instructions	Should not be used with other tobacco products owing to risk of nicotine toxicity Tobacco-use cessation, with or without nicotine replacement, may require adjustment of doses of other medications
Nicotine polacrilex gum				
Nicotine polacrilex	Nicorette, Nicorette DS; Nicorette Plus [CAN]	As part of a comprehensive behavioral tobacco-use cessation program to relieve nicotine withdrawal symptoms	Depending on stage of treatment and patient's health, weight and level of nicotine dependence, dosage can range from 2 to 4 mg/dose, taken whenever the urge to smoke or chew tobacco occurs Typically, 9-12 pieces/day, not to exceed 96 mg/day Should be chewed until tingling is felt (which means nicotine is being released); when tingling stops, chewing can be resumed See manufacturer's instructions	Should not be used with tobacco products owing to risk of nicotine toxicity Tobacco-use cessation, with or without nicotine replacement, may require adjustment of doses of other medications Coffee, colas and fruit juices taken immediately before or during use of polacrilex may decrease salivary pH and thereby decrease absorption of nicotine; therefore, use of gum should be delayed for at least 15 min after consumption of food or beverages

[CAN] indicates a drug available only in Canada.

Continued on next page

Table 29.1 (cont.)

General Information: Tobacco-Use Cessation Drugs

Generic name	Brand name(s)	Indications/uses	Dosage range	Interactions with other agents
Transdermal nicotine system				
Nicotine trans-dermal patches*	Habitrol, NicoDerm, Nicotrol, Prostep	As part of a comprehensive behavioral tobacco-use cessation program to relieve nicotine withdrawal symptoms	Depending on stage of treatment and patient's health, weight and level of nicotine dependence, dosage can range from 5 to 22 mg/day Entire course of nicotine substitution and gradual withdrawal takes between 6 and 20 w, depending on brand and size of initial dose See manufacturer's instructions	Should not be used with other tobacco products owing to risk of nicotine toxicity Tobacco-use cessation, with or without nicotine replacement, may require adjustment of doses of other medications Following agents may require decreased dose of nicotine on cessation of tobacco-use: acetaminophen, adrenergic antagonists (for example, prazosin and labetalol), caffeine, imipramine, insulin, oxazepam, pentazocine, propranolol, theophylline Adrenergic agonists (for example, isoproterenol and phenylephrine) may require increased dose on cessation of tobacco use

* See Table 29.2 for further information on transdermal patches.

Special Dental Considerations

Drug Interactions of Dental Interest

Centrally acting non-nicotine agent: bupropion HCl

Bupropion HCl (Zyban), is used in tobacco-use cessation programs as a centrally acting non-nicotine agent. Its interactions with many drugs—including alcohol, antipsychotic agents, hepatic enzyme inducers and inhibitors, levodopa and MAO inhibitors—are of concern, as many of these potentiate the risk of seizures. The use of Zyban is contraindicated for patients who are being treated with Wellbutrin (which is also bupropion), antipsychotics, antidepressants, theophylline or systemic steroids, as well as for patients who abruptly discontinue use of a benzodiazepine or another agent that lowers the seizure threshold.

Nicotine replacement systems

Tobacco-use cessation, with or without nicotine replacement, may alter the pharmacokinetics of certain concomitantly administered medications. Use of tobacco-use cessation products may require a simultaneous decrease in dose of certain medications, such as acetaminophen, caffeine, imipramine, oxazepam, pentazocine, propranolol, theophylline, insulin and adrenergic antagonists (for example, prazosin and labetalol). However, it may require an increase in dose of others, such as adrenergic agonists (for example, isoproterenol and phenylephrine).

Table 29.2

Transdermal Nicotine Patches: Dosage Information

Brand name	Usual initial dose	Adjusted initial dose*	First weaning dose	Second weaning dose	Sample instructions	Plasma nicotine concentration from maximum dose
Habitrol	21 mg/day for 4-8 w (recommended duration: 6 w)	14 mg/day for 4-8 w (recommended duration: 6 w)	14 mg/day for 2-4 w (recommended duration: 2 w)	7 mg/day for 2-4 w (recommended duration: 2 w)	Prescription: Habitrol 21 mg/day, box of 30, apply one patch daily upon awakening	**Minimum:** 9 ng/mL **Average:** 13 ng/mL **Maximum:** 17 ng/mL
NicoDerm CQ	21 mg/day for 4-8 w (recommended duration: 6 w)	14 mg/day for 4-8 w (recommended duration: 6 w)	14 mg/day for 2-4 w (recommended duration: 2 w)	7 mg/day for 2-4 w (recommended duration: 2 w)	Over the counter: NicoDerm CQ 21 mg/day, 1-2 box(es) of 14, apply one patch daily upon awakening	**Minimum:** 11 ng/mL **Average:** 17 ng/mL **Maximum:** 23 ng/mL
Nicotrol	15 mg/day for 4-12 w (recommended duration: 12 w)	None recommended	None recommended	None recommended	Over the counter: Nicotrol 15 mg/day, 1-2 box(es) of 14, apply one patch daily upon awakening and remove patch at bedtime	**Minimum:** 3 ng/mL **Average:** 9 ng/mL **Maximum:** 13 ng/mL
Prostep	22 mg/day for 4-8 w	11 mg/day for 4-8 w	11 mg/day for 2-4 w	None recommended	Prescription: Prostep 22 mg/day, 1-4 box(es) of 7, apply one patch daily upon awakening	**Minimum:** 5 ng/mL **Average:** 11 ng/mL **Maximum:** 16 ng/mL

* Adjusted for patients weighing < 100 lb, patients who have cardiovascular disease or patients who smoke < half pack of cigarettes/day.

Transdermal systems relieve withdrawal symptoms by release of nicotine into the bloodstream via skin, while nicotine polacrilex products release nicotine into the bloodstream via the oral mucosa. Possible advantages of transdermal nicotine patches vs. gums for use in cessation programs include control of dose and the lack of issues related to unpleasant taste, gastrointestinal distress or mandibular stress. Importantly, both treatments result in about one-quarter the nicotine plasma concentration found in smokers; furthermore, nicotine does not produce carbon monoxide and other toxic pyrrolates of tobacco smoke products that are linked with cardiovascular disease and cancer risks. This statement does not imply that smokeless tobacco may be safer than smoked tobacco products. It is clear that both types of tobacco are detrimental.

Special Patients

Pregnant women

Bupropion is in pregnancy risk category B. It crosses the placenta barrier; thus precautions should be used in administering this drug to women who are pregnant or planning to have children. In addition, bupropion and its metabolites pass into breast milk and thus is contraindicated for patients who are breastfeeding children. (There is potential for adverse reactions—such as seizures—in infants.)

There is some evidence that smoking during pregnancy builds nicotine tolerance in the fetus. Although bupropion has a low abuse potential and there is no evidence that it harms the fetus, every effort should be made to help pregnant women quit without the assistance of this or any other FDA-approved pharmaceutical agent for smoking cessation.

Geriatric and pediatric patients

Older people are more sensitive to the anticholinergic, sedative and cardiovascular side effects of antidepressants. In addition, they often have age-related renal and hepatic problems that may require dose adjustment.

All nicotine replacement products deliver nicotine at levels that are lower than self-administered nicotine via tobacco products. There is no evidence that age is itself a consideration in establishing dosing strengths and schedules.

Use of tobacco-use cessation medications with children has not been evaluated.

Adverse Effects, Precautions and Contraindications

It is imperative for a dentist who is involved directly in providing tobacco-use cessation programs for patients to understand the positive and negative features of such a program. Table 29.3 lists adverse effects associated with tobacco-use cessation drugs; Table 29.4 lists precautions and contraindications for their use. Please note, as stated in Table 29.4, that nicotine drugs are contraindicated for patients who have malignant hypertension and for patients in the immediate postmyocardial infarct period.

Table 29.3

Tobacco-Use Cessation Drugs: Adverse Effects

Body system	Centrally acting non-nicotine agent	Nicotine inhalation system	Nicotine nasal spray	Nicotine polacrilex gum	Transdermal nicotine systems
CV	*Hypertension*	Edema, cardiac irritability, *hypertension*	Edema, cardiac irritability, *hypertension*	Edema, cardiac irritability, hypertension	*Hypertension*

Italics indicate information of major clinical significance.

Continued on next page

Table 29.3 (cont.)

Tobacco-Use Cessation Drugs: Adverse Effects

Body system	Centrally acting non-nicotine agent	Nicotine inhalation system	Nicotine nasal spray	Nicotine polacrilex gum	Transdermal nicotine systems
CNS	*Insomnia, seizures,* (related to dose)	Anorexia, dizziness, *headache,* insomnia	Anorexia, dizziness, *headache,* insomnia	Anorexia, dizziness, *headache,* insomnia	Dizziness, *headache,* insomnia, abnormal dreams
EENT	None of significance to dentistry	*Pharyngitis* During first w, local irritant effects, including nasal irritation, runny nose, throat irritation, watering eyes, sneezing, coughing	*Pharyngitis* During first week, local irritant effects, including nasal irritation, runny nose, throat irritation, watering eyes, sneezing, coughing	*Pharyngitis,* hoarseness	None of significance to dentistry
Endoc	None of significance to dentistry	Dysmenorrhea	Dysmenorrhea	Dysmenorrhea	Dysmenorrhea
GI	Altered appetite	*GI upset, nausea, vomiting, eructation, increased appetite*	*GI upset, nausea, vomiting, eructation, increased appetite*	*GI upset, nausea, vomiting, eructation, increased appetite*	Diarrhea, dyspepsia, nausea, GI upset, *increased appetite*
Integ	None of significance to dentistry	Erythema, flushing, itching, rash, hypersensitivity	Erythema, flushing, itching, rash, hypersensitivity	Erythema, flushing, itching, rash, hypersensitivity	Cutaneous hypersensitivity, rash, increased sweating, erythema
Musc	None of significance to dentistry	None of significance to dentistry	None of significance to dentistry	Muscle pain	Arthralgia, back pain
Oral	Xerostomia	Xerostomia, increased susceptibility to oral fungal infections	Xerostomia, increased susceptibility to oral fungal infections	Aphthous ulcers, altered taste, excess salivation, glossitis, *jaw ache,* hiccups	Altered taste, xerostomia
Resp	None of significance to dentistry	None of significance to dentistry	None of significance to dentistry	None of significance to dentistry	Chest pain, increased cough

Italics indicate information of major clinical significance.

Table 29.4

Tobacco-Use Cessation Drugs: Precautions and Contraindications

Drug	Precautions	Contraindications
Centrally acting non-nicotine agent: bupropion HCl	Associated with dose-dependent risk of seizures; risk related to patient factors, clinical situation and concurrent medication, all of which should be considered before prescription is given Dose should not be > 300 mg/day for tobacco-use cessation	Contraindicated for patients with anorexia or bulimia nervosa, bipolar disorders, CNS tumor, head trauma, history of drug abuse, hepatic or renal function impairment, recent history of myocardial infarct, unstable heart disease, psychosis, seizure disorders Contraindicated for simultaneous use with monoamine oxidase inhibitors Contraindicated for patients with sensitivity to bupropion (Wellbutrin)
Nicotine inhalation system	Can be toxic and addictive Should be kept out of reach of children and pets Patient should stop smoking completely on initiating therapy Treatment should be discontinued if patient experiences severe or persistent local skin reactions at the site of application Should be used with caution and only when the benefits of use (including nicotine replacement in a smoking cessation program) outweigh risks for patients with following conditions: coronary heart disease, serious cardiac arrhythmias, renal or hepatic impairment, hyperthyroidism, pheochromocytoma, insulin-dependent diabetes and active peptic ulcers Not recommended for use with children or for patients with history of drug abuse and dependence, because of nicotine's addictive nature As with many other inhalers, may increase susceptibility to oral fungal infections	Contraindicated for continuous use of > 6 mo Contraindicated for patients who have asthma or chronic nasal disorders Contraindicated for patients during immediate postmyocardial infarction period, patients with serious arrhythmias or severe or worsening angina pectoris, pregnant women Contraindicated for patients who have hypersensitivity or allergy to nicotine or to any component of therapeutic system
Nicotine nasal spray	See note above As with many other nasal sprays, may increase susceptibility to oral fungal infections	Contraindicated for continuous use of > 3 mo Contraindicated for patients who have asthma or chronic nasal disorders Contraindicated for patients during immediate postmyocardial infarction period, patients with serious arrhythmias or severe or worsening angina pectoris, pregnant women Contraindicated for patients who have hypersensitivity or allergy to nicotine or to any component of therapeutic system

Continued on next page

Table 29.4 (cont.)

Tobacco-Use Cessation Drugs: Precautions and Contraindications

Drug	Precautions	Contraindications
Nicotine polacrilex gum	Can be toxic and addictive Should be kept out of reach of children and pets Patient should stop smoking completely on initiating therapy Treatment should be discontinued if patient experiences severe or persistent local skin reactions at the site of application Should be used with caution and only when the benefits of use (including nicotine replacement in a smoking cessation program) outweigh risks for patients with following conditions: coronary heart disease, serious cardiac arrhythmias, renal or hepatic impairment, hyperthyroidism, pheochromocytoma, insulin-dependent diabetes and active peptic ulcers Not recommended for use with children or for patients with history of drug abuse and dependence, because of nicotine's addictive nature As with many other inhalers, may increase susceptibility to oral fungal infections May have oral side effects, including interactions with restorative materials, xerostomia and pharyngeal and oral inflammation	Contraindicated for patients who are nonsmokers, are in immediate postmyocardial infarction period, have severe or worsening angina pectoris, have active temporomandibular joint disease or are pregnant Contraindicated for patients with active temporomandibular joint disorders, history of GI disorders Contraindicated for patients who wear dentures Contraindicated for patients who have hypersensitivity or allergy to nicotine or to any component of therapeutic system
Transdermal nicotine system	See note above, with exception of final paragraph (on oral side effects)	Contraindicated for continuous use of > 3 mo Contraindicated for patients during immediate postmyocardial infarction period, patients with serious arrhythmias or severe or worsening angina pectoris, pregnant women Contraindicated for patients who have hypersensitivity or allergy to nicotine or to any component of therapeutic system

Pharmacology

Centrally Acting Non-nicotine Agent: Bupropion HCl

We are rapidly developing an understanding of the brain's molecular and cellular function related to exposure to various addictive substances. All drugs of dependence seem to work in the same area of the mesolimbic system, although each uses slightly different mechanisms at the neuronal synaptic junction.

This is important, as bupropion HCl appears to act on the two critical centers involved: the nucleus accumbens for dopamine release/reward signals and the locus caeruleus for penalty/withdrawal signals.

Bupropion is primarily metabolized to hydroxybupropion by the CYP2B6 isoenzyme. Therefore, the potential exists for a drug interaction between Zyban and drugs that affect the CYP2B6 isoenzyme metabolism, such as orphenadrine and cyclophosphamide.

No systemic data have been collected on the metabolism of Zyban after concomitant administration with other drugs or, alternatively, the effect of concomitant administration of Zyban on the metabolism of other drugs. The metabolism of bupropion may be induced by some drugs—such as carbamazepine, phenobarbital and phenytoin—and inhibited by others, such as cimetidine.

Nicotine replacement systems

Nicotine, through interactions that occur via nicotine-specific receptors, is a potent ganglionic and CNS stimulant. Therefore, the rationale for using all nicotine replacement agents is to slowly decrease the serum levels of nicotine and thereby prevent withdrawal symptoms and, ultimately, stop the smoking behavior. Also, the change to replacement agents from inhaled nicotine results in lower and slower activity doses of nicotine. Moreover, this method eliminates exposure to associated carcinogens and gases of smoke.

Nicotine inhalation systems

These systems deliver nicotine at low concentrations, in vapor form (via a cartridge attached to a mouthpiece); absorption occurs mainly through oral and pharyngeal mucosa.

Nicotine nasal spray

Nasal spray delivers nicotine more rapidly than gum or transdermal systems. The rationale behind the nasal spray system is that the more rapid rise in nicotine concentration that it provides, analogous to that derived from smoking, may help patients who have not been successful with other programs.

However, some initial studies suggest that the spray is addictive.

Nicotine polacrilex gum

Nicotine gum releases nicotine into the bloodstream via the oral mucosa.

Nicotine transdermal systems

Nicotine patches release nicotine into the bloodstream via the skin.

Suggested Readings

The Smoking Cesation Clinical Practice Guideline Panel and Staff. The Agency for Health Care Policy and Research smoking cessation clinical practice guideline. JAMA 1996;275:1270-80.

Christen AG, McDonald JL, Klein JA, Christen JA, Guba CJ. A smoking cessation program for the dental office (monograph). Indianapolis: Indiana University School of Dentistry; 1994.

Fiester S, Goldstein M, Resnick M, et al. Practice guideline for the treatment of patients with nicotine dependence. Am J Psychiatry 1996; 153(10) (Supplement 31).

Fiore MC, Bailey WE, Cohen SJ, et al. Smoking cessation. Clinical practice guideline no. 18. Rockville, Md.: U.S. Department of Health and Human Services, 1996. AHCPR publication no. 96-0692.

Research, Science and Therapy Committee. Position paper: tobacco use and the periodontal patient. J Periodontol 1996;67:51-6.

Henningfield J. Nicotine medications for smoking cessation. N Engl J Med 1995;333:1196-1202.

Mecklenburg RE, Christen AG, Gerbert B, et al. How to help your patients stop using tobacco: a national cancer institute manual for the oral health team. Bethesda, Md.: U.S. Department of Health and Human Services, National Institutes of Health, 1993. NIH publication no. 93-31391.

Ostrowski DJ, DeNelsky GY. Pharmacologic management of patients using smoking cessation aids. Dent Clin North Am 1996;40:779-801.

Schneider NG, Olmstead R, Nilsson F, Vaghaiwalla-Mody F, Franzon M, Doan K. Efficacy of a nicotine inhaler in smoking cessation: a double-blind, placebo-controlled trial. Addiction 1996;9:1293-1306.

Chapter 30.

Substance Abuse

Linda Kittelson, M.S., R.N.

This chapter offers information to help practitioners safely manage patients who have or are suspected of having substance abuse problems.

Consider the following points:

- Without some intelligent skepticism, a dentist can become an easy target for someone seeking to exploit a health care provider who has a license to prescribe controlled substances.
- Without appropriate protections, dental offices can be vulnerable to theft of medications, nitrous oxide, needles and syringes and prescription pads.
- Without some understanding of drug dependence, dentists may prescribe inappropriately for an active user or mismanage analgesia for a recovering addict or alcoholic.

Defining Addiction

In 1986, the ADA House of Delegates adopted the ADA Policy Statement on Chemical Dependency (Resolution 64H-1986), the opening statement of which is "The ADA recognizes that chemical dependency is a disease that affects all of society."

"Addiction" is defined by the American Society of Addiction Medicine as "a disease process characterized by the continued use of a specific psychoactive substance despite physical, psychological or social harm." Addiction is not a result of moral failing, poor upbringing or indulgent or unfortunate circumstances. Characteristics of addiction are as follows:

- The use of the substance may be continuous or periodic.
- The addict experiences impaired control over the use, meaning that there is an inability to limit the use of the substance or of the quantity and/or frequency of use, and predictability of the behavioral consequences of use.
- Preoccupation is manifested in excessive, focused attention on the substance—its acquisition, its effects and its use—often to the exclusion of other issues that are more important.
- The addict experiences physical, psychological or social consequences that are substance-related problems such as withdrawal syndromes; liver disease; neurological impairment; gastritis; impaired cognition; mood lability or alteration; problems with anger control or anxiety management; occupational impairment; marital/relationship dysfunction; and/or legal, financial, and spiritual problems.
- The addict expresses denial, a hallmark of addiction, representing a range of psychological maneuvers designed to eliminate or reduce awareness of problems with the substance.

The incidence of addiction in the general population is commonly thought to be about 10%. Here are some guiding principles to keep in mind:

- People who have one or more close family members with an addiction are at significantly greater risk of developing the disease themselves.

- Men have a higher rate of addiction than women.
- Addicts come from all racial and ethnic groups, from all socioeconomic groups and from all educational levels. While some will look unkempt, most will come to a dental office looking like the professionals, laborers, teachers, students, PTA members or card-carrying senior citizens that they are.

The Dentist's Role with Addicted Patients

In 1989, the ADA House of Delegates augmented its 1986 statement with a policy statement on provision of dental care for patients who are or have been chemically dependent. The statement read in part, "The use of certain therapeutic agents in dental treatment may have effects on the health and relapse potential of the recovering chemically dependent patient." Furthermore, the statement read, "It is the professional responsibility of the practicing dentists in the United States to be aware of chemical dependency as an illness and to address the issues of appropriate dental care in the chemically dependent population."

It is important that the dentist be aware of a patient's substance use history. It should be noted that the use of this information will be subject to state confidentiality law, and may also be subject to federal, state and local antidiscrimination laws.

Key Points Dentists Should Remember

- Patients with a history of addiction are likely to need more analgesia than those without such a history.
- Obtaining an appropriate medical history is one of the best protections against being manipulated by patients. It is a good idea to ask specific questions about prescriptions obtained from other providers (dentists or physicians), including how much of the prescription is left and the condition for which it is being taken.

- Patients who use nonprescribed substances (over-the-counter or illicit) may experience adverse reactions from concomitant use of prescribed substances.
- The use of some substances is contraindicated in patients recovering from substance dependence. Tramadol and butorphanol, for example, while not scheduled drugs, have abuse potential in patients with a history of substance dependence. Patients expect their health providers to know their history and to prescribe safely for them.
- Patients taking disulfiram will experience an adverse reaction, potentially life-threatening, upon exposure to alcohol in any form.
- Patients receiving opioid antagonist therapy (naltrexone) will have an altered response to analgesia.

Table 30.1 provides a summary of some prescribing considerations for dentists who have patients with a history of substance abuse/dependency.

Recognizing Addicted Patients

Some addicted patients may not reveal their history of substance abuse. To arm themselves for dealing with patients such as these, dentists should become aware of the symptoms of substance abuse.

The symptoms of substance dependence will vary with the substance used. Substances of abuse can be grouped into 11 categories: alcohol, amphetamines, caffeine, cannabis (marijuana), cocaine, hallucinogens, inhalants, nicotine, opioids, phencyclidine hydrochloride (PCP) and sedatives/hypnotics/anxiolytics.

Symptoms of dependence

Alcohol dependence is one of the more prominent forms of dependence. Its symptoms include the following:

- **Physical:** Tremors, facial "spider veins," blackouts (temporary amnesia induced by consumption of a large quantity of alcohol), gastritis, esophagitis, liver disease, elevated blood pressure, weight gain or loss, neglect of physical appearance, bruises or other

Table 30.1

Substances of Abuse: Dental Implications

Abused substance	Facts to aid in diagnosis	Drugs that may interact	Dental implications
Alcohol	Patient may appear drunk or drowsy and have slurred speech Odor of alcohol may be present Patient may have difficulty maintaining position of head	Other central nervous system depressants (such as opioid analgesics) enhance alcohol-induced respiratory depression Metronidazole interacts with alcohol to produce flushing, hypotension, nausea and vomiting	Alcohol-containing mouthrinses and liquid medications that contain high concentrations of alcohol should be avoided in dental treatment of recovering alcoholics Recovering alcoholics with liver disease may require a lower dose of medications containing acetaminophen
Amphetamines	Patient may act jittery, irritable, unable to sit still Patient may exhibit tremors, dilated pupils, increased blood pressure and heart rate	Intravascular injection of local anesthetics containing vasoconstrictors may enhance amphetamine-induced increase in blood pressure	Measure blood pressure preoperatively; if high (diastolic >110 mm), reschedule procedure Methamphetamine users have been reported to have high caries index
Barbiturates	Patient may appear drunk or drowsy and have slurred speech Patient may have difficulty maintaining position of head	Other CNS depressants (such as opioid analgesics) may enhance barbiturate-induced respiratory depression	Dose of opioids should be reduced to avoid enhanced respiratory depression
Benzodiazepines	These CNS depressants are favorites among drug abusers	Other CNS depressants (such as opioid analgesics) may enhance benzodiazepine-induced respiratory depression	Dose of opioids should be reduced to avoid enhanced respiratory depression Xerostomia is a frequent side effect and may lead to increased caries
Cocaine	Patient may act jittery, irritable, unable to sit still Patient may exhibit tremors, dilated pupils, increased blood pressure and heart rate	Intravascular injection of local anesthetics containing vasoconstrictors may enhance cocaine-induced increase in blood pressure and heart rate; cardiac arrest	Avoid local anesthetics containing vasoconstrictors; local anesthetics without vasoconstrictors may be used

Continued on next page

Note: As a general rule, patients in recovery from chemical dependency, including alcohol, should not be given any psychoactive drug, such as nitrous oxide or benzodiazepines.
Source: Hal Crossley, D.D.S., Ph.D.

Table 30.1 (cont.)

Substances of Abuse: Dental Implications

Abused substance	Facts to aid in diagnosis	Drugs that may interact	Dental implications
Inhalants	Most, if not all, inhalants are excreted via the lungs Patient who has abused an inhalant within a few hours will have an odor on breath	Most inhalants are CNS depressants Other CNS depressants (such as opioid analgesics) may enhance inhalant-induced respiratory depression	Chronic inhalant abuse may cause liver damage, decreasing rate of inactivation of prescribed or over-the-counter drugs such as acetaminophen and thus increasing their toxicity
Lysergic acid diethylamide (LSD)	Patient may appear disoriented and confused Patient may exhibit dilated pupils, increased blood pressure and heart rate	No confirmed interactions with dental drugs	None of significance to dentistry
Marijuana	Patient may appear sedated and lethargic and have bloodshot eyes Heart rate may be increased but blood pressure will be decreased	No confirmed interactions with dental drugs	None of significance to dentistry
Nicotine	Patient may have history of use Patient may exhibit staining of teeth and oral tissues, malodor characteristic of smokers	No confirmed interactions with dental drugs	See Chapter 29, Cessation of Tobacco Use
Opioids	Patient may appear drowsy, lethargic, disoriented and confused Pupils may be constricted Arms may exhibit scars from previous injuries or needle marks	Other CNS depressants (such as sedatives or hypnotics) may enhance opioid-induced respiratory depression Patients taking naltrexone, an opioid antagonist, during recovery may exhibit decreased effect of opioid analgesics	Opioid users in recovery or actively using drugs may require increased dose of opioid analgesics to achieve analgesia Avoid prescribing opioid-type analgesics postoperatively in patients recovering from opioid addiction Opioid users may exhibit profound xerostomia with increased craving for sweets, resulting in rampant caries
Phencyclidine hydrochloride (PCP)	This anesthetic agent may program CNS depression with paradoxical CNS excitation accompanied by hallucinations	Other CNS depressants may enhance PCP-induced respiratory depression	None of significance to dentistry

Note: As a general rule, patients in recovery from chemical dependency, including alcohol, should not be given any psychoactive drug, such as nitrous oxide or benzodiazepines.
Source: Hal Crossley, D.D.S., Ph.D.

injuries, odor of alcohol on breath at inappropriate times.

- **Emotional/psychological:** Mood swings, irritability, depression, remorse, resentfulness, defensiveness about or denial of a problem, difficulty in concentration, chronic anger.
- **Social/behavioral:** Unpredictability, unreliability, arrests for driving under the influence (DUI) and other legal problems, conflict with significant others, family members adapting behaviors to accommodate drinking, financial problems and occupational impairment.

Many of the aforementioned symptoms will also be apparent in the abuse of other substances. Table 30.2 is included as a reference for the uses and effects of controlled substances which, by definition, have abuse potential.

Drug-seeking behaviors

Drug-seeking patients use various techniques and manipulations to acquire substances or prescriptions:

- They may contact the dentist at inopportune times—such as at the end of the day or on a weekend—when it is impossible or inconvenient for the dentist to conduct a complete examination.
- They may say they are from out of town, "just passing through," or that they are in the middle of a procedure with a dentist in another town and forgot to bring their prescription medications.
- Addicts are likely to appear very knowledgeable about their dental conditions and about which pain medications are and are not effective for them.
- They may request an antibiotic first, then follow up with a request for pain medication.
- They may engage the dentist in what may seem to be an innocent conversation about drug supplies or prescribing practices, the effects of nitrous oxide, security procedures or similar topics.

- Addicts may ask for pharmaceutical samples in addition to prescriptions.
- An abuser may call with a story about a lost prescription.

Guarding Against Drug Theft

A number of safeguards can be implemented in the office to help protect the dentist from being targeted as a source of controlled substances. These measures should be implemented subject to applicable laws, including those regarding confidentiality. Suggestions include the following:

- Store narcotics in locked cabinets away from patient areas and well out of view of patients.
- Never leave medications unattended in a room, regardless of whether or not a patient is present.
- Keep prescription pads out of sight and, preferably, in a locked cabinet.
- When writing prescriptions, give quantities in words as well as numbers (for example, if writing for 12 Tylenol no. 3, specify "twelve Tylenol no. 3" as well).
- Do not use prescription blanks preprinted with your U.S. Drug Enforcement Agency (DEA) number.
- Be suspicious of patients who request specific medications.
- Use the lowest effective doses and noncontrolled substances as much as possible (it is important, however, to manage acute pain aggressively enough that patients experience relief).

Prescribe in small quantities—a 2- to 3-day supply should be adequate for most dental procedures.

Keep a tally in the patient record of quantities of controlled substances prescribed so as not to exceed a reasonable cutoff point.

- Maintain strict inventory control of any controlled substances stored in the office, and do not keep substances in stock that are not used in the office.
- Keep stocks of syringes out of view of patients.

Table 30.2

Controlled Substances: Uses and Effects

Drugs	CSA Schedules	Trade or Other Names	Medical Uses	Physical Dependence
Narcotics				
Heroin	I	Diacetylmorphine, Horse, Smack	None in U.S., analgesic, antitussive	High
Morphine	II	Duramorph, MS-Contin, Roxanol, Oramorph SR	Analgesic	High
Codeine	II,III,V	Tylenol w/Codeine, Empirin w/Codeine, Robitussin A-C, Fiorinal w/Codeine, APAP w/Codeine	Analgesic, antitussive	Moderate
Hydrocodone	II,III	Tussionex, Vicodin, Hycodan, Lorcet	Analgesic, antitussive	High
Hydromorphone	II	Dilaudid	Analgesic	High
Oxycodone	II	Percodan, Percocet, Tylox, Roxicet, Roxicodone	Analgesic	High
Methadone and LAAM	I,II	Dolophine, Methadose, Levo-alpha-acetylmethadol, Levomethadyl acetate	Analgesic, treatment of dependence	High
Fentanyl and analogs	I,II	Innovar, Sublimaze, Alfenta, Sufenta, Duragesic	Analgesic, adjunct to anesthesia, anesthetic	High
Other narcotics	II,III,IV,V	Percodan, Percocet, Tylox, Opium, Darvon, Talwin*, Buprenorphine, Meperidine (Pethidine), Demerol	Analgesic, antidiarrheal	High-Low
Depressants				
Chloral hydrate	IV	Noctec, Somnos, Felsules	Hypnotic	Moderate
Barbiturates	II,III,IV	Amytal, Florinal, Nembutal, Seconal, Tuinal, Phenobarbital, Pentobarbital	Anesthetic, anticonvulsant, sedative hypnotic, veterinary euthanasia agent	High-Moderate
Benzodiazepines	IV	Ativan, Dalmane, Diazepam, Librium, Xanax, Serax, Valium, Tranxene, Verstran, Versed, Halcion, Paxipam, Restoril	Antianxiety, sedative, anticonvulsant, hypnotic	Low
Glutethimide	II	Doriden	Sedative, hypnotic	High
Other depressants	I,II,III,IV	Equanil, Miltown, Noludar, Placidyl, Valmid, Methaqualone	Antianxiety, sedative, hypnotic	Moderate
Stimulants				
Cocaine**	II	Coke, Flake, Snow, Crack	Local anesthetic	Possible
Amphetamine/methamphetamine	II	Biphetamine, Desoxyn, Dexedrine, Obetrol, Ice	Attention deficit disorder, narcolepsy, weight control	Possible
Methylphenidate	II	Ritalin	Attention deficit disorder, narcolepsy	Possible
Other stimulants	I,II,III,IV	Adipex, Didrex, lonamin, Melfiat, Plegine, Captagon, Sanorex, Tenuate, Tepanil, Prelu-2, Preludin	Weight control	Possible

*Designated a narcotic under the Controlled Substances Act (CSA).
** Not designated a narcotic under the CSA.

Psychological Dependence	Tolerance	Duration (Hours)	Usual Method	Possible Effects	Effects of Overdose	Withdrawal Syndrome
Narcotics						
High	Yes	3-6	Injected, sniffed, smoked	Euphoria	Slow and shallow breathing	Watery eyes
High	Yes	3-6	Oral, smoked, injected	Drowsiness	Clammy skin	Runny nose
Moderate	Yes	3-6	Oral, injected	Respiratory depression	Convulsions	Yawning
				Constricted pupils	Coma	Loss of appetite
				Nausea	Possible death	Irritability
High	Yes	3-6	Oral			Tremors
High	Yes	3-6	Oral, injected			Panic
High	Yes	4-5	Oral			Cramps
						Nausea
High	Yes	12-72	Oral, injected			Chills and sweating
High	Yes	10-72	Injected, transdermal patch			
High-Low	Yes	Variable	Oral, injected			
Depressants						
Moderate	Yes	5-8	Oral	Slurred speech	Shallow respiration	Anxiety
High-Moderate	Yes	1-16	Oral, injected	Disorientation	Clammy skin	Insomnia
Low	Yes	4-8	Oral, injected	Drunken behavior without odor of alcohol	Dilated pupils	Tremors
					Weak and rapid pulse	Delirium
					Coma	Convulsions
Moderate	Yes	4-8	Oral		Possible death	Possible death
Moderate	Yes	4-8	Oral			
Stimulants						
High	Yes	1-2	Sniffed, smoked, injected	Increased alertness	Agitation	Apathy
High	Yes	2-4	Oral, injected, smoked	Excitation	Increased body temperature	Long periods of sleep
High	Yes	2-4	Oral, injected	Euphoria	Hallucination	Irritability
High	Yes	2-4	Oral, injected	Increased pulse rate & blood pressure	Convulsions	Depression
				Insomnia	Possible death	Disorientation
				Loss of appetite		

Continued on next page

Table 30.2 (cont.)

Controlled Substances: Uses and Effects

Drugs	CSA Schedules	Trade or Other Names	Medical Uses	Physical Dependence
Cannabis				
Marijuana	I	Pot, Acapulco Gold, Grass, Reefer, Sinsemilla, Thai Sticks	None	Unknown
Tetrahydrocannabinol	I,II	THC, Marinol	Antinauseant	Unknown
Hashish and hashish oil	I	Hash, Hash Oil	None	Unknown
Hallucinogens				
LSD	I	Acid, Microdot	None	None
Mescaline and peyote	I	Mescal, Buttons, Cactus	None	None
Amphetamine variants	I	2, 5-DMA, STP, MDA, MDMA, Esctasy, DOM, DOB	None	Unknown
Phencyclidine and analogs	I,II	PCE, PCPy, TCP, PCP, Hog, Loveboat, Angel Dust	None	Unknown
Other hallucinogens	I	Bufotenine, Ibogaine, DMT, DET, Psilocybin, Psilocyn	None	None
Anabolic Steroids				
Testosterone (cypionate, enanthate)	III	Depo-Testosterone, Delatestryl	Hypogonadism	Unknown
Nandrolone (decanoate, phenpropionate)	III	Nortestosterone, Durabolin, Deca-Durabolin, Deca	Anemia, breast cancer	Unknown
Oxymetholone	III	Anadrol-50	Anemia	Unknown

Source: Drugs of Abuse, 1996 edition. Washington, D.C.: U. S. Department of Justice, Drug Enforcement Administration; 1996.

Psychological Dependence	Tolerance	Duration (Hours)	Usual Method	Possible Effects	Effects of Overdose	Withdrawal Syndrome
Cannabis						
Moderate	Yes	2-4	Smoked, oral	Euphoria	Fatigue	Occasional reports of insomnia
Moderate	Yes	2-4	Smoked, oral	Relaxed inhibitions Increased appetite	Paranoia Possible psychosis	Hyperactivity
Moderate	Yes	2-4	Smoked, oral	Disorientation		Decreased appetite
Hallucinogens						
Unknown	Yes	8-12	Oral	Illusions and hallucinations	Longer	Unknown
Unknown	Yes	8-12	Oral	Altered perception of time and distance	More intense "trip" episodes	
Unknown	Yes	Variable	Oral, injected		Psychosis	
High	Yes	Days	Oral, smoked		Possible death	
Unknown	Possible	Variable	Smoked, oral, injected, sniffed			
Anabolic Steroids						
Unknown	Unknown	14-28 days	Injected	Virilization	Unknown	Possible depression
Unknown	Unknown	14-21 days	Injected	Acne Testicular atrophy		
Unknown	Unknown	24	Oral	Gynecomastia Aggressive behavior Edema		

- If you or your office staff phone in prescriptions to the pharmacy, do so out of hearing range of patients in the office or waiting room. Information that can be gleaned, and possibly exploited, by eavesdropping includes the staff member's name, brand name, dosage, and quantity of drug in a usual prescription, the dentist's DEA number, whether refills are authorized, and anything else typically included in phone orders from a particular office.
- Follow appropriate procedures for securing nitrous oxide tanks.
- Do not prescribe medications over the phone for unknown patients.
- Investigate suspicious stories, such as treatment begun by another dentist in another community, by calling the other dentist.
- When treating patients who are recovering from substance abuse, coordinate their pain management with their primary physicians.

Actions Dentists Should Take on Recognizing Addicted Patients

When a dentist suspects a substance abuse problem in a patient, the appropriate response will vary, depending on the patient and the situation. It is important to keep in mind the obligation to practice within ethical guidelines and legal mandates, and also to protect one's practice and professional license from exploitation or abuse. Some of the possible actions to take, subject to applicable confidentiality and other laws, are as follows:

- Express concern to a patient and provide him or her with phone numbers for a local treatment facility, community mental health center or substance abuse counselor.
- Express concern to a family member and offer to be of support in urging the patient to seek help.
- Notify local pharmacies of any suspicions of prescription abuse.
- Contact local police about suspicious behavior, such as requests made of you to prescribe illegally.
- If appropriate, share concerns with your patient's physician.

Suggested Readings

American Dental Association Transactions 1986:519, Resolution 64H-1986.

American Dental Association. ADA policy statement on provision of dental care for patients who are or have been chemically dependent. Chicago: American Dental Association; 1989.

American Psychiatric Association. Diagnostic and statistical manual of mental disorders, fourth edition. Washington, D.C.: American Psychiatric Association; 1994.

Drugs of Abuse, 1996 Edition. Washington, D.C.: U.S. Department of Justice, Drug Enforcement Administration; 1996.

Glick M. Medical considerations for dental care of patients with alcohol-related liver disease. JADA 1997;128(1):61-70.

Steindler ES. Addiction. In: Principles of addiction medicine. Chevy Chase, Md.: American Society of Addiction Medicine; 1994.

Williams AG. Dentistry faces addiction: How to be part of the solution. St. Louis: Mosby Year-Book; 1992.

Chapter 31.

Legal Implications of Using Drugs in Dental Practice

Kathleen M. Todd, J.D.; Jill Wolowitz, J.D.

Editor's note: This chapter is based on a 1992 article by Linda M. Wakeen, J.D., that originally appeared in the *Journal of Public Health Dentistry.*[1]

Dentists often fear that they need a law license to practice their profession successfully in today's climate of excessive federal regulation and burgeoning litigation. This fear is sometimes manifested when doctors face difficult choices about the types of drugs they prescribe in their practices.

Two types of approval processes can assist dentists in making difficult choices: the federal Food, Drug, and Cosmetic Act approval process, and the American Dental Association's Seal of Acceptance Program. Overall, a dentist who prescribes a drug approved by the U.S. Food and Drug Administration in a manner that is consistent with the label approved by the FDA—according to the approved directions for dosage, indications for usage and so forth—can feel relatively confident that the drug is safe and effective for its approved uses. Similarly, products that bear the ADA's Seal have been found by the ADA Council on Scientific Affairs to meet ADA guidelines for safety and effectiveness. An FDA-approved, ADA-accepted drug is a wise choice.

However, the wise choice may not always be the reasonable choice. In court, a doctor will be judged according to the applicable standard of care. Generally, doctors are judged according to a reasonableness standard; in a malpractice action, courts look to see how a reasonably prudent doctor would have acted in the same or similar circumstances. This means the doctor must be able to show at all times that his or her decision about which drug to prescribe was reasonable.

For example, it would be unreasonable to prescribe a drug approved for pain relief to a patient who has no pain. Although the safety and efficacy of the drug may be well established by the FDA, prescribing the drug for a pain-free patient would be inappropriate and might well constitute a breach of the standard of care.

Conversely, there may be instances in which it is reasonable for a doctor to prescribe an approved drug for a nonapproved use or even to prescribe a non–FDA-approved drug. In this situation, in the absence of state regulations that might prohibit the use of a non–FDA-approved drug, the doctor's actions will be judged primarily by the same standard of reasonableness that would be used in a typical dental or medical malpractice action. However, the analysis is trickier, because some jurisdictions have found that use of nonapproved drugs or use of approved drugs in nonapproved ways is prima facie negligence—in other words, negligence on the face of it. Such a finding places the burden on the doctor to justify the scientific basis for his or her decision, to show that a reasonably prudent doctor acting in the same or similar circumstances would have made the same decision. In some situations, it may be appropriate to obtain specific informed consent for the use prescribed.

Overall, the law defers to the doctor's need and ability to exercise independent professional judgment in the prescription of all drugs but holds doctors accountable for the results of negligent decisions. This chapter will discuss the legal ramifications of various decisions that are made in the context of making difficult prescription choices.

Use of FDA-Approved Drugs for Unapproved Uses

Generally, the FDA does not regulate dentists and physicians.[2,3] Thus, if an approved drug is shipped in interstate commerce with an approved package insert, and neither the shipper nor the recipient intends that it be used for an unapproved purpose, all requirements of the Food, Drug, and Cosmetic Act (the Act) are satisfied. Once the drug is in a local pharmacy, a dentist or physician may lawfully prescribe a different dosage for his or her patient, or may otherwise vary the conditions of use from those approved in the package insert, without informing or obtaining the approval of the FDA.[2,3]

The FDA has itself explained that Congress did not intend the FDA to interfere with medical practice or to regulate the practice of medicine between the doctor and the patient. Congress recognized that patients have the right to seek civil damages in the courts if there should be evidence of malpractice and declined to place any legislative restrictions on the medical profession.[2,4,5] (The FDA stated in an issue of FDA Drug Bulletin, "Accepted medical practice often includes drug use that is not reflected in approved drug labeling."[4] And in Chaney vs. Heckler, the court stated, "Congress would have created havoc in the medical profession had it required physicians to follow the expensive and time-consuming

procedure of obtaining FDA approval before putting drugs to new uses."[5]) These pronouncements also should apply to the practice of dentistry, although the FDA has not made any specific statements to that effect.

Determining Liability in Malpractice Cases

Although FDA does not regulate the prescription by doctors of FDA-approved drugs, doctors are subject to civil liability for their actions. Thus, while it is not uncommon for doctors to prescribe approved drugs for unapproved purposes, in doing so they take upon themselves the burden of justifying their actions and assume potential liability if a mistake is made. In a typical dental or medical malpractice case, the plaintiff must prove these elements[6]:

- the existence of a duty, created by a doctor-patient relationship between the plaintiff and defendant;
- evidence of the standard of care owed by the defendant doctor to the plaintiff;
- evidence that the standard of care was violated or breached;
- proof that the breach of the standard of care was the proximate cause of the plaintiff's injury.

Generally, the standard of care in a malpractice case must be established through the use of expert testimony. The rationale for this rule is that laypeople (in other words, jurors) cannot comprehend technical information without expert assistance.[7-9]

Courts have relied heavily on FDA-approved uses for approved drugs as evidence of the standard of care. In a malpractice action involving administration of a drug, some courts have gone so far as to hold that a drug manufacturer's clear and explicit instructions regarding the proper manner of administering a drug, accompanied by specific warnings of the hazards encountered in its improper administrations, are prima facie evidence of the standard of care. Under these decisions, no expert testimony is needed for the plaintiff to show the standard of care.

For example, in Haught vs. Maceluch,[10] the Physicians Desk Reference (PDR), which publishes drug manufacturers' instructions and package inserts, was cited as independent evidence of the medical standard for the administration of the drug oxytocin (Pitocin). This drug induces or augments labor. In the Haught case, the plaintiff claimed the defendant physician was negligent for failing to recognize well-established signs of fetal distress and to take appropriate action, and that the defendant negligently administered Pitocin. At trial, the court accepted evidence directly from the PDR that specifically contraindicated the use of Pitocin when fetal distress is suspected. The court held that the PDR established the standard because the physician ignored two important indicators of fetal distress.

In another case, a physician was found to have ignored the manufacturer's instructions for the intravenous injection of promazine hydrochloride (Sparine), as well as the warnings about complications that would arise from its improper administration.[11] The court relied directly on the FDA-approved manufacturer's instructions as evidence of the standard of care. The court held that where a drug manufacturer recommends to the medical profession the conditions under which its drug should be prescribed, the disorders it is designed to relieve, and the precautionary measures that should be observed and warns of the dangers inherent in its use, a doctor's deviation from such recommendations is prima facie evidence of negligence.[11,12] This evidence creates a reputable presumption that the doctor acted negligently and requires the doctor to come forward at trial with evidence as to why he or she was not negligent in deviating from the instructions.

Is it sufficient to follow manufacturer's instructions?

These cases represent an extreme view. Other cases, even from the same jurisdictions as the cases discussed above, have been careful to require that the manufacturer's instructions be absolutely clear and explicit before the courts will presume negligence. In Young vs. Cerniak,[13] for example, the defendant physicians were accused of deviating from the standard of care in failing to administer a proper dosage of the anticoagulant heparin. The plaintiff had an expert witness who relied at trial not on the manufacturer's instructions about the appropriate dosage, but on texts and treatises of experts in the field. The manufacturer's instructions were not, in the appellate court's opinion, explicit about the proper dosage and method of administration of the drug, and did not contain warnings about undesirable results if the physician deviated from the precise instructions. Moreover, the defendant physicians' experts testified that the manufacturer's recommendations contained one acceptable procedure for determining dosage, but the defendants followed an equally acceptable alternative method. The appellate court held that the manufacturer's instructions were not evidence of the standard of care, and the trial court had erred by telling the jury that the drug company's recommendations were a standard against which defendant's conduct was to be measured.

Similarly, in Nicolla vs. Fasulo,[14] an oral surgeon was sued for injuries allegedly resulting from his prescribing the drug oxycodone and acetaminophen (Percodan). The plaintiff asked the court to instruct the jury that the defendant would be prima facie negligent if the defendant deviated from the manufacturer's recommendations contained in the PDR. The appellate court held that the trial judge acted appropriately by refusing the request, because there was no clear and explicit contraindication or warning about Percodan in the PDR from which the defendant deviated.

Product inserts and expert testimony

An even more common approach is to allow product inserts and their parallel PDR references into evidence to show the standard of care, but only if expert testimony is also presented to explain the standard to the jury. This rule was followed in the case of Morlino vs. Medical Center of Ocean County.[15,16] In Morlino, a physician prescribed the antibiotic ciprofloxacin hydrochloride to the plaintiff, who was 8 mo pregnant and suffering from acute pharyngitis. Earlier treatment with another antibiotic had been ineffective. The plaintiff's fetus died 1 day after she ingested the drug. Experts for the plaintiff testified that a reasonable and prudent physician would not have used ciprofloxacin in a pregnant patient and pointed to the explicit warning in the PDR against such use. The defendant physician acknowledged that he was familiar with the PDR warning but produced an expert who testified that the suspected infectious agent (*Haemophilus influenzae*) was much more risky to the mother and the developing fetus than ciprofloxacin. The defendant argued that it was reasonable for him to prescribe ciprofloxacin in these circumstances.

The jury rendered a verdict for the defendant, and the plaintiff appealed. On appeal, the plaintiff argued that the jury should have been allowed to find that the physician was prima facie negligent for deviating from the PDR warning, without reference to conflicting expert testimony. The appellate court disagreed. It reasoned that to have allowed the jury to find that failure to follow the PDR warning alone was negligence would force a physician to follow the PDR directives or automatically suffer the consequences of a malpractice action. The court pointed out the differences between a package insert and accepted medical practice. The former is based on the rigorous proof a regulatory agency demands, the latter on the clinical judgment of a doctor based on the doctor's training, experience and skill and the specific needs of the individual patient. The court (quoting Peter H. Rheinstein, Drug Labeling as Standard for Medical Care, 4 J. Legal Med. 22, 24 [1976]) held that one cannot be taken as a standard for the other.[15]

The cases discussed above deal with the use of FDA-approved drugs for unapproved purposes, or the simple use of drugs in a manner inconsistent with the manufacturer's instructions. There are no reported cases discussing a dentist's use of an ADA-accepted drug. It is logical to assume, however, that if the dentist used the drug in the manner recommended by the manufacturer, the dentist would certainly try to introduce testimony about the product's acceptance by the ADA as evidence of the reasonableness of the dentist's action. When the ADA accepts a dental product, all of the claims made by the manufacturer about the product are also reviewed and approved. In fact, attorneys representing dentists frequently contact the ADA to find out whether a product used by a dentist bears the ADA Seal.

In summary, dentists and physicians may prescribe and use FDA-approved drugs in ways that differ from the uses approved by the FDA. Doctors should always base these decisions on sound professional judgment and should recognize that the decisions may need to be justified if the doctor is accused of malpractice.

Failure to Obtain Adequate Informed Consent

A related issue that needs to be considered is whether a doctor must obtain a special informed consent from a patient if the doctor prescribes an FDA-approved drug for a nonapproved purpose. A doctor's failure to obtain adequate informed consent can form a basis of liability to a patient that is separate and distinct from a negligence claim.

Traditionally, the standard of disclosure has been based on the customary practice of the community. Thus, courts look at what risks of treatment a reasonably prudent doctor would disclose in similar circumstances.[17,18] A more contemporary approach focuses on a lay standard of disclosure. While this approach varies by jurisdiction, courts generally look at what information a reasonable patient would consider material to the decision about whether or not to undergo treatment or diagnosis.[19-23]

The case of Reinhardt vs. Colton[24] is informative on the issue of informed consent in the context of using FDA-approved drugs for unapproved uses. In this case, the plaintiff's physician prescribed the drug penicillamine for the treatment of rheumatoid arthritis. At the time the drug was prescribed for her, it was used by other doctors to treat rheumatoid arthritis, but it was not approved by the FDA for this purpose. Penicillamine has the potential to cause many side effects, including destruction of the capacity to make red blood cells, which causes aplastic anemia. The plaintiff developed aplastic anemia after using penicillamine and brought suit against her physician.

One of the theories on which she based her lawsuit was a theory of "negligent nondisclosure of risk." Under this theory (a contemporary version of lack of informed consent), the plaintiff was required to prove that the physician had a duty to know of a risk or alternative treatment plan, that the physician had a duty to disclose the risk or alternative, that the duty was breached and that the plaintiff was harmed because of the nondisclosure of the risk. The standard used to judge the duty to disclose was based on the significance that a reasonable person in the plaintiff's position would have attached to the risk or the alternative in deciding whether to consent to treatment.

At trial, there was conflicting testimony about whether the plaintiff was informed that the use of penicillamine for rheumatoid arthritis was not approved by the FDA. However, the important testimony was the doctor's own statement about the risks of aplastic anemia associated with using the drug, the wide recognition of this risk in the medical community and other testimony about whether the patient had been sufficiently warned about this risk. The court held that this testimony was sufficient to create an issue that had to be decided by the jury.

The case shows that standard principles of informed consent, just like standard principles of negligence, govern the doctor's treatment decisions. It may not be necessary always to disclose whether a particular drug or device has been approved by the FDA. The overall analysis will focus on the total circumstances, as well as on whether the doctor acted within the applicable standard of care and informed the patient of risks and alternatives in a manner consistent with the standard applicable in the doctor's jurisdiction.

Use of Drugs Not Approved by the FDA

As discussed in the previous section, the FDA does not generally have jurisdiction over the practice of dentistry or medicine. Therefore, the FDA cannot, as a general rule, take action against a dentist or physician who prescribes drugs that do not have FDA approval.

Pharmacy as Manufacturer

An exception to this general principle arises if a dentist or physician places bulk orders from a pharmacy for unapproved prescription drugs. In this situation, the doctor may not be exempt from regulation by the FDA. For example, the FDA has stated that the dental drug called Sargenti Paste, Sargenti Compound, or N2 is an unapproved new drug (letter from Carl C. Peck, M.D., director, Center for Drug Evaluation and Research, Food and Drug Administration, to Newell Yaple, D.D.S., secretary, Ohio State Dental Board, Aug. 12, 1991).[25] Single prescriptions for individual patients may be lawfully prepared by pharmacies according to the Food, Drug, and Cosmetic Act, but bulk shipments by pharmacists to dentists are not permitted. The maximum amount of the formulation that the FDA permits to be dispensed is five grams (letter from Carl C. Peck, M.D., to Newell Yaple, D.D.S., Aug. 12, 1991). Conceivably, the FDA could take enforcement action against a dentist who ordered Sargenti Paste in bulk from a pharmacy.

A note about the above situation: Under the "pharmacy" exception to the Act, pharmacies are exempt from regulation under the act if they are regularly engaged in dispensing prescription drugs or devices, on prescriptions of practitioners licensed to administer such drugs or devices to patients under the care of such practitioners in the course of their professional practice, and if they do not manufacture, prepare, propagate, compound, or process drugs or devices for sale other than in the regular course of their business of dispensing or selling drugs or devices at retail. On the other hand, where a pharmacy compounds drugs in bulk, and sells them at wholesale prices with nationwide distribution, the pharmacy becomes a "manufacturer" under the act and is subject to FDA regulation. Relevant factors used to determine whether a pharmacy qualifies for the "pharmacy" exception to the Act are

- whether particular drugs are being compounded on a regular basis, as opposed to periodic compounding of different drugs,
- whether drugs are being compounded primarily for individual patient prescriptions as opposed to orders contemplating larger amounts for office use,
- the geographic area of distribution,
- whether any form of advertising or promotion is being used,
- the percentage of gross income received from sales of particular compounded drugs, and
- whether particular compounded drugs are being offered at wholesale prices.[26]

A dentist's use of non–FDA-approved drugs could conceivably also be limited by state law or by rules issued by a state licensing board. Some years ago, the Ohio State Dental Board considered a rule that would have prohibited dentists in that state from using any drug or medication not approved by the FDA in the treatment of patients. The rule was not adopted.

Use of Drugs Not Accepted by the ADA

The American Dental Association does not require its members to use only products that bear the ADA Seal of Acceptance. This policy reflects the voluntary nature of the ADA's Seal Program.

While the Seal is an important indicator that a product meets ADA guidelines for safety and efficacy, the fact that a product has not been evaluated by the ADA Council on Scientific Affairs does not necessarily mean the product is unsafe or ineffective. Therefore, while a dentist may rely on the existence of the Seal as an indicator of safety and efficacy, lack of the Seal should not be used to create any presumptions about the safety or efficacy of the unaccepted product.

Unproven Reliability and Effectiveness

Potential civil liability in a malpractice suit remains the most significant legal consequence of using a non–FDA-approved drug. In this area of inquiry, the existence of informed consent can be crucial, but will not always be enough to protect a doctor from later claims of negligence. Another crucial fact is whether alternative drugs of known effectiveness and proven reliability were available. In some cases, the outcome seems to depend upon the apparent egregiousness of the doctor's conduct.

The case of Sullivan vs. Henry illustrates the problems that can arise when a doctor prescribes a non–FDA-approved drug.[27] Sullivan involved a general physician who diagnosed his patient with cancer, determined it could not be treated with conventional cancer therapies and suggested that the patient try amygdalin (Laetrile). Use of Laetrile was not approved by the FDA except for investigational use by experts qualified by scientific training and experience to investigate the safety and efficacy of the drug. The doctor in this case was not participating in such an investigation.

The patient was informed about the

experimental nature of her treatment with Laetrile and knew that the drug was not approved by the FDA. The key issue was whether the physician acted negligently in choosing this course of treatment. The defendant asserted that he should win as a matter of law because he acted reasonably and within the standard of care. In opposition to that claim, the plaintiffs (the patient's family) produced affidavits from expert witnesses stating that Laetrile was not listed in the PDR, was a known poison with no known benefits and was unsafe at any dosage. Another expert for the plaintiffs expressed the opinion that the defendant doctor did not fully explore the nature of the patient's malignancy. This raised questions about the doctor's conclusion that conventional cancer therapies, such as chemotherapy and radiotherapy, were not suitable for this patient's cancer. These facts created a jury question as to whether the defendant was negligent.

It is interesting to note that the plaintiffs' expert in Sullivan focused on the potential that experimental treatment was unnecessary. Failure to prescribe a drug of known effectiveness and proven reliability, which could have been used instead of a non–FDA-approved drug, may constitute a breach of the standard of care. This occurred in Blanton vs. U.S.,[28] in which the plaintiff was asked to participate in an experiment to test whether the drug $Rh_0(D)$ immune globulin (HypRho-D) had effectiveness beyond its FDA-approved shelf life. The plaintiff, a hospital patient, refused to participate in the experiment, but she received the drug anyway by mistake.

The court noted that this was not a simple case of the plaintiff receiving one drug that was inaccurately represented as another. Rather, the drug was in effect a "new drug" that was not FDA-approved, and "it was administered despite the availability of a drug of known effectiveness and proven reliability." The court held that the hospital, by administering the drug to plaintiff without her consent, violated "accepted medical standards."[28 (at 362)] While this case involved a hospital's conduct, not that of a physician or dentist, the rationale could be extended to a health professional as well.

Duty of Disclosure

In truly egregious cases, courts may look beyond a negligence theory to impose liability on doctors who act improperly in prescribing non–FDA-approved therapies. For example, in Nelson vs. Gaunt, the plaintiff received from the defendant a series of silicone injections for breast augmentation.[29] The uncontested evidence showed that at the time the plaintiff received the injections, the FDA considered silicone injections dangerous for use in human body tissues, and only persons who obtained a special permit to administer the injections under scientific circumstances could use silicone for this purpose. The defendant physician not only had no such permit, but he told the plaintiff that the substance was safe, inert and had absolutely no side effects. He did not tell her the name of the substance, the fact that it could be used only for the purposes of scientific research, that even under those conditions its use required state or federal approval, and that he did not have a permit to perform the injections.

These facts, the court found, went beyond an ordinary negligence theory and even beyond a claim of battery, which would exist if, for example, a doctor performed an operation without the patient's consent. The theory applicable on these facts was fraud, based on the physician's fiduciary duty to disclose information to the patient that may be relevant to a meaningful decision-making process and necessary to form the basis of an intelligent consent by the patient to the proposed treatment. In this case, the court found, the doctor provided the patient with false and misleading information and knowingly concealed information that was material to the cause of the plaintiff's injuries.[29 (at Cal Rptr 174)]

The fact that a doctor is participating in an FDA-approved clinical investigation is not in itself sufficient to protect the doctor from claims of negligence. In a case involving use of a medical device, Daum vs. Spinecare Medical Group, Inc.,[30] a physician was required to defend himself against the charge that he failed to obtain the patient's informed consent to use the investigational device—a metal screw—in spinal fusion surgery. Applicable federal and state laws incorporated in the manufacturer's protocol for clinical trials required that patients be informed of the device's investigational status, give written consent to participate in the trial and be provided with a copy of their consent form.

The patient claimed that he was not told that the device was investigational or provided with the consent form until he was sedated and on a gurney being wheeled to the operating room; this raised an issue of whether the patient's consent was truly informed. However, the immediate question for the appellate court was whether the jury could find that simple failure to comply with the rules for conduct of the clinical trial, including the rule on informed consent, was negligence per se. The court held that it could, reasoning that the physician was not required to participate in the clinical trials but that once he did, he was required to abide by its rules. The jury was entitled to consider the physician's failure to comply with the rules on informed consent as evidence of negligence per se, shifting to the physician the burden of proving that he did what might reasonably be expected of a person of ordinary prudence, acting under similar circumstances who desired to comply with the law. There is no reason to believe that the court would not apply the same rule to a new drug.

Conclusion

Dentists, in using drugs in their practices, need to be cognizant of the status of those agents within the FDA and the ADA. However, the more important concern is to exercise sound professional judgment in making choices and to be sure that patients are fully cognizant of material information concerning their treatments and the alternatives available to them.

1. Wakeen LM. Legal implications of using drugs and devices in the dental office. J Public Health Dent 1992;52(6):403-8.
2. See 21 U.S.C.A. §360(g) (West 1972 and Supp. 1997).
3. See also 21 CFR Part 130, Legal Status of Approved Labeling for Prescription Drugs; Prescribing for Uses Unapproved by the Food and Drug Administration, Aug. 15, 1972.
4. See also "Use of Approved Drugs for Unlabeled Indications," 12 FDA Drug Bulletin 4 (April 1982).
5. See also Chaney vs. Heckler, 718 F.2d 1174, 1180 (D.C. App. 1983), rev'd on other grounds, 470 U.S. 821 (1985).
6. See, e.g., Winkjer vs. Herr, 277 N.W.2d 579, 583 (N.D. 1979).
7. See, e.g., Blackwell vs. Hurst, 46 Cal.App.4th 939, 942 (Cal. App. 1996).
8. See, e.g., Rallings vs. Evans, 930 S.W.2d 259, 262 (Texas Ct. App. 1996).
9. See, e.g., Ellis vs. Oliver, 323 S.C. 121, 125 (1996).
10. Haught vs. Maceluch, 681 F.2d 291 (5th Cir. 1982).
11. Ohligschlager vs. Proctor Community Hospital, 303 N.E.2d 392 (Ill. 1973).
12. See also Mulder vs. Parke Davis & Company, 181 N.W.2d 882 (Minn. 1970).
13. See Young vs. Cerniak, 467 N.E.2d 1045 (Ill. App. 1984).
14. See Nicolla vs. Fasulo, 557 N.Y.S.2d 539 (App. Div. 1990).
15. Morlino vs. Medical Center of Ocean County, 295 N.J.Super. 113, 122 (1996).
16. See also Ramon vs. Farr, 770 P.2d 131 (Utah 1989).
17. See, e.g., Ross vs. Hodges, 234 So.2d 905 (Miss. 1970).
18. See, e.g., Aiken vs. Clary, 396 S.W.2d 668 (Mo. 1965).
19. See, e.g., Cobbs vs. Grant, 502 P.2d 1 (Cal. 1972).
20. See, e.g., Wilkinson vs. Vesey, 295 A.2d 676 (R.I. 1972).
21. See also Pa. Stat. Ann. Tit. 40, §1301.103 (Purdon Supp. 1997).
22. See also R.I. Gen. Laws §9-19-32 (1996).
23. See also Wash. Rev. Code Ann.§7.70.050(1)(c) (West Supp. 1997).
24. Reinhardt vs. Colton, 337 N.W.2d 88 (Minn. 1983).
25. See 21 U.S.C. §360(g)(1).
26. See Cedars North Towers Pharmacy, Inc. vs. United States of America, 824 CCH Food-Drug-Cosmetics Law Reporter par 38,200 (S.D.Fla. 1978).
27. Sullivan vs. Henry, 287 S.E.2d 652 (Ga.App. 1982).
28. Blanton vs. United States, 428 F.Supp. 360 (D.D.C. 1977).
29. Nelson vs. Gaunt, 125 Cal.App.3d 623 (1981).
30. Daum vs. Spinecare Medical Group, Inc., 52 Cal. App.4th 1285 (Cal.App.1997).

Appendixes

U.S. and Canadian Schedules for Controlled Substances

U.S. Classifications

Schedule	Definition
I	No recognized legal medical use; used in research with appropriate registration
II	Most stringent classification for drugs; these drugs have legitimate medical use and very high abuse potential; inventory and distribution are tightly controlled; prescriptions not refillable
III	Significant abuse potential, but less than Schedule II; up to 5 authorized refills within 6 months
IV	Abuse potential lower than Schedule III; up to 5 authorized refills within 6 months
V	Lowest abuse potential; prescriber may authorize as many refills as desired; some drugs in this class may be available without a prescription

Canadian Classifications

Schedule	Definition
N (Narcotics)	Products containing narcotics; depending on the preparation, may be subject to strict or lesser regulatory controls
C (Controlled Drugs, Controlled Drugs Preparations)	Non-narcotic preparations with abuse potential (includes schedules E, F, G, H); depending on content, various regulatory controls apply

Schedules for Controlled Substances

Drug	United States	Canada
Heroin, LSD, peyote, marijuana, mescaline, phencyclidine	Schedule I (CI)	Schedule H
Opium, fentanyl, morphine, meperidine, methadone, oxycodone (and combinations), hydromorphone, codeine (single-drug entity), cocaine	Schedule II (CII)	Schedule N
Short-acting barbiturates	Schedule II	Schedule C
Amphetamine, methylphenidate	Schedule II	Schedule G
Codeine combinations, hydrocodone combinations, glutethimide, paregoric, phendimetrazine, thiopental, testosterone, other androgens	Schedule III (CIII)	Schedule F
Benzodiazepines (e.g., diazepam, midazolam), chloral hydrate, meprobamate, phenobarbital, propoxyphene (and combinations), pentazocine (and combinations), methohexital	Schedule IV (CIV)	Schedule F
Antidiarrrheals and antitussives with opioid derivatives	Schedule V (CV)	

U.S. Food and Drug Administration Pregnancy Classifications

Classification	Definition
A	No risk demonstrated to the fetus in any trimester
B	No adverse effects in animals; no human studies available
C	Only given after risks to the fetus are considered; animal studies have shown adverse reactions; no human studies available
D	Definite fetal risks; may be given in spite of risks if needed in life-threatening situations
X	Absolute fetal abnormalities; not to be used at any time during pregnancy

Appendix C.

Teratogens and Toxicological Agents That Affect the Fetus

Angelo J. Mariotti, D.D.S., Ph.D.

A teratogen is a drug or chemical that induces alterations in the formation of cells, tissues and organs and thus creates physical defects in a developing embryo or fetus. Teratogens act via a number of diverse mechanisms to ultimately damage the developing fetus. Drug-induced teratogenic changes can occur only during organogenesis; however, drug-induced toxicological changes affect the fetus after completion of tissue or organ formation because these drugs induce degenerative changes in formed tissue or organs. Unfortunately, the teratogenic or toxicological potential of many drugs has not been evaluated in utero.

To be safe, drugs that are known to be innocuous to the embryo or fetus should be the drugs of choice in the dental management of pregnant women. Drugs with unknown teratogenic or toxicological potential should be prescribed in consultation with the patient's obstetrician and used sparingly. Drugs with known teratogenic or toxicological effects should not be considered for use during dental procedures.

To aid health care providers, the U.S. Food and Drug Administration has developed a rating system for drugs that affect the fetus. The five categories the FDA uses to evaluate drug effects during pregnancy are shown in Appendix B.

The first list below comprises drugs that require special precautions when used during pregnancy. Many of these drugs are not teratogenic, but the potential side effect of each agent may affect the embryo or fetus; therefore, each drug should be carefully investigated. If you have questions about any drug that might cause problems during pregnancy, contact an obstetrician or the Pregnancy Risk Line (1-801-328-2229) for agencies in your region that deal with potential harmful drugs to pregnant women.

The second list is of drugs that are excreted in breast milk.

Pregnancy Caution Information List

Alprazolam (systemic)	Bupivacaine (parenteral-local)
Amitriptyline (systemic)	Butabarbital, alone and in combinations (systemic)
Amobarbital (systemic)	Butorphanol (systemic)
Aprobarbital (systemic)	Caffeine (systemic)
Ascorbic acid (systemic)	Calcium carbonate (oral-local)
Aspirin, alone and in combination (systemic)	Carbamazepine (systemic)
Atropine (systemic)	Cefoxitin (systemic)

Continued on next page

Chloral hydrate (systemic)

Chloramphenicol (systemic)

Chlordiazepoxide, alone and in combination (systemic)

Ciprofloxacin (ophthalmic)

Clarithromycin (systemic)

Clonazepam (systemic)

Clonidine (systemic)

Clorazepate (systemic)

Clotrimazole

Codeine

Cortisone (systemic)

Cyanocobalamin Co 57 (systemic)

Demeclocycline (systemic)

Desoximetasone

Dexamethasone

Diclofenac (systemic)

Diflunisal

Epinephrine

Erythromycin estolate

Ethchlorvynol (systemic)

Etidocaine (parenteral-local)

Etodolac (systemic)

Fenoprofen (systemic)

Fentanyl (systemic)

Fluconazole (systemic)

Flurazepam (systemic)

Flurbiprofen (systemic)

Griseofulvin (systemic)

Halazepam (systemic)

Haloperidol (systemic)

Halothane (systemic)

Hydralazine (systemic)

Hydrocodone (systemic)

Hydrocortisone (systemic)

Hydromorphone (systemic)

Hyoscyamine (systemic)

Ibuprofen (systemic)

Indomethacin (systemic)

Iodine (topical)

Ketazolam (systemic)

Ketoprofen (systemic)

Ketorolac (systemic)

Labetalol (systemic)

Lidocaine (parenteral-local)

Lorazepam (systemic)

Meclizine (systemic)

Meclofenamate (systemic)

Mefenamic acid (systemic)

Meperidine (systemic)

Methadone (systemic)

Metronidazole (systemic)

Miconazole (vaginal)

Minocycline (systemic)

Morphine (systemic)

Naproxen (systemic)

Neomycin (oral-local)

Nicotine (systemic)

Nitrous oxide (systemic)

Norfloxacin (systemic)

Ofloxacin (ophthalmic)

Orphenadrine, aspirin and caffeine (systemic)

Oxazepam (systemic)

Oxycodone (systemic)

Oxytetracycline (systemic)

Paregoric (systemic)

Penbutolol (systemic)

Pentazocine (systemic)

Phenobarbital (systemic)

Phenylbutazone (systemic)

Prednisone (systemic)

Procaine (parenteral-local)

Promazine (systemic)

Promethazine (systemic)

Propoxyphene (systemic)

Pseudoephedrine (systemic)

Rifampin (systemic)

Salicylic acid (topical)

Salsalate (systemic)

Secobarbital (systemic)

Sufentanil (systemic)

Sulindac (systemic)

Tetracaine (parenteral-local)

Tetracycline (systemic)

Triamcinolone (systemic)

Triazolam (systemic)

Vitamin A (systemic)

Source: United States Pharmacopeial Convention, Inc. Drug information for the health care professional. Vol. I. 1995: Rockville, Md.: United States Pharmacopeial Convention, Inc.; 1995:3027-32.

Drugs Excreted in Breast Milk

Ampicillin	Meperidine
Antihistamines*	Meprobamate
Aspirin	Methacycline
Atropine	Methadone
Barbiturates	Morphine
Cephalexin*	Narcotics
Cephalothin*	Oxacillin*
Chloral hydrate	Penicillins*
Chloramphenicol	Pentazocine*
Codeine	Phenobarbital
Corticosteroids	Propantheline bromide*
Demeclocycline*	Propoxyphene
Diazepam	Salicylates
Diphenhydramine*	Scopolamine*
Erythromycin*	Streptomycin
Fluorides*	Tetracyclines*
Lincomycin*	Thiopental sodium*

No adverse effects reported.

Prevention of Bacterial Endocarditis

Prevention of Bacterial Endocarditis: A Statement for the Dental Profession

ADA Council on Scientific Affairs

The new American Heart Association (AHA) recommendations for the prevention of bacterial endocarditis represent a substantial departure from past guidelines. The new recommendations reflect a better understanding of the disease and its potential prevention. Major changes involve the indications for prophylaxis, antibiotic choice and dosing, ancillary procedures that may reduce bacteremic risk, a detailed discussion of mitral valve prolapse and greater attention to the medicolegal aspects of endocarditis.

Previously, antibiotic prophylaxis was suggested for dental procedures associated with any amount of bleeding. Now, only those that are associated with significant bleeding are recommended for prophylaxis as dictated by clinical judgment. This allows for a substantial number of dental procedures to be eliminated from the prophylaxis recommendation. A table is provided that delineates dental treatment procedures into those that may be associated with significant bleeding and those that pose negligible or no bacteremic risk. Recommended antibiotic prophylaxis regimens now consist of a single preprocedural dose; no second dose

is recommended. If the clinical decision is made not to premedicate and significant unanticipated bleeding occurs, the dental professional may then begin the antibiotic and continue the procedure. A gentle prerinse with chlorhexidine can be employed, but gingival (subgingival) irrigation is not recommended due to conflicting data on efficacy in bacteremia reduction, the lack of data establishing that gingival irrigation will reduce endocarditis, its own potential for causing bacteremias and the lack of any standardized regimen.

It is recommended that all identified at-risk patients be strongly encouraged to maintain good oral health via professional and home care and plaque control procedures. This is particularly true for patients prior to cardiovascular surgical procedures. It is acknowledged that plaque control may induce bacteremias, but with much less or negligible risk as compared to a mouth with ongoing inflammation. The recommendations identify at-risk patients both medically and dentally.

Importantly, the medicolegal aspects of bacterial endocarditis are thoroughly addressed in the new recommendations, particularly regarding causation. The incubation period for most cases of endocarditis is defined, as are several factors that must be considered before attempting to attribute cause and effect to a given invasive procedure. It is acknowledged that most endocarditis is not associated with invasive procedures and that professional dental care is responsible for only a small percentage of endocarditis cases. However, antibiotic prophylaxis is still recommended prior to dental procedures associated with significant bleeding in high- and moderate-risk patients who are at a much greater risk of endocarditis than the general population. These recommendations are not intended as the standard of care, and practitioners should use their own clinical judgment in individual cases or special circumstances.

The new AHA recommendations for the prevention of bacterial endocarditis better define at-risk patients and the dental procedures to be covered by antibiotic prophylaxis. As a result, these new recommendations should aid in both patient and practitioner compliance, and diminish the adverse effects of prophylaxis including its role in promoting the development of microbial antibiotic resistance.

Prevention of Bacterial Endocarditis: Recommendations by the American Heart Association

The following tables are reprinted with permission of the publisher from Dajani AS, Taubert KA, Wilson W, et al. Prevention of Bacterial Endocarditis: Recommendations by the American Heart Association. JAMA 1997; 277:1794-801.

Cardiac Conditions Associated With Endocarditis.[1-21]

Endocarditis Prophylaxis Recommended
High-risk category

Prosthetic cardiac valves, including bioprosthetic and homograft valves

Previous bacterial endocarditis

Complex cyanotic congenital heart disease (e.g., single ventricle states, transposition of the great arteries, tetralogy of Fallot)

Surgically constructed systemic pulmonary shunts or conduits

Moderate-risk category

Most other congenital cardiac malformations (other than above and below)

Acquired valvar dysfunction (e.g., rheumatic heart disease)

Hypertrophic cardiomyopathy

Mitral valve prolapse with valvar regurgitation and/or thickened leaflets

Endocarditis Prophylaxis Not Recommended
Negligible-risk category (no greater than the general population)

Isolated secundum atrial septal defect

Surgical repair of atrial septal defect, ventricular septal defect, or patent ductus arteriosus (without residua beyond 6 mo)

Previous coronary artery bypass graft surgery

Mitral valve prolapse without valvar regurgitation

Physiologic, functional or innocent heart murmurs

Continued on next page

Cardiac Conditions Associated With Endocarditis[1-21] (cont.)

Endocarditis Prophylaxis Not Recommended (cont.)

Previous Kawasaki disease without valvar dysfunction

Previous rheumatic fever without valvar dysfunction

Cardiac pacemakers (intravascular and epicardial) and implanted defibrillators

1. Steckelberg JM, Wilson WR. Risk factors for infective endocarditis. Infect Dis Clin North Am. 1993;7:9-19.
2. Saiman L, Prince A, Gersony WM. Pediatric infective endocarditis in the modern era. J Pediatr. 1993;122:847-853.
3. Gersony WM, Hayes CJ, Driscoll DJ, et al. Bacterial endocarditis in patients with aortic stenosis, pulmonary stenosis, or ventricular septal defect. Circulation. 1993;87(suppl I):121-126.
4. Prabhu SD, O'Rourke RA. Mitral valve prolapse. In: Braunwald E, series ed, Rahimtoola SH, volume ed. *Atlas of Heart Diseases: Valvular Heart Disease Vol XI.* St. Louis, Mo: Mosby-Year Book Inc;1997:10.1-10.18.
5. Boudoulas H, Wooley CF. Mitral valve prolapse. In: Emmanouilides GC, Riemenschneider TA, Allen HD, Gutgesell HP, eds. *Moss and Adams Heart Disease in Infants, Children, and Adolescents Including the Fetus and Young Adult.* 5th ed. Baltimore, Md: Williams & Wilkins; 1995; 1063-1086.
6. Carabello BA. Mitral valve disease. Curr Probl Cardiol. 1993;7:423-478.
7. Devereux RB, Hawkins I, Kramer-Fox R, et al. Complications of mitral valve prolapse: disproportionate occurrence in men and older patients. Am J Med. 1986; 81:751-758.
8. Danchin N, Briancon S, Mathieu P, et al. Mitral valve prolapse as a risk factor for infective endocarditis. Lancet. 1989;1:743-745.
9. MacMahon SW, Roberts JK, Kramer-Fox R, et al. Mitral valve prolapse and infective endocarditis. Am Heart J. 1987;113:1291-1298.
10. Marks AR, Choong CY, Sanfilippo AJ, Ferre M, Weyman AE. Identification of high-risk and low-risk subgroups of patients with mitral-valve prolapse. N Engl J Med. 1989;320:1031-1036.
11. Devereux RB, Frary CJ, Kramer-Fox R, Roberts RB, Ruchlin HS. Cost-effectiveness of infective endocarditis prophylaxis for mitral valve prolapse with or without a mitral regurgitant murmur. Am J Cardiol. 1994;74:1024-1029.
12. Zuppiroli A, Rinaldi M, Kramer-Fox R, Favili S, Roman MJ, Devereux RB. Natural history of mitral valve prolapse. Am J Cardiol. 1995;75:1028-1032.
13. Wooley CF, Baker PB, Kolibash AJ, et al. The floppy, myxomatous mitral valve, mitral valve prolapse, and mitral regurgitation. Prog Cardiovasc Dis. 1991;33:397-433.
14. Morales AR, Romanelli R, Boucek RJ, Tate LG, Alvarez RT, Davis JT. Myxoid heart disease: an assessment of extravalvular cardiac pathology in severe mitral valve prolapse. Human Pathol. 1992;23:129-137.
15. Weissman NJ, Pini R, Roman MJ, Kramer-Fox R, Andersen HS, Devereux RB. In vivo mitral alve morphology and motion in mitral valve proplapse. Am J Cardiol. 1994;73:1080-1088.
16. Nishimura RA, McGoon MD, Shub C, et al. Echocardiographically documented mitral-valve prolapse. N Engl J Med. 1985;313:1305-1309.
17. McKinsey DS, Ratts TE, Bisno AL. Underlying cardiac lesions in adults with infective endocarditis. Am J Med. 1987;82:681-688.
18. Devereux RB, Kramer-Fox R, Kligfield P. Mitral valve prolapse: causes, clinical manifestations, and management. Ann Intern Med. 1989;111:305-317.
19. Stoddard MF, Prince CR, Dillon S, Longaker RA, Morris GT, Liddell NE. Exercise-induced mitral regurgitation is a predictor of morbid events in subjects with mitral valve prolapse. J Am Coll Cardiol. 1995;25:693-699.
20. Awadallah SM, Kavey REW, Byrum CJ, Smith FC, Kveselis DA, Blackman MS. The changing pattern of infective endocarditis in childhood. Am J Cardiol. 1991;68:90-94.
21. Durack DT. Prevention of infective endocarditis. N Engl J Med 1995;332:38-44.

Reprinted with permission of the publisher from Dajani AS, Taubert KA, Wilson W, et al. Prevention of Bacterial Endocarditis: Recommendations by the American Heart Association. JAMA 1997;277:1794-801.

Dental Procedures and Endocarditis Prophylaxis.[1-4]

Endocarditis Prophylaxis Recommended*

Dental extractions

Periodontal procedures including surgery, scaling and root planing, probing and recall maintenance

Dental implant placement and reimplantation of avulsed teeth

Endodontic (root canal) instrumentation or surgery only beyond the apex

Subgingival placement of antibiotic fibers or strips

Initial placement of orthodontic bands but not brackets

Intraligamentary local anesthetic injections

Prophylactic cleaning of teeth or implants where bleeding is anticipated

Endocarditis Prophylaxis Not Recommended

Restorative dentistry† (operative and prosthodontic) with or without retraction cord‡

Local anesthetic injections (nonintraligamentary)

Intracanal endodontic treatment; post placement and buildup

Placement of rubber dams

Postoperative suture removal

Placement of removable prosthodontic or orthodontic appliances

Taking of oral impressions

Fluoride treatments

Taking of oral radiographs

Orthodontic appliance adjustment

Shedding of primary teeth

Prophylaxis is recommended for patients with high- and moderate-risk cardiac conditions.
† This includes restoration of decayed teeth (filling cavities) and replacement of missing teeth.
‡ Clinical judgment may indicate antibiotic use in selected circumstances that may create significant bleeding.

1. Durack DT. Prevention of infective endocarditis. N Engl J Med 1995;332:38-44.
2. Pallasch TJ, Slots J. Antibiotic prophylaxis and the medically compromised patient. Periodontol 2000. 1996;10:107-138.
3. Bender IB, Naidorf IJ, Garvey GJ. Bacterial endocarditis: a consideration for physicians and dentists. J Am Dent Assoc. 1984;109:415-420.
4. Guntheroth WG. How important are dental procedures as a cause of infective endocarditis? Am J Cardiol. 1984;54:797-801.

Reprinted with permission of the publisher from Dajani AS, Taubert KA, Wilson W, et al. Prevention of Bacterial Endocarditis: Recommendations by the American Heart Association. JAMA 1997;277:1794-801.

Prophylactic Regimens for Dental, Oral, Respiratory Tract, or Esophageal Procedures.[1-4]

Situation	Agent	Regimen*
Standard general prophylaxis	Amoxicillin	**Adults:** 2.0 g **Children:** 50 mg/kg orally 1 hour before procedure
Unable to take oral medications	Ampicillin	**Adults:** 2.0 g intramuscularly (IM) or intravenously (IV) **Children:** 50 mg/kg IM or IV within 30 minutes before procedure
Allergic to penicillin	Clindamycin OR	**Adults:** 600 mg **Children:** 20 mg/kg orally 1 hour before procedure
	Cephalexin† or cefadroxil† OR	**Adults:** 2.0 g **Children:** 50 mg/kg orally 1 hour before procedure
	Azithromycin or clarithromycin	**Adults:** 500 mg **Children:** 15 mg/kg orally 1 hour before procedure
Allergic to penicillin and unable to take oral medications	Clindamycin OR	**Adults:** 600 mg **Children:** 20 mg/kg IV within 30 minutes before procedure
	Cefazolin†	**Adults:** 1.0 g **Children:** 25 mg/kg IM or IV within 30 minutes before procedure

* Total children's dose should not exceed adult dose.
† Cephalosporins should not be used in individuals with immediate-type hypersensitivity reaction (urticaria, angioedema, or anaphylaxis) to penicillins.

1. Dajani AS, Bisno AL, Chung KJ, et al. Prevention of bacterial endocarditis. JAMA. 1990;264:2919-2922.
2. Durack DT. Prevention of infective endocarditis. N Engl J Med 1995;332:38-44.
3. Dajani AS, Bawdon RE, Berry MC. Oral amoxicillin as prophylaxis for endocarditis: what is the optimal dose? Clin Infect Dis. 1994;18:157-160.
4. Rouse MS, Steckelberg JM, Brandt CM, Patel R, Miro JM, Wilson WR. Efficacy of azithromycin or clarithromycin for the prophylaxis of viridans streptococcal experimental endocarditis. Antimicrob Agents Chemother. In press.

Reprinted with permission of the publisher from Dajani AS, Taubert KA, Wilson W, et al. Prevention of Bacterial Endocarditis: Recommendations by the American Heart Association. JAMA 1997;277:1794-801.

Appendix E.

Antibiotic Prophylaxis for Dental Patients With Total Joint Replacements

Advisory Statement: Antibiotic Prophylaxis for Dental Patients With Total Joint Replacements

American Dental Association; American Academy of Orthopaedic Surgeons

Approximately 450,000 total joint arthroplasties are performed annually in the United States. Deep infections of these total joint replacements usually result in failure of the initial operation and the need for extensive revision. Due to the use of perioperative antibiotic prophylaxis and other technical advances, deep infection occurring in the immediate postoperative period resulting from intraoperative contamination has been markedly reduced in the past 20 years.

Patients who are about to have a total joint arthroplasty should be in good dental health prior to surgery and should be encouraged to seek professional dental care if necessary. Patients who already have had a total joint arthroplasty should perform effective daily oral hygiene procedures to remove plaque (for example, by using manual or powered toothbrushes, interdental cleaners or oral irrigators) to establish and maintain good oral health. The risk of bacteremia is far more substantial in a mouth with ongoing inflammation than in one that is healthy and employing these home oral hygiene devices.[1]

Bacteremias can cause hematogenous seeding of total joint implants, both in the early postoperative period and for many years following implantation.[2] It appears that the most critical period is up to 2 years after joint placement.[3] In addition, bacteremias may occur in the course of normal daily life and concurrently with dental and medical procedures.[4-6] It is likely that many more oral bacteremias are spontaneously induced by daily events than are dental treatment-induced.[6] Presently, no scientific evidence supports the position that antibiotic prophylaxis to prevent hematogenous infections is required prior to dental treatment in patients with total joint prostheses.[1] The risk/benefit[7,8] and cost/effectiveness[7,9] ratios fail to justify the administration of routine antibiotic prophylaxis. The analogy of late prosthetic joint infections with infective endocarditis is invalid, as the anatomy, blood supply, microorganisms and mechanisms of infection are all different.[10]

It is likely that bacteremias associated with acute infection in the oral cavity,[11,12] skin, respiratory, gastrointestinal and urogenital systems and/or other sites can and do cause late implant infection.[12] Any patient with a total joint prothesis with acute orofacial infection should be vigorously treated as any other patient with elimination of the source of the infection (incision and drainage, endodontics, extraction) and appropriate therapeutic antibiotics when indicated.[1,12] Practitioners should maintain a high index of suspicion for any unusual signs and symptoms (such as fever, swelling, pain, joint that is warm to touch) in patients with total joint prostheses.

Antibiotic prophylaxis is not indicated for dental patients with pins, plates and screws, nor is it routinely indicated for most dental patients with total joint replacements. This position agrees with that taken by the ADA Council on Dental Therapeutics[13] and the American Academy of Oral Medicine,[14] and is similar to that taken by of the British Society for Antimicrobial Chemotherapy.[15] There is limited evidence that some immunocompromised patients with total joint replacements

(Box, "Patients at Potential Increased Risk of Hematogenous Total Joint Infection") may be at higher risk for hematogenous infections.[12,16-21] Antibiotic prophylaxis for such patients undergoing dental procedures with a higher bacteremic risk (as defined in the box "Incidence Stratification of Bacteremic Dental Procedures") should be considered using an empirical regimen (Box, "Suggested Antibiotic Prophylaxis Regimens"). In addition, antibiotic prophylaxis may be considered when the higher-risk dental procedures (again, as defined in the box "Incidence Stratification...") are performed on dental patients within 2 years post-implant surgery,[3] on those who have had previous prosthetic joint infections and on those with some other conditions (Box, "Patients at Potential Increased Risk...").

Patients at Potential Increased Risk of Hematogenous Total Joint Infection.*

Immunocompromised/immunosuppressed patients

Inflammatory arthropathies: rheumatoid arthritis, systemic lupus erythematosus

Disease-, drug- or radiation-induced immunosuppression

Other patients

Insulin-dependent (Type 1) diabetes

First 2 years following joint placement

Previous prosthetic joint infections

Malnourishment

Hemophilia

---

* Based on Ching and colleagues,[12] Brause,[16] Murray and colleagues,[17] Poss and colleagues,[18] Jacobson and colleagues,[19] Johnson and Bannister,[20] and Jacobson and colleagues.[21]

Incidence Stratification of Bacteremic Dental Procedures.*

Higher incidence†

Dental extractions

Periodontal procedures including surgery, subgingival placement of antibiotic fibers/strips, scaling and root planing, probing, recall maintenance

Dental implant placement and reimplantation of avulsed teeth

Endodontic (root canal) instrumentation or surgery only beyond the apex

Initial placement of orthodontic bands but not brackets

Intraligamentary local anesthetic injections

Prophylactic cleaning of teeth or implants where bleeding is anticipated

Lower incidence‡

Restorative dentistry§ (operative and prosthodontic) with/without retraction cord**

Local anesthetic injections (nonintraligamentary)

Intracanal endodontic treatment; post placement and buildup

Placement of rubber dam

Postoperative suture removal

Placement of removable prosthodontic/orthodontic appliances

Taking of oral impressions

Fluoride treatments

Taking of oral radiographs

Orthodontic appliance adjustment

Adapted with permission of the publisher from Dajani AS, Taubert KA, Wilson W, et al.[22]
† Prophylaxis should be considered for patients with total joint replacement that meet the criteria in the box "Patients at Potential Increased Risk of Hematogenous Total Joint Infection." No other patients with orthopedic implants should be considered for antibiotic prophylaxis prior to dental treatment/procedures.
‡ Prophylaxis not indicated.
§ This includes restoration of carious (decayed) or missing teeth.
*** Clinical judgment may indicate antibiotic use in selected circumstances that may create significant bleeding.*

Suggested Antibiotic Prophylaxis Regimens.*

Patient type	Regimen
Patients not allergic to penicillin: cephalexin, cephradine or amoxicillin	2 grams orally 1 hour prior to dental procedure
Patients not allergic to penicillin and unable to take oral medications: cefazolin or ampicillin	Cefazolin 1 g or ampicillin 2 g intramuscularly or intravenously 1 hour prior to the procedure
Patients allergic to penicillin: clindamycin	600 milligrams orally 1 hour prior to the dental procedure
Patients allergic to penicillin and unable to take oral medications: clindamycin	600 mg IM/IV 1 hr prior to the procedure

No second doses are recommended for any of these dosing regimens.

Occasionally, a patient with a total joint prosthesis may present to the dentist with a recommendation from his or her physician that is not consistent with these guidelines. This could be due to lack of familiarity with the guidelines or to special considerations about the patient's medical condition that are not known to the dentist. In this situation, the dentist is encouraged to consult with the physician to determine if there are any special considerations that might affect the dentist's decision on whether or not to premedicate, and may wish to share a copy of these guidelines with the physician if appropriate. After this consultation, the dentist may decide to follow the physician's recommendation or, if in the dentist's professional judgment antibiotic prophylaxis is not indicated, may decide to proceed without antibiotic prophylaxis. The dentist is ultimately responsible for making treatment recommendations for his or her patients based on the dentist's professional judgment. Any perceived potential benefit of antibiotic prophylaxis must be weighed against the known risks of antibiotic toxicity; allergy; and development, selection and transmission of microbial resistance.

This statement provides guidelines to supplement practitioners in their clinical judgment regarding antibiotic prophylaxis for dental patients with a total joint prosthesis. It is not intended as the standard of care nor as a substitute for clinical judgment as it is impossible to make recommendations for all conceivable clinical situations in which bacteremias originating from the oral cavity may occur. Practitioners must exercise their own clinical judgment in determining whether or not antibiotic prophylaxis is appropriate. ∎

The ADA/AAOS Expert Panel consisted of Robert H. Fitzgerald Jr., M.D.; Jed J. Jacobson, D.D.S., M.S., M.P.H.; James V. Luck Jr., M.D.; Carl L. Nelson, M.D.; J. Phillip Nelson, M.D.; Douglas R. Osmon, M.D.; and Thomas J. Pallasch, D.D.S. The staff liaisons were Clifford W. Whall Jr., Ph.D., for the ADA, and William W. Tipton Jr., M.D., for the AAOS.

1. Pallasch TJ, Slots J. Antibiotic prophylaxis and the medically compromised patient. Periodontology 2000 1996;10:107-38.
2. Rubin R, Salvati EA, Lewis R. Infected total hip replacement after dental procedures. Oral Surg Oral Med Oral Pathol 1976;41(1):13-23.
3. Hansen AD, Osmon DR, Nelson CL. Prevention of deep prosthetic joint infection. Am J Bone Joint Surg 1996;78-A (3):458-71.
4. Bender IB, Naidorf IJ, Garvey GJ. Bacterial endocarditis: a consideration for physicians and dentists. JADA 1984;109:415-20.
5. Everett ED, Hirschmann JV. Transient bacteremia and endocarditis prophylaxis: a review. Medicine 1977;56:61-77.
6. Guntheroth WG. How important are dental procedures as a cause of infective endocarditis? Am J Cardiol 1984;54:797-801.
7. Jacobsen JJ, Schweitzer SO, DePorter DJ, Lee JJ. Antibiotic prophylaxis for dental patients with joint prostheses? A decision analysis. Int J Technol Assess Health Care 1990;6:569-87.
8. Tsevat J, Durand-Zaleski I, Pauker SG. Cost-effectiveness of antibiotic prophylaxis for dental procedures in patients with artificial joints. Am J Public Health 1989;79:739-43.
9. Norden CW. Prevention of bone and joint infections. Am J Med 1985;78(6B):229-32.
10. McGowan DA. Dentistry and endocarditis. Br Dent J 1990;169:69.
11. Bartzokas CA, Johnson R, Jane M, Martin MV, Pearce PK, Saw Y. Relation between mouth and haematogenous infections in total joint replacement. Br Med J 1994;309:506-8.
12. Ching DWI, Gould IM, Rennie JAN, Gibson PII. Prevention of late haematogenous infection in major prosthetic joints. J Antimicrob Chemother 1989;23:676-80.
13. Council on Dental Therapeutics. Management of Dental patients with prosthetic joints. JADA 1990;121:537-8.
14. Eskinazi D, Rathbun W. Is systematic antimicrobial prophylaxis justified in dental patients with prosthetic joints? Oral Surg Oral Med Oral Pathol 1988;66:430-1.
15. Cawson RA. Antibiotic prophylaxis for dental treatment: for hearts but not for prosthetic joints. Br Dent J 1992;304:933-4.
16. Brause BD. Infections associated with prosthetic joints. Clin Rheum Dis 1986;12:523-35.
17. Murray RP, Bourne MH, Fitzgerald RH Jr. Metachronous infection in patients who have had more than one total joint arthroplasty. J Bone Joint Surg [Am] 1991;73(10):1469-74.

18. Poss R, Thornhill TS, Ewald FC, Thomas WH, Batte NJ, Sledge CB. Factors influencing the incidence and outcome of infection following total joint arthroplasty. Clin Orthop 1984;182:117-26.

19. Jacobson JJ, Millard HD, Plezia R, Blankenship JR. Dental treatment and late prosthetic joint infections. Oral Surg Oral Med Oral Pathol 1986;61:413-17.

20. Johnson DP, Bannister GG. The outcome of infected arthroplasty of the knee. J Bone Joint Surg [Br] 1986;68(2):289-91.

21. Jacobson JJ, Patel B, Asher G, Wooliscroft JO, Schaberg D. Oral *Staphylcoccus* in elderly subjects with rheumatoid arthritis. J Am Geriatr Soc 1997;45:1-5.

22. Dajani AS, Taubert KA, Wilson W, et al. Prevention of bacterial endocarditis: Recommendations by the American Heart Association. From the Committee on Rheumatic Fever, Endocarditis and Kawasaki Disease, Council on Cardiovascular Disease in the Young. JAMA 1997;277:1794-1801. Also in Circulation. July 1, 1997;96 (in press). Copyright © American Medical Association.

A Legal Perspective on Antibiotic Prophylaxis

Kathleen M. Todd, J.D.

The Advisory Statement on Antibiotic Prophylaxis for Dental Patients with Total Joint Replacements reflects growing concern about the development of microbial resistance owing to the inappropriate use of antibiotics and recognizes that there are risks as well as benefits involved in the use of antibiotics. It delineates the limited circumstances in which antibiotic prophylaxis should be considered for dental patients who have had total joint replacements and cautions physicians and dentists to weigh the perceived potential benefits of antibiotic prophylaxis against the known risks of antibiotic toxicity, allergies and the development of microbial resistance.

But what should the dentist do if the patient brings to the appointment a recommendation for premedication from his or her physician with which the dentist disagrees? Should the dentist ignore the physician's rec-ommendation or simply defer to the physician's judgment?

Neither approach is prudent from a risk management perspective. On the one hand, the physician's recommendation may be based on facts about the patient's medical condition that are not known to the dentist. On the other, the physician may not be familiar with this advisory statement or that premedication may be indicated for some dental procedures but not for others. The careful dentist will attempt to ascertain the basis for the physician's recommendation and to acquaint the physician with the reasons why the dentist disagrees. Ideally, consensus can be reached. Most dentists would be uncomfortable with the thought of the physician's testifying in a malpractice suit that the dentist failed to follow the physician's treatment recommendation. However, the dentist who blindly follows the physician's recommendation, even though it conflicts with the dentist's professional judgment, will not be able to defend himself or herself by claiming "the devil made me do it" if the patient sues. The courts recognize that each independent professional is ultimately responsible for his or her own treatment decisions.

The answer to this dilemma may lie in the concept of informed consent, which acknowledges the patient's right to autonomous decision making. Informed consent usually can be relied on to protect from legal liability the practitioner who respects the patient's wishes, as long as the practitioner is acting within the standard of care. However, for informed consent to be legally binding, it is incumbent on the practitioner to inform the patient of all reasonable treatment options and the risks and benefits of each. In the situation in question, the dentist would be prudent to inform the patient when the dentist's treatment recommendations differ from those of the patient's physician and even encourage the patient to discuss the treatment options with his or her physician before making a decision. All discussions with the patient and the patient's physician should be well-documented. Of course, allowing the patient to choose assumes that both the dentist's and the physician's treatment recommendations are acceptable.

Dentists are not obligated to render treatment that they deem not to be in the patient's best interest, simply because the patient requests it. In such circumstances, referral to another practitioner may be the only solution. ■

The above information should not be construed as legal advice or a standard of care. A dentist should always consult his or her own attorney for answers to the dentist's specific legal questions.

The material in this appendix first appeared in the following two sources:

American Dental Association and American Academy of Orthopaedic Surgeons. Advisory statement: antibiotic prophylaxis for dental patients with total joint replacements. JADA 1997;128:1004-7.

Todd K. A legal perspective on antibiotic prophylaxis. JADA 1997;128:1007-8.

Appendix F.

Antibiotic Use in Dentistry

ADA Council on Scientific Affairs

Microbial resistance to antibiotics is increasing at an alarming rate. In the last few years, penicillin resistance in *Streptococcus pneumoniae* has risen from virtually zero to 25-60% of all isolates. Such penicillin resistance is increasing in viridans streptococci, and a significant number of *Prevotella* and *Porphyromonas* isolates exhibit β-lactamase production. Hospital epidemics of vancomycin-aminoglycoside-methicillin–resistant staphylococci and vancomycin-resistant, β-lactamase–producing enterococci contribute significantly to the 150,000 annual deaths in United States hospitals that result from nosocomial septicemias.

The major cause of this public health problem is the use of antibiotics in an inappropriate manner, leading to the selection and dominance of resistant microorganisms and/or the increased transfer of resistance genes from antibiotic-resistant to antibiotic-susceptible microorganisms. Inappropriate antibiotic use includes faulty dosing (too low a dose, too long a duration), wrong choice of antibiotic (microorganisms not likely to be sensitive), improper combination of antibiotics and therapeutic or prophylactic use in unwarranted and unproven clinical situations.

Antibiotics are properly employed only for the management of active infectious disease or the prevention of metastatic infection (such as infective endocarditis) in medically high-risk patients. Antibiotic prophylaxis to prevent medical perioperative surgical infections is documented effective in high-risk surgical procedures (cardiovascular, neurological, orthopedic) when the antibiotics are employed intraoperatively (begun shortly before and terminated shortly after the surgery). The use of antibiotics after routine dental treatment to prevent infection has generally not been proven effective. However, the use of antimicrobial therapy may be of benefit in selective surgical procedures and their postoperative management on an empirical basis, and further research in this area is encouraged.

Dentistry has been relatively conservative with antibiotic use and has likely not contributed greatly to the worldwide problems of antibiotic microbial resistance. Adherence to the above principles of antibiotic use will continue and even improve our record of judicious use of antibiotics. Antibiotics are one of the few kinds of drugs that affect not only a single patient but entire populations of individuals through their collective effects on microbial ecology. Our responsibility lies not only with our own patients but with a world of such patients.

This statement was adopted by the Council on Scientific Affairs in September 1996. It first appeared in ADA Council on Scientific Affairs. Antibiotic use in dentistry. JADA 1997;128:648.

Nitrous Oxide
in the Dental Office

ADA Council on Scientific Affairs;
ADA Council on Dental Practice

The safe use of nitrous oxide in the dental office has been an issue the ADA has monitored for many years. In 1977, an ad hoc committee convened by the Association published a report on the potential health hazards of trace anesthetics in dentistry.[1] Also in 1977, the National Institute of Occupational Safety and Health (NIOSH) reported that, by using several control measures, nitrous oxide levels of approximately 50 parts per million were achievable in dental operatories during routine dental anesthesia/analgesia.[2] A few years later, in 1980, the ADA Council on Dental Materials, Instruments and Equipment recommended that effective scavenging devices be installed and monitoring programs be instituted in dental offices in which nitrous oxide is used, and the council indicated that using these methods or devices would assist in keeping the levels of nitrous oxide at the lowest possible level.[3]

NIOSH continued its activities relating to nitrous oxide concentrations in the dental office and, in 1994, published an alert called "Request for Assistance in Controlling Exposures to Nitrous Oxide During Anesthetic Administration."[4] In the same year, NIOSH also reported on field evaluations and laboratory studies evaluating nitrous oxide scavenging systems and modifications in attempts to achieve the current NIOSH recommended exposure limit of 25 ppm during administra-

tion. NIOSH concluded that nitrous oxide levels may be controlled to about 25 ppm by maintaining leak-free delivery systems and using proper exhaust rates, better-fitting masks and auxiliary exhaust ventilation.[5]

In 1995 the ADA Council on Scientific Affairs convened an expert panel to review scientific literature on nitrous oxide and to revise recommendations on controlling nitrous oxide concentrations in the dental office. What follows is an overview of the conclusions reached by that panel.

Conclusions and Recommendations of the Expert Panel

Nitrous oxide continues to be a valuable agent for the control of pain and anxiety. However, chronic occupational exposure to nitrous oxide in offices not using scavenging systems may be associated with possible deleterious neurological and reproductive effects on dental personnel. Limited studies show that as little as three to five hours per week of unscavenged nitrous oxide exposure could result in adverse reproductive effects. In contrast, in dental offices using nitrous oxide scavenging systems, there has been no evidence of adverse health effects.[6] It is strongly recommended, therefore, that while there is no consensus on a recommended exposure limit to nitrous oxide, appropriate scavenging systems and methods of administration should be adopted. A protocol for controlling nitrous oxide is outlined below.

Recommendations for Controlling Nitrous Oxide Exposure

The expert panel identified a number of recommendations that are important to consider in the safe and effective use of nitrous oxide:

- The dental office should have a properly installed nitrous oxide delivery system. This includes appropriate scavenging equipment with a readily visible and accurate flow meter (or equivalent measuring device), a vacuum pump with the capacity for up to 45 L of air per min per workstation, and a variety of sizes of masks to ensure proper fit for individual patients.
- The vacuum exhaust and ventilation exhaust should be vented to the outside (for example, through the vacuum system) and not in close proximity to fresh-air intake vents.
- The general ventilation should provide good room air mixing.
- Each time the nitrous oxide machine is first turned on and every time a gas cylinder is changed, the pressure connections should be tested for leaks. High-pressure–line connections should be tested for leaks on a quarterly basis. A soap solution may be used to test for leaks. Alternatively, a portable infrared spectrophotometer can be used to diagnose an insidious leak.
- Prior to first daily use, all nitrous oxide equipment (reservoir bag, tubings, mask, connectors) should be inspected for worn parts, cracks, holes or tears. Replace as necessary.
- The mask may then be connected to the tubing and the vacuum pump turned on. All appropriate flow rates (that is, up to 45 L/min or per manufacturer's recommendations) should be verified.
- A properly sized mask should be selected and placed on the patient. A good, comfortable fit should be ensured. The reservoir (breathing) bag should not be over- or underinflated while the patient is breathing oxygen (before administering nitrous oxide).
- The patient should be encouraged to minimize talking and mouth breathing while the mask is in place.
- During administration, the reservoir bag should be periodically inspected for changes in tidal volume and the vacuum flow rate should be verified.
- On completing administration, 100% oxygen should be delivered to the patient for 5 min before removing the mask. In this way, both the patient and the system will be purged of residual nitrous oxide. Do not use an oxygen flush.
- Periodic (semiannual interval is suggested) personal sampling of dental personnel, with emphasis to chairside personnel exposed to nitrous oxide, should be conducted (for example, use of diffusive sampler [dosimeters] or infrared spectrophotometer).

Research Priorities

The expert panel identified a number of areas that require high-priority research:

- the elucidation of biological mechanisms that result in the adverse health effects associated with exposure to nitrous oxide;
- studies to gain a full understanding of the potential health effects of chronic low-level exposure to nitrous oxide, with emphasis on prospective studies that use direct nitrous oxide exposure measurement;
- the investigation of possible cognitive effects related to exposure to low levels of nitrous oxide;
- the development of equipment to evaluate and control exposure to nitrous oxide;
- the study of ventilation systems and air-exchange mechanisms for dental office designs;
- the evaluation of advantages associated with the use of nitrous oxide in combination with other sedative drugs.

The councils will continue to work with industry and the research community to address research and development needs that will further reduce occupational exposure to nitrous oxide.

1. ADA Ad Hoc Committee on Trace Anesthetics as Potential Health Hazard in Dentistry. Reports of subcommittees of the ADA Ad Hoc Committee on Trace Anesthetics as Potential Health Hazard in Dentistry: review and current status of survey. JADA 1977;95(10):787-90.
2. Whitcher CE, Zimmerman DC, Piziali RL. Control of occupational exposure to N2O in the dental operatory. Cincinnati: National Institute of Occupational Safety and Health, 1977; DHEW publication no. (NIOSH) 77-171.
3. Council on Dental Materials, Instruments and Equipment. Council position on nitrous oxide scavenging and monitoring devices. JADA 1980;101(1):62.
4. Alert: request for assistance in controlling exposures to nitrous oxide during anesthetic administration. Cincinnati: U.S. Department of Health and Human Services, Public Health Service, Centers for Disease Control, National Institute of Occupational Safety and Health, 1994; DHHS publication no. (NIOSH) 94100.
5. Technical report: control of nitrous oxide in dental operatories. Cincinnati: U.S. Department of Health and Human Services, Public Health Service, Centers for Disease Control and Prevention, National Institute of Occupational Safety and Health, Division of Physical Sciences and Engineering, Engineering Control Technology Branch, 1994; DHHS publication no. (NIOSH) 94-129.
6. Rowland AS, Baird DD, Weinberg CR, Shore DL, Shy CM, Wilcox AJ. Reduced fertility among women employed as dental assistants exposed to high levels of nitrous oxide. N Engl J Med 1992;327:993-7.

This material first appeared in ADA Council on Scientific Affairs and ADA Council on Dental Practice. Nitrous oxide in the dental office. JADA 1997; 128:864-5.

Appendix H.

Normal Laboratory Values

Hematologic Examinations

Examination	Range
Blood cells	

Erythrocytes (per mm^3)
  Men 4,100,000-5,900,000
  Women 3,800,000-5,500,000

Leukocytes (per mm^3) 4,100-12,300

Differential leukocytes (per mm^3)
  Segmented neutrophils 2,500-6,000 (40-60%)
  Band neutrophils 0-500 (0-5%)
  Juvenile neutrophils 0-100 (0-1%)
  Myelocytes 0 (0%)
  Lymphocytes 1,000-4,000 (15.5-46.6%)
  Monocytes 200-800 (2.8-12.9%)
  Eosinophils...50-300 (0-6%)
  Basophils 0-100 (0-2.3%)

Platelets (per mm^3)..140,000-450,000

Hemoglobin (g/100 mL)
  Men 13-17.5
  Women 11.6-16.2

Hematocrit (percentage)
  Men 40-52
  Women 35-47

Erythrocyte sedimentation rate (mm/h)
  Men 1-13
  Women 1-20

Coagulation screening tests

Bleeding time ....3-9 min

Coagulation time (Lee-White) (glass)..5-15 min

Prothrombin time ....less than 2 s deviation from control

Partial thromboplastin time (PTT) (activated) ....25-37 s

Chemical Constituents of Blood

Constituent	Range
Proteins (g/100 mL)	
Total serum protein	6.0-8.4
Albumin, serum	3.5-5.0
Globulin, serum	2.3-3.5
A/G ratio	1.5:1-3.1
Lipids (mg/100 mL)	
Cholesterol, total	
Men	140-284
Women	140-252
Triglycerides	30-170
Enzymes	
Amylase	4-25 U/mL
Creatine phosphokinase—CPK (mU/mL)	
Men	5-55
Women	5-35
Lactate dehydrogenase—LDH (IU/L)	
Men	86-272
Women	82-249
Phosphatase (alkaline)	31-121 IU/L
Transaminases	
Serum glutamate-oxaloacetate transaminase—SGOT (IU/L)	
Men	6-37
Women	5-37
Serum glutamate-pyruvate transaminase—SGPT (IU/L)	
Men	6-46
Women	6-37
Urea nitrogen—BUN	
Urea nitrogen—BUN	4-24 mg/100 mL
Uric acid	
Men	2.4-8.7
Women	2.1-6.9
Creatinine (mg/100 mL)	
Men	0.5-1.3
Women	0.4-1.2
BUN/Creatinine	
BUN/creatinine	7-20
Oxygen saturation (arterial)	
Oxygen saturation (arterial)	96-100%
PO_2	
PO_2	75-100 mm Hg
PCO_2	
PCO_2	35-45 mm Hg
CO_2 combining power	
CO_2 combining power	24-34 mEq/L

Continued on next page

Chemical Constituents of Blood (cont.)

Constituent	Range
pH	
pH	7.35-7.45
Electrolytes and inorganic constituents	
Chloride (Cl-serum)	94-111 mEq/L
Sodium (serum)	135-145 mEq/L
Potassium (serum)	3.5-5.0 mEq/L
Calcium (serum)	9-11 mg/100 mL
Phosphorus (serum) (mg/100 mL)	
Adults	2.3-5.1
Children	4-6.5
Iron, total	50-150 µg/100 mL
Total base	143-155 mEq/L
Glucose, fasting	
Glucose, fasting	70-110 mg/100 mL
Bilirubin (mg/100 mL)	
Total	0.3-1.2
Direct	0.0-0.2
Bromsulfalein (BSP)	Less than 5% retention (45 min)

Urine Analysis

Component	Range
Macroscopic (fresh specimen)	
Color	clear yellow
Specific gravity	1.010-1.025
pH	4.8-7.5
Microscopic	
Bacteria	0 (single specimen)
Leukocytes	0-few (single specimen) up to 1,800,000/24 h
Erythrocytes	0-few (single specimen) up to 500,000/24 h
Casts (hyaline)	0 (single specimen) up to 5,000/24 h
Chemical components	
Glucose	0 (single specimen) less than 100 mg/100 mL (24-h specimen)
Albumin	0 (single specimen) 10-150 mg/24 h
Ketones	0 (single specimen) less than 50 mg/24 h
Creatinine clearance	150-180 L/day/1.73 m^2 surface area

Weights and Measures

Common Metric Measurements and Their Abbreviations

Metric measurement	Abbreviation
Weight	
gram	g
kilogram	kg
milligram	mg
microgram	µg
Volume	
liter	L
milliliter	mL
microliter	µL

Measures of Weight

Metric	Apothecary
1 gram (g)	15 grains (gr)
4 g	60 gr 1 dram
30 g	1 ounce (oz)
1 kilogram (kg)	2.2 pounds (lb)
60 milligram (mg)	1 gr

Measures of Volume

Metric	Apothecary
5 milliliters (mL)	1 dram 1 teaspoonful
30 mL	1 fluid ounce
480 mL	1 pint
960 mL	1 quart

Common Metric Equivalents

Weight	
0.000001 gram (g)	1 microgram (µg)
0.001 g	1 milligram (mg)
1 g	1,000 milligrams (mg) 1,000,000 µg
1 kg	1,000 g
Volume	
0.001 milliliter (mL)	1 microliter (µL)
1 mL	0.001 liter (L)
1,000 mL	1 L

Calculation of Local Anesthetic and Vasopressor Dosages

Stanley F. Malamed, D.D.S.

Local Anesthetic Dosages

Percentage concentration	= mg/mL	x 1.8 = mg/cartridge
0.5	5	9
1	10	18
1.5	15	27
2	20	36
3	30	54
4	40	72

Vasopressor Concentrations (Equivalency Formula and Use)

Dilution OR	mg/mL x 1.8	= mg/cartridge	Recommended use
1:1,000	1.0		Anaphylaxis (IM, SC)
1:10,000	0.1		Cardiac arrest (IV)
1:20,000	0.05	0.09	Local anesthesia; levonordefrin
1:50,000	0.02	0.036	Local anesthesia; epinephrine
1:80,000	0.0125	0.0225	Local anesthesia; epinephrine (UK)
1:100,000	0.01	0.018	Local anesthesia; epinephrine
1:200,000	0.005	0.009	Local anesthesia; epinephrine

Appendix K.

HIV and Common Antiretroviral Medications

Michael Glick, D.M.D.

Treatment regimens for human immunodeficiency (HIV) disease are accompanied by a long list of prophylactic and maintenance medications. Prophylactic medications are usually indicated when the patient's immune system has deteriorated to a point at which opportunistic infections can be expected. The more common medications include anti–*Pneumocystis-carinii*-pneumonia (PCP) agents such as trimethoprim sulfamethoxazole; anticytomegalovirus agents such as oral ganciclovir; antifungal medications such as itraconazole and fluconazole; and antimycobacteria agents such as rifampin and isoniazid. Many of these medications interact with other medications commonly used in dentistry.

However, the fastest progress in treatment for HIV disease is in the field of antiretroviral medications. These medications directly or indirectly inhibit HIV replication through different mechanisms. Nucleoside reverse transcriptase inhibitors (NRTIs) and non-nucleoside reverse transcriptase inhibitors (NNRTIs) act as competitive inhibitors to an enzyme, reverse transcriptase, that the virus carries for the purpose of transcribing the viral RNA into viral DNA. The newest group is protease inhibitors. These medications prevent breakdown of proteins, produced by the HIV-infected cell, into appropriate sizes for viral production. Continuous development of antiretroviral medications will challenge all health care workers treating HIV-infected patients to keep apprised of new agents that usually are associated with a high degree of toxicity.

The table below presents antiretroviral medications used for HIV disease, which may interact with a number of drugs prescribed by dentists.

Common Antiretroviral Medications: Dental Considerations

Generic name	Brand name	Toxicity relevant to dentistry	Interactions with medications used in dentistry
Nucleoside reverse transcriptase inhibitors (NRTIs)			
Didanosine (ddI)	Videx	Peripheral neuropathy, xerostomia	Reduces efficacy of itraconazole and ketoconazole, so these drugs should be administered within 2 h of ddI administration
			Reduces efficacy of quinolone and tetracyclines, so these should be administered 2 h before or 6 h after ddI administration

Continued on next page

Common Antiretroviral Medications: Dental Considerations (cont.)

Generic name	Brand name	Toxicity relevant to dentistry	Interactions with medications used in dentistry
Nucleoside reverse transcriptase inhibitors (NRTIs) (cont.)			
Lamivudine (3TC)	Epivir	None noted	No data available
Stavudine (d4T)	Zerit	Peripheral neuropathy	No data available
Zalcitabine (ddC)	HIVID	Peripheral neuropathy, oral ulcerations	No data available
Zidovudine (AZT, ZDV)	Retrovir	Anemia, neutropenia	No data available
Non-nucleoside reverse transcriptase inhibitors (NNRTIs)			
Delavirdine	Rescriptor	None noted	Inhibits cytochrome p 450 enzymes
			Levels decreased by phenobarbitol
			Increases levels of clarithromycin, dapsone
			Administration of buffered medications should be avoided within 2 h of delavirdine administration
			Contraindicated for concomitant administration with midazolam
Nevirapine	Viramune	None noted	Induces cytochrome p 450 enzymes
Protease inhibitors			
Indinavir	Crixivan	Thrombocytopenia	Inhibits cytochrome p 450 enzymes
			Avoid concurrent use with midazolam and triazolam
			Levels increased by ketaconazole
Nelfinavir	Viracept	None noted	Inhibits cytochrome p 450 enzymes
			Avoid concurrent use with midazolam and triazolam
Ritonavir	Norvir	Dysgeusia	Inhibits cytochrome p 450 enzymes (potent)
			Decreases levels of clarithromycin
			Contraindicated for concomitant administration with diazepam, meperidine, midazolam, piroxicam, propoxyphene
Saquinavir	Invirase	None noted	Inhibits cytochrome p 450 enzymes
			Levels decreased by dexamethasone

Appendix L.

Sample Prescriptions and Prescription Abbreviations

Sample Prescriptions

The following prescriptions are not all-inclusive; they are provided only as examples of prescriptions commonly written by dentists. Drugs are listed by generic name in these examples. Those listed as drug combinations are available under a variety of brand names. Selection of any particular drug for inclusion in these examples in no way indicates recommendation of that agent over another. Abbreviations are presented for prescription directions. However, if in doubt, write the directions out.

Antibiotic for Patients Requiring Antibiotic Premedication

Drug	#	Directions	Abbreviated directions
Penicillin			
Amoxicillin capsules 500 mg	4	Sig: 4 capsules 1 hour before procedure	Sig: 4 caps 1 h ā procedure
For patients allergic to penicillins			
Clindamycin 150 mg	4	Sig: 4 capsules 1 hour before procedure	Sig: 4 caps 1 h ā procedure
Cephalexin capsules 500 mg	4	Sig: 4 capsules 1 hour before procedure	Sig: 4 caps 1 h ā procedure

To Reduce Excess Salivation

Drug	#	Directions	Abbreviated directions
Propantheline bromide	6	Sig: 1-2 tablets 1/2 hour before procedure	Sig: 1-2 tab 1/2 h ā procedure
Atropine sulfate 0.3 mg	9	Sig: 2-3 tablets 1/2 hour before procedure	Sig: 2-3 tab 1/2 h ā procedure

Continued on next page

To Increase Salivation

Drug	#	Directions	Abbreviated directions
Pilocarpine 5 mg	30	Sig: 1-2 tablets three times daily	Sig: 1-2 tab tid

To Relax a Patient Before a Dental Procedure

Drug	#	Directions	Abbreviated directions
Diazepam 5 mg	12	Sig: 1 tablet 1 hour before sleep; 1 tablet 1 hour before procedure	Sig: 1 tab 1 hs; 1 tab 1 h ā procedure
Hydroxyzine pamoate 50 mg	10	Sig: 2 tablets 1 hour before sleep; 1-2 tablets 1 hour before procedure	Sig: 2 tab 1 hs; 1-2 tab 1 h ā procedure
Secobarbital sodium 100 mg	10	Sig: 1 capsule 1 hour before sleep; 1 tablet 1 hour before procedure	Sig: 1 cap 1 hs; 1 tab 1 h ā procedure

For Pain Relief

Drug	#	Directions	Abbreviated directions
For mild to moderate pain			
Ibuprofen 400 mg	15	Sig: 1 tablet every 4-6 hours as needed; maximum daily dose 6 tablets	Sig: 1 tab q 4-6 h prn pain MDD 6 tab
Codeine phosphate 30 mg	15	Sig: 1-2 tablets every 4 hours as needed for pain; maximum daily dose 8 tablets	Sig: 1-2 tab q 4 h prn pain MDD 8 tab
Propoxyphene napsylate 100 mg with acetaminophen 650 mg	16	Sig: 1 tablet every 4 hours as needed	Sig: 1 tab q 4 h prn pain
For moderate to severe pain			
Pentazocine HCl 50 mg	12	Sig: 1 tablet every 4 hours; maximum daily dose 6 tablets	Sig: 1 tab q 4 h MDD 6
Hydrocodone bitartrate 5 mg and acetaminophen 500 mg or 750 mg	12	Sig: 1 tablet every 4 hours; maximum daily dose 6 tablets	Sig: 1 tab q 4 h MDD 6
Oxycodone HCl 5 mg and acetaminophen 325 mg or 500 mg	12	Sig: 1 tablet every 6 hours; maximum daily dose 4 tablets	Sig: 1 tab q 6 h MDD 4

For Pain Relief (cont.)

Drug	#	Directions	Abbreviated directions
For severe pain			
Meperidine HCl 50 mg	12	Sig: 1 tablet every 4 hours; maximum daily dose 6 tablets	Sig: 1 tab q 4 h MDD 6
Hydromorphone HCl 2 mg	12	Sig: 1 tablet every 5-6 hours as needed for pain; maximum daily dose 7 tablets	Sig: 1 tab q 6 h prn pain MDD 7
Methadone HCl 5 mg	12	Sig: 1 tablet every 4 hours; maximum daily dose 6 tablets	Sig: 1 tab q 4 h MDD 6

For Infections in the Mouth and Adjacent Tissues

Drug	#	Directions	Abbreviated directions
Penicillin V 250 mg or amoxicillin 250 mg	30	Sig: 2 tablets initially, 1-2 tablets every 4 hours to finish	Sig: 2 tab stat, 1 tab qid
Erythromycin 250 mg	30	Sig: 2 tablets initially, 1 tablet every 4 hours to finish	Sig: 2 tab stat, 1 tab qid
Minocycline HCl 100 mg	15	Sig: 2 capsules initially, 1 capsule twice daily to finish	Sig: 2 cap stat, 1 cap bid
Tetracycline HCl 250 mg	30	Sig: 2 capsules initially, 1 capsule every 4 hours	Sig: 2 cap stat, 1 cap qid
Cephalexin 250 mg	30	Sig: 2 capsules initially, 1 capsule every 4 hours to finish	Sig: 2 cap stat, 1 cap qid

For Oral Candidiasis

Drug	#	Directions	Abbreviated directions
Nystatin 400,000 units	480 mL	Sig: Rinse and swallow 4 cc four times daily until symptoms disappear	Sig: 4 cc qid, rinse and swallow
0.12 % chlorhexidine	16 oz	Sig: 1/2 oz twice a day as a rinse until symptoms disappear	Sig: 0.5 oz bid
Clotrimazole troche 10 mg	70	Sig: 1 troche by mouth five times daily	Sig: 1 troche po 5 times d

For Mild to Moderate Desquamative Gingivitis and Lichen Planus

Drug	#	Directions	Abbreviated directions
Fluocinonide	60 g	Sig: Apply with cotton swab to affected areas 4 times daily	Sig: Apply c̄ cotton swab qid

For Mild Allergic Reactions

Drug	#	Directions	Abbreviated directions
Diphenhydramine HCl 50 mg	30	Sig: 1 tablet every 4 hours as needed	Sig: 1 tab qid prn

Prescription Abbreviations

Abbreviation	Term
ā	before
ac	before meals
aq, H₂O	water
bid	2 times a day
c̄, c	with
cap	capsule
d	day
gtt	drops
h	hour
hs, HS, hor som	at bedtime
non rep, nr, NR	do not repeat
pc	after eating
po	by mouth
prn	as needed
qh	each hour
qid	4 times a day
s̄, sine	without
sig	write on the label
s̄s̄, ss	one-half
stat	immediately
tab	tablet
tid	3 times a day
aw	week

MEDWATCH Form

MEDWATCH
THE FDA MEDICAL PRODUCTS REPORTING PROGRAM

For **VOLUNTARY** reporting by health professionals of adverse events and product problems

Page ____ of ____

Form Approved: OMB No. 0910-0291 Expires: 4/30/96
See OMB statement on reverse

FDA Use Only
Triage unit sequence #

A. Patient information

1. Patient identifier
2. Age at time of event:
   or _____
   Date of birth:
   In confidence
3. Sex
   ☐ female
   ☐ male
4. Weight
   ____ lbs
   or
   ____ kgs

B. Adverse event or product problem

1. ☐ Adverse event and/or ☐ Product problem (e.g., defects/malfunctions)

2. Outcomes attributed to adverse event (check all that apply)
   ☐ death _____ (mo/day/yr)
   ☐ life-threatening
   ☐ hospitalization – initial or prolonged
   ☐ disability
   ☐ congenital anomaly
   ☐ required intervention to prevent permanent impairment/damage
   ☐ other: _____

3. Date of event (mo/day/yr)
4. Date of this report (mo/day/yr)

5. Describe event or problem

6. Relevant tests/laboratory data, including dates

7. Other relevant history, including preexisting medical conditions (e.g., allergies, race, pregnancy, smoking and alcohol use, hepatic/renal dysfunction, etc.)

PLEASE TYPE OR USE BLACK INK

C. Suspect medication(s)

1. Name (give labeled strength & mfr/labeler, if known)
   #1
   #2

2. Dose, frequency & route used
   #1
   #2

3. Therapy dates (if unknown, give duration) from/to (or best estimate)
   #1
   #2

4. Diagnosis for use (indication)
   #1
   #2

5. Event abated after use stopped or dose reduced
   #1 ☐ yes ☐ no ☐ doesn't apply
   #2 ☐ yes ☐ no ☐ doesn't apply

6. Lot # (if known)
   #1
   #2

7. Exp. date (if known)
   #1
   #2

8. Event reappeared after reintroduction
   #1 ☐ yes ☐ no ☐ doesn't apply
   #2 ☐ yes ☐ no ☐ doesn't apply

9. NDC # (for product problems only)
   ___ – ___ – ___

10. Concomitant medical products and therapy dates (exclude treatment of event)

D. Suspect medical device

1. Brand name

2. Type of device

3. Manufacturer name & address

4. Operator of device
   ☐ health professional
   ☐ lay user/patient
   ☐ other:

6. model # _____
   catalog # _____
   serial # _____
   lot # _____
   other #

5. Expiration date (mo/day/yr)

7. If implanted, give date (mo/day/yr)

8. If explanted, give date (mo/day/yr)

9. Device available for evaluation? (Do not send to FDA)
   ☐ yes ☐ no ☐ returned to manufacturer on _____ (mo/day/yr)

10. Concomitant medical products and therapy dates (exclude treatment of event)

E. Reporter (see confidentiality section on back)

1. Name & address | phone #

2. Health professional? ☐ yes ☐ no
3. Occupation
4. Also reported to
   ☐ manufacturer
   ☐ user facility
   ☐ distributor

5. If you do NOT want your identity disclosed to the manufacturer, place an " X " in this box. ☐

FDA

Mail to: MEDWATCH
5600 Fishers Lane
Rockville, MD 20852-9787

or FAX to:
1-800-FDA-0178

FDA Form 3500 1/96   Submission of a report does not constitute an admission that medical personnel or the product caused or contributed to the event.

Continued on next page

ADVICE ABOUT VOLUNTARY REPORTING

Report experiences with:
- medications (drugs or biologics)
- medical devices (including in-vitro diagnostics)
- special nutritional products (dietary supplements, medical foods, infant formulas)
- other products regulated by FDA

Report SERIOUS adverse events. An event is serious when the patient outcome is:
- death
- life-threatening (real risk of dying)
- hospitalization (initial or prolonged)
- disability (significant, persistent or permanent)
- congenital anomaly
- required intervention to prevent permanent impairment or damage

Report even if:
- you're not certain the product caused the event
- you don't have all the details

Report product problems – quality, performance or safety concerns such as:
- suspected contamination
- questionable stability
- defective components
- poor packaging or labeling
- therapeutic failures

How to report:
- just fill in the sections that apply to your report
- use section C for all products except medical devices
- attach additional blank pages if needed
- use a separate form for each patient
- report either to FDA or the manufacturer (or both)

Important numbers:
- 1-800-FDA-0178 to FAX report
- 1-800-FDA-7737 to report by modem
- 1-800-FDA-1088 to report by phone or for more information
- 1-800-822-7967 for a VAERS form for vaccines

If your report involves a serious adverse event with a device and it occurred in a facility outside a doctor's office, that facility may be legally required to report to FDA and/or the manufacturer. Please notify the person in that facility who would handle such reporting.

Confidentiality: The patient's identity is held in strict confidence by FDA and protected to the fullest extent of the law. The reporter's identity, including the identity of a self-reporter, may be shared with the manufacturer unless requested otherwise. However, FDA will not disclose the reporter's identity in response to a request from the public, pursuant to the Freedom of Information Act.

The public reporting burden for this collection of information has been estimated to average 30 minutes per response, including the time for reviewing instructions, searching existing data sources, gathering and maintaining the data needed, and completing and reviewing the collection of information. Send comments regarding this burden estimate or any other aspect of this collection of information, including suggestions for reducing this burden to:

DHHS Reports Clearance Office
Paperwork Reduction Project (0910-0291)
Hubert H. Humphrey Building, Room 531-H
200 Independence Avenue, S.W.
Washington, DC 20201

"An agency may not conduct or sponsor, and a person is not required to respond to, a collection of information unless it displays a currently valid OMB control number."

Please do NOT return this form to either of these addresses.

U.S. DEPARTMENT OF HEALTH AND HUMAN SERVICES
Public Health Service • Food and Drug Administration

FDA Form 3500-back   **Please Use Address Provided Below – Just Fold In Thirds, Tape and Mail**

**Department of
Health and Human Services**
Public Health Service
Food and Drug Administration
Rockville, MD 20857

Official Business
Penalty for Private Use $300

NO POSTAGE
NECESSARY
IF MAILED
IN THE
UNITED STATES
OR APO/FPO

BUSINESS REPLY MAIL
FIRST CLASS MAIL   PERMIT NO. 946   ROCKVILLE, MD

POSTAGE WILL BE PAID BY FOOD AND DRUG ADMINISTRATION

MEDWATCH

**The FDA Medical Products Reporting Program
Food and Drug Administration
5600 Fishers Lane
Rockville, MD 20852-9787**

Indexes

General Index

This index has been alphabetized strictly according to letter, disregarding punctuation. Therefore, drugs that begin with a hyphenated prefix, for example, are alphabetized as if the hyphen was not there: Novo-Chlorpromazine is followed by Novoclens Topical Solution, which in turn is followed by Novo-Clopate.

Page numbers listed in **boldface** type indicate where basic information about a generic or brand-name drug or other entry can be found. Such information includes usage and dosage, as well as interactions, cross-sensitivity, pharmacology, adverse effects and precautions and contraindications.

Page numbers listed in *italic* type indicate where to find the oral manifestations of the drug.

Drugs often come in many forms, but all of those forms are listed under one main entry.

The ★ symbol indicates a product bearing the ADA Seal of Acceptance. When the symbol appears in parentheses (★), it means that there may be several brand names subsumed under the one listing and among those, one or more of the brands bears the Seal of Acceptance.

A

Abbokinase (urokinase), **395**
Absorbable gelatin sponge, **108-116**
Accu-Gard Vinyl Examination (non-latex patient-care gloves), **496**
Accupril (quinapril), **310**, 457, *486*
Accutane (isotretinoin), 467, 469, *482*
Acebutolol, **305-308**
Acenocoumarol [CAN], **386**, **389-391**
Acetaminophen, 38, **96-107**, 126, **432-440**
Acetazolam (acetazolamide), **343**
Acetazolamide, **342-346**

Acetohexamide, 456, *476*
Acetohexamine, **404**, **409**, **410**
Acetophenazine, **367-374**, 465, *476*
Achromycin V (tetracycline), **148**, **440**, 459, 461, *487*
Acidulated phosphate fluoride rinses and solutions, **218-225**
Acidulated sodium fluoride gel, **218-225**
Act Fluoride Anti-Cavity Dental Rinse ★ (fluoride), **202-203**
Act for Kids Fluoride Anti-Cavity Treatment ★ (fluoride), **202-203**
Actifed (triprolidine/pseudoephedrine), 472, *488*
Actinomycosis, 165
Activase (recombinant alterplase), **395**
Activus ★ (topical stannous fluoride gel), **221**
Acute myocardial infarction, emergency management of, **291-292**
Acyclovir, **171-174**, **432-440**
Adactazide (spironolactone + HCTZ), **304**
Adalat (nifedipine), **309**
Adapin (doxepin), 471, *480*
Addiction, **517-518**
Addicts, drug or alcohol, **517-526**
Adipex-P (phentermine), 469, *485*
Adrenalin (epinephrine), 255
Adrenergic blocking agents, 5, 14, 62, **305-308**, **314-317**
Adrucil (5-fluorouracil), 460, *480*
Advanced Formula Plax (prebrushing rinse), **203**
Advil ★ (ibuprofen), **101**, **436**, 455, 469, 475, *482*
AeroBid (flunisolide), **320**
Aerosol reduction system, **491-492**, **493-495**
Agranulocytosis, 453, 463-464
A-hydroCort (hydrocortisone sodium succinate), 250
Aid Premium Latex Examination ★ (nonsterile latex examination gloves), **495**

Aim (★) (caries or calculus prevention dentifrices), **209**, **210**
Aim Safe (recapping device), **503**
Air/water syringe tips, disposable, **491-492**, **493-495**
Akineton (biperiden), **347**, 473, *477*
Akorazol [CAN] (ketoconazole), **166**
Aladan Classic Latex Examination ★ (nonsterile latex examination gloves), **495**
Albert Glyburide (glyburide), **409**
Albuterol, 247, **321-323**, 474, *476*
Alcohol abuse, 519
Alcohol, 4, 28, 38, 51, 53, 54, 62, 93, 104, 238
Aldactone (spironolactone), **303**, 461, *487*
Aldehydes, **180-185**
Aldomet (methyldopa), **312**, 465, 466, 468, 472, *484*
Aleve (naproxen), **101**, **438**, 455, 475, *484*
Alfenta (alfentanil), **42**
Alfentanil, **40-47**
Alkaban-AQ (vinblastine), 468
Alkeran (melphalan), **444**
All-Bond DS Desensitizer (methacrylate polymer bonding agent), **230**
Allay (hydrocodone bitartrate with acetaminophen), **84**
Allergen avoidance/chemicals to denature allergens, **324**, **325**
Allergy, emergency management of, **287-289**
Allerjoy Latex Examination ★ (nonsterile latex examination gloves), **495**
Allopurinol, 459, *476*
α-adrenergic blockers, 5, 62, 195
Alpha-Baclofen (baclofen), **350**
Alphacaine (lidocaine hydrochloride or lidocaine hydrochloride with epinephrine), **3**

Alpha-Dent ★ (topical stannous fluoride gel), **221**

Alphaderm HC (hydrocortisone [cortisol] [low potency]), **131**

Alpha-Tamoxifen (tamoxifen), **444**

Alphatrex (betamethasone), 420

Alprazol (alprazolam), **358, 376**

Alprazolam, 18-30, **358-360, 374, 376-378,** 470, *476*

Alprazolam Intensol (alprazolam), **358, 376**

Altace (ramipril), **310,** 457, *486*

Altered consciousness, emergency management of, **283-284**

Alternagel (aluminum salts), 335

Alterplase, recombinant, **394-395**

Alu-Cap (aluminum salts), 335

Alu-Tab (aluminum salts), 335

Aludrox (magnesium salts and aluminum salts), 335

Aluminum combinations, **116-117**

Aluminum Hydroxide Gel (aluminum salts), 335

Aluminum oxalate, **226-232**

Aluminum salts, **333-337**

Alupent (metaproterenol sulfate), 322

Alurate (aprobarbital), **35**

Amantadine, **347-350**

Ambenonium, 62, **346-347**

Ambien (zolpidem), **27, 377**

Amcill (ampicillin), **137**

Amen (medroxyprogesterone), 410

Amerglo Deluxe Latex ★ (nonsterile latex examination gloves), 495

Amicar (aminocaproic acid), 392

Amidate (etomidate), **59**

Amides, 1, 6

Amiloride and amiloride + hydrochlorothiazide (HCTZ), **303, 304**

Aminocaproic acid, **388, 392**

Aminoglycosides, 62, 74, 455

Aminophyllin (theophylline ethylenediamine-xanthine), phyllocontin, somophyllin-DF, somophyllin, dyphylline, parolon [CAN], **322**

Amiodarone, 4, 62, **296-298**

Amitriptyline, 5, 14, **360-366,** 458, 471, *476*

Amitriptyline/perphenazine, 471, 473, *476*

Amobarbital, **32-40,** 464, *476*

Amoxapine, **360-366,** 465, 471, 476

Amoxicillin and amoxicillin/clavulanic acid, **134-142, 432-440,** 455, 458, *476,* 546

Amoxil (amoxicillin), **137, 434,** 455, 458, *476*

Amphetamine abuse, 519

Amphetamine variants, **524-525**

Amphetamine/methamphetamine, **522-523**

Amphetamines, 14, 93

Amphojel (aluminum salts), **335**

Amphotericin B, 75, 126, **164-171,** 460, *476*

Ampicillin, **134-142, 432-440,** 467, *476,* 546

Amrinone, 460, *476*

Amytal (amobarbital), **34,** 464, *476*

Amytal [CAN] (amobarbital), **34**

Ana-Guard (epinephrine), 244

Anabolic steroids, 126

Anacin (salicylates), **439,** *476*

Anacobin (cyanocobalamin), 394

Anadrol-50 (oxymetholone), **402**

Anafranil (clomipramine), 364

Anapolon 50 (oxymetholone), **402**

Anaprox (naproxen), **101, 438,** 455, 475, *484*

Anaspaz (hyoscyamine), 470, *481*

Anbesol (benzocaine and benzocaine combinations), **12**

Anbocaine (benzocaine), **12**

Ancalixir (phenobarbital), 344

Andro (testosterone), **402**

Androgens, 126, **400-401, 402, 412-413, 414-415**

Android-F (fluoxymesterone), **402**

Android-10 (methyltestosterone), **402**

Andryl 200 (testosterone), **402**

Anectine (succinylcholine chloride), **72**

Anesthetic mouthrinse, **199-207**

Anesthetics
    general, 4, **56-69**
    hydrocarbon inhalation, 5, 14
    injectable, **1-9**
    local, 62, 74
    topical, 6, 7-8, **10-16**
    volatile inhalation, 75

Anexsia (hydrocodone bitartrate with acetaminophen), **84**

Angina pectoris, 299-300
    emergency management of, **290-291**

Angioedema, 452, 457

Angiotensin-converting enzyme inhibitors, 62

Anhydron (cyclothiazide), **303**

Anisindione, **386, 389-391**

Anistreplase, **394-395**

Ankylosing spondylitis, 418

Anolar DH5 (hydrocodone bitartrate with acetaminophen), **84**

Anorex (phendimetrazine), 469, *485*

Ansaid (flurbiprofen), **100,** 465, *481*

Anspor (cephradine), **139**

Antacids, 126, 190

Antianemic agents, **386, 387-388, 396-397, 398-399**

Antianginal drugs, **299-301**

Antianxiety agents, **17-55, 358-360, 379-382, 383-385**

Antiarrhythmic drugs, 4, **296-298**

Antibiotic prophylaxis with prosthetic joint replacements, 547-552

Antibiotics, use in dentistry, 553

Anticholinergic drugs, **186-193,** 195, **323, 326-327, 328**

Anticholinesterases, 74

Anticoagulant agents, 38, 51, 53, 94, **386, 389-391, 396-397, 398-399**

Anticonvulsant drugs, **342-346, 352-354, 355**

Antidepressant agents, 4, 53, 62, **360-366**

Antidiabetic agents, 126

Antidiarrheal agents, 93, 190, **330-331, 338-340, 341**

Antifibrinolytic agent, **388, 392, 396-397, 398-399**

Antifungal agents, **164-171**

Antiglaucoma agents, 4

Antihistamines, 4, 62

Antihypertensive drugs, 45, 93, 104, **301-313**
    centrally acting, 4, 62, **311, 312, 314-317**

Antihypoglycemics (orange juice, nondiet soft drinks), 247

Antimanic/bipolar disorder drugs, **366-367, 379-382, 383-385**

Antimuscarinic agents, **186-193**

Antimyasthenic agents, 4, 74, 190, 195, **346-347, 352-354, 355**

Antimyasthenic cholinesterase inhibitors, 62

Antineoplastic agents, **441-449**

Antiparkinsonism drugs, 190, 195, **347-350, 352-354, 355**

Antipsychotic agents, 4, 5, 62, 190, 195, **367-374, 379-382, 383-385**

Antiretraction valve, **491-492, 493-495**

Antiseptics, **178-180**

Antisialogogues, **186-193**

Antispastic drugs, **350**

Antithrombotic agents, **392-394, 396-397, 398-399**

Antivert (meclizine), **473,** *483*

Antiviral agents, **171-174**

Anusol-HC (hydrocortisone [cortisol] [low potency]), **131**

Anxanil (hydroxyzine), **359**

Anxiety control, **17-55**

Anxiety, 358

Aparkane (trihexphenidyl), **348**

Aphthous ulcers, 172

Apo-Acetazolamide [CAN] (acetazolamide), **343**

Apo-Alpraz [CAN] (alprazolam), **20**, **358**, **376**

Apo-Amitriptyline [CAN] (amitriptyline), **364**

Apo-Amoxi [CAN] (amoxicillin), **434**

Apo-Ampi [CAN] (ampicillin), **434**

Apo-Atenol [CAN] (atenolol), **305**

Apo-Benztropine [CAN] (benztropine), **347**

Apo-Carbamazepine [CAN] (carbamazepine), **343**, **367**, **372**

Apo-Chlorazepate [CAN] (clorazepate), **358**

Apo-Chlordiazepoxide [CAN] (chlordiazepoxide), **20**, **358**

Apo-Chlorthalidone [CAN] (chlorthalidone), **303**

Apo-Clorazepate [CAN] (clorazepate), **20**

Apo-Diazepam [CAN] (diazepam), **21**, **343**, **359**, **376**

Apo-Diclo [CAN] (diclofenac sodium), **100**

Apo-Dipyridamole [CAN] (dipyridamole), **393**

Apo-Ferrous Gluconate [CAN] (ferrous gluconate), **387**

Apo-Ferrous Sulfate [CAN] (ferrous sulfate), **388**

Apo-Flurazepam [CAN] (flurazepam), **23**, **376**

Apo-Flurbiprofen [CAN] (flurbiprofen), **100**

Apo-Folic [CAN] (folic acid), **394**

Apo-Glyburide [CAN] (glyburide), **409**

Apo-Haloperidol [CAN] (haloperidol), **368**

Apo-Hydro [CAN] (hydrochlorothiazide), **303**

Apo-Hydroxyzine [CAN] (hydroxyzine), **359**

Apo-Ibuprofen [CAN] (ibuprofen), **101**

Apo-Imipramine [CAN] (imipramine), **365**

Apo-Indomethacin [CAN] (indomethacin), **99**

Apo-Keto [CAN] (ketoprofen), **101**

Apo-Keto-E [CAN] (ketoprofen, sustained relief), **101**

Apo-Lorazepam [CAN] (lorazepam), **23**, **359**, **376**

Apo-Meprobamate [CAN] (meprobamate), **54**

Apo-Methyldopa [CAN] (methyldopa), **312**

Apo-Metoprolol [CAN] (metoprolol), **305**

Apo-Napro-Na [CAN] (naproxen sodium), **101**

Apo-Naproxen [CAN] (naproxen), **101**

Apo-Nifed [CAN] (nifedipine), **309**

Apo-Oxazepam [CAN] (oxazepam) **26**, **359**

Apo-Piroxicam [CAN] (piroxicam), **100**

Apo-Prednisone [CAN] (prednisone), **125**

Apo-Primidone [CAN] (primidone), **345**

Apo-Propranolol [CAN] (propranolol), **305**, **349**

Apo-Sulin [CAN] (sulindac), **99**

Apo-Tamox [CAN] (tamoxifen), **444**

Apo-Thioridazine [CAN] (thioridazine), **370**

Apo-Timol [CAN] (timolol), **305**

Apo-Tolbutamide [CAN] (tolbutamide), **409**

Apo-Triazo [CAN] (triazolam), **27**, **377**

Apo-Trihex [CAN] (trihexphenidyl), **348**

Apo-Trimip [CAN] (trimipramine), **365**

Apresoline (hydralazine), **308**

Aprobarbital, **32-40**

Aquachloral Supprettes (chloral hydrate), **50**

Aquaflow (hands-free faucet), **494**

Aquafresh ★ (caries or calculus prevention dentifrices), **209**, **210**, **221**

Aquafresh Sensitive Teeth (sodium fluoride and potassium nitrate combination), **233**

AquaMephyton (vitamin K, or phytonadione), **111**

Aquaphyllin (theophylline, theophylline sodium glycinate), **323**

Aquatensen (methyclothiazide), **303**

Aquest (estrone), **403**

Arbor ★ (caries prevention dentifrice), **209**

Arduan (pipecuronium bromide), **72**

Arestocaine (mepivacaine hydrochloride), **3**

Aristocort (triamcinolone acetonide [medium potency]), **132**, **421**

Arm & Hammer (caries prevention dentifrices), **209**

Arm & Hammer Dentacare (sodium fluoride and potassium nitrate combination), **233**

Arm-a-Med Isoetharine (isoetharine hydrochloride/isoetharine mesylate), **322**

Arm-a-Med (isoproterenol), **474**

Armour Thyroid (thyroid), **411**

Aromatic ammonia, **254**

Artane (trihexphenidyl), **348**, **473**, *488*

Articaine hydrochloride with epinephrine [CAN], **1-9**

A.S.A. (aspirin), *476*

Ascomp with codeine (codeine with aspirin, caffeine and butalbitol), **83**

Ascriptin (aspirin), *476*

Asendin (amoxapine), **364**, **465**, **471**, *476*

Asep-Gluv (heavy utility gloves), **496**

Aseptex Fluid Resistant (mask, single retention band), **497**

Asepti-IDC (iodophor), **502**

Asepti-phene 128 (water-based tri-phenolics), **502**

Asepti-Steryl (alcohol-based phenolics), **502**

Asepticare TB (alcohol-based quaternary ammonium compound), **502**

Aseptiwater system (sterile water delivery system), **494**

Aspergum (aspirin), *476*

Aspirin, **102**, **104**, **419**, **424-425**, **427**, **455**, **469**, *476*

Aspiritab (salicylates), **439**

Assert Spore vials/Incubator (spore testing equipment), **501**

Assure Plus Self-sealing ★ (sterilization pouch), **498**

Assure Self-sealing ★ (sterilization pouch), **498**

Astemizole, **471**, *476*

Astra Pro Disposable Latex Exam ★ (nonsterile latex examination gloves), **495**

Astramorph PF (morphine and morphine sulfate), **43**, **91**, **248**, **260**, **438**

Astringadent ★ (ferric sulfate), **116**

Astringents, **116-117**

Atarax (hydroxyzine), **359**, **473**, *481*

Aternolol, **305-308**

ATI (process indicator), **500**

ATI Self-sealing (sterilization pouch), **498**

Ativan (lorazepam), **23**, **359**, **376**, **437**, **458**, **470**, *483*

Ativan [CAN] (lorazepam), **23**

Atracurium besylate, **70-79**

Atretol (carbamazepine), **367**, **372**

Atromid-S (clofibrate), **460**, **467**, *478*

Atropine sulfate, **186-193**, **254**, **255**, **470**, *476*

Atropisol (atropine), **470**, *476*

Atrovent (ipratropium bromide), **323**

Attention deficit disorder, **374**

Attention deficit drugs, **374**, **375**, **379-382**, **383-385**

Attest Spore vials/Incubator (spore testing equipment), **500**

Audra Latex Examination ★ (nonsterile latex examination gloves), **495**

Augmentin (amoxicillin/clavulanic acid), **137**, **435**, **458**, *476*

Auralate (gold salts), **419**

Auranofin, 457, 459, 467, *476*

Aurothioglucose, 459, 467, **477**

Automatic Faucet (infrared) (hands-free faucet), **494**

Aventyl (nortriptyline), **365**, 471, *484*

Avirax [CAN] (acyclovir), **172**

Axid (nizatidine), **336**

Aygestin (norethindrone), **410**

Azalides, 142

Azathioprine (prednisone), **332**, 460, 468, **477**

Azithromycin, **142-146**, 546

Azmacort (triamcinolone), **320**, 456, *488*

Azoles, 164, 165, 168

Azulfidine (sulfasalazine), **332**

B

Baby Orabase ★ (benzocaine), **12**

Baby Oragel [CAN] (benzocaine), **12**

Bacampicillin, **134-142**

Baclofen (lioresal), **350**, 461, *482*

Bacterial endocarditis, 542-546

Bactocill (oxacillin), **138**

Bactrim (trimethoprim and sulfamethoxazole), **161**

Baldur Latex Examination ★ (nonsterile latex examination gloves), **495**

Bancap-HC (hydrocodone bitartrate with acetaminophen), **84**

Banflex (orphenadrine), **348**, **429**

Banicide (glutaraldehyde liquid sterilant), **500**

Banthine (methantheline), **189**, 470, *483*

Barbita (phenobarbital), **36-37**, **344**, 439

Barbiturate abuse, 519

Barbiturates, 4, **32-40**, 62, 63, 93, **522-523**

Barrier Dental Sealant (sodium fluoride varnish), **229**

Barrier protective wear (infection control products), **497**

Bayer (salicylates), **439**, *476*

Bayer Select Ibuprofen (ibuprofen), **101**

Beclomethasone dipropionate, **320**, 456, **477**

Beclovent (beclomethasone dipropionate), **320**

Beconase (beclomethasone dipropionate), 456, **477**

Bedoz (cyanocobalamin), **394**

Beepen-VK (penicillin V potassium), **439**

Belladonna alkaloids, 190, 470, **477**

Bellergal (belladonna alkaloids), 470, **477**

Benadryl (diphenhydramine), 245, **347**, 472, *479*

Benazepril, **310-311**, 457, **477**

Bendroflumethiazide, **301-304**

Benemid (probenecid), **420**

Benisone (betamethasone [medium to high potency]), **131**

Bentyl (dicyclomine), 470, *479*

Benuryl [CAN] (probenecid), **420**

Benzocaine and benzocaine combinations, 6, **10-16**

Benzodent ★ (benzocaine), **12**

Benzodiazepine abuse, 519

Benzodiazepines, 4, **18-30**, 28, 45, 62, **358-359**, **379-382**, **383-385**, **522-523**
  antagonist, **30-32**

Benzthiazide, **301-304**

Benztropine mesylate, **347-350**, 473, 477

Benzylpenicillin (penicillin G benzathine suspension), **138**

Bepadin (bepridil), **309**

Bepridil, **309-310**

β-adrenergic agonists, 126, **321-322**, **326-327**, 328

β-adrenergic blocking agents, 4, 5, 14, 62, 74

Beta-Val (betamethasone [medium to high potency]), **131**

Betadine (iodophors), **177**, **179**

Betalol (metoprolol), **305**

Betamethasone, **124-130**, **129-133**, **420-422**, 457, **477**

Betapace (sotalol), **297**, **305**

Betapen-K (phenoxymethyl-penicillin), **138**

Betapen-VK (penicillin V potassium), **439**

Betaxolol, **301**, **305-308**

Bethanechol, 195, 467, **477**

Betnelan [CAN] (betamethasone), **125**

BiArrest-2 (water-based dual phenolics), **502**

Biaxin (clarithromycin), **144**, 459, *478*

Bicillin L-A (penicillin G), **439**

BiCNU (carmustine), **444**, 468, *478*

Bio-Flex Dental Examination ★ (nonsterile latex examination gloves), **495**

Biocef (cephalexin), **139**

Biocide (iodophor), **502**

Biohazard bags, **492-493**, **503-504**

Biohazard communication, **492-493**, **504**

Biological monitoring, **492**, **501**

Biosign Spore vials/Incubator (spore testing equipment), **501**

Biosonic Ultrasonic Cleaner (mechanical instrument cleaner), **498**

Biozyme (enzymatic solution), **498**

Biperiden, **347-350**, 473, **477**

Bipolar disorder drugs, **366-367**, **379-382**, **383-385**

Birex_se (water-based dual phenolics), **502**

Bismatrol Extra Strength (bismuth subsalicylate), **330**

Bismuth subsalicylate, **330-331**

Bisoprolol, **306**

Bitolterol, **321-323**

Black hairy tongue, 452-453, 458

Blanex (chlorzoxazone), **429**

Bleaching agents, 235-239

Blenoxane (bleomycin), 460, *477*

Bleomycin, 460, **477**

Blocadren (timolol), **305**

Blood, chemical constituents of normal laboratory values for, 558-559

Bonding agents, desensitizing, **226-232**

Bone marrow transplantation, 442

Brethaire (terbutaline), **322**

Brethine (terbutaline), **322**

Bretylate (bretylium), **297**

Bretylium tosylate, 258, **296-298**, 460, **477**

Bretylol (bretylium), 258, **297**, 460, **477**

Brevibloc (esmolol), 251, **305**

Brevicon (ethinyl estradiol/norethindrone), **407**, 459, 469, *480*

Brevital (methohexital Na), **60**

BrianCare Antimicrobial Skin Cleanser ★ (chlorhexidine gluconate solution), **177**

Bricanyl (terbutaline), **322**

Brietal [CAN] (methohexital Na), **60**

Bromazepam, **18-30**, **358-360**, 374, **376-378**

Bromides, 75

Bromocriptine, **347-350**

Brompheniramine and combinations, 471, **477**

Bronalide [CAN] (flunisolide), **320**

Bronchodilators, **321-323**, **326-327**, 328

Bronchospasm, emergency management of, **286**

Bronkaid Mist (epinephrine or epinephrine combinations), **321**

Bronkodyl (theophylline, theophylline sodium glycinate), **323**

Bronkometer (isoetharine hydrochloride/isoetharine mesylate), **322**

Bronkosol (isoetharine hydrochloride/isoetharine mesylate), **322**

Brooks (★) (caries prevention dentifrice), **209**

Bruxism, nocturnal, 357

Buckley's Formo Cresol ★ (formocresol), **181**

Budesonide, **320-321**

Bufferin (aspirin), *476*

Bumethanide, **301-304**

Bumex (bumethanide), **302**

Bupivacaine hydrochloride with epinephrine, **1-9**

Buprenorphine, **40-47**

Bupropion, 360-366, 508-516

Buscopan [CAN] (scopolamine butylbromide), 189

Busodium (butabarbital), 35

BuSpar (buspirone), 359

Buspirone, 358-360

Busulphan, 468, 477

Butabarbital, 32-40

Butalan (butabarbital), 35

Butalbitol compound with codeine (codeine with aspirin, caffeine and butalbitol), 83

Butamben, 6

Butazolidin (phenylbutazone), 461, 462, 464, 466, 475, 485

Butinal with codeine (codeine with aspirin, caffeine and butalbitol), 83

Butisol (butabarbital), 35

Butler (disposable prophy angles), 495

Butler (fluoride prophylaxis paste), 220

Butorphanol, 40-47, 93
agonist-antagonist, 80-96

C

C-Lexin (cephalexin), 435

Cafergot (ergotamine tartrate and caffeine), 351

Caffree (cosmetic dentifrice), 210

Calan (verapamil), 259, 309

Calciclean (heparin), 390

Calciparine (heparin), 390

Calcium channel blockers, 62, 74, 309-310

Calcium chloride, 261

Calcium hydroxide, 180-185

Calcium salts, 333-337

Camalox (calcium salts), 335

Camphorated parachlorophenol (CPC), 180-185

Camphorated Parachlorophenol, U.S.P. ★ (CPC), 184

Cancer therapy, oral complications of, 441-443

Candidiasis, oral, 165, 567

Canesten [CAN] (clotrimazole), 166

Cannabis, 524-525

Cantil (mepenzolate bromide), 335

Capital with Codeine (codeine with acetaminophen), 82

Capoten (captopril), 310, 457, 460, 465, 468, 472, 477

Capreomycin, 62, 74

Capsaicin, 417-420, 424-425, 427

Captopril, 310-311, 457, 460, 465, 468, 472, 477

Carafate (sucralfate), 336

Carbamazepine, 38, 62, 93, 190, 195, 342-346, 367-374, 432-440, 460, 462, 470, 477

Carbamide peroxide, 235-239

Carbenicillin, 137

Carbidopa/levodopa, 347-350, 473, 477

Carbocaine ★ (mepivacaine hydrochloride), 3

Carbocaine with Neo-Cobefrin ★ (mepivacaine hydrochloride with levonordefrin), 3

Carbolith (lithium), 367

Carbonic anhydrase inhibitors, 75, 126

Carboplatin, 468, 477

Cardene (nicardipine), 309

Cardiac glycosides, 299

Cardilate (erythrityl tetranitrate), 300

Cardiovascular drugs, 295-318

Cardizem (diltiazem), 309, 461, 463, 479

Cardoquin (quinidine gluconate or sulfate), 296

Care-4 ★ (topical acidulated phosphate fluoride), 220

Carerite Nylon ★ (sterilization pouch), 498

Carisoprodol, 428-431

Carmustine (nitrosourea), 444, 468, 478

Carteolol, 305-308

Cartol (carteolol), 305

Cassettes (sterilization packaging), 498

Cataflam (diclofenac), 100, 455, 479

Catapres (clonidine), 312, 472, 479

Catecholamine, 51

Cavicide (alcohol-based quaternary ammonium compound), 502

Ceclor (cefaclor), 138, 435, 455, 478

CeeNU (lomustine), 468, 483

Cefaclor, 134-142, 432-440, 455, 478

Cefadroxil, 134-142, 546

Cefamandol, 459, 478

Cefanex (cephalexin), 139

Cefazolin, 546

Cefixime, 134-142

Ceftin (cefuroxime), 139

Cefuroxime, 134-142

Celestone (betamethasone), 125, 422, 457

Celestone [CAN] (betamethasone), 125

Celontin (methsuximide), 344

Centrax (prazepam), 26, 359, 470, 486

Cepacol (cosmetic mouthrinse), 201

Cephalexin, 134-142, 432-440, 546

Cephalosporins, 134-142, 455

Cephradine, 134-142

Cetacaine ★ (benzocaine, butamben and tetracaine hydrochloride), 12

Charcoal, 38

Chateau (★) (caries prevention dentifrices), 209

Check valve (antiretraction valve), 494

Chemical indicators, 492, 500

Chemical mediator inhibitors, 320-321, 326-327, 328

Chemical vapor sterilizer, unsaturated, 500

Chemotherapy and dental management, 443

Chest pain, emergency management of, 290-292

Chewing gum, fluoridated, 216

Chlor-Pro 10 (chlorpheniramine), 245

Chlor-Trimeton (chlorpheniramine), 245, 472, 478

Chloral hydrate, 49-52, 432-440, 522-523

Chloramphenicol, 38, 463, 478

Chloraseptic (benzocaine or benzocaine and menthol anesthetic mouthrinse), 12, 201

Chlordiazepoxide, 18-30, 358-360, 432-440, 470, 478

Chlordiazepoxide/clidinium, 470, 478

Chlorhexidine or chlorhexidine combination, 175-178, 199-207, 461, 478

Chlorine-based surface disinfectants, 492, 502

Chlormycetin, 463, 478

Chlorofon-F (chlorzoxazone), 429

Chloroprocaine, 6

Chlorostat Antimicrobial Skin Cleanser ★ (chlorhexidine gluconate solution), 177

Chlorothiazide, 301-304, 474, 478

Chlorox (sodium hydrochloride), 182

Chlorpheniramine, 245, 472, 478

Chlorpromanyl (chlorpromazine), 370

Chlorpromazine, 28, 367-374, 463, 465, 473, 478

Chlorpropamide, 404, 409, 410, 456, 462, 465, 478

Chlorprothixene, 367-374, 463, 465, 478

Chlorthalidone, 301-304

Chlortrianisene, 401, 403

Chlorzoxazone, 428-431

Choledyl (theophylline), 323

Cholestyramine, 330-331, 460, 478

Choline and magnesium trisalicylate, 96-107

Cholinergic antiglaucoma drugs, 195

Cholinergic drugs, 194-196
antagonists, 186-193

Cholinesterase inhibitors, 4

Cibalith-S (lithium), 367

Cida-Stat Antimicrobial Solution ★ (chlorhexidine gluconate solution), 177

Cida-Steryl Plus (glutaraldehyde liquid sterilant), 500

Cidex Plus (glutaraldehyde liquid sterilant), 500

Cidex Plus test strips (glutaraldehyde concentration monitor), 501

Cimetidine, 4, 28, 333-337

Cinquin (quinidine gluconate or sulfate), 296

Cipro (ciprofloxacin), 157, 456, 486

Dipridacot (dipyridamole), **393**

Diprivan (propofol), **60**

Diprosone (betamethasone [medium to high potency]), **131,** 420

Dipyridamole, **392-394,** 454, 461, *480*

DisCide (alcohol-based phenolics), **502**

Disalcid (salsalate), **102**

DisCide-TB (alcohol-based quaternary ammonium compound), **502**

Disinfectants
see Infection control techniques and products

Disipal (orphenadrine), **348**

Disodium cromoglycate/cromolyn, **320-321**

Disopyramide, **296-298**

Dispatch (chlorine-based surface disinfectant), **502**

Disposable clothing, **489-497**

Disposable Face Shield (faceshield), **497**

Disposable Gowns (disposable clothing), **497**

Disposable Protectors (surface covers), **502**

Disposable Side Shields (clip-on side shields), **497**

Disposable Sleeves (surface covers), **502**

Disposa Chain (disposable napkin chains), **495**

Dispos-a Med (isoetharine hydrochloride/isoetharine mesylate), **322**

Disposa-Shield (surface covers), **502**

Dispos-a-Trap (disposable vacuum traps), **495**

DisposiNeedle System (sharps containers), **503**

Disulfiram, **28**

Ditropan (oxybutynin), 470, *485*

Diucardin (hydroflumethiazide), **303**

Diuchlor H (hydrochlorothiazide), **303**

Diulo (metolazone), **303**

Diuretics, 45, 62, 75, 104, 126, **301-304,** 314-317

Diuril (chlorothiazide), **303,** 474, *478*

Divalproex, **366-367**

Dixarit (clonidine), **312**

DNase inhibitors (Dornase alfa), **324, 325**

Dolacet (hydrocodone bitartrate with acetaminophen), **84**

Dolagesic (hydrocodone bitartrate with acetaminophen), **84**

Dolgesic (ibuprofen), **101**

Dolobid (diflunisal), **102,** 455, 465, 475, *479*

Donnatal (hyoscyamine/atropine/phenobarbital/scopolamine), 470, *481*

Dopamine, 14

Dopar (levodopa), **348,** 460, 465, 473, *482*

Doral (quazepam), **27, 376**

Doryx (doxycycline hyclate), **148, 436**

Doxacurium chloride, **70-79**

Doxapram, 62

Doxepin, 5, 14, **360-366,** 471, *480*

Doxy-Caps (doxycycline), **436**

Doxycin (doxycycline hyclate), **148**

Doxycycline, 38, **146-150, 432-440,** 456

Doxy Film (doxycycline), **436**

Doxylin (doxycycline hyclate), **148**

Dramamine (dimenhydrinate), 473, *480*

Dri-Clave (non-enzymatic solution), **498**

Dronabinol, 190, 195

Droperidol-type opioids, 63

Droperidol/fentanyl citrate, **56-69**

Drug Emporium (★) (caries prevention dentifrice), **209**

Drug resistance, 171

Drug-seeking behaviors, 521

Drug theft, 521, 526

Dry-dose (isoetharine hydrochloride/isoetharine mesylate), **322**

Dry heat sterilizers, 492, **498-501**

Dry socket, 453, 459

Dual-X (water-based dual phenolics), **502**

Dulcets (trimethadione), **345**

Duocet (hydrocodone bitartrate with acetaminophen), **84**

Duotrate (pentaerythritol tetranitrate), **300**

Durabolin (nandrolone), **402**

Dura-Estrin (estradiol), **403**

DuraFit Powder-Free Latex Procedural Exam ★ (nonsterile latex examination gloves), **495**

Duraflor (sodium fluoride varnish), **220, 229**

Duragen (estradiol), **403**

Duralith (lithium), **367**

Duramorph (morphine or morphine sulfate), **43, 91,** 248, 260, **438**

Duranest with Epinephrine ★ (etidocaine hydrochloride with epinephrine), **3**

Duraphat (fluoride-containing varnish), **220, 229**

Duraquin (quinidine gluconate or sulfate), **296**

Duratest (testosterone), **402**

Durathate-200 (testosterone), **402**

Duretic (methyclothiazide), **303**

Duricel (cefadroxil), **139**

Durules (metoprolol), **305**

D-Val (diazepam), **21,** 247, **343,** 359, **376, 436**

D-Val [CAN] (diazepam), **343,** 359, **376, 436**

Dyazide (triamterene/HCTZ), **303,** 474, *488*

Dycil (dicloxacillin), **138**

Dyclone ★ (dyclonine hydrochloride), **13**

Dyclonine hydrochloride, **10-16**

Dyflex (aminophyllin [theophylline ethylenediamine-xanthine], phyllocontin, somophyllin-DF, somophyllin, dyphylline, parolon [CAN]), **322**

Dymelor (acetohexamine), **409,** 456, *476*

Dyna-Hex Antimicrobial Skin Cleanser ★ (chlorhexidine gluconate solution), **177**

Dynacin (minocycline hydrochloride), **148**

DynaCirc (isradipine), **309**

Dynapen (dicloxacillin), **138**

Dyrenium (triamterene), **303,** 474, *488*

Dysgeusia, 453, 459-461

E

Eagle Sterilizer (steam autoclave), **499**

Ear Loop Face and Procedure (mask, earloop), **496**

Easy-Gel (topical stannous fluoride gel), **221**

EC-Naprosyn (naproxen), **438**

Ecotrin (aspirin), *476*

E-Cypionate (estradiol), **403**

Edercin (ethacrynic acid), **302**

EDTAC (EDTA), **182**

E.E.S. (erythromycin ethylsuccinate), **144,** *480*

Effexor (venlafaxine), **362**

Egg phosphatide (lecithin), 63

Elavil (amitriptyline), **364,** 458, 471, *476*

Eldepryl (selegiline), **348**

E-Lor (propoxyphene hydrochloride with acetaminophen), **86**

Eltroxin (levothyroxine), **411**

Emergencies, medical, **240-278, 279-292**
see also specific types of emergencies

Emergency drugs, **240-278**

Emergency equipment, 242

Emergency procedures (P,A,B,C,D), 240, 279-281

Emergency situations, incidence of, 280

Eminase (anistreplase), **395**

Empirin (codeine with aspirin), **82,** **439,** *476*

E-Mycin (erythromycin base), **144,** **436,** *480*

Enalapril, **310-311,** 461, 472, *480*

Enamelon (caries prevention dentifrice), **209**

Enanthate, **524-525**

Encaid (encainide), **297**

Encainide, **296-298**

Endep (amitriptyline), **364**, 471, *476*

Endocet (oxycodone with aceta-minophen), **85**

Endocrine/hormonal drugs, **400-415**, **412-413, 414-415**

Endogenous catecholamine: epinephrine, **244**

Enduron (methyclothiazide), **303**

Enflurane, 5, 14, **56-69**

Entertainer's Secret (saliva substitute), **197**

Enzol (enzymatic solution), **498**

Enzymatic instrument cleaning solution, **492, 498-501**

EpiAdrenalin (epinephrine or epinephrine combinations), **321**

Epiclase (phenacemide), **344**

Epimorph [CAN] (morphine or morphine sulfate), **43, 91**, 248, 260

Epinephrine and epinephrine combinations, 14, 255, **321-323**

EpiPen Auto-Injector (epinephrine or epinephrine combinations), 244, **321**

Epitol (carbamazepine), **343, 367**, 372

Epival [CAN] (divalproex), **367**

Epivir, **564**

Epoetin alfa, **386, 387-388, 396-397, 398-399**

Epogen (epoetin alfa), **387**

Eprex (epoetin alfa), **387**

Equanil (meprobamate), **54**, 467, 470, *483*

Equanil [CAN] (meprobamate), **54**

Equate ★ (caries prevention denti-frices), **209**

Ercaf (ergotamine tartrate and caffeine), **351**

Ergocaff (ergotamine tartrate and caffeine), **351**

Ergomar (ergotamine tartrate), **351**

Ergostat (ergotamine tartrate), **351**

Ergotamine combinations, **350-352**

Eryc (erythromycin), *480*

Erypar (erythromycin stearate), **144**

Eryped (erythromycin ethylsucci-nate), **144**

Ery-Tab (erythromycin base), **144, 436**

Erythema multiforme, 418, 453, 461-462

Erythrityl tetranitrate, **299-301**

Erythro (erythromycin ethylsuccinate), **144, 436**

Erythrocin (erythromycin stearate), **144, 436**

Erythrocot (erythromycin stearate), **144**

Erythromycin base and erythromycin combinations, **142-146**

Erythromycin Base Filmtab (erythro-mycin base), **144**

Erythromycin, 28, **432-440**, 455, *480*

Esidrix (hydrochlorothiazide), **303**, 474, *481*

Eskalith (lithium), **367**, 460, 466, 473, *483*

Esmolol, 251, **305-308**

Estazolam, **18-30, 374, 376-378**

Esterified estrogens, **403**

Esters, 1, 6

Estinyl (ethinyl estradiol) **403**, 459, 469, *480*

Estrace (estradiol), **403**

Estraderm (estradiol), **403**

Estradiol, **400-401, 403**

Estragyn (estrone or estradiol), **403**

Estra-L 40 (estradiol), **403**

Estratab (esterified estrogens), **403**

Estro-A (estrone), **403**

Estro-Cyp (estradiol), **403**

Estrofem (estradiol), **403**

Estrogens, **401, 403, 412-413, 414-415**

Estroject-LA (estradiol), **403**

Estro-L.A. (estradiol), **403**

Estrone, **403**

Estropipate, **400-401, 403**

Estro-Span (estradiol), **403**

Estrovis (quinestrol), **403**

Ethacrynic acid, **301-304**

Ethchlorvynol, **52-53**

Ethinyl estradiol and combinations, **401, 403, 404, 407-408**, 459, 469, *480*

Ethopropazine, **347-350**, 473, *480*

Ethosuximide, **342-346**

Ethotoin, **342-346**

Ethrane (enflurane), **58**

Ethyl alcohol, **178-180**

Ethylenediamine-tetra-acetic acid (EDTA), **180-185**

Ethynodiol and ethinyl estradiol, **404, 407-408**, 459, 469, *480*

Etidocaine hydrochloride with epinephrine, **1-9**

Etodolac, **96-107**, 455, *480*

Etomidate, **56-69**

Etrafon (amitriptyline/perphenazine), 471, *476*

Eugenol U.S.P. ★ (eugenol), **184**

Eugenol, **180-185**

Euglucon (glyburide), **409**

Evacuation Screens (disposable vacuum traps), **495**

Evacuation systems, **491-492, 493-495**

Evacuation tips and saliva ejector tips, high volume disposable **491-492, 493-495**

Evacuator/Ejector Tips (disposable high volume evacuation tips and saliva ejector tips), **494**

Everone (testosterone), **402**

E-Vista (hydroxyzine), **359**

Excedrin IB (ibuprofen), **101, 436**

Excell Antimicrobial Skin Cleanser ★ (chlorhexidine gluconate solution), **177**

Exna (benzthiazide), **303**

Extended insulin zinc, **401, 404, 405-406**

External bleaching, 235-236

Eye Clasps (disposable eyewear), **494**

Eye drops, 74

Eyeglasses, **492, 496-497**

Eyesaver glasses (eyeglasses), **497**

Eyewear, protective, **492, 493-495, 497**

F

Faceshields, **492, 495-497**

Famotidine, **333-337**

Fastin (phentermine), 469, *485*

Feldene (piroxicam), **100**, 455, 475, *486*

Felodipine, **309-310**

Femiron (ferrous fumarate), **387**

Femogex (estradiol), **403**

Fenfluramine, 469, *480*

Fenoprofen, **96-107**, 475, *480*

Fentanyl and analogs, **40-47, 522-523**

Fentanyl-type opioids, 63

Feosol (ferrous sulfate), **388**, *482*

Feostat (ferrous fumarate), **387**

Fergon (ferrous gluconate), **387**

Fer-In-Sol (ferrous sulfate), **388**

Fero-Fradumet (ferrous sulfate), **388**

Fero-Grad (ferrous sulfate), **388**

Ferospae (ferrous sulfate), **388**

Ferralet (ferrous gluconate), **387**

Ferralyn (ferrous sulfate), **388**

Ferra-TD (ferrous sulfate), **388**

Ferric oxalate, **226-232**

Ferric sulfate, **116-117**

Ferrous fumarate, **386, 387-388**

Ferrous gluconate, **386, 387-388**

Ferrous sulfate, **386, 387-388**

Fertinic (ferrous gluconate), **387**

File-EZE (EDTA), **182**

Finast ★ (caries prevention dentifrice), **209**

Fiorinal (codeine with aspirin, caffeine and butalbitol), **83**

5-fluorouracil, 460, *480*

Flagyl (metronidazole), **153, 332, 437**, 459, *484*

Flaxedil (gallamine triethiodide), **71**

Flecainide, **296-298**

Flexaphen (chlorzoxazone), **429**

Flexeril (cyclobenzaprine hydro-chloride), **429**, 458, 474, *479*

Flexoject (orphenadrine), **348**

Flexon (orphenadrine), **429**

Flora, resident (colonizing) and tran-sient (contaminating), 175-176

Florentine II ★ (topical stannous fluoride gel), **221**

Floricet #3 (codeine with acetamino-phen, caffeine and butalbitol), **82**

Fluanoxol Depot [CAN] (molindone), **370**

H

Habitrol (nicotine transdermal patch), 461, 475, *484*, **510, 511**
Halazepam, **18-30,** 358-360
Halcinonide, 420-422
Halcion (triazolam), **27, 377, 440,** 475, *488*
Haldol (haloperidol), **368,** 463, 466, 473, *481*
Hallucinogens, 524-525
Halog Cream (halcinonide), 420
Halogenated hydrocarbons, 63
Haloperidol, 5, **367-374,** 463, 466, 473, *481*
Halotestin (fluoxymesterone), **402**
Halothane, 5, 14, **56-69**
Haltran (ibuprofen), **101**
Hands-free faucets, **491-492, 493-495**
Handwashing agents, **175-178**
Hannaford ★ (caries prevention dentifrice), **209**
Harken Assure Self-seal ★ (sterilization pouch), **498**
Harmonyl (deserpidine), **312**
Harvey Chemiclave (chemical vapor sterilizer, unsaturated), **500**
Hashish and hashish oil, 524-525
Health-Dent Desensitizer (strontium chloride), **227**
Health Sonics Ultrasonic Cleaner (mechanical instrument cleaner), **498**
Heat Sealer and Cutter (heat sealer), **499**
Heat sealers (sterilization packaging), **492, 498-501**
Heavy Duty Nitrile (heavy utility gloves), **496**
Heavy utility gloves, **492, 495-497**
Hema-Glu Desensitizer (strontium chloride), **227**
Hematologic drugs, **386-399, 396-397, 398-399**
Hematologic examination normal laboratory values, 557
Hemocyte (ferrous fumarate), **387**
Hemodent (retraction cord, plain), **118**
Hemodent ★ (aluminum chloride), **116**
Hemodent ★ (retraction cord with aluminum chloride), **118**
Hemodent-PS (ferric sulfate), **116**
Hemodettes (aluminum chloride), **116**
Hemogin-L (aluminum chloride), **116**
Hemostasis, abnormal, 452, 454-455
Hemostatics, **108-116**
Henry Schein Ultrasonic Cleaner (mechanical instrument cleaner), **498**
Hepalean (heparin), **390,** 454, *481*
Heparin Leo (heparin), **390**
Heparin, 104, **386, 389-391,** 454, *481*

Hepatic disease, therapeutics in, **432-440**
Hepatic enzyme inducers, 62, 126
Heroin, 522-523
Hexafluorenium, 74
Hismanal (astemizole), 471, *476*
Histerone (testosterone), **402**
Histoplasmosis, 165
HIVID, **564**
Homebest ★ (caries prevention dentifrice), **209**
Honvol (diethylstilbestrol), **403**
Host resistance, altered, 452, 455-457
Human immunodeficiency virus (HIV) treatment, 563-564
Humulin (extended insulin zinc, insulin, insulin zinc or isophane insulin), **405, 406,** 456, *482*
Hurricaine ★ (benzocaine), **12**
Hybolin (nandrolone), **402**
Hycomed (hydrocodone bitartrate with acetaminophen), **84**
Hyco-pap (hydrocodone bitartrate with acetaminophen), **84**
Hydantoins, 38
Hydralazine, **308**
Hydrea (hydroxyurea), 468, *481*
Hydrex (benzthiazide), **303**
Hydro-chlor (hydrochlorothiazide), **303**
Hydrochlorothiazide, **301-304,** 474, *481*
Hydrocodone bitartrate with acetaminophen, 80-96
Hydrocodone, **40-47,** 522-523
Hydrocortisone sodium succinate (low potency), **129-133,** 250, 420-422
Hydro-D (hydrochlorothiazide), **303**
HydroDIURIL (hydrochlorothiazide), **303,** 474, *481*
Hydroflumethiazide, **301-304**
Hydrogen peroxide, **180-185, 235-239**
Hydrogesic (hydrocodone bitartrate with acetaminophen), **84**
Hydromorphone, **40-47, 80-96,** 522-523
Hydromox (quinethazone), **304**
Hydroset (hydrocodone bitartrate with acetaminophen), **84**
Hydrostat IR (hydromorphone hydrochloride), **89**
Hydroxacen (hydroxyzine), **359**
Hydroxychloroquine, **417-420, 424-425, 427**
Hydroxyprogesterone, **410-411**
Hydroxyurea, **468,** *481*
Hydroxyzin (hydroxyzine), **359**
Hydroxyzine, 94, **358-360,** 472, 473
Hy/Gestrone (hydroxyprogesterone), **410**
Hygroton (chlorthalidone), **303**
Hylorel (guanadrel), **313**
Hylutin (hydroxyprogesterone), **410**

Hyoscyamine and combinations, 470, *481*
Hyperactivity disorder drugs, **374, 375, 379-382, 383-385**
Hyperactivity disorders, 374
Hyperglycemia, signs of, 404
Hypertension, 301
Hy-phen (hydrocodone bitartrate with acetaminophen), **84**
Hypnotics (sedative), 94
Hypogen (sodium hydrochloride), **183**
Hypoglycemia, signs of, 404
Hypoglycemics (oral), 104
Hypotension-producing drugs, 62
Hytone (hydrocortisone [cortisol] [low potency]), **131**
Hytrin (α-1 selective) (terazosin), **306**
Hy-Vee ★ (caries prevention dentifrice), **209**
Hyzine-50 (hydroxyzine), **359**

I

Ibu (ibuprofen), **101**
Ibuprin (ibuprofen), **101, 436**
Ibuprofen, **96-107, 432-440,** 455, 465, 469, 475, *482*
Ibuprohm (ibuprofen), **101**
Idenal with codeine (codeine with aspirin, caffeine and butalbital), **83**
Imipramine, 5, 14, 28, **360-366,** 471, *482*
Imitrex (sumatriptan succinate), **351**
Immunosuppressive agents (methotrexate), **324, 325**
Imodium A-D (loperamide), **331,** 471, *483*
Imovane [CAN] (zopicione), **377**
Impril (imipramine), **365**
IMS instrument processing products, **498, 500**
Imuran (azathioprine), **332,** 460, 468, *477*
Indandione-derivative anticoagulants, 51
Inderal (propranolol), **305, 349**
Indinavir, 563-564
Indocid [CAN] (indomethacin), **99**
Indocin (indomethacin and indomethacin, sustained release), **99,** 455, 469, *482*
Indomethacin, **96-107,** 455, 469, *482*
Infection control techniques and products
  aseptic **491-492, 493-495**
  barrier, **492, 495-497**
  instrument processing, **492, 498-501**
  surface asepsis, **492, 502**
  waste management, **492-493, 503-504**

Libritabs (chlordiazepoxide), **20, 358, 435**

Librium (chlordiazepoxide), **20, 358, 435,** 470, *478*

Lichen planus, 130, 418, **568**

Lichenoid lesions, 453, 465

Lidex (fluocinonide [high potency]), **131**

Lidex Gel (flucinonide), 420

Lidocaine (cardiac), **296-298**

Lidocaine and lidocaine combinations, **1-9, 10-16,** 256

Lightly Powdered Latex Exam ★ (nonsterile latex examination gloves), **495**

Lignospan (lidocaine hydrochloride), 3

Lignospan Forte ★ (lidocaine hydrochloride with epinephrine), 3

Lignospan Standard ★ (lidocaine hydrochloride with epinephrine), 3

Lincocin (lincomycin), 459, *482*

Lincomycin, 74, 459, *482*

Lioresal (baclofen), 350, 461, *482*

Liothyronine, 5, 14, **411**

Liotrix, **411**

Liquaemin (heparin), **390**

Liquid Pred (prednisone), **125, 332**

Lisinopril, **310-311,** 472, *483*

Listerine ★ (phenolic compound mouthrinse, preprocedure antimicrobial), 203, **493**

Listermint (cosmetic mouthrinses), 201

Lithane (lithium), 367

Lithium, 74, 104, **366-367,** 460, 466, 473, *483*

Lithizine (lithium), 367

Lithobid (lithium), 367

Lithonate (lithium), 367

Lithotabs (lithium), 367

Lobac (chlorzoxazone), **429**

Local anesthetic overdose, emergency management of, **289-290**

Local anesthetics
dosage calculation, 562
injectable, **1-9**
topical, 6, 7-8, **10-16**

Locomot (diphenoxylate hydrochloride and atropine sulfate), 331

Lodine ★ (etodolac), 99, 455, *480*

Loestrin (ethinyl estradiol/norethindrone), **408,** 459, *480*

Lofene (diphenoxylate hydrochloride and atropine sulfate), 331

Loftran (ketazolam), 359

Loftran [CAN] (ketazolam), 23

Logen (diphenoxylate hydrochloride and atropine sulfate), 331

Lomotil (diphenoxylate hydrochloride and atropine sulfate), 331, 471, *479*

Lomustine, 468, *483*

Longs ★ (caries prevention dentifrice), 209

Loniten (minoxidil), 308

Lonox (diphenoxylate hydrochloride and atropine sulfate), 331

Lo/Ovral (ethinyl estradiol/norgestrel, norgestrel or norethindrone), **408,** 459, 469, *480*

Loperamide, 330-331, 471, *483*

Lopressor (metoprolol), **305,** 472, *484*

Loratadine, 472, *483*

Lorazepam, **18-30, 358-360, 374, 376-378, 432-440,** 458, 470, *483*

Lorazepam Intensol (lorazepam), **359, 376**

Lorcet (hydrocodone bitartrate with acetaminophen), 84

Lortab (hydrocodone bitartrate with acetaminophen), 83, 84

Losartan, **310-311**

Lotensin (benazepril), **310,** 457, *477*

Lotrimin (clotrimazole), 166

Loxapac [CAN] (loxapine), 369

Loxapine, 367-374, 466, 473, *483*

Loxitane (loxapine), 369, 466, 473, *483*

Lu Fyllin (aminophylline [theophylline ethylenediamine-xanthine], phyllocontin, somophyllin-DF, somophyllin, dyphylline, parolon [CAN]), 322

Ludiomil (maprotiline), **364,** 471, *483*

Luminal (phenobarbital), **36-37, 344,** 462, 464, *485*

Lupus erythematosus, 417, 418

Luride Lozi-Tabs (topical neutral or acidulated sodium fluoride gel), 220

Luride Lozi-Tabs ★ (systemic sodium fluoride), 217

Luroscrub Antimicrobial Skin Cleanser ★ (chlorhexidine gluconate solution), 177

Lurosep Antimicrobial Lotion Soap (chloroxylenol), 177

Luvox (fluvoxamine), 363

Lysatec (recombinant alterplase), 395

Lysergic acid diethylamide (LSD), 520, **524-525**

Lysol I.C. (water-based dual phenolics or alcohol-based phenolics), 502

Lysol I.C. Antimicrobial Soap (triclosan or irgasan), 177

M

Maalox (loperamide or magnesium salts and aluminum salts), 331, 335

Macrodantin (nitrofurantoin), 458, *484*

Macrolides, **142-146,** 455

Magill intubation, 242

Magnesium salts and aluminum salts, 74, **333-337**

Majeptil [CAN] (thioproperazine), **371**

Malaytex Latex Examination ★ (nonsterile latex examination gloves), **495**

Malogen (testosterone), **402**

Malpractice cases, 528-530

Mandol (cefamandol), 459, *478*

Maprotiline, 5, **360-366,** 471, *483*

Marbaxin (methocarbamol), **429**

Marblen (calcium salts), 335

Marcaine with Epinephrine ★ (bupivacaine hydrochloride with epinephrine), 3

Marflex (orphenadrine), **348, 429,** 473, *485*

Margesic-H (hydrocodone bitartrate with acetaminophen), 84

Marijuana, **524-525**
abuse, 520

Marplan (isocarboxazid), **363,** 471, *482*

Marsin Latex Examination ★ (nonsterile latex examination gloves), **495**

Marvelon (ethinyl estradiol/desogestrel), **407**

Masks, earloop, single retention band or tie-on, **492, 496-497**

Masnasil (fluoride prophylaxis paste), 220

Maxair (pirbuterol acetate), 322

MaxiCide (glutaraldehyde liquid sterilant), **500**

Maxiclens ★ (chlorhexidine gluconate solution), 177

Maxizyme (enzymatic solution), **498**

Maxzide (triamterene/HCTZ), 474, *488*

M.C.P. Root Canal Dressing ★ (parachlorophenol [PCP]), 184

Mebaral (mephobarbital), **35, 344,** 464, *483*

Mebenol (tolbutamide), **409**

Mechanical instrument cleaners, **492, 498-501**

Meclizine, 473, *483*

Meclofenamate, **96-107,** 455, *483*

Meclomen (meclofenamate), **98,** 455, *483*

Medihaler (epinephrine or epinephrine combinations), 321

Medihaler Ergotamine (ergotamine tartrate), 351

Medi-Plus Self-sealing ★ (sterilization pouch), 498

Medi-Plus Sterilization ★ (sterilization pouch), 498

Medipren (ibuprofen), **101**

Medrol (methylprednisolone), 422, 457, *484*

Medroxyprogesterone, **410-411**

MEDWATCH form (for reporting adverse effects of medications), 569-570

Mefenamic acid, **96-107**, 455, *483*

Megace (megestrol), **410**

Megestrol, **410-411**

Meijer ★ (caries prevention dentifrice), **209**

Mellaril (thioridazine), **370**, 464, 466, 474, *487*

Melphalan (nitrogen mustard), **441-449**

Menadiol sodium diphosphate or vitamin K, **108-116**

Menaval-20 (estradiol), **403**

Menest (esterified estrogens), **403**

Mentadent ★ (caries prevention dentifrice), **209**, 221

Mepenzolate bromide, **333-337**

Meperidine, **40-47**, **80-96**, **432-440**, 474, *483*

Mephenytoin, **342-346**

Mephobarbital, **32-40**, **342-346**, 464, *483*

Mephyton (vitamin K, or phytona-dione), **111**

Mepivacaine hydrochloride and mepivacaine hydrochloride with levonordefrin, **1-9**

Meprobamate, **53-55**, 467, 470, *483*

Meprospan (meprobamate), **54**

Meprospan 400 [CAN] (meproba-mate), **54**

Mercaptopurine, 468, *483*

Mercury, 468, *483*

Mesantoin (mephenytoin), **344**

Mescaline, **524-525**

M-Eslon [CAN] (morphine sulfate), **91**

Mesoridazine, **371**, 463, 466, *483*

Mestinon (pyridostigmine), **346**

Metaformin, 456, *483*

Metandren (methyltestosterone), **402**

Metaprel (metaproterenol sulfate), **322**

Metaproterenol sulfate, **321-323**

Methacrylate polymer bonding agent, **226-232**

Methadone, **41**

Methadone and LAAM, **522-523**

Methantheline, **186-193**, 470, 483

Metharbitol, **342-346**

Methimazole, 460, *484*

Methocarbamol, **428-431**

Methohexital, 45, **56-69**

Metholazone, **301-304**

Methotrexate, 104, **324**, **325**, **417-420**, **424-425**, 427, **441-449**, 460, 468, *484*

Methotrimeprazine, 74, **367-374**

Methoxamine, **249**

Methoxyflurane, 39, **56-69**

Methscopolamine, **333-337**, 470, *484*

Methsuximide, **342-346**

Methyclothiazide, **301-304**

Methydrin (trichloromethiazide), **304**

Methyldopa, 5, 14, **311**, **312**, 465, 466, 468, 472, *484*

Methylphenidate, 14, **374**, **375**, **522-523**

Methylprednisolone, 420-422, 457, *484*

Methyltestosterone, **400-401**, **402**

Methylxanthines, **62**

Methysergide maleate, **350-352**

Meticorten (prednisone), **125**, 332

Metoclopramide, 94, 190, **333**, **334**, **333-337**

Metocurine iodide, **70-79**

Metoprolol, **305-308**, 472, *484*

Metric 21 (metronidazole), **332**, 437

MetriCide (glutaraldehyde liquid sterilant), **500**

MetriGuard (alcohol-based quaternary ammonium compound), **502**

MetriZyme (enzymatic solution), **498**

Metronidazole, 39, **152-155**, **331-333**, **432-440**, 459, *484*

Metroprolol, **4**

Metubine Iodide (metocurine iodide), **71**

Mexiletine, 4, **296-298**

Mexitil (mexiletine), **296**

Micro prime (methacrylate polymer bonding agent), **230**

Micro-Touch Latex Surgical (sterile latex gloves), **496**

Microfibrillar collagen hemostat, **108-116**

Micronase (glyburide), **409**

Micronor (norethindrone), **410**

Midamor (amiloride), **303**

Midazolam, **18-30**, 457, *484*

Midmark (steam autoclave), **499**

Midol (ibuprofen), **101**

Midrin (isometheptene mucate, dichlorphenazone, aceta-minophen), **351**

Miflex (chlorzoxazone), **429**

Milk of Magnesia (magnesium salts and aluminum salts), **335**

Milk, fluoridated, **216**

Milontin (phensuximide), **345**

Miltown (meprobamate), **54**, 470, *483*

Miltown [CAN] (meprobamate), **54**

Minestrin (ethinyl estradiol/norethin-drone acetate), **408**

Mini-Ovral (ethinyl estradiol/levonorgestrel), **407**

Minipress (α-1 selective) (prazosin), **306**, 472, *486*

Minocin (minocycline), **148**, **437**, 467, *484*

Minocycline, **146-150**, **432-440**, 467, *484*

Minoxidil, **308**

Miradon (anisindione), **389**

Mirtazapine, **360-366**

Misoprostol, **333-337**

Mivacron (mivacurium chloride), **71**

Mivacurium chloride, **70-79**

Moban (molindone), **370**, 473, *484*

Modecate (fluphenazine), **371**

ModiCon (ethinyl estradiol/norethin-drone), **407**

Moditen (fluphenazine), **371**

Moduretic (amiloride/HCTZ), **304**

Mogadon (nitrazepam), **26**

Mogadon [CAN] (nitrazepam), **26**, 376

Moi-Stir (saliva substitute), **197**

Mol-iron (ferrous sulfate), **388**

Molded face (mask, single retention band), **497**

Molindone, **367-374**, 473, *484*

Monitan (acebutolol), **306**

Monitoring Services (mail-in spore testing service), **501**

Monoamine oxidase inhibitors, 14, 39, 45, 94

Monodox (doxycycline hyclate), **148**, **436**

Monopril (fosinopril), **310**, 457, *481*

Monotray (recapping device), **503**

Morlutate (norethindrone), **410**

Morphine Extra-Forte (morphine sulfate), **248**, **260**

Morphine Extra-Forte [CAN] (mor-phine or morphine sulfate), **43**, **91**

Morphine Forte [CAN] (morphine or morphine sulfate), **43**, **91**, **248**, **260**

Morphine H.P. (morphine sulfate), **248**, **260**

Morphine HP [CAN] (morphine or morphine sulfate), **43**, **91**

Morphine hydrochloride or morphine sulfate, **40-47**, **80-96**, **248**, **260**, **432-440**, 474, *484*, **522-523**

Morphitec (morphine hydro-chloride), **90**

M.O.S. [CAN] (morphine hydro-chloride), **90**

Motrin (ibuprofen), **101**, **436**, 455, 465, 469, 475, *482*

Mouth Kote (caries prevention denti-frice), **209**

Mouthkote (saliva substitute), **197**

Mouthrinses, **199-207**

preprocedure antimicrobial, **491-492**, **493-495**

Movement disorders, 453-454, 465-466

MS Contin (morphine), **438**, 474, *484*

MSIR (morphine sulfate), **91**

MS/L (morphine sulfate), **91**

Mucositis, **442**

Multipax [CAN] (hydroxyzine), **359**

Mus-Lac (chlorzoxazone), **429**

Muscle paralysis reversal drugs, **4**

Muscle relaxants, centrally acting, 4, 62

Musculoskeletal relaxant drugs, **428-431**

Mycelex (clotrimazole), **166**

Pro-Dentx ★ (topical acidulated phosphate fluoride or stannous fluoride gel), **220, 221**
Pro-Depo (hydroxyprogesterone), **410**
Prodrox (hydroxyprogesterone), **410**
ProE-Vac (evacuation system cleaner), **493**
ProEZ (enzymatic solution), **498**
Progesterone, **410-411**
Progestins, **410-411, 412-413, 414-415**
Proglycem (diazoxide), **456**, *479*
Prolixin (fluphenazine), **371, 463, 466**, *480*
Proloid (thyroglobulin), **411**
Promazine, **367-374, 464, 466, 473**, *486*
Promethazine, **472**, *486*
Promine (procainamide), **296**
Prompt insulin zinc, **401, 404, 405-406**
Pronestyl (procainamide), **257, 296**
Proof Plus Spore vials/Incubator (spore testing equipment), **501**
ProPak Nylon Sterilization (nylon tubing sterilization packaging), **499**
Propantheline bromide, **186-193, 333-337, 470**, *486*
ProPhene (water-based dual phenolics), **502**
Prophy (fluoride prophylaxis paste), **220**
Prophy angles, disposable, **491-492, 493-495**
Propofol, **56-69**
Propoxyphene Compound-65 (propoxyphene hydrochloride with aspirin and caffeine), **87**
Propoxyphene hydrochloride combinations, **80-96**
Propoxyphene, **432-440**
Propranolol, 4, 5, 14, **305-308, 347-350**
Propulsid (cisapride), **334**
ProSom (estazolam), **23, 376**
Pro-Sonic (non-enzymatic solution), **498**
Pro-Sonic Cleaning System (mechanical instrument cleaner), **498**
Pro-Span (hydroxyprogesterone), **410**
ProSpec protective wear (infection control products), **497**
ProSpray (water-based dual phenolics), **502**
Prostaphlin (oxacillin), **138**
Prostep (nicotine transdermal patch), **510, 511**
Prostigmin (neostigmine), **346**
Protect (potassium oxalate), **228**
Protect ★ (topical acidulated phosphate fluoride or fluoride-containing dentifrice), **220, 221**
Protect Sensitive Teeth ★ (sodium fluoride and potassium nitrate combination), **210, 233**
Protective clothing, **492, 495-497**

ProTector infection control products, **503, 504**
Protocream-HC (hydrocortisone [cortisol] [low potency]), **131**
Protophylline [CAN] (aminophyllin [theophylline ethylenediamine-xanthine], phyllocontin, somo-phyllin-DF, somophyllin, dyphylline, parolon [CAN]), **322**
Protostat (metronidazole), **153, 332, 437**
ProTouch gloves), **495, 496**
ProView Sterilization ★ (sterilization pouch), **498**
Prozac (fluoxetine), **363, 471**, *480*
Psoriasis, **417-418**
Psychoactive drugs, **356-385**
Pulmicort [CAN] (budesonide), **320**
Pulmozyme (dornase alfa), **324**
Pulpdent Temp Canal (calcium hydroxide), **181**
Purevac (evacuation system cleaner), **493**
Purinethol (mercaptopurine), **468**, *483*
Pyribenzamine (PBZ) (tripelennamine), *472*, *488*
Pyridostigmine, 62, **346-347**

Q
Q-profen (ibuprofen), **101**
QualiTouch Latex ★ (nonsterile latex examination gloves), **495**
Quality Choice ★ (caries prevention dentifrices), **209**
Quanethidine, **466**, *486*
Quantrex Ultrasonic Cleaner (mechanical instrument cleaner), **498**
Quantum Latex Examination ★ (nonsterile latex examination gloves), **495**
Quaternary ammonium compound, **492, 502**
Quazepam, **18-30, 374, 376-378**
Quelicin (succinylcholine chloride), **72**
Questran (cholestyramine), **331, 460**, *478*
Quibron-T (theophylline, theophylline sodium glycinate), **323**
Quiess (hydroxyzine), **359**
Quinalan (quinidine gluconate or sulfate), **296**
Quinamm (quinine), **463**, *486*
Quinapril, **310-311, 457**, *486*
Quinestrol, **401, 403**
Quinethazone, **301-304**
Quinidex (quinidine gluconate or sulfate), **296**
Quinidine gluconate or sulfate, 39, 74, 190, 195, **296-298**

Quiniglute (quinidine gluconate or sulfate), **296**
Quinine, **463**
Quinolones, **155-159**, *486*
Quinora (quinidine gluconate or sulfate), **296**

R
R-Cord (retraction cord with aluminum sulfate or racemic epinephrine), **119**
Racord (retraction cord with racemic epinephrine), **119**
Radant (fluoride prophylaxis paste), **220**
Raley's ★ (caries prevention dentifrice), **209**
Ramipril, **310-311, 457**, *486*
Ranitidine, **333-337**
Rastringent (aluminum chloride), **116**
Raudixin (rauwolfia serpentina), **313**
Rauval (rauwolfia serpentina), **313**
Rauverid (rauwolfia serpentina), **313**
Rauwolfia serpentina, **312-313**
RC Prep ★ (EDTA), **182**
Reach (fluoride), **202-203**
Reach Act (★) (sodium fluoride rinses), **221**
Recapping devices, **492-493, 503-504**
Reclomide (metoclopramide hydrochloride), **334**
REDTA (EDTA), **182**
Redwood Latex Examination ★ (nonsterile latex examination gloves), **495**
Regitine (phentolamine), **306**
Reglan (metoclopramide hydrochloride), **334**
Regonol (pyridostigmine), **346**
Regular Iletin (insulin), **405**
Regular Insulin (insulin), **405**
Reiter's syndrome, **417-418**
Relafen (nabumetone), **102**
Rembrandt (cosmetic dentifrice), **210**
Rembrandt Lighten Bleaching Gel ★ (carbamide peroxide), **237**
Rembrandt Mouth Refreshing Rinse (cosmetic mouthrinse), **201**
Rembrandt Whitening Sensitive (sodium monofluorophosphate and potassium nitrate combination), **210, 233**
Remeron (mirtazapine), **362**
Renal impairment, therapeutics in, **432-440**
Renedil (felodipine), **309**
Renese (polythiazide), **304**
Renin-angiotensin system drugs, **310-311, 314-317**
Renoquid (sulfacytine), **462, 464**, *487*
Rescriptor, **564**

Topex ★ (benzocaine), **12**
Topicaine [CAN] (benzocaine), **12**
Topical local anesthetics, 6, 7-8, **10-16**
Topicale ★ (benzocaine), **12**
Topicort (desoximetasone), 420
Topol Smoker's ★ (caries prevention dentifrices), **209**
Toprol XL (metoprolol), 305
Toradol (ketorolac), **99**, 455, 469, *482*
Tornalate (bitolterol), **321**
Totcillin (ampicillin), **434**
Tourniquets, 242
Tower Dual Peel Self-sealing ★ (sterilization pouch), **498**
Toxicological agents in pregnancy and breast-feeding, 539
Tracrium (atracurium besylate), **71**
Tramadol, 80
Trancot (meprobamate), **54**
Trandate (labetalol), 253, **306**
Transderm-Scop (scopolamine), 470, *487*
Transene-SD (clorazepate), 358
Transport containers, **491-492, 493-495**
Tranxene (clorazepate), **21**, 358
Tranxene [CAN] (clorazepate), **21**
Tranylcypromine, 363, *471*, *488*
Trasicor (oxprenolol), 305
Trazodone, 360-366, *471*, *488*
Trazon (trazodone), 363
Trendar (ibuprofen), **101**
Triadapin (doxepin), 364
Trialodine (trazodone), 363
Triamcinolone acetonide or triamcinolone acetonide with nystatin (medium potency), **129-133, 320-321**, 420-422, 456, *488*
Triamterene and triamterene/hydrochlorothiazide (HCTZ), 104, **303, 304**, *474*, *488*
Triavil (amitriptyline/perphenazine), *473, 476*
Triazolam, **18-30**, 374, **376-378, 432-440**, *475*, *488*
Trichlorex (tricloromethiazide), 304
Tri-Cide (water-based tri-phenolics), **502**
Tri-Clean 110 Latex Exam ★ (nonsterile latex examination gloves), **495**
Tricloromethiazide, **301-304**
Triclosan or irgasan, **175-178**, 207-208
Tri-Cyclen (ethinyl estradiol/norgestimate), **408**
Tricyclic antidepressants, 5, 14, 190, 195
Tridil (nitroglycerin), **300**
Tridione (trimethadione), 345
Triflex (non-latex patient-care gloves), **496**

Trifluoperazine, **367-374**, 464, 466, *488*
Triflupromazine, **367-374**
Trihexane (trihexphenidyl), **348**
Trihexphenidyl, **347-350**
Trihexy (trihexyphenidyl), **348**
Trihexyphenidyl, 473, *488*
Trilafon (perphenazine), **371**, 463, 466, *485*
Tri-Levlen (ethinyl estradiol/levonorgestrel), **407**, 459, 469, *480*
Trilisate (choline and magnesium trisalicylate), **102**
Trimethadione, **342-346**
Trimethoprim and sulfamethoxazole, **159-163**, 563
Trimipramine, **360-366**
Trimox (amoxicillin), **137, 434**
Tri-Norinyl (ethinyl estradiol/norethindrone), **407**
Tripelennamine, 472, *488*
Triphasil (ethinyl estradiol/levonorgestrel), **407**, 459, 469, *480*
Triprolidine/pseudoephedrine, 472, *488*
Triptil [CAN] (protriptyline), 365
Triquilar (ethinyl estradiol/levonorgestrel), **407**
Troleandomycin, 28
Tronex Latex Examination—Lightly Powdered ★ (nonsterile latex examination gloves), **495**
Tru-Touch Stretch Vinyl (non-latex patient-care gloves), **496**
Trymex (triamcinolone acetonide), 421
Tubarine [CAN] (tubocurarine chloride), **73**
Tubing sterilization packaging, nylon, **492, 498-501**
Tubocurarine chloride, **70-79**
Tuinal (secobarbital and amobarbital), 37
Tums (calcium salts), **335**
Turbo-Vac (evacuation system cleaner), **493**
Tuttnauer (steam autoclave), **499**
Tuttnauer Ultrasonic Cleaner (mechanical instrument cleaner), **498**
Tylenol (acetaminophen), **98, 434**
Tylenol (codeine with acetaminophen), 81
Tylox (oxycodone with acetaminophen), 85

Ultra Brite (caries prevention dentifrices), **209**
Ultra Fresh Fluoride ★ (caries prevention dentifrice), **209**
Ultracaine (articaine hydrochloride with epinephrine [CAN]), **3**
Ultracaine Forte (articaine hydrochloride with epinephrine [CAN]), **3**
Ultracef (cefadroxil), **139**
UltraClean (non-enzymatic solution), **498**
Ultralente (extended insulin zinc), **405**
Ultram (tramadol), 80
Ultrapak (retraction cord, plain), **118**
UltraSafe Aspirating Syringe (safety syringes), **503**
Ultrasonic Cleaning System (mechanical instrument cleaner), **498**
Unconsciousness, emergency management of, **282-283**
UniBraid (retraction cord with potassium aluminum sulfate), **119**
Unipen (nafcillin), **138**
Uniphyl (theophylline, theophylline sodium glycinate), **323**
Unipro (fluoride prophylaxis paste), **220**
Uniseal Latex Examination ★ (nonsterile latex examination gloves), **495**
Urdon (chlorthalidone), **303**
Urecholine (bethanechol), *467, 477*
Urine analysis, normal laboratory values for, 559
Uritol (furosemide), **302**
Urokinase, **394-395**
Urozide (hydrochlorothiazide), **303**

Valrelease (diazepam, extended release capsule), **22**

Valu-Rite ★ (caries prevention dentifrice), **209**

Vanacet (hydrocodone bitartrate with acetaminophen), **84**

Vanceril (beclomethasone dipropionate), **320**

Vapo-Iso (isoproterenol), 474

Vaponefrin [CAN] (epinephrine or epinephrine combinations), **321**

Vapor Line (integrator for steam sterilization), **500**

Vapor Phase (rust inhibitor), **498**

Varnishes, desensitizing, **226-232**

Vascular headache suppressants, **350-352, 352-354, 355**

Vasoconstrictors, 1, 2, 5, 8, 9

Vasodilators, 62, 93
    direct acting, **308**

Vasopressors, dosage calculation, 562

Vasotec (enalopril), **310**, 461, 472, *480*

Vasoxyl (methoxamine), 249

Vecuronium bromide, **70-79**

Veetids (penicillin), **138**, 461

Velosef (cephradine), **139**

Velosulin Human (insulin), **405**

Vendone (hydrocodone bitartrate with acetaminophen), **84**

Venlafaxine, **360-366**

Ventolin (albuterol), 247, **321**, 474, *476*

Verapamil, 39, 259, **309-310**

Verelan (verapamil), **309**

Versed (midazolam), **24-26**, 457, *484*

Vesprin (triflupromazine or prochlorperazine), **371**

VI-Atro (diphenoxylate hydrochloride and atropine sulfate), **331**

Viadent (plaque prevention dentifrices), **211**

Viadent Oral Rinse (sanguinarine), **204**

Vibra-tabs (doxycycline hyclate), **148**

Vibramycin (doxycycline), **148, 436,** 456, *487*

Vibratabs (doxycycline), **436**

Vicodin ★ (hydrocodone bitartrate with acetaminophen), **84**

Videx (didanosine [ddI]), **563**

Vincristine, 460, 468, *488*

Vinlon IM (testosterone), **402**

Vinylite (non-latex patient-care gloves), **496**

Viracept, **564**

Viramune, **564**

Vironex (chloroxylenol), **177**

ViscoStat (ferric sulfate), **116**

Visken (pindolol), **305**

Vistaject (hydroxyzine), **359**

Vistaril (hydroxyzine), **359**, 472, 473, *481*

Vistazine-50 (hydroxyzine), **359**

Vital Defense protective wear (infection control products), **495, 496, 502**

Vital Shield Gold Non-Sterile Medical Examination ★ (nonsterile latex examination gloves), **495**

Vitamin K (menadiol or menadione sodium diphosphate or phytonadione), **108-116**

Vitamin supplements, 126

Vivactil (protriptyline), **365**

Vivol [CAN] (diazepam), **21, 343,** **359, 376**

Volatile anesthetics, 62, 63

Voltaren (diclofenac), **100**, 455, *479*

Vytone (hydrocortisone with iodoquinolone [low potency]), **132**

W

Walgreens Sodium Fluoride ★ (caries prevention dentifrice), **209**

Warfarin, **386, 389-391**, 454, 467, *488*

Warfilone (warfarin), **391**

Waste disposal, **492-493, 503**

Waterforde Hypoallergenic Latex Examination ★ (nonsterile latex examination gloves), **495**

Waterline filters, **491-492, 493-495**

WaterSense controller (hands-free faucet), **494**

Wegmans Fluoride ★ (caries prevention dentifrice), **209**

Wehgen (estrone), **403**

Weights and measures, 560-561

Weis Quality ★ (caries prevention dentifrices), **209**

Wellbutrin (bupropion), **362**

Wellcovorin (leucovorin), **392**

Westhroid (thyroid), **411**

Wet-Grip Latex Exam ★ (non-sterile latex examination gloves), **495**

Wigraine (ergotamine tartrate and caffeine), **351**

Winpred [CAN] (prednisone), **125**

Winstrol (stanozolol), **402**

Wolfina (rauwolfia serpentina), **313**

Wraps, sterilization, **492, 498-501**

Wycillin (penicillin G), **439**, 459, *486*

Wygesic (propoxyphene hydrochloride with acetaminophen), **86**

Wymox (amoxicillin), **434**

Wytensin (guanabenz), **312**

X

Xanax (alprazolam), **20, 358, 376,** 470, *476*

Xanax [CAN] (alprazolam), **20**

Xanthines, **222-223, 226-227, 228**

Xero-Lube (saliva substitute), **197**

Xerostomia, 442, 454, **469-475**

Xylocaine (★) (lidocaine or lidocaine hydrochloride), **3, 13**, 256, **296**

Xylocaine Viscous ★ (lidocaine hydrochloride), **13**

Xylocaine with Epinephrine ★ (lidocaine hydrochloride with epinephrine), **3**

Xylocard (lidocaine), **296**

Xylonor (benzocaine), **12**

Y

Young (disposable prophy angles), **495**

Z

Zafirlukast (Accolate) (leukotrine antagonists and inhibitors), **324**

Zalcitabine (ddC), **563-564**

Zanaflex (tizanidine-hydrochloride), **350**

Zantac (ranitidine), **336**

Zarontin (ethosuximide), **343**

Zaroxolyn (metolazone), **303**

Zebeta (bisoprolol), **306**

Zemuron (rocuronium bromide), **72**

Zerit, **564**

Zestril (lisinopril), **310**, 472, *483*

Zetran (diazepam), **22, 343, 359, 376**

Zidovudine (AZT, ZDV), **563-564**

Zilactin-B (benzocaine), **12**

Zileuton (Zyflo) (leukotrine antagonists and inhibitors), **324**

Zinc oxide and zinc oxide-eugenol preparations, **180-185**

Zinc Oxide, U.S.P. ★ (zinc oxide), **183**

Zircon F (fluoride prophylaxis paste), **220**

Ziroxide (fluoride prophylaxis paste), **220**

Zithromax (azithromycin), **144**

Zoloft (sertraline), **363**, 471, *487*

Zolpidem, **18-30, 374, 376-378**

Zopicione [CAN], **374, 376-378**

Zorprin, *476*

Zostrix-OTC (capsaicin), **419**

Zovirax (acyclovir), **172, 434**

Zyban (bupropion hydrochloride), **508**

Zydone (hydrocodone bitartrate with acetaminophen), **84**

Zyloprim (allopurinol), **459**, *476*

Zyprexa (olanzapine), **369**

Dental Indications Index

A

Abscesses
    tetracyclines, 146-150
Actinomycosis
    antifungal agents, 164-171
    penicillin G benzathine
      suspension, 134-142
    tetracyclines, 146-150
Allergic reactions
    chlorpheniramine, 245
    diphenhydramine, 245
    sample prescription, 568
Allergic reactions, mild systemic skin
    management, 287-288
Allergic reactions, severe or
    incapacitating
    hydrocortisone sodium succi-
      nate, 250
Altered consciousness, 283-284
Anaerobic bacilli, gram negative
    metronidazole, 152-155
Anaerobic bacterial infection
    clindamycin, 150-152
Anaerobic cocci, obligate gram positive
    metronidazole, 152-155
Analgesia
    acetaminophen, 96-107
    chloral hydrate, 49-52
    droperidol/fentanyl, 56-69
    enflurane, 56-69
    methoxyflurane, 56-69
    nitrous oxide, 56-69
    nonsteroidal anti-inflammatory
      drugs, 96-107
    opioids, 40-47, 80-96
    propofol, 56-69
    thiopental, 56-69
Analgesia adjunct
    chloral hydrate, 49-52
Anaphylaxis or anaphylactic shock
    chlorpheniramine, 245
    diphenhydramine, 245
    epinephrine, 244

Anesthesia
    anesthetic mouthrinse, 199-207
    general anesthetics, 56-69
    injectable local anesthetics, 1-9
    topical local anesthetics, 10-16
    vasoconstrictors, 2, 5-9
Anesthesia adjuncts
    barbiturates, 32-40
    opioids, 40-47
    scopolamine hydrobromide,
      186-193
Angina pectoris
    antiangina drugs, 299-301
    calcium channel blockers, 309-310
    management, 290-291
    nitroglycerin, 246, 298
Angioedema
    chlorpheniramine, 245
    diphenhydramine, 245
Antibiotic premedication/prophylaxis
    bacterial endocarditis, 542-546
    sample prescriptions, 565
    with prosthetic joint replacements,
      547-552
Anxiety
    barbiturates, 32-40
    benzodiazepines, 18-30, 356-360
    conscious sedation and agents
      for control of, 17
    general anesthetic, 56-69
    meprobamate, 53-55
    nitrous oxide, 56-69
Aphthous ulcers
    amlexanox, 172
    topical corticosteroids, 129-133,
      420-422
Aspergillosis
    systemic antifungal agents, 164-171
Asthma
    bronchodilators, 319-323
    corticosteroids, 124-135
Autoimmune disease
    corticosteroids, 122-133

B

Bacterial endocarditis
    recommendations for prevention,
      542-546
Benzodiazepine overdose
    flumazenil, 30-32, 263
β-lactamase–producing oral
    bacteria
    amoxicillin/clavulanic acid,
      134-142
    cloxacillin, 134-142
    dicloxacillin, 134-142
    oxacillin, 134-142
    tetracyclines, 146-150
Blastomycosis
    systemic antifungal agents, 164-171
Blood pressure support and
    maintenance
    methoxamine, 249
Bradycardia, severe
    atropine, 254, 255
Bronchospasm in reversible
    obstructive airway disease
    albuterol, 247
    epinephrine, 244
Bronchospasm, exercise induced
    albuterol, 247
Bruxism, nocturnal
    psychoactive drugs, 357-385

C

Calcium channel blocker toxicity
    calcium chloride, 261
Calculus
    dentifrices, 207-213
Cancer pain
    long-acting opioid analgesics,
      80-96
Cancer therapy, oral complications
    associated with
    dental management, 441-449

Candidiasis, oral
    antifungal agents, 164-171
    sample prescriptions, 567
Cardiac arrest
    adrenalin, 255
Cardiac arrhythmia
    antiarrhythmic agents, 296-298
    atropine, 254
    lidocaine, 256
Caries prevention
    dentifrices, 207-213
    home use desensitizing products,
        232-234
    in-office fluoride desensitizing
        agents, 226-232
    mouthrinses, 199-207
    systemic fluorides, 215-218
    topical fluorides, 218-225
Caries treatment
    topical fluorides, 218-225
Carious lesions, prevention or
        remineralization
    mouthrinses, 199-207
Chest pain
    management, 290-292
Chronic nonmalignant pain
    long-acting opioid analgesics,
        80-96
Clostridium difficile
    metronidazole, 152-155
Coccidioidomycosis
    systemic antifungal agents,
        164-171
Convulsive seizures
    diazepam, 247
Cryptococcosis
    systemic antifungal agents,
        164-171
Dental abscesses
    tetracyclines, 146-150
Dentinal sensitivity
    dentifrices, 207-213
    topical fluorides, 218-225
Denture irritation
    topical local anesthetics, 10-16
Dry mouth/dry throat
    saliva substitutes, 196-198

E

Endocrine disorders
    corticosteroids, 122-133
Endodontic therapy
    root canal medications/dress-
        ings, 180-185
Erythema multiforme
    connective-tissue disorder drugs,
        418-427

F

Facial pain
    vascular headache suppressants,
        350-351
Fear of dental treatment
    see Anxiety
Fever
    aspirin, 96-107
    ibuprofen, 96-107
    naproxen, 96-107
Fungal infections
    antifungal agents, 164-171

G

Gagging
    topical local anesthetics, 10-16
Gingival retraction
    astringents, 116-117
    gingival retraction cord, 117-121
Gingivitis
    dentifrices, 207-213
    mouthrinses, 199-207
    topical fluorides, 218-225
Gingivitis, acute necrotizing ulcerative
    penicillins and cephalosporins,
        134-142
    tetracyclines, 146-150
Gingivitis, desquamative
    topical corticosteroids, 129-133
    sample prescription, 568

H

Halitosis
    mouthrinses, 199-207
Hand-foot-and-mouth disease
    antiviral agents, 171-174
Hemostasis
    absorbable gelatin sponge, 108, 110
    aluminum salts, 116-117
    astringents, 116-117
    collagen absorbable hemostat,
        109, 110
    hemostatics, 108-116
    iron salts, 116-117
    microfibrillar collagen hemostat,
        109, 110
    oxidized cellulose, 108-110
    oxidized regenerated cellulose,
        109, 110
    thrombin, 109, 112, 113
    vitamin K, 109, 111
Herpangina
    antiviral agents, 171-174
Herpes labialis
    acyclovir, 171-174
Herpes simplex virus–associated
        lesions
    antiviral agents, 171-174

Histoplasmosis
    antifungal agents, 164-171
HIV disease
    antiretroviral medications,
        563-564
Hypersensitivity reaction
    endogenous catecholamine:
        epinephrine, 244
Hypertension
    antihypertensive drugs, 301-318
    minimizing rebound in dental
        patients, 295
Hypertension, intra- or postoperative
    esmolol, 251, 252
Hypoglycemia
    antihypoglycemics (orange
        juice, nondiet soft drinks),
        247, 404-410
    dextrose, 250
    glucagon hydrochloride, 249

I

Immunosuppression
    corticosteroids, 122-133
Infection control
    clothing, equipment, procedures,
        489-504
    handwashing agents, 175-178
Infections, bacterial
    amoxicillin, 134-142
    ampicillin, 134-142
    azithromycin, 142-146
    ciprofloxacin, 155-159
    clarithromycin, 142-146
    clindamycin, 150-152
    erythromycin, 142-146
    metronidazole, 152-155
    phenoxymethyl-penicillin
        (penicillin V), 134-142
    tetracyclines, 146-150
Infections, fungal
    antifungal agents, 164-171
Infections, mouth and adjacent tissues
    sample prescriptions, 567
Infections, viral
    antiviral agents, 171-174
Inflammation
    corticosteroids, 122-133
Insomnia
    barbiturates, 32-40
    benzodiazepines, 18-30
Irrigation, endodontic
    root canal medications/
        dressings, 180-185

L

Lichen planus
    connective-tissue disorder

Lichen planus (cont.)
   drugs, 418, 427
   sample prescription, 568
   topical corticosteroids, 129-133
Lupus erythematosus
   connective-tissue disorder drugs,
      417, 427

M

Mechanical ventilation management
   neuromuscular blocking drugs,
      70-79
Meningococcal meningitis
   penicillin G benzathine suspen-
      sion, 134-142
Metabolic acidosis
   sodium bicarbonate, 259, 279
Microbial load reduction, skin and
      oral mucosa
   skin and mucosal antiseptics,
      175-180
Mucous membrane inflammation
   mouthrinses, 199-207
Muscle spasm
   benzodiazepines, 18
   neuromuscular blocking drugs,
      70-79
   skeletal muscle relaxants, 428-431
Myocardial infarction, acute, 248,
      290-292

O

Opioid overdosage, acute
   naloxone, 47-49, 262-263
Oral inflammation, nonviral
   topical corticosteroids, 129-133
Orofacial pain, acute
   codeine (in combination prepara-
      tions), 80-96
   dihydrocodeine (in combination
      preparations), 80-96
   hydrocodone (in combination
      preparations), 80-96
   nonsteroidal anti-inflammatory
      drugs, 96-107
   oxycodone (in combination
      preparations), 80-96
Orofacial pain, chronic
   nonsteroidal anti-inflammatory
      drugs, 96-107
   psychoactive drugs, 356-385
   vascular headache suppressants,
      350-351

P

Pain, mild to moderate
   acetaminophen, 96-107
   nonsteroidal anti-inflammatory
      drugs, 96-107

Pain, moderate to moderately severe
   opioid combination analgesics,
      80-87
   opioids, 40-46
Pain, postoperative, dental
   codeine (in combination prepara-
      tions), 80-96
   dihydrocodeine (in combination
      preparations), 80-96
   hydrocodone (in combination
      preparations), 80-96
   oxycodone (in combination
      preparations), 80-96
Pain associated with acute myocardial
      infarction
   morphine sulfate, 248
Pain of inflammatory origin
   nonsteroidal anti-inflammatory
      drugs, 96-107
Pain relief
   sample prescriptions, 566-567
Pain unresponsive to nonnarcotic
      analgesics
   morphine sulfate, 248
Pemphigoid
   systemic corticosteroids, 122-133,
      418-427
Pemphigus
   systemic corticosteroids, 122-133,
      418-427
Penicillin hypersensitivity
   azithromycin, 142-146
   clarithromycin, 142-146
   clindamycin, 150-152
   erythromycin, 142-146
Periodontal care
   periodontal dressings, 183-184
Periodontitis, refractory, adult
   clindamycin, 150-152
   tetracyclines, 146-150
Periodontitis, refractory, juvenile
   tetracyclines, 146-150
Plaque
   dentifrices, 207-213
   mouthrinses, 199-207
Prosthetic joint replacement
   antibiotic prophylaxis, 547-552
Psoriasis
   methotrexate, 419
Pulse rate, sudden decrease in
   atropine, 254, 255

R

Relaxation before a dental procedure
   sample prescriptions, 566
Respiratory depression
   respiratory stimulants, 254
Respiratory distress
   oxygen, 245

Respiratory distress due to
      bronchospasm
   epinephrine, 244
   management, 285-287
Reversal of pharmacological effects
   of anesthetic, 289-290
   of benzodiazepines, 30-32, 263
   of opioids, 47-49, 262, 263
Rheumatologic disorders
   connective-tissue disorder drugs,
      418-427
Root canal therapy
   root canal medications/dress-
      ings, 180-185
Root surface sensitivity
   home use desensitizing products,
      232-234
   in-office desensitizing agents,
      226-232

S

Salivation control
   anticholinergic and antisialogogic
      agents, 186-193
   atropine, 254, 255
   cholinergic drug (pilocarpine),
      194-196
   saliva substitutes, 196-198
   sample prescriptions, 565-566
Sedation
   barbiturates, 32-40
   benzodiazepines, 18-30
   droperidol/fentanyl, 56-69
   enflurane, 56-69
   ethchlorvynol, 52-53
   methoxyflurane, 56-69
   nitrous oxide, 56-69
   propofol, 56-69
   thiopental, 56-69
Sedation, nocturnal or preoperative
   chloral hydrate, 49-52
   scopolamine hydrobromide,
      186-193
Seizures
   management, 284-285
Septicemia
   clindamycin, 150-152
   metronidazole, 152-155
Shock unresponsive to conventional
      therapy
   hydrocortisone sodium succi-
      nate, 250
Skeletal muscle relaxation (during
      general anesthesia)
   neuromuscular blocking drugs,
      70-79
Sleep disorders
   benzodiazepines, 18, 376-378
   ethchlorvynol, 52-53

Comments and Suggestions

Your *ADA Guide to Dental Therapeutics* is scheduled to be updated every 2 years. To ensure that future versions of the *Guide* are as useful to you as possible, we would appreciate your comments and suggestions on this, the first edition of the book. Please be sure to tell us what you would like added to or changed in the second edition.

You have several options for communicating your thoughts to us. Either copy this page and mail it to us after writing your comments below, or write to us at one of our various addresses as follows:

ADA ONLINE
http://www.ada.org/adapco/adapco.html

E-mail
adapco@ada.org

U.S. mail
ADA Publishing Co., Inc.
Suite 2010
211 East Chicago Avenue
Chicago, IL 60611

Comments: